Series Editor: Richard Riegelman

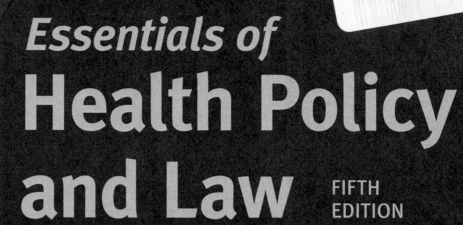

Essentials of
Health Policy
and Law

FIFTH EDITION

ESSENTIAL PUBLIC HEALTH

Sara E. Wilensky, JD, PhD

Department of Health Policy and Management
Milken Institute School of Public Health
The George Washington University

Joel B. Teitelbaum, JD, LLM

Department of Health Policy and Management
Milken Institute School of Public Health
The George Washington University

JONES & BARTLETT
LEARNING

World Headquarters
Jones & Bartlett Learning
25 Mall Road
Burlington, MA 01803
978-443-5000
info@jblearning.com
www.jblearning.com

Jones & Bartlett Learning books and products are available through most bookstores and online booksellers. To contact Jones & Bartlett Learning directly, call 800-832-0034, fax 978-443-8000, or visit our website, www.jblearning.com.

Substantial discounts on bulk quantities of Jones & Bartlett Learning publications are available to corporations, professional associations, and other qualified organizations. For details and specific discount information, contact the special sales department at Jones & Bartlett Learning via the above contact information or send an email to specialsales@jblearning.com.

24749-7

Production Credits
Vice President, Product Management: Marisa R. Urbano
Vice President, Content Strategy and Implementation: Christine Emerton
Director of Product Management: Matthew Kane
Product Manager: Sophie Fleck Teague
Director, Content Management: Donna Gridley
Manager, Content Strategy: Carolyn Pershouse
Content Strategist: Sara Bempkins
Director, Project Management and Content Services: Karen Scott
Manager, Project Management: Jessica deMartin
Project Manager: Jennifer Risden
Digital Project Manager: Angela Dooley
Senior Marketing Manager: Susanne Walker
Content Services Manager: Colleen Lamy
VP, Manufacturing and Inventory Control: Therese Connell
Composition: Straive
Cover Design: Michael O'Donnell
Media Development Editor: Faith Brosnan
Rights & Permissions Manager: John Rusk
Rights Specialist: Maria Leon Maimone
Cover Image (Title Page, Part Opener, Chapter Opener): © Bill Perry/ Shutterstock
Printing and Binding: LSC Communications

Library of Congress Cataloging-in-Publication Data
Names: Wilensky, Sara E., author. | Teitelbaum, Joel Bern, author.
Title: Essentials of health policy and law / Sara E. Wilensky, JD, PhD, Department of Health Policy and Management, Milken Institute School of Public Health, The George Washington University, Joel B. Teitelbaum, JD, LLM, Department of Health Policy and Management, Milken Institute School of Public Health, The George Washington University.
Description: Fifth edition. | Burlington, Massachusetts: Jones & Bartlett Learning, [2023] | Includes bibliographical references and index. |
Identifiers: LCCN 2021043276 | ISBN 9781284247459 (paperback)
Subjects: LCSH: Medical policy—United States—Textbooks. | BISAC: MEDICAL / Health Policy
Classification: LCC RA395.A3 T45 2023 | DDC 362.10973--dc23/eng/20211021
LC record available at https://lccn.loc.gov/2021043276

6048

Printed in the United States of America
26 25 24 23 22   10 9 8 7 6 5 4 3 2

Brief Contents

Contents

PART I Setting the Stage: An Overview of Health Policy and Law   1

Chapter 1 Understanding the Role of and Conceptualizing Health Policy and Law.   3

Chapter 2 Policy and the Policymaking Process.   11

Chapter 3 Law and the Legal System.   33

Chapter 4 Overview of the Healthcare System   49

Chapter 5 What Is Public Health? . . .83

PART II Essential Issues in Health Policy and Law   111

Chapter 6 Individual Rights in Health Care and Public Health . . .113

Chapter 7 Structural and Social Drivers of Health and the Role of Law in Optimizing Health 137

Chapter 12 Healthcare Quality Policy and Law. 297

Chapter 13 What Is Public Health Emergency Preparedness?. 319

PART III Basic Skills in Health Policy Analysis   337

Chapter 14 The Art of Structuring and Writing a Health Policy Analysis. 339

THE ESSENTIAL PUBLIC HEALTH SERIES

From the impact of COVID-19 to the cost of health care, this unique series will introduce you to the full range of issues that impact the public's health.

Current and Forthcoming Titles in the Essential Public Health Series:

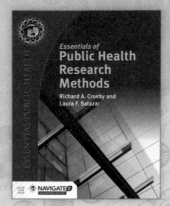

Essentials of
**Public Health
Research
Methods**

Richard A. Crosby and
Laura F. Salazar

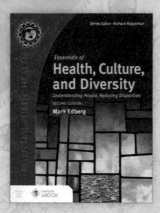

Essentials of
**Health, Culture,
and Diversity**

Understanding People, Reducing Disparities

SECOND EDITION

Mark Edberg

Essentials of
**Public Health
Ethics**

Ruth Gaare Bernheim, James F. Childress
Richard J. Bonnie, Alan L. Melnick

Essentials of
**Health
Information
Systems and
Technology**

Jean Balgrosky

Essentials of
**Health
Economics**

Second Edition

Diane M. Dewar

Essentials of
**Public Health
Communication**

Claudia Parvanta, David E. Nelson,
Sarah A. Parvanta, and Richard N. Harner

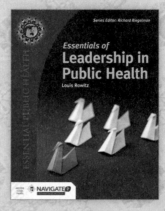

Essentials of
**Leadership in
Public Health**

Louis Rowitz

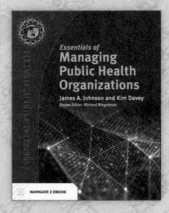

Essentials of
**Managing
Public Health
Organizations**

James A. Johnson and Kim Davey

SECOND EDITION

Essentials of
**Public Health
Preparedness
and Emergency
Management**

Rebecca Katz
James Banaski, Jr.

Essential
**Case Studies
in Public Health**

Putting Public Health into Practice

Katherine L. Hunting and Brenda L. Gleason

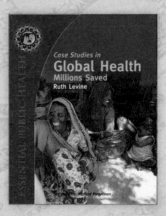

Case Studies in
Global Health

Millions Saved
Ruth Levine

ABOUT THE EDITOR

Richard K. Riegelman, MD, MPH, PhD, is Professor of Epidemiology-Biostatistics, Medicine, and Health Policy, and Founding Dean of The George Washington University Milken Institute School of Public Health in Washington, DC. He has taken a lead role in developing the Educated Citizen and Public Health initiative which has brought together arts and sciences and public health education associations to implement the Institute of Medicine of the National Academies' recommendation that "…all undergraduates should have access to education in public health." Dr. Riegelman also led the development of The George Washington's undergraduate major and minor and currently teaches "Public Health 101" and "Epidemiology 101" to undergraduates.

www.EssentialPublicHealth.com

Editor's Preface

The fifth edition of *Essentials of Health Policy and Law* describes and analyzes, through the lenses of policy and law, the transformations taking place across the United States healthcare delivery and public health systems. Building on the core content and engaging style of earlier editions, this edition is by necessity influenced by the shifts occurring as a result of the 2020 election cycle, including the ways in which the Patient Protection and Affordable Care Act (commonly known as the ACA) is being interpreted and implemented.

Professors Sara Wilensky and Joel Teitelbaum have deep experience analyzing and communicating about the ACA and many other aspects of health policy and law, and this edition benefits from their combined 40 years in the field. Capitalizing on this expertise, *Essentials of Health Policy and Law, Fifth Edition* takes a broad approach to the study of health policy and law and provides a coherent framework for grappling with important healthcare and public health issues in the United States.

Health policies and laws are an inescapable and critical component of our everyday lives. Scores of important issues—from the accessibility, cost, and quality of health care; to the country's preparedness for natural disasters and pandemics; to the effects that structural and social determinants of health have on individual and community health; to the right to make individual decisions about one's own medical care—fall under the health policy and law umbrella. Health policies and laws have a strong and lasting effect on the quality of our lives as individuals, and on our safety, health, and well-being as a nation.

Professors Wilensky and Teitelbaum do a marvelous job of succinctly describing the nation's policy- and law-making machinery, the always-evolving healthcare and public health systems, the ways in which policy and law affect essential healthcare and public health concerns, and methods of advocacy for those individuals and organizations that aim to promote health through policy and legal reform. Both authors have a unique ability to make complex issues accessible to a wide range of readers, including those without a background in health care or public health. Their training as policy analysts and lawyers shines through as they systematically describe and analyze the complex field of health policy and law, and provide vivid examples to help make sense of it all.

Equally apparent is their wealth of experience teaching health policy and law at both the undergraduate and graduate levels. Between them, they have designed and taught many different health policy and/or law courses, designed and directed a bachelor of science degree program in public health, and received multiple teaching awards for their efforts in the classroom. Readers of this text are the beneficiaries of their experience, enthusiasm, and commitment, as you will see in the pages that follow.

I am pleased that *Essentials of Health Policy and Law* is a part of the Essential Public Health series. From the earliest stages of the series' development, Professors Wilensky and Teitelbaum have played a central role. They have closely coordinated efforts with other series authors to ensure that the series provides a comprehensive approach with only intended overlap. This is well illustrated by the numerous additions and revisions, which are described in the Preface, that have taken place with the publication of this latest edition.

I am confident that you will enjoy reading and greatly benefit from *Essentials of Health Policy and Law*. Whether you are studying public health, public policy, healthcare administration, or a field within the clinical health professions, this text is a key component of your education.

—*Richard Riegelman, MD, MPH, PhD, editor, Essential Public Health Series*

Authors' Preface

In the preface to the fourth edition of this text, we described several significant changes that had transpired across the healthcare and public health landscapes in the 13 years since we authored the very first edition: passage and implementation of the Patient Protection and Affordable Care Act (commonly known as the Affordable Care Act, or ACA); a new, national focus on the ways in which myriad social determinants of health affect individual and population health and well-being; shifts in public health education; and a mainly unanticipated election at the very top of the national ticket in 2016, a result that dramatically altered the trajectory of federal health policy. To this list we now add two key events that have taken place since we wrote the fourth edition manuscript in 2018. First, we note the protracted federal election cycle of 2020, which bled into early 2021 due to runoff races for both of Georgia's Senate seats and which again dramatically shifted the balance of power over federal policymaking. After all the votes were counted, Democrats emerged in control of the presidency and, by the slimmest of margins, both houses of Congress. What effects this will have on federal health policy and law, at least until the midterm elections in 2022—which could again easily reshape the Senate and/or the House of Representatives—remains to be seen, but expectations are high that Democrats will use their rare control of all the levers of federal policymaking to enact new health-related programs and policies, and to enforce existing ones with gusto. Of course, Democrats' legislative power is not completely unfettered, owing in large part to Senate filibuster rules. Whatever the case, we do our best in this edition to describe the key health policy and legal changes brought about by the Biden administration and the Democrat-controlled Congress as of the time of this writing, in August 2021.

The second addition to the list is, of course, the COVID-19 pandemic and its many devastating and intertwined health, economic, and social consequences. While it will take years to truly comprehend all of the national and global ramifications of the pandemic, and many more to adjust to and recover from them, it is fair to say this much about COVID-19 in the United States as of mid-2021: While it has affected all segments of the population, it has been particularly deadly and damaging to groups who have been racially minoritized in society, people living in poverty situations, older persons, persons with disabilities, LGBTQ+ populations, youth, and indigenous peoples; it has deepened long-standing inequalities across a range of subjects and sectors; it has caused record levels of unemployment and business closures, and it will have major long-term repercussions on the economy and on consumer behavior; it is likely to alter the nature of work and education, and the role of technology in them; it has seemingly exacerbated a deep-seated lack of societal cohesion; it has taken a toll on the nation's mental health and well-being, particularly among young people; and, if not properly addressed through policy and law, the triple crises of the pandemic—health, economic, and social—will likely increase inequity, inequality, social deprivation, and exclusion in the long term.

Yet for all of the extant and potential consequences of COVID-19, it does not receive deep treatment in this text. This text aims to provide readers with a broad understanding of some of the most essential topics and tools in health policy and law, so that when students consider a major health event like COVID-19, they can do so using policy and law lenses. However, COVID-19 is used to illuminate discussions about various aspects of our political and legal landscape: the U.S. political system, including federalism and the politicization of the judicial branch of government; legal doctrines that are remnants of century-old judicial decisions; the organization and financing of American health care, including the public and private health insurance systems; the state of the public health workforce; structural discrimination and myriad social determinants of health; ways to advocate for change; and more. Thus, while readers may only periodically encounter content that specifically calls out COVID-19, in many respects you are reading about the policies and laws and concepts that either allow the nation to respond well and equitably to events like COVID-19, or that drive the country to a response that leaves tens of millions of people in harm's way. We turn now to brief summaries of some other key events and frameworks that have animated this book across several editions.

Implementation of the Affordable Care Act

Now hailed as the most important set of changes to health insurance since the 1965 enactment of Medicare and Medicaid, the ACA was signed into law by President Barack Obama in March of 2010. Since that time, the ACA itself has been on quite a journey, given the policy shifts and legal challenges it has undergone in a relatively short time. Broadly speaking, the ACA represents two landmark achievements in health policy: major reform of the private health insurance market and, relatedly, a redistribution of resources to groups and individuals who, by virtue of indigence and/or illness, have historically been excluded from the health insurance market and/or healthcare system. Additionally, the law includes dozens of other important reforms and programs unrelated to insurance. For example, more efficient and higher-quality health care, population health, healthcare access, long-term care, the health workforce, health disparities, community health centers, healthcare fraud and abuse, comparative effectiveness research, health information technology, and more all receive attention by the ACA. Indeed, it is fair to say that a fully implemented ACA would move the nation toward a more affordable, equitable, and stable insurance system, not only for the millions of individuals who have and are expected to gain insurance, but also for the tens of millions of people who no longer face the threat of a loss or lapse of coverage.

Yet, full implementation of the ACA is still just a goal, as many federal and state policymakers and a substantial bloc of the voting public continue their efforts to undermine, if not totally destroy, the law. To understand these efforts, readers must understand that many ACA reforms required a reordering of the relationships that lie at the heart of the nation's healthcare and public systems. Individuals, providers, insurers, employers, governments, and others were forced to alter once-normative behaviors in response to the policy and legal decisions underpinning the law. These types of major policy and legal shifts—such as, in the case of the ACA, the creation of the "individual insurance mandate," new prohibitions that prevent private insurers from using discriminatory enrollment practices, the creation of new health insurance exchanges, and the expansion of Medicaid eligibility standards—are basically destined to create backlash, given the very nature of how people respond to change and the vast amounts of money that, for some industries, are at stake. Add to this the fact that the ACA bill that eventually became law passed in Congress by the slimmest of margins after months of rancorous debate, and fully half the states in the United States actively opposed the ACA's implementation after its passage. Even now, more than a decade since the ACA became law, courts across the country have ACA-related cases on their dockets and the law continues to be used as a cudgel on the campaign trail. Needless to say, the outcomes of these lawsuits and policy debates will no doubt be discussed in both the national media and in the health policy and law courses in which you register, and they will be devoted space in the pages of this text in future editions.

Shifts in Public Health Education

Several important shifts in public health education have taken place since 2007. One change that is particularly relevant to this text (and to the entire Essential Public Health series, of which this text is a part) is the effort undertaken by the Association of American Colleges and Universities (AAC&U) and the Association of Schools and Programs of Public Health (ASPPH) to develop the Educated Citizen and Public Health Initiative. This initiative seeks to integrate public health perspectives into a comprehensive liberal education framework and to develop and organize publications, presentations, and resources to help faculty develop public health curricula in the nation's colleges and universities. As a result, public health perspectives generally, and health policy and law specifically, are increasingly being integrated into courses as diverse as political science, history, sociology, public policy, and a range of courses that prepare students for the health professions. Furthermore, the most recent accreditation standards from the Council on Education for Public Health (CEPH) requires that Master of Public Health students learn to "advocate for political, social or economic policies and programs that will improve health in diverse populations" (see https://storage.googleapis.com/media.ceph.org/wp_assets/2016.Criteria.pdf), and this edition responds to that call with a brand-new chapter on health advocacy. We are proud that this text has played a role in shaping (and supplying) the market for health policy and law education as part of a liberal education framework, and we aim with this *Fifth Edition* to make the material as accessible as possible to diverse audiences. Indeed, we know from user surveys that this text is used across several disciplines (public health, health administration, medicine, health, other public policy, etc.) and degree levels (bachelor, master, doctoral), and as a result we attempt to strike a balance on the topics that are covered, the depth of the content covered, and the overall length of the text. We recognize that certain educators and programs wish that we would alter our approach to at least one of those three things, but we ask for your understanding as we aim to satisfy multiple audiences.

Addressing Complex Health Policy Challenges

Some health policy concerns are exceedingly complex. On this topic we offer four factors for your consideration as you delve into the chapters that follow. First, like most challenging public policy problems, pressing health policy questions simultaneously implicate politics, law, ethics, and social mores, all of which come with their own set of competing interests and advocates. Second, health policy debates often involve deeply personal matters pertaining to one's quality—or very definition—of life, philosophical questions about whether health care should be a market commodity or a social good, or profound questions about how to appropriately balance population welfare with closely guarded individual freedoms and liberties. Third, it is often not abundantly clear how to begin tackling a particular health policy problem. For example, is it one best handled by the medical care system, the public health system, or both? Which level of government—federal or state—has the authority or ability to take action? Should the problem be handled legislatively or through regulatory channels? The final ingredient that makes health policy problems such a complex stew is the rapid developments often experienced in the areas of healthcare research, medical technology, and public health threats. Generally speaking, this kind of rapid evolution is a confounding problem for the usually slow moving American policy- and lawmaking machinery.

Furthermore, the range of topics fairly included under the banner of "health policy and law" is breathtaking. For example, what effect is healthcare spending having on national and state economies? How should finite financial resources be allocated between health care and public health? How can we ensure that the trust funds established to account for Medicare's income and disbursements remain solvent in the future as an enormous group of baby boomers becomes eligible for program benefits? What kind of return (in terms of quality of individual care and the overall health of the population) should we expect from the staggering amount of money we collectively spend on health? Should individuals have a legal entitlement to health insurance? How should we attack extant health disparities based on race, ethnicity, and socioeconomic status? What policies will best protect the privacy of personal health information in an increasingly electronic medical system? Can advanced information technology systems improve the quality of individual and population health? Should the right to have an abortion continue to be protected under the federal Constitution? Should physician assistance in dying be promoted as a laudable social value? Will mapping the human genome lead to discrimination based on underlying health status? How prepared is the country for natural and man-made catastrophes, like pandemic influenza or bioterrorism attacks? What effect will chronic diseases, such as diabetes and obesity-related conditions, have on healthcare delivery and financing? How should we harness advancing scientific findings for the benefit of the public's health?

As seen from even this partial list of questions, the breadth of issues encountered in the study of health policy and law is virtually limitless, and we do not grapple in this text with all of the preceding questions. We do, however, introduce you to many of the policies, laws, and concepts that give rise to them; provide an intellectual framework for thinking about how to address them going forward; and direct you to additional relevant readings. Given the prominent role played by policy and law in the health of all Americans, and the fact that the Health and Medicine Division of the National Academies recommends that students of public health and other interdisciplinary subjects (for example, public policy or medicine) receive health policy and law training, the aim of this text is to help you understand the broad context of American health policy and law, the essential issues impacting and flowing out of the healthcare and public health systems, and how health policies and laws are influenced and formulated. Broadly speaking, the goal of health policy is to promote and protect the health of individuals and of populations bound by common circumstances. Because the legal system provides the formal structure through which public policy—including health policy—is debated, effected, and interpreted, law is an indispensable component of the study of health policy. Indeed, law is inherent to the expression of public policy: Major changes to policies often demand the creation, amendment, or rescission of laws. As such, students studying policy must learn about policymaking *and* the law, legal process, and legal concepts.

About the *Fifth Edition*

As a result of the changes described earlier, and in response to comments we received from users of the previous edition of *Essentials of Health Policy and Law*, this edition includes a brand-new chapter; renovations and updates to several existing chapters; updated figures, tables, and discussion questions; and updated references and readings. Specifically, there is new or updated content in the areas of national and state health reform; the healthcare delivery and public health systems; the policymaking process; the ACA's effect on Medicaid, Medicare, and CHIP; individual rights in health care; structural and social drivers of health; and health advocacy, a topic that now lays claim to its own chapter. In addition, there is a new feature—specialized text boxes. Text boxes are now color-coded and divided into Discussion Questions, Special Topics, and Technical Spotlights, allowing instructors to select the content most appropriate for their courses.

Part I

Part I of this text includes five preparatory chapters. **Chapter 1** describes generally the influential role of policy and law in health care and public health and introduces various conceptual frameworks through which the study of health policy and law can take place. The chapter also illustrates why it is important to include policy and law in the study of health care and public health. However, an advanced exploration of health policy and law in individual and population health necessitates both a basic and practical comprehension of policy and law in general—including the policymaking process and the workings of the legal system—and an understanding of the nation's rather fragmented healthcare and public health systems. Thus, **Chapter 2** discusses both the meaning of policy and the policymaking process, including the basic functions, structures, and powers of the legislative and executive branches of government and the respective roles of the federal and state governments in policymaking. **Chapter 3** describes the meaning and sources of law and several key features of the American legal system, including the separation of

powers doctrine, federalism, the role of courts, and due process. **Chapter 4** provides an overview of the healthcare system, including basic information on healthcare finance, access, and quality and examples of how the U.S. system differs from those in other developed nations. Part I closes with an overview, in **Chapter 5**, of the public health system, including its origins, evolution, core functions, and contributions.

Part II

Part II offers several chapters focusing on key substantive health policy and law issues. **Chapter 6** examines the ways in which the law creates, protects, and restricts individual rights in the contexts of health care and public health, including a discussion of laws (such as Medicaid and Medicare) that aim to level the playing field where access to health care is concerned. The chapter also introduces the "no-duty-to-treat" principle, which rests at the heart of the legal framework pertaining to healthcare rights and duties and holds that there is no general legal duty on the part of healthcare providers to render care. **Chapter 7** describes how structural and social factors play a critical role in the attainment (or not) of health equity and of individual and population health, discusses the ways in which law can both exacerbate and ameliorate negative social determinants of health, and introduces readers to the concept of health and social services integration. **Chapters 8** and **9** cover the fundamentals of health insurance and health economics, respectively, and set up a subsequent thematic discussion in **Chapters 10** and **11**. Specifically, **Chapter 8** describes the function of risk and uncertainty in health insurance, defines the basic elements of health insurance, discusses important health policy issues relating to health insurance, and more; **Chapter 9** explains why it is important for health policymakers to be familiar with basic economic concepts; the basic tenets of supply, demand, and markets; and the way in which health insurance affects economic conditions.

Chapter 10 explains how federal and state policymakers have created health insurance programs for individuals and populations who otherwise might go without health insurance coverage. The basic structure, administration, financing, and eligibility rules of the three main U.S. public health insurance programs—Medicaid, the Children's Health Insurance Program, and Medicare—are discussed, as are key health policy questions relating to each program. **Chapter 11** focuses on health reform and the ACA. This chapter discusses the reasons why for decades the United States failed to achieve significant national health reform in the 50 years prior to the ACA, how and why the ACA passed given this history, and what the ACA aims to achieve. Part II then moves to a discussion of healthcare quality in **Chapter 12**, which reflects on several important policy and legal questions in the areas of provider licensure and accreditation of health facilities (both of which represent quality control through regulation), the evolution of the standard of care, tort liability for healthcare providers and insurers, preventable medical errors, and, with the ACA as the focal point, efforts to improve healthcare quality through quality improvement and provider incentive programs. Part II concludes with **Chapter 13**, which focuses on public health emergency preparedness, including discussions about the role of public health in emergency preparedness, the concept of the "whole community" approach to preparedness and response, and the types of legal issues that arise in the context of emergency preparedness.

Part III

The text concludes in Part III with two chapters that cover the basic skills of health policy analysis and health advocacy, respectively. The substance of health policy can be understood only as the product of an infinite number of policy choices regarding whether and how to intervene in many types of health policy problems. **Chapter 14** explains how to structure and write a short health policy analysis, which is a tool frequently used by policy analysts when they assess policy options and discuss rationales for their health policy recommendations. Finally, **Chapter 15** examines the role of advocacy in health policymaking and the key tools used by health policy advocates, and it also includes a roadmap for developing a health advocacy campaign.

Additional learning resources can be found in the Navigate eBook that accompanies this text. These materials include an interactive glossary, flashcards, chapter review slides, end-of-chapter quizzes to assess learning, and an interactive timeline. These materials are available by redeeming the access code found on the card inside this book.

Resources for instructors are also available and include slides in PowerPoint format, a test bank, midterm and final exam, and sample syllabus.

Pedagogical Features

Learning Objectives

Learning objectives at the start of each chapter give you a preview of the topics to be covered in the chapter.

LEARNING OBJECTIVES

By the end of this chapter you will be able to:

1. Understand the role of risk and uncertainty in insurance
2. Define the basic elements of health insurance
3. Differentiate various insurance products
4. Discuss incentives created for providers and patients in various types of insurance arrangements
5. Discuss health policy issues relating to health insurance

Box 8.9 DISCUSSION QUESTIONS

In terms of containing healthcare costs and improving healthcare quality, do you think healthcare consumers and professionals need even more restrictions than are currently used in managed care? Are there any reasons to revert back to the FFS system, even knowing its inflationary qualities? If you think that managed care is not the answer to our still-rising healthcare costs and quality concerns, what other tools might help lower costs and improve the quality of care? Should any tools be imposed by government regulation or agreed to voluntarily by insurers and the insured?

Discussion Question Boxes

Discussion Question boxes found throughout the text promote critical thinking, classroom discussion, and enhanced student learning.

Box 10.4   Special Topic

Federal Poverty Level

Federal poverty guidelines are determined annually and calculated based on the number of individuals in a family. The guidelines are commonly referred to as the *federal poverty level*, but the U.S. Department of Health and Human Services (HHS) discourages the use of this term because the Census Bureau also calculates, using different methods, a figure referred to as the *federal poverty threshold*. However, because the term *federal poverty level* is still commonly used when discussing eligibility for federal and state programs, we use it here. The poverty guidelines are somewhat higher for Alaska and Hawaii due to administrative procedures adopted by the Office of Economic Opportunity.

Special Topics

Special Topics boxes provide more detailed information on key topics throughout.

Vignettes

Vignettes featured throughout help readers apply key concepts and bring topics to life.

Technical Spotlight

Technical Spotlight boxes highlight the more complex and technical details of various policies and key topics for additional student learning.

Box 10.11   Technical Spotlight

Alternative Benefit Plan (Section 1937 Plan) Requirements

- Align with an approved benchmark or benchmark equivalent
- Provide essential health benefits
- Include early and periodic screening, diagnosis, and treatment for children up to age 21 years
- Cover federally qualified health center/rural healthcare services
- Cover nonemergency transportation to medical care
- Cover family planning services and supplies
- Comply with mental health parity law
- Comply with traditional Medicaid cost-sharing rules
- Do not cover care for beneficiaries in institutions for mental diseases
- Exempt certain medically frail populations from benefit limits

---

Box 8.1 VIGNETTE

William owns a small farm that raises chickens and goats. He has nine employees and has always made it a priority to offer competitive benefits, including health insurance. Unfortunately, last year one of his employees was diagnosed with cancer, which he continues to fight. Due to the sharp increase in use of health services by his employee group, the insurance company doubled his group premiums for the upcoming year. When William contacted other carriers, several of them would not consider insuring his group, and most of the others gave him quotes that were just as expensive as his current carrier. One company gave him a lower quote, but it covered only catastrophic care; his employees would have to pay for the first $5000 of care out of their own pockets. After reviewing his company's finances, William is left with several unattractive options: stop offering health insurance; offer comprehensive health insurance but pass on the cost increase to his employees, which would make it unaffordable for most of them; offer the bare-bones catastrophic plan only; or significantly lower wages and other benefits to defray the rising health insurance costs. In addition to wanting to offer competitive benefits, William is concerned that adopting any of these options will cause his employees to leave and make it hard to attract others, threatening the sustainability of his company.

The 2010 health reform law (ACA) attempts to help small businesses like William's by creating state health insurance exchanges. Starting in 2014, these exchanges offered a variety of plans to individuals and small businesses that otherwise might not be able to afford health insurance coverage. By creating large groups of purchasers through the exchanges, it is possible to pool risk and keep prices lower than if individuals or small businesses were attempting to purchase insurance coverage on their own.

Unsuccessful Attempts to Pass National Health Insurance Reform

Since the early 1900s, when medical knowledge became advanced enough to make health care and health insurance desirable commodities, there have been periodic attempts to implement universal coverage through national health reform. The Socialist Party was the first U.S. political party to support health

Timeline

Noted with a clock icon, these key milestones in U.S history are identified at relevant points throughout the text. These milestones are also included in the Interactive Timeline available in the enriched eBook.

Please refer to the interactive timeline that can be found inside the Navigate eBook that accompanies this text. Simply redeem the access code found at the front of the book at www.jblearning.com.

---

overthrow it (Starr, 1982, p. 243). In 1912, Progressive Party candidate Theodore Roosevelt supported a social insurance platform modeled on the European

Additional Materials Available in the Accompanying Navigate eBook

Your new copy of *Essentials of Health Policy and Law, Fifth Edition* includes complimentary access to the accompanying Navigate eBook (see access code card at the front of the book). This resource provides you with the complete text in an easy-to-read, digital format for convenient online or offline access from your computer, tablet, or mobile device.

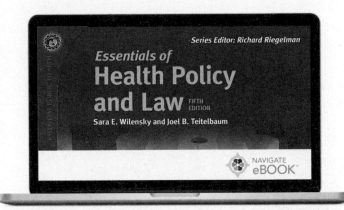

The Navigate eBook includes several additional learning resources including an interactive glossary, flashcards, chapter review slides, and student quizzes for each chapter.

The Navigate eBook also includes an interactive timeline that looks at key milestones in U.S. history as they relate to health policy. This interactive enrichment contains four timelines in one that outline:

- The political party in power in the federal government including the president, the House of Representatives, and the Senate

- Major social and political events such as the #MeToo movement, the Great Recession, the Progressive Era, and the Cold War Era

- Important developments in health and medicine such as the founding of the American Medical Association, the opening of the first school of nursing, and the establishment of the role of nursing during the Civil War

- Key federal legislative proposals/laws and key legal decisions such as the Affordable Care Act, the Health Insurance Portability and Accountability Act, and the Social Security Act

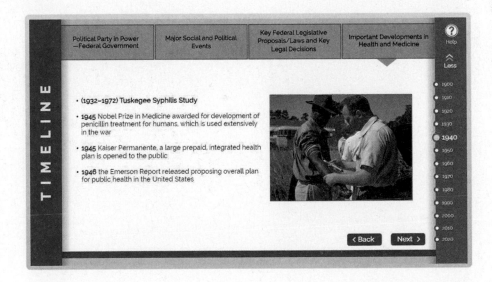

To redeem your code and gain access to your Navigate eBook, log on to **www.jblearning.com**

Acknowledgments

We are grateful to the many people who generously contributed their guidance, assistance, and encouragement to us during the writing of the several editions of this textbook. At the top of the list is Dr. Richard Riegelman, founding dean of the Milken Institute School of Public Health at the George Washington University and professor of epidemiology and biostatistics, medicine, and health policy. The Essential Public Health series was his brainchild, and his stewardship of the project as series editor made our involvement in it both enriching and enjoyable. We are indebted to him for his guidance and friendship.

We single out one other colleague for special thanks. Sara Rosenbaum, the Harold and Jane Hirsh Professor of Health Law and Policy and a past chair of the George Washington University's Department of Health Policy and Management, has been a wonderful mentor, colleague, and friend for decades. We are indebted to her for supporting our initial decision to undertake the writing of this textbook.

During the writing of the various editions of this book, we have been blessed by the help of several stellar research assistants. The first edition could not have been completed without V. Nelligan Coogan, Mara B. McDermott, Sarah E. Mutinsky, Dana E. Thomas, and Ramona Whittington; Brittany Plavchak and Julia Roumm were essential to the completion of the second edition; Jacob Alexander's assistance was key to the third edition; Joanna Theiss was instrumental in updating the fourth edition; and Layna Teitelbaum provided invaluable research assistance for the current edition. To all of them, we send our deep appreciation for their help and steady supply of good cheer.

Our gratitude extends also to Mike Brown, former publisher for Jones & Bartlett Learning, for his then-visionary decision to include a policy and law textbook in the earliest set of books that would become the Essential Public Health series. Similarly, we are indebted to the entire team at Jones & Bartlett Learning—particularly Sophie Teague, Sara Bempkins, and Susanne Walker—for their support, confidence, patience, and expertise.

Finally, we wish to thank those closest to us. Sara gives special thanks to Trish Manha, her wife, sounding board and constant supporter, and to Sophia and William, budding authors in their own right who make life fun, surprising, and ever-changing. Joel sends special thanks to his family: Laura Hoffman, Jared Teitelbaum, and Layna Teitelbaum, his favorite people and unending sources of joy and laughter.

About the Authors

Sara Wilensky, JD, PhD, is assistant dean for undergraduate education at the Milken Institute School of Public Health (SPH) at the George Washington University (GW) in Washington, D.C., and special services faculty for undergraduate education in its Department of Health Policy and Management.

Dr. Wilensky has taught a health policy analysis course and health systems overview course that is required of all students in the Master of Public Health–Health Policy degree program, as well as the health policy course required of all undergraduate students majoring in public health. She has been the principal investigator or co-principal investigator on numerous health policy research projects relating to a variety of topics, such as Medicaid coverage, access and financing, community health centers, childhood obesity, HIV preventive services, financing of public hospitals, and data sharing barriers and opportunities between public health and Medicaid agencies.

As the assistant dean for undergraduate education Dr. Wilensky is responsible for overseeing all undergraduate programs and cocurricular activities in SPH, sets the strategic vision for the undergraduate programs, and works with campus partners and outside stakeholders to improve undergraduate public health education.

Dr. Wilensky is involved with several GW service activities: She has taught a service learning in public health course in the undergraduate program; she has been heavily involved in making GW's Writing in the Disciplines program part of the undergraduate major in public health; and she is the advisor to students receiving a master in public policy or a master in public administration with a focus on health policy from GW's School of Public Policy and Public Administration. She also serves on the publications board for the American Public Health Association.

Prior to joining GW, Dr. Wilensky was a law clerk for federal Judge Harvey Bartle III in the Eastern District of Pennsylvania and worked as an associate at the law firm of Cutler and Stanfield, LLP, in Denver, Colorado.

Joel Teitelbaum, JD, LLM, is professor of health policy, director of the Hirsh Health Law and Policy Program, and codirector of the National Center for Medical-Legal Partnership at the George Washington University Milken Institute School of Public Health in Washington, D.C. He also carries a faculty appointment in the GW School of Law, and for 11 years served as vice-chair for academic affairs for the Department of Health Policy and Management.

Professor Teitelbaum has taught law, graduate, or undergraduate courses on healthcare law, healthcare civil rights, public health law, minority health policy, and long-term care law and policy. He was the first member of the School of Public Health faculty to receive the University-wide Bender Teaching Award, he has received the School's Excellence in Teaching Award, and he is a member of the University's Academy of Distinguished Teachers and the School's Academy of Master Teachers. He has authored or coauthored dozens of peer-reviewed articles and reports in addition to many book chapters, policy briefs, and blogs on law and social drivers of health, health equity, civil rights issues in health care, health reform and its implementation, medical–legal partnership, and insurance law and policy, and he has delivered more than 100 invited lectures/presentations at leading universities and national conferences. In addition to *Essentials of Health Policy and Law,* he is coauthor of *Essentials of Health Justice: A Primer.* In 2000, Professor Teitelbaum was corecipient of The Robert Wood Johnson Foundation Investigator Award in Health Policy Research, which he used to explore the creation of a new framework for applying Title VI of the 1964 Civil Rights Act to the modern healthcare system.

Among other organizations, Professor Teitelbaum is a member of Delta Omega, the national honor society recognizing excellence in the field of public health; the ASPH/Pfizer Public Health Academy of Distinguished Teachers; and the Society for American Law

Teachers. In 2016, during President Obama's second term, Professor Teitelbaum became the first lawyer named to the U.S. Department of Health and Human Services Secretary's Advisory Committee on National Health Promotion and Disease Prevention Objectives (a.k.a. "Healthy People"), the national agenda aimed at improving the health of all Americans over a 10-year span. He serves as a member of the board of advisors of PREPARE, a national advanced care planning organization, and on multiple committees of the American Bar Association: as a liaison to the Task Force on Eviction, Housing Stability, and Equity; as an advisor to the Coordinating Committee on Veterans Benefits and Services; and as a member of the Advisory Board of the Public Health Legal Services Research Project in the Center for Human Rights.

Contributors

Chapter 5: What Is Public Health?

Guthrie S. Birkhead, MD, MPH; Cynthia B. Morrow, MD, MPH; and Sylvia Pirani, MS, MPH
University at Albany, Albany, New York (Dr. Birkhead)
Virginia Tech Carilion School of Medicine, Roanoke, Virginia (Dr. Morrow)
Public Health Practice Consultant, New York, New York (Ms. Pirani)

Chapter 13: What Is Public Health Emergency Preparedness?

Suzet McKinney, DrPH, MPH, and Mary Elise Papke, DrPH, MPH, MA
Illinois Medical District, Chicago, Illinois (Dr. McKinney)
University of Wisconsin-Milwaukee, Milwaukee, Wisconsin (Dr. Papke)

Chapter 15: Federal Policy Advocacy: Advancing Policy Goals

Katie Horton, RN, MPH, JD, and Naomi Seiler, JD
The George Washington University
Washington, D.C.

Setting the Stage: An Overview of Health Policy and Law

Part I of this textbook includes five contextual chapters aimed at preparing you for the substantive health policy and law discussions in Chapters 6–13 and for the skills-based discussion of policy analysis in Chapters 14 and 15. Chapter 1 generally describes the role of policy and law in health care and public health and introduces conceptual frameworks for studying health policy and law. Chapter 2 describes the meaning of *policy* and also the policymaking process itself. Chapter 3 provides an overview of the meaning and sources of law and of several important features of the legal system. Part I closes with overviews of the U.S. healthcare system and public health system, in Chapter 4 and Chapter 5, respectively.

CHAPTER 1

Understanding the Role of and Conceptualizing Health Policy and Law

LEARNING OBJECTIVES

By the end of this chapter you will be able to:

1. Describe generally the important role played by policy and law in the health of individuals and populations
2. Describe three ways to conceptualize health policy and law

Introduction

In this chapter, we introduce the role played by policy and law in the health of individuals and populations and describe various conceptual frameworks with which you can approach the study of health policy and law. In the chapters that follow, we build on this introduction to provide clarity in areas of health policy and law that are neither readily discernable—even to those who use and work in the healthcare and public health systems—nor easily reshaped by those who make, apply, and interpret policy and law.

The goals of this chapter are to describe why it is important to include policy and law in the study of health care and public health and how you might conceptualize health policy and law when undertaking your studies. To achieve these goals, we first briefly discuss the vast influence of policy and law in health care and public health. You will have a much better feel for how far policy and law reach into these areas as you proceed through this text, but we dedicate a few pages here to get you started. We then describe three ways to conceptualize health policy and law.

Role of Policy and Law in Health Care and Public Health

The forceful influence of policy and law on the health and well-being of individuals and populations is undeniable. Policy and law have always been fundamental in shaping the behaviors of individuals and industries, the practice of health care, and the environments in which people live and work. They have also been vital in achieving both everyday and landmark public health improvements.

For example, centuries-old legal principles have, since this country's inception, provided the bedrock on which healthcare quality laws are built, and today the healthcare industry is regulated in many different ways. Indeed, federal and state policy and law shape virtually all aspects of the healthcare system, from structure and organization, to service delivery, to financing, to administrative and judicial oversight. Whether pertaining to the accreditation and certification of individual or institutional healthcare providers, requirements to provide care under certain circumstances, the creation of public insurance programs, the regulation of private insurance systems, or any other number of issues, policy and law drive the healthcare system to a degree unknown by most people.

In fact, professional digests that survey and report on the subjects of health policy and law typically include in their pages information on topics like the advertising and marketing of health services and products, the impact of health expenditures on federal and state budgets, antitrust concerns, healthcare contracting, employment issues, patents, taxation, healthcare discrimination and disparities, consumer protection, bioterrorism, health insurance, prescription drug regulation, death-with-dignity laws, biotechnology, human subject research, patient privacy and confidentiality, organ availability and donation, and more. Choices made by policymakers and decisions handed down through the judicial system influence how we approach, experience, analyze, and research all of these and other specific aspects of the healthcare system. Once you have read the next four preparatory chapters—one on policy and the policymaking process, one on law and the legal system, and one each covering the structure and organization of the healthcare and public health systems—and begin to digest the substantive chapters that follow them, the full force of policy and law in shaping the individual healthcare system will unfold. For now, simply keep in the back of your mind the fact that policy and law heavily influence the way in which overall health and well-being are achieved (or not), health care is accessed, medicine is practiced, treatments are paid for, and much more.

The role of policy and law in public health is no less important than in individual health care, but their influence in the field of public health is frequently less visible and articulated. In fact, policy and law have long played a seminal role in everyday public health activities. Think, for example, of food establishment inspections, occupational safety standards, policies related to health services for persons with chronic health conditions such as diabetes, and policies and laws affecting the extent to which public health agencies are able to gauge whether individuals in a community suffer from certain health conditions. Similarly, policy and law have been key in many historic public health accomplishments such as

water and air purification, reduction in the spread of communicable diseases through compulsory immunization laws, reduction in the number of automobile-related deaths through seat belt and consumer safety laws, and several other achievements.[a] Public health professionals and students quickly learn to appreciate that combating public health threats requires both vigorous policymaking and adequate legal powers. Indeed, in recent years, enhanced fears about bioterrorism and newly emerging infectious diseases have increased the public's belief that policy and law are important tools in creating an environment in which people can achieve optimal health and safety.

Of course, policies and laws do not always cut in favor of what many people believe to be in the best interests of public health and welfare. A policy or law might, for example, favor the economic interests of a private, for-profit company over the personal interests of residents of the community in which the company is located.[b] Such situations occur because one main focus of public health policy and law is on locating the appropriate balance between public regulation of private individuals and corporations and the ability of those same parties to exercise rights that allow them to function free from overly intrusive government intervention. Achieving this balance is not easy for policymakers, as stakeholders disagree on things like the extent to which car makers should alter their operations to reduce environmentally harmful vehicle emissions, or the degree to which companies should be limited in advertising cigarettes, or whether gun manufacturers should be held liable in cases where injuries or killings result from the negligent use of their products.

How do policymakers and the legal system reach a (hopefully) satisfactory balance of public health and private rights? The competing interests at the heart of public health are mainly addressed through two types of policies and laws: those that define the functions and powers of public health agencies and those that aim to directly protect and promote health.[c] State-level policymakers and public health officials create these types of policies and laws through what are known as their *police powers*. These powers represent the inherent authority of state and local governments to regulate individuals and private business in the name of public health promotion and protection. The importance of police powers cannot be overstated; it is fair to say that they are the most critical aspect of the sovereignty that states retained at the founding of the country, when the colonies agreed to a governmental structure consisting of a strong national government. Furthermore, the reach of police powers should not be underestimated: They give government officials the authority—in the name of public health and welfare—to coerce private parties to act (or refrain from acting) in certain ways. However, states do not necessarily need to exercise their police powers in order to affect or engage in public health–related policymaking. Because the public's health is impacted by many social, economic, and environmental factors, public health agencies also conduct policy-relevant research, disseminate information aimed at helping people engage in healthy behaviors, and establish collaborative relationships with healthcare providers and purchasers and with other government policymaking agencies.

Federal policy and law also play a role in public health. Although the word *health* does not appear in the U.S. Constitution, the document confers powers on the federal government—to tax and spend, for example—that allow it to engage in public health promotion and disease prevention activities. For example, the power to tax (or establish exemptions from taxation) allows Congress to incentivize healthy behaviors, as witnessed by the heavy taxes levied on packages of cigarettes; the power to spend enables Congress to establish executive branch public health agencies and to allocate public health–specific funds to states and localities.

Conceptualizing Health Policy and Law

Having just read about the importance of taking policy and law into account when studying health care and public health, the next step is to begin thinking about how you might conceptually approach the study of health policy and law.

There are multiple ways to conceptualize the many important topics that fall under the umbrella of health policy and law. We introduce three conceptual frameworks in this section: one premised on the broad topical domains of health policy and law, one based on prevailing historical factors, and one focused on the individuals and entities impacted by a particular policy or legal determination (**Box 1.1**).

We draw on these frameworks to various degrees in this text. For example, the topical domain approach of Framework 1 is on display in the sections about individual rights in health care and public health and healthcare quality policy and law. Framework 2's focus on historical perspectives is highlighted in the chapters on health reform and government health insurance programs. Finally, Framework 3, which approaches the study of health policy and law from

---

Box 1.1 Three Conceptual Frameworks for Studying Health Policy and Law

Framework 1. Study based on the broad topical domains of:

a. Health care
b. Public health
c. Bioethics

Framework 2. Study based on historically dominant social, political, and economic perspectives:

a. Professional autonomy
b. Social contract
c. Free market

Framework 3. Study based on the perspectives of key stakeholders:

a. Individuals
b. The public
c. Healthcare professionals
d. Federal and state governments
e. Managed care and traditional insurance companies
f. Employers
g. Healthcare industries (e.g., the pharmaceutical industry)
h. The research community
i. Interest groups
j. Others

---

the perspectives of key stakeholders, is discussed in the policy and policymaking process section and also in the chapter dedicated to the structural and social determinants of health. We turn now to a description of each framework.

The Three Broad Topical Domains of Health Policy and Law

One way to conceptualize health policy and law is as consisting of three large topical domains. One domain is reserved for policy and law concerns in the area of *health care*, another for issues arising in the *public health* arena, and the last for controversies in the field of *bioethics*. As you contemplate these topical domains, bear in mind that they are not individual silos whose contents never spill over into the others. In fact, spillage of one domain's contents into another domain is common (and, as noted in the Preface, it is one reason why fixing health policy problems can be terribly complicated). We briefly touch on each domain.

Healthcare Policy and Law

In the most general sense, this domain is concerned with an individual's access to care (e.g., What policies and laws impact an individual's ability to access needed care?), the quality of the care the person receives (e.g., Is it appropriate, cost-effective, and adequate?), and how the person's care will be financed (e.g., Is the person insured?). However, "access," "quality," and "financing" are themselves rather large subdomains, with their own sets of complex policy and legal issues; in fact, it is common for students to take semester-long policy and/or law courses focused on just one of these subdomains.

Public Health Policy and Law

The second large topical domain is that of public health policy and law. A central focus here is on why and how the government regulates private individuals and corporations in the name of protecting the health, safety, and welfare of the general public. Imagine, for example, that the federal government is considering a blanket policy decision to vaccinate individuals across the country against the deadly smallpox disease, believing that the decision is in the best interests of national security. Would this decision be desirable from a national policy perspective? Would it be legal? If the program's desirability and legality are not immediately clear, how would you go about analyzing and assessing them? These are the kinds of questions with which public health policy and law practitioners and scholars grapple.

Bioethics

Finally, there is the *bioethics* domain to health policy and law. Strictly speaking, the term *bioethics* is used to describe ethical issues raised in the context of medical practice or biomedical research. More comprehensively, bioethics can be thought of as the point at which public policy, law, individual morals, societal values, and medicine intersect. The bioethics domain houses some of the most explosive questions in health policy, including the morality and legality of abortion, conflicting values around the meaning of death and the rights of individuals nearing the end of life, and the policy and legal consequences of mapping the human genetic code.

Social, Political, and Economic Historical Context

Dividing the substance of health policy and law into broad topical categories is only one way to conceptualize them. A second way to consider health policy and law is in historical terms, based on the social, political, and economic views that dominate a particular era.[d] Considered this way, health policy and law have been influenced over time by three perspectives, all of which are technically active at any given time, but each of which has eclipsed the others during specific periods in terms of political, policy, and legal outcomes. These perspectives are termed *professional autonomy*, *social contract*, and *free market*.[e]

Professional Autonomy Perspective

The first perspective, grounded in the notion that the medical profession should have the authority to regulate itself, held sway from approximately 1880 to 1960, making it the most dominant of the three perspectives in terms of both the length of time it held favored status and its effect in the actual shaping of health policy and law. This model is premised on the idea that physicians' scientific expertise in medical matters should translate into legal authority to oversee essentially all aspects of delivering health care to individuals; in other words, according to proponents of the physician autonomy model, legal oversight of the practice of medicine should be delegated to the medical profession itself. During the period that this perspective remained dominant, policymakers and lawmakers were generally willing to allow physicians to control the terms and amounts of payments for rendered healthcare services, the standards under which medical licenses would be granted, the types of patients they would treat, the type and amount of information to disclose to patients, and the determination as to whether their colleagues in the medical profession were negligent in the treatment of their patients.

Social Contract Perspective

The second perspective that informs a historical conceptualization of health policy and law is that of the "modestly egalitarian social contract" (Rosenblatt et al., 1997, p. 2; the authors write that the American social contract lags behind those of other developed countries, and thus use the phrase "modestly egalitarian" in describing it). This paradigm overshadowed its competitors, and thus guided policymaking, from roughly 1960 to 1980, a time notable in U.S. history for social progressiveness, civil rights, and racial inclusion. At the center of this perspective is the belief that complete physician autonomy over the delivery and financing of health care is potentially dangerous in terms of patient care and healthcare expenditures, and that public policy and law can and sometimes should enforce a "social contract" at the expense of physician control. Put differently, this perspective sees physicians as just one of several stakeholders (including but not limited to patients, employers, and society more broadly) that lay claim to important rights and interests in the operation of the healthcare system. Health policies and laws born of the social contract era centered on enhancing access to health care (e.g., through what is now called the Examination and Treatment for Emergency Medical Conditions and Women in Labor Act, the debate around which began in the early 1980s), creating new health insurance programs (Medicare and Medicaid were established in 1965), and passing antidiscrimination laws (one of the specific purposes of Title VI of the federal 1964 Civil Rights Act was wiping out healthcare discrimination based on race).

Free Market Perspective

The final historical perspective—grounded in the twin notions of the freedom of the marketplace and of market competition—became dominant in the 1990s and continues with force today (though one could argue that the Patient Protection and Affordable Care Act [ACA] evidences a curbing of the free market perspective and an episodic elevation of the social contract perspective). The free market perspective contends that the markets for healthcare services and for health insurance operate best in a deregulated environment, and that commercial competition and consumer empowerment will lead to the most efficient healthcare system. Regardless of the validity of this claim, this perspective argues that the physician autonomy model is falsely premised on the idea of scientific expertise, when in fact most healthcare services deemed "necessary" by physicians have never been subjected to rigorous scientific validation (think of the typical treatments for the common cold or a broken leg). It further argues that even the modest version of the social contract theory that heavily influenced health policy and law during the civil rights generation is overly regulatory. Furthermore, market competition proponents claim that both other models are potentially inflationary: In the first case, self-interest will lead autonomous physicians to drive up the cost of their services, and in the second instance, public insurance programs like Medicare would lead individuals to seek unnecessary care.

To tie a couple of these historical perspectives together and examine (albeit in somewhat oversimplified fashion) how evolving social and economic mores have influenced health policy and law, consider the

example of Medicaid, the joint federal–state health insurance program for low-income individuals. In 1965, Medicaid was born out of the prevailing societal mood that it was an important role of government to expand legal rights for the poor and needy. Its creation exemplified a social contract perspective, which in the context of health, promotes the view that individuals and society as a whole are important stakeholders in the healthcare and public health systems. Medicaid entitled eligible individuals to a set of benefits that, according to courts during the era under consideration, was the type of legal entitlement that could be enforced by beneficiaries when they believed their rights under the program were infringed.

These societal expectations and legal rights and protections withstood early challenges during the 1970s, as the costs associated with providing services under Medicaid resulted in state efforts to roll back program benefits. Then, in the 1980s, Medicaid costs soared higher, as eligibility reforms nearly doubled the program's enrollment and some providers (e.g., community health centers) were given higher payments for the Medicaid services they provided. Still, the social contract perspective held firm, and the program retained its essential egalitarian features.

As noted, however, the gravitational pull of the social contract theory weakened as the 1980s drew to a close. This, coupled with the fact that Medicaid spending continued to increase in the 1990s, led to an increase in the number of calls to terminate program members' legal entitlement to benefits.[f] Also in the 1990s, federal and state policymakers dramatically increased the role of private managed care companies in both Medicaid and Medicare, an example of the trend toward free market principles.

Key Stakeholders

A third way to conceptualize health policy and law issues is in terms of the stakeholders whose interests are impacted by certain policy choices or by the passage or interpretation of a law. For example, imagine that in the context of interpreting a state statute regulating physician licensing, your state's highest court ruled that it was permissible for a physician to not treat a patient who was in urgent need of care, even though the doctor had been serving as the patient's family physician. What stakeholders could be impacted by this result? Certainly the patient, as well as other patients whose treatment may be colored by the court's decision. Obviously the doctor and other doctors practicing in the same state could be impacted by the court's conclusion. What about the state legislature? Perhaps it unintentionally drafted the licensing statute in an ambiguous fashion, which led the court to determine that the law conferred no legal responsibility on the physician to respond to a member of a family that was part of the doctor's patient load. Or maybe the legislature is implicated in another way—maybe it drafted the law with such clarity that no other outcome was likely to result, but the citizenry of the state became outraged because its elected officials created public policy that is out of step with constituents' values. Note how this last example draws in the perspective of another key stakeholder—the broader public.

Of course, patients, healthcare providers, governments, and the public are not the only key stakeholders in important matters of health policy and law. Managed care and traditional insurance companies, employers, private healthcare industries, the research community, interest groups, and others all may have a strong interest in various policies or laws under debate.

Conclusion

The preceding descriptions of the roles played by policy and law in the health of individuals and populations, and of the ways to conceptualize health policy and law, were cursory by design. But what we hope is apparent to you at this early stage is the fact that the study of policy and law is essential to the study of both health care and public health. Consider the short list of major problems with the U.S. health system as described in a book edited and written by a group of leading scholars: the coverage and financing of health care, healthcare quality, health disparities, and threats to population health (Mechanic et al., 2005, p. 10). All of the responses and fixes to these problems—and to many other healthcare- and public health–related concerns—will invariably and necessarily involve creative policymaking and rigorous legal reform (and indeed, the ACA, about which you will read in various sections, addressed each of these topics to one degree or another). This fact is neither surprising nor undesirable: Policy and law have long been used to effect positive social change, and neither the healthcare nor public health field should be immune to these efforts. Thus, going forward, there is little reason to expect that policy and law will not be two of the primary drivers of health-related reform.

Policy and legal considerations are not relevant only in the context of major healthcare and public health transformations, however—they are critical to the daily functioning of the health system, and to the health and safety of individuals and communities across a range of everyday life events. Think about pregnancy and childbirth, for example. There are approximately 10,200 births each day in this country, and thus society views pregnancy and childbirth as more or less normal and unremarkable events. In fact, the process of becoming pregnant, accessing and receiving high-quality prenatal health care, and experiencing a successful delivery is crucial not only to the physical, mental, and emotional health and well-being of individuals and families, but to the long-term economic and social health of the nation. It also implicates a dizzying number of interesting and important policy questions. Consider the following questions:

- Should there be a legal right to health care in the context of pregnancy, and, if so, should that right begin at the point of planning to get pregnant, at the moment of conception, at the point of labor, or at some other point?
- Regardless of legal rights to care, how should the nation finance the cost of pregnancy care? Should individuals and families be expected to save enough money to pay out-of-pocket for what is a predictable event? Should the government help subsidize the cost of prenatal care? If so, in what way? Should care be subsidized at the same rate for everyone, or should subsidy levels be based on financial need?
- Regarding the quality of care, what is known about the type of obstetrical care women should receive, and how do we know they are getting that care? Given the importance of this type of care, what policy steps are taken to ensure that the care is sound? What should the law's response be when a newborn or pregnant woman is harmed through an act of negligence? When should clinician errors be considered preventable and their commission thus tied to a public policy response? And what should the response be?
- What should the legal and social response be to prospective parents who act in ways that are risky to the health of a fetus? Should there be no societal response because the prospective parents' actions are purely a matter of individual right? Does it depend on what the actions are?
- Is it important to track pregnancy and birth rates through public health surveillance systems? Why or why not? If it is an important function, should the data tracking be made compulsory or voluntary?

- How well does the public health system control known risks to pregnancies, both in communities and in the workplace?
- Finally, who should answer these questions? The federal government? States? Individuals? Should courts play a role in answering some or all of them, and, if so, which ones? Whose interests are implicated in each question, and how do these stakeholders affect the policymaking process?

There are scores of topics—pregnancy and child-birth among them, as you can see—that implicate a range of complex health policy questions, and these are the types of questions this text prepares you to ask and address. Before you turn your attention to the essential principles, components, and issues of health policy and law, however, you must understand something about policy and law generally, and about the organization and purposes of the healthcare and public health systems. The next two chapters provide a grounding in policy and law and supply the basic information needed to study policy and law in a health context. In those chapters, we define policy and law, discuss the political and legal systems, introduce the

administrative agencies and functions at the heart of the government's role in health care and public health, and more. With this information at your disposal, you will be better equipped to think through some of the threshold questions common to many policy debates, including the following questions: Which sector—public, private, or not-for-profit (or some combination of them)—should respond to the policy problem? If government responds, at what level—federal or state—should the problem be addressed? What branch of government is best suited to address, or is more attuned to, the policy issue? When the government takes the lead in responding to a policy concern, what is the appropriate role of the private and not-for-profit sectors in also attacking the problem? What legal barriers might there be to the type of policy change being contemplated? Once you have the knowledge to critically assess these types of questions, you will be able to focus more specifically on how the healthcare and public health systems operate in the United States, and on the application of policy and law to critical issues in health care and public health.

References

Mechanic, D., Rogut, L. B., Colby, D. C., & Knickman, J. R. (Eds.). (2005). *Policy challenges in modern health care.* Rutgers University Press.

Rosenblatt, R. E., Law, S. A., & Rosenbaum, S. (1997). *Law and the American health care system.* The Foundation Press.

Endnotes

a. See, for example, Parmet, W. E. (2007). Introduction: The interdependency of law and public health. In R. A. Goodman, R. E. Hoffman, W. Lopez, G. W. Matthews, M. A. Rothstein, & K. L. Foster (Eds.), *Law in public health practice* (2nd ed., pp. xxvii–xxvii). New York, NY: Oxford University Press.

b. For a nonfictional and utterly engrossing example of the ways in which law and legal process might stand in the way of effective public health regulation, we recommend Harr, J. (1995). *A civil action.* New York, NY: Vintage Books.

c. See, for example, Gostin, L. O., Thompson, F. E., & Grad, F. P. (2007). The law and the public's health: The foundations.

In R. A. Goodman, R. E. Hoffman, W. Lopez, G. W. Matthews, M. A. Rothstein, & K. L. Foster (Eds.), *Law in public health practice* (2nd ed., pp. 25–44). New York, NY: Oxford University Press.

d. The particular historical framework described here was developed to apply to health care rather than to public health. We do not mean to imply, however, that it is impossible to consider public health from a historical, or evolutionary, vantage point. In fact, it is fair to say that public health practice may have just entered its third historical phase. Throughout the 1800s and most of the 1900s, protection of the public's health occurred mainly through direct regulation of private behavior. In the latter stages of the 20th century, strict reliance on regulation gave way to an approach that combined regulation with chronic disease management and public health promotion, an approach that necessitated a more active collaboration between public health agencies and healthcare providers and purchasers. Now, it appears that public health professionals are adding to this revised practice model another strategic initiative: building collaborative relationships with policymaking agencies whose responsibilities are not directly related to public health—for example, agencies whose primary fields are housing, transportation, or agriculture.

e. The discussion of these perspectives is guided by Rosenblatt, R. E., Law, S. A., & Rosenbaum, S. (1997). *Law and the American health care system*. Westbury, CT: The Foundation Press, pp. 24–35; Rosenblatt, R. E. (2004). The four ages of health law. *Health Matrix: Journal of Law-Medicine, 14*(1), 155–196.

f. By 2005, proponents of weakening Medicaid-enrolled persons' entitlement to program benefits had made significant strides: Congress passed a law called the Deficit Reduction Act that, among other things, granted states the ability to redefine the benefits and services to which Medicaid beneficiaries are entitled.

CHAPTER 2

Policy and the Policymaking Process

LEARNING OBJECTIVES

By the end of this chapter you will be able to:

1. Describe the concepts of policy and policymaking
2. Describe the basic function, structure, and powers of the legislative branch of government
3. Describe the basic function, structure, and powers of the executive branch of government
4. Explain the role of federal and state governments in the policymaking process
5. Explain the role of interest groups in the policymaking process

Introduction

The first steps for any student of health policy are to gain a general understanding what policy is and to learn about the policymaking process. It is vital to consider policy questions in the particular context in which they arise, both in terms of the general politics of the issue and the values and powers of the policymaker. As you will discover, there is no single definition of policy. Even so, this chapter arms you with the information needed to know what issues to consider when thinking about a public policy problem, how to account for a variety of competing policy views, and what policy options are possible given the political process in the United States.

The chapter first defines what policy is and then moves to a discussion of the policymaking process by examining the roles and powers of two of the political branches of government—the legislative and executive branches. As part of this discussion, we introduce you to the federal and state agencies that make up the healthcare and public health bureaucracy. We conclude with a discussion about the roles of interest

groups in policymaking and the influence they wield in the policymaking process.

Defining Policy

In this section we consider various aspects of what we mean by the term *policy*. Before delving into the policymaking process, we identify which issues fall within the realm of a public policy decision and, generally, what kinds of decisions might be made by policymakers.

Identifying Public Problems

Scholars have defined policy in many different ways. Consider just a few definitions, as listed here:

- Authoritative decisions made in the legislative, executive, or judicial branches of government that are intended to direct or influence the actions, behaviors, and decisions of others (Longest, 2016, p. 10).
- A course of action adopted and pursued by a government, party, statesman, or other individual

or organization (Subcommittee on Health and Environment, 1976, p. 124).

- Authoritative decisions and guidelines that direct human behavior toward specific goals either in the private or the public sector (Hanley, 1999, p. 125).

The differences in these definitions raise several important issues. The first question to consider is whether private actors make policy or whether policymaking is an activity for the government exclusively. The first definition refers only to governmental policymakers, the second definition allows for both public and private policymakers, and the third definition is unclear on this issue. Of course, the government is a key player in any policy field, and it is certainly true that decisions by government entities represent public policy. However, in this text we also focus on private actors who make policy, such as commercial insurance companies, private employers, influential individuals, and others who can all be part of health policy. For example, when a major health insurance company decides to cover obesity prevention measures, or when the Bill and Melinda Gates Foundation provides grants to develop crops that are high in essential vitamins and minerals to improve the nutrition of people in developing countries, they are making health policy decisions.

Regardless of whether the policymaker is a public or private figure, it is necessary that the decision being made is an *authoritative* decision. An authoritative decision is one that is made by an individual or group that has the power to implement the decision. There are a variety of levels where these kinds of decisions can take place. For example, within government, authoritative decisions may be made by the president, cabinet officials, agency heads, members of Congress, governors, state legislatures, public health commissioners, and many others.

All decisions by public and private individuals or entities are not necessarily policy decisions. The key issue in determining whether a "decision" represents a "policy" is whether the question at hand is an individual concern or a public policy problem. A public policy problem goes beyond the individual sphere and affects the greater community. Whereas an individual might decide to take advantage of employer-sponsored health insurance, a public policy question is whether all employers should be required to offer health insurance to their employees. Whereas an individual might decide to purchase a generic (as opposed to a brand name) drug to save money, a public policy question is whether patients should be induced to buy less expensive generic drugs. When deciding whether something is a public policy decision, the focus is not

only on who is making a decision, but also on what kind of decision is being made.

Furthermore, just because a problem is identified as a public policy problem does not necessarily mean the only solution involves government intervention. For example, consider the problem of an influenza vaccine shortage. Although there are government-oriented solutions to this problem, such as expanding public research and development or creating production incentives (through tax cuts or subsidies) to encourage private manufacturers to produce more vaccine, other solutions may rely solely on private actors. Private companies may decide to invest in the research and development of new ways to produce vaccines or to build new plants to increase production capacity, because they believe they can make a profit in the long run. Just as private individuals and entities can make policy decisions for their own benefit, they can also play a central role in solving public policy problems. Operation Warp Speed was an example of a public–private initiative to develop, manufacture, and distribute a COVID-19 vaccine. The Department of Health and Human Services (HHS), the Department of Defense (DoD), and other federal agencies provided funding to several private pharmaceutical companies, accelerated clinical trials, and shortened the planning and distribution process to "accelerate vaccine development and mitigate risk" (Government Accountability Office, 2021). A lengthier discussion about options for solving public policy problems and the arguments for and against government intervention is found in a review of health economics.

Structuring Policy Options

Considered broadly, there are different ways to approach public policy problems. For example, some policy options are voluntary, whereas others are mandatory. It is important to recognize that authoritative decisions do not always *require* others to act or refrain from acting in a certain way. Some of the most important and effective policies are those that provide incentives to others to change their behavior. Indeed, the power of persuasion is very important to public officials, particularly those working for the federal government, which is limited in its ability to force states and individuals to take certain actions. This restriction stems from the fact that the 10th Amendment of the U.S. Constitution limits Congress and the executive branch to specific powers and reserves all other powers for the states. However, members of the federal government may use their enumerated powers, such as those to tax and spend, to persuade states and others to act in desired ways.

For example, the Constitution does not give the legislative or executive branches the power to protect the public's health, meaning that this area is primarily within the purview of states to regulate. As a result, Congress and the president cannot require states to create emergency preparedness plans. Yet, Congress may provide incentives to states to do so by offering them federal money in return for state preparedness plans that meet certain criteria established by the federal government. As illustrated by the federal response to the COVID-19 pandemic, however, a number of laws give the federal government the power to protect the public's health during times of emergency (see Chapter 13, "What Is Public Health Emergency Preparedness?").

In addition, it is important to remember that inaction can also be a policy decision. Deciding to do nothing may be a decision to keep a prior decision in place or not to engage in a new issue. For example, a governor could decide against trying to change a restrictive abortion law, or a state legislature could choose not to pass a law expanding the allowable scope of practice for nurse practitioners. Both of these inactions result in important policy decisions that will affect the choices and opportunities available to individuals, advocacy organizations, and others.

This brief discussion about policy has raised several important issues to consider when identifying policy options. In the next section we discuss the policymaking process in detail, providing you with the background knowledge necessary to identify and understand the roles and powers of various policymakers.

Public Policymaking Structure and Process

The public policymaking structure refers to the various branches of government and the individuals and entities within each branch that play a role in making and implementing policy decisions. In this section, we review the structure, powers, and constituency of these branches, with a focus on the U.S. House of Representatives, the U.S. Senate, and various commissions and agencies that assist Congress, the president, White House staff, and federal executive branch administrative agencies. In addition to reviewing the policymaking structure, we discuss the processes used by these various individuals and entities for making public policy decisions.

State-Level Policymaking

The federal government does not have a monopoly on policymaking. Indeed, important policy decisions are regularly made at the state level as well, especially in the healthcare arena (**Box 2.1**). However, because state governments are similar to the federal government in many ways, the policymaking duties and powers presented in the following discussion can often be applied to a state-level analysis. At the same time, there is a significant amount of variation in how states structure their legislative and executive branches, agencies, and offices, and it is not possible to review the differences that exist among all 50 states. Accordingly, after a brief discussion of state-level policymaking, this chapter focuses primarily on the federal policymaking structure and process.

Like the federal government, each state has three branches of government. State legislatures pass laws, appropriate money within the state, and conduct oversight of state programs and agencies. States also have their own judiciary, with trial and appellate courts. The governor is the head of the state executive branch and can set policy, appoint cabinet members, and use state administrative agencies to issue regulations that implement state laws. Although there are limits to a state's power to regulate healthcare issues, state regulation is an extremely important aspect of health policy. Just a few examples of the healthcare matters states can regulate include provider licensing,

---

💡 Box 2.1 DISCUSSION QUESTIONS

The COVID-19 pandemic illustrated the tensions and consequences of our federalist system. At the outset of the pandemic, the federal government used its emergency powers to restrict economic and personal liberty through a national lockdown. As the lockdown was lifted, state governments became the locus of decision-making for continued responses to the pandemic. At times, governors and state legislatures had opposing views about which restrictions to impose in their state and disputes had to be resolved by the courts. As a result, where one lived determined everything from whether face coverings were mandatory, to whether schools were open for children, to when COVID-19 vaccines became available. Because COVID-19 is a communicable disease, the decisions in one state to loosen restrictions could affect citizens in other states.

Where do you think the decision-making power should rest in a pandemic? How long should the federal government maintain the power to impose national restrictions? Should the states have the flexibility to respond to the politics and circumstances in their area? Does your answer depend on what type of national emergency exists?

accreditation, some aspects of health insurance, and most public health concerns.

Although state governments share these general characteristics, it is important to realize that not all state governments are exactly alike. The governor has more power in some states than in others, agencies are combined in different ways among the states, state legislatures may meet annually or biannually, state legislators may be full-time or part-time employees, and so on. Because these differences exist, it is essential for policy analysts to understand the specific structure of the state in which their client resides.

Furthermore, there are important differences between the federal government and state governments. Unlike the federal government, almost all states are required to have a balanced budget, and most states cannot borrow money for operating expenses. These rules mean that states must act to raise revenue or cut programs if they project that their budget will be in deficit by the end of the fiscal year. In addition, 28 states have at least one tax and expenditure limit rule that restricts the growth of government revenues or spending to a fixed numerical target, sometimes using changes in population level or the inflation rate as guideposts (Rueben & Randall, 2017). Furthermore, 16 states require a legislative supermajority or voter approval to raise taxes (a supermajority means that more than a simple majority—over 50%—is required; for example, a two-thirds majority vote could be required) (Center on Budget and Policy Priorities, 2018). As a result, state officials may be more likely than federal officials to make the difficult choice to either limit programs or cut resources from one program to fund another.

As is evident from this brief discussion, state-level policymaking is both a rich area for discussion and a difficult area to make generalizations about because each state is unique. Having highlighted some of the key differences and similarities among the states and between the state and the federal governments, we now turn to the legislative and executive branches of the federal government.

The Federal Legislative Branch

Article I of the U.S. Constitution makes Congress the lawmaking body of the federal government by granting it "all legislative powers" and the right to enact "necessary and proper laws" to effect its prerogatives (U.S. Const. art. I, § 1; U.S. Const. art. I, § 8). Congressional responsibilities are fulfilled by the two chambers of Congress, the Senate and the House of Representatives ("the House"). The Constitution grants specific powers to Congress, including but not limited to the power to levy taxes, collect revenue, pay debts, provide for the general welfare, regulate interstate and foreign commerce, establish federal courts inferior to the Supreme Court, and declare war (U.S. Const. art. I, § 1). The Senate has the specific power to ratify treaties and confirm nominations of public officials.

The Senate consists of two elected officials from each state, for a total of 100 senators.[a] Each senator is elected in a statewide vote for a 6-year term, whereas representatives in the House sit for 2-year terms. Due to the lengthy term of its members, the Senate is considered less volatile and more concerned with long-term issues than the House. A senator must be at least 30 years old, a U.S. citizen for at least 9 years, and a resident of the state they are seeking to represent (U.S. Const. art. I, § 3).

The House includes 435 members allocated proportionally based on the population of the 50 states, with each state guaranteed at least one representative.[b] For example, in 2020, California was allotted 53 representatives, while Vermont had only 1. Due to the proportionality rule, members from larger states dominate the House and often hold leadership positions. Members of the House are elected by voters in congressional districts and serve 2-year terms. They must be at least 25 years old, a U.S. citizen for at least 7 years, and a resident of the state where the election takes place (U.S. Const. art. I, § 2).

Leadership Positions

Leadership roles in Congress are determined by political party affiliation, with the party in the majority gaining many advantages. The vice president of the United States is also the president of the Senate and presides over its proceedings. In the vice president's absence, which is common given the other obligations of the office, the president *pro tempore*, a mostly ceremonial position, presides over the Senate. In most cases the vice president is not a major player in Senate voting, but with the power to break a tie vote, the vice president wields an important power. Indeed, after the 2020 elections, the Democrats and Republicans each held 50 seats in the Senate. As a result, Vice President Harris gave the Democrats the majority by virtue of holding the tie-breaking vote in the Senate. The Speaker of the House ("Speaker") presides over that chamber and has the authority to prioritize and schedule bills, refer bills to committees, and name members of joint and conference committees. Other than the vice president's senatorial role, leadership positions in Congress are not determined by the voters; instead, they are determined by the members of the party who have been elected to Congress. Other key congressional leadership positions include the following:

- **Senate majority leader:** Speaks on behalf of the majority party, schedules floor action and bills, works on committees, directs strategy, and tries to keep the party united.
- **House majority leader:** Works with the Speaker to direct party strategy and set the legislative schedule.
- **House and Senate minority leaders:** Speak on behalf of the minority party, direct strategy, and try to maintain party unity; as members of the minority, they do not have the legislative duties of the majority leader/Speaker.
- **House and Senate majority and minority whips:** Track important legislation, mobilize members to support leadership positions, keep a count of how party members are planning to vote, and generally assist their leaders in managing their party's legislative priorities.

Committees

Committees have been referred to as the "workhorses" of Congress; they are where many key decisions are made and legislative drafting takes place. Given the vast array of issues that Congress contends with in any given legislative session, it is impossible for every member to develop expertise on every issue. Although members vote on bills that cover a wide range of issues, members often concentrate on the areas relevant to the committees on which they serve.

Committees have a variety of important roles, including drafting and amending legislation; educating members on key issues; shepherding the committee's legislation on the floor when it goes before a vote by all the members of one chamber; working with the president, the president's administration, and lobbyists to gain support for a bill; holding hearings; and conducting oversight of executive branch departments, agencies, commissions, and programs within their purview. Committee members often gain expertise in the areas covered by their committees, and other members often rely on their advice when making voting decisions.

Standing committees are generally permanent committees with specified duties and powers. There are 20 standing committees in the House and 16 in the Senate. House committees tend to be larger than those in the Senate, with about 40 members per committee. Some committees have *authorization* jurisdiction, allowing them to create programs and agencies. Other committees have *appropriation* authority, meaning

they are responsible for funding various programs and agencies. Standing committees also have *oversight* authority, meaning they monitor how programs are run and funds are spent. Each chamber of Congress has established specific oversight committees for some programs and issues that cut across committee jurisdiction, as well as committees that review the efficiency and economy of government actions (Heitshusen, 2018).

Not surprisingly, some of the most powerful and popular committees are those that deal with appropriating money. These include the following:

- **House Ways and Means and Senate Finance Committees:** These committees have jurisdiction over legislation concerning taxes, tariffs, and other revenue-generating measures, and over entitlement programs such as Medicare and Social Security. The Constitution requires all taxation and appropriations bills to originate in the House, and House rules require all tax bills to go through the Ways and Means Committee.
- **House and Senate Appropriations Committees:** These committees have responsibility for writing federal spending bills.
- **House and Senate Budget Committees:** These committees are tasked with creating the overall budget plan that helps guide tax and appropriation committee work.
- **House Rules Committee:** This committee has jurisdiction over the rules and order of business in the House, including rules for the floor debates, amendments, and voting procedures. Unlike in the Senate, all House bills must go to the House Rules Committee before reaching the House floor for a vote by all representatives.

Table 2.1 identifies the key health committees and subcommittees and their health-related jurisdictions.

Congressional Commissions and Staff Agencies

Although the committee system helps members of Congress focus on particular areas, members often need assistance with in-depth research and policy analysis. Commissions and staff agencies provide members with information they might not otherwise have the time to gather and analyze. There are too many commissions and agencies to list here, but a few key ones include the following:

- **Congressional Budget Office:** An agency that provides Congress with cost estimates of bills and federal mandates to state and local governments,

Table 2.1 Key Health Committees and Subcommittees

Committee/Subcommittee	Health-Related Jurisdiction
Senate Finance Committee	

■ Subcommittee on Health Care	■ Department of Health and Human Services
	  • Centers for Medicare and Medicaid Services (includes Children's Health Insurance Program [CHIP])
	  • Administration for Children and Families
	■ Department of the Treasury
	  • Group health plans under the Employee Retirement Income Security Act (ERISA)

Senate Appropriations Committee	
■ Subcommittee on Labor, Health and Human Services, Education, and Related Agencies	■ Department of Health and Human Services • All areas except Food and Drug Administration, Indian Health Service, and construction activities
■ Subcommittee on Agriculture, Rural Development, Food and Drug Administration, and Related Agencies	■ U.S. Department of Agriculture (except Forest Service) • Includes child nutrition programs; food safety and inspections; nutrition program administration; special supplemental nutrition program for Women, Infants, Children (WIC); and Supplemental Nutrition Assistance Program (SNAP) ■ Food and Drug Administration

■ Subcommittee on Interior, Environment, and Related Agencies	■ Department of Health and Human Services
	  • Indian Health Service
	  • Agency for Toxic Substances and Disease Registry

Senate Health, Education, Labor, and Pensions Committee	
■ Subcommittee on Children and Families ■ Subcommittee on Primary Health and Retirement Security	■ Occupational safety and health, public health, Health Resources and Services Act, substance abuse and mental health, oral health, healthcare disparities, ERISA
Senate Committee on Agriculture, Nutrition, and Forestry	
■ Subcommittee on Food and Nutrition, Specialty Crops, Organics, and Research	■ Food from fresh waters; SNAP; human nutrition; inspection of livestock, meat, and agricultural products; pests and pesticides; school nutrition programs; other matters related to food, nutrition, and hunger
Senate Committee on Environment and Public Works	

■ Subcommittee on Clean Air, Climate, and Nuclear Safety
  • Chemical Safety, Waste Management, Environmental Justice, and Regulatory Oversight
  • Fisheries, Water, and Wildlife
	■ Air pollution, environmental policy, research and development, water pollution, nonmilitary control of nuclear energy, solid waste disposal and recycling

House Committee on Ways and Means	
■ Subcommittee on Health	■ Programs providing payments for health care, health delivery systems, and health research ■ Social Security Act ■ Maternal and Child Health Block Grant ■ Medicare ■ Medicaid ■ Peer review of utilization and quality control of healthcare organizations

(continues)

Table 2.1 Key Health Committees and Subcommittees ___ *(continued)*

Committee/Subcommittee	Health-Related Jurisdiction
	■ Tax credit and deduction provisions of the Internal Revenue Service relating to health insurance premiums and healthcare costs
■ Subcommittee on Worker and Family Support	■ Social Security Act • Public assistance provisions • Supplemental Security Income provisions • Mental health grants to states
House Committee on Appropriations	
■ Subcommittee on Labor, Health and Human Services, Education, and Related Agencies	■ Department of Health and Human Services • Administration for Children and Families • Administration for Community Living • Agency for Healthcare Research and Quality • Centers for Disease Control and Prevention • Centers for Medicare and Medicaid Services • Health Resources Services Administration • National Institutes of Health • Substance Abuse and Mental Health Services • Federal Mine Safety and Health Review Commission • Medicaid and CHIP Payment and Access Commission • Medicare Payment Advisory Committee • National Council on Disability • Occupational Safety and Health Review Commission • Social Security Administration
■ Subcommittee on Agriculture, Rural Development, Food and Drug Administration, and Related Agencies	■ Food and Drug Administration ■ Department of Agriculture (except Forestry)
■ Subcommittee on Energy and Water Development, and Related Agencies	■ Department of Energy • National Nuclear Strategy Administration • Federal Energy Regulatory Commission ■ Department of Interior ■ Bureau of Reclamation ■ Defense Nuclear Facilities Safety Board ■ Nuclear Regulatory Commission
■ Subcommittee on Interior, Environment, and Related Agencies	■ Department of Interior (except Bureau of Reclamation and Central Utah Project) ■ Environmental Protection Agency ■ Indian Health Service ■ National Institute of Environmental Health Sciences ■ Chemical Safety and Hazard Investigation Board
House Committee on Agriculture	
■ Subcommittee on Nutrition, Oversight, and Department Operations	■ Nutrition programs, including SNAP
■ Subcommittee on Biotechnology, Horticulture, and Research	■ Policies and statutes relating to horticulture, bees, organic agriculture, pest and disease management, bioterrorism, biotechnology
■ Subcommittee on Livestock and Foreign Agriculture	■ Policies and statutes relating to inspections of livestock, dairy, poultry, and seafood; aquaculture; animal welfare

as well as forecasts economic trends and spending levels.

- **Government Accountability Office:** An independent, nonpartisan agency that studies how federal tax dollars are spent and advises Congress and executive agencies about more efficient and effective ways to use federal resources.
- **Congressional Research Service:** The public policy research service that conducts nonpartisan, objective research on legislative issues.
- **Medicare Payment Advisory Commission:** An independent federal commission that gives Congress advice on issues relating to the Medicare program, including payment, access to care, and quality of care.

How Laws Are Made

One way that members of Congress indicate their policy preferences is by passing laws that embody their values and the values of their constituents. This is a lengthy process, with many steps along the way that could derail a bill (**Figure 2.1**).

Before a committee considers a bill, it must be introduced by a member of Congress. Once this occurs, the Speaker refers the bill to one or more committees in the House, and the majority leader does the same in the Senate. The bill may die in committee if there is not sufficient support for it, although there are rarely invoked procedures that allow a bill to be reported to the full chamber even without committee approval. While the bill is in committee, members may hold hearings on it or "mark up" the bill by changing or deleting language in the proposed bill or by adding amendments to it. If a majority of the committee members approves a bill, it goes to the full chamber (House or Senate, depending on where the bill originated).

The full House or Senate then debates the merits of the bill and puts it to a vote. If a majority does not support the bill, it dies on the chamber floor. If a majority supports the bill, it is sent to the other chamber for consideration. The second chamber may pass the exact same bill or a different version of the bill. If the second chamber does not pass any version of the bill, it dies on the chamber floor and no version of the bill moves forward. If the second chamber passes an identical bill, it goes directly to the president for consideration.

If there are differences in the bills passed by the House and Senate, the two chambers must reach a consensus through an exchange of amendments for the bill to have a chance of becoming law. Consensus building is facilitated by a "conference committee" made up of members from both chambers. If the committee cannot reach a consensus, the bill dies. If the committee reaches a consensus, the bill is sent back to each chamber for a vote on the new version of the bill. If either chamber does not approve it, the bill dies at that point. If both the House and the Senate pass the new version, it is sent to the president for consideration.

The president may choose to sign the bill into law, or the president may choose to veto the bill. If the president chooses not to sign the bill while Congress is in session, the bill becomes law after 10 days; if Congress is not in session and the bill goes unsigned, the bill dies (this is referred to as a "pocket veto"). If the president vetoes the bill, Congress may override the veto with approval of a two-thirds majority in each chamber.

Congressional Budget and Appropriations Process

Although the budget and appropriations process may sound dry, it is about much more than numbers and charts. If you take a close look at budget documents, they include narratives that discuss why certain programs are being funded and what the government hopes to achieve by doing so. In many ways, this process is a key policy tool for members of Congress and the president; they are able to show which programs and issues have their support through their funding decisions.

Given both the amount of money involved in running the United States ($4.4 trillion in 2019) and the various jurisdictions of congressional committees, it is not surprising that the federal budget process is fairly complex. The Congressional Budget and Impoundment Control Act of 1974 ("Budget Act") and subsequent amendments were passed by Congress to create a process that brings together the numerous committees involved in crafting an overall budget plan. The budget process works in concert with the appropriations process, which involves congressional passage of bills from each of the appropriations committees to distribute the funds provided for in the overall budget (House Committee on the Budget Majority Caucus, 2001; Senate Committee on the Budget, 1998).

The president is required to submit a budget proposal to Congress by the first Monday in February. This proposal is the administration's request; it is not binding on Congress. Each chamber then passes a *budget resolution*, identifying how the chamber would spend federal money delineated by different categories of

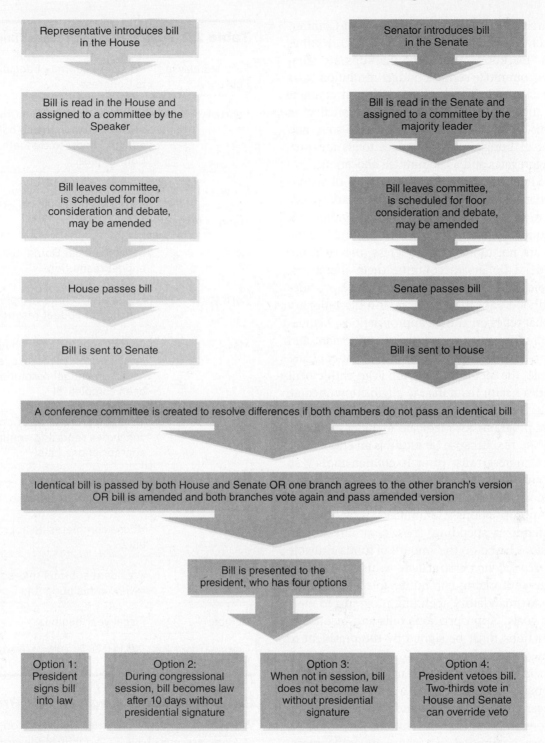

Figure 2.1 How a Bill Becomes a Law

spending (e.g., defense, agriculture, transportation). Members from each chamber then meet to develop a single *conference report* reflecting a consensus agreement on the overall budget. Congress then passes a *concurrent budget resolution*, which is binding upon the House and Senate as a blueprint for revenue collection and spending. However, it is not a law and the president is not bound by the budget resolution.

Over the 6 weeks subsequent to the passage of the concurrent budget resolution, the House and

Senate Budget Committees hold hearings to discuss the budget, and other committees review the budget as it pertains to their jurisdiction. The latter committees supply the Budget Committees with their "views and estimates" of appropriate spending and/or revenue levels for the upcoming year. In addition, the Congressional Budget Office provides the Budget Committees with its budget and economic outlook reports and gives the Budget and Appropriations Committees its analysis of the president's proposal.

In March, the House and Senate Budget Committees each craft a budget plan during public meetings known as "markups." When the markups are complete, each committee sends a budget resolution to its respective chamber. The budget resolution contains a budget total, spending breakdown, reconciliation instructions, budget enforcement mechanisms, and statements of budget policy. Budget totals are provided as aggregates and as committee allocations.

The federal budget includes two types of spending: *discretionary* and *mandatory*. Discretionary spending refers to money that is set aside for programs that must be funded annually in order to continue. If the programs are not funded by Congress, they will not receive federal dollars to continue their operations. For example, the Head Start program, which provides early childhood education services, is a discretionary program that relies on annual appropriations. Mandatory spending refers to spending on entitlement and other programs that must be funded as a matter of law. For example, the Medicaid program is an entitlement that provides health insurance to eligible low-income individuals. The *authorizing legislation* (the law that created the program) for Medicaid includes eligibility rules and benefits. Because Medicaid is an entitlement program, Congress must provide enough money so the Medicaid agency can meet the obligations found in the authorizing legislation.

The Appropriations Committees write bills to cover discretionary spending. These committees make their decisions based on the amount of funds available and any *reconciliation instructions*, which direct the appropriate authorizing committee to make changes in the law for mandatory spending programs to meet budgetary goals. Appropriations bills and reconciliation instructions must be signed by the president to become law.

Members of the House and Senate have the opportunity to make changes to the work of the Budget Committees. Once the House and Senate pass their own versions of the budget resolution, they establish a conference committee to resolve any differences. Once the differences are resolved, each full chamber votes on the compromise budget.

Congress often does not meet Budget Act deadlines (shown in **Table 2.2**). If the appropriations bills are not passed by every October 1—the beginning of the fiscal year—Congress may pass a *continuing resolution* that allows the government to continue to spend money. If Congress does not pass a continuing resolution or if the president vetoes it, all nonessential activities of federal agencies must stop until additional funds are provided.

Table 2.2 **Federal Budget Process Timeline**

First Monday in February	President submits budget proposal to Congress.
February 15	Congressional Budget Office submits economic and budget outlook report to Budget Committees.
Six weeks after president submits budget	Committees submit views and estimates to Budget Committees.
April 1	Senate Budget Committee reports budget resolution.
April 15	House and Senate complete concurrent budget resolution.
May 15	Annual appropriations bills may be considered in the House, even if action on budget resolution has not been completed.
June 10	House Appropriations Committee concludes reporting annual House appropriations bills.
June 15	If necessary, Congress completes reconciliation legislation.
June 30	House completes its appropriations bills.
July 15	President submits mid-session review of his budget to Congress.
October 1	Fiscal year begins.

Congressional Research Service. (2008, March 20). *The congressional budget process timetable.* https://fas.org/sgp/crs/misc/98-472.pdf

Constituents of Legislative Branch

With the wide array of issues they take on, members of Congress may have an equally wide array of constituents to be concerned about when making policy decisions. Clearly, members are concerned about pleasing the voters who elect them. Even though there may be a variety of policy views to consider, members often prioritize their home constituents. In addition to courting their home-state voters, members often try to court independents or voters from the opposing party in their home state to strengthen their appeal. High approval ratings deter challengers from trying to take an incumbent's congressional seat and allow members of Congress more leeway to pursue their goals and policies.

Although concern for their home-state base may be their first priority, representatives and senators often need to be concerned about supporting their party's position on issues. Today, elected federal politicians are usually affiliated with the Democratic or Republican Party, and voters may be influenced by the party's stance on issues. In fact, "ticket splitting"—voting for one party's candidate for president and the other party's candidate for Congress—is increasingly rare. In the 2020 election, Maine was the only state where the winning senator (Collins, R-ME) and the winning presidential candidates were from different parties (Rakich & Best, 2020). Also, if the balance of power between the two parties is close in Congress, the parties usually cannot afford to have members defect from their party's positions. Members' concern regarding keeping their party strong is magnified if they hold leadership positions in Congress or are considering running for national office.

Finally, the views of the president may be important for members to consider, depending on whether the member and the president share the same party, the particular issue involved, and the president's popularity. Members who are in the same party as the sitting president have incentive to help the president remain popular because they will likely advance many of the same policies. In addition, presidents are often prodigious fundraisers and campaigners who may be able to assist members during election season. Even when members disagree with the president, the president's power to affect their influence in Congress may be a deterrent to opposing the president. Of course, if the president is exceedingly popular, it is difficult for members of either party to oppose presidential policy goals.

The Federal Executive Branch

Article II of the U.S. Constitution establishes the executive branch and vests executive power in the most well-known member of the branch, the president (U.S. Const. art. II, § 1). Of course, the president does not act alone in running the executive branch. Presidents rely on Executive Office agencies and staff such as the Council of Economic Advisors and Office of Management and Budget, as well as policy development offices such as the National Security Council and Domestic Policy Council (see **Box 2.2** for a description of one such office). In addition, there are 15 cabinet departments led by individuals selected by the president (subject to Senate confirmation) and additional non–cabinet-level agencies, all of which are responsible for, among other duties, interpreting

Box 2.2 Office of Management and Budget

The Office of Management and Budget (OMB) reports directly to the president and plays an important role in policy decisions. OMB is responsible for preparing the presidential budget proposal, which includes reviewing agency requests, coordinating agency requests with presidential priorities, working with Congress to draft appropriation and authorization bills, and working with agencies to make budget cuts when needed. In addition to these budgetary functions, OMB provides an estimate of the cost of regulations, approves agency requests to collect information, plays a role in coordinating domestic policy, and may act as a political intermediary on behalf of the president. OMB also has an oversight and evaluation function over select federal agencies as a result of the Government Performance and Results Act, which requires agencies to set performance goals and have their performance evaluated.

and implementing the laws passed by Congress. All of these advisors identify issues to be addressed and formulate policy options for the president to consider. In theory, all of these parts of the executive branch work in furtherance of the goals set by the president.

The Presidency

The president is the head of the federal executive branch. As powerful as that may sound, the country's founders created three distinct branches of government and limited the president's power in order to ensure that no single individual gained too much control over the nation. As you will see, in some ways the president is very powerful, and in other ways the president's power is quite limited.

Although there have been third-party candidates for president in the past, generally speaking, the United States operates with a two-party system, with the Democratic and Republican parties as the major parties. Each party selects a candidate for president who represents the party in the election. Presidents (and their vice presidents) are elected through a nationwide vote to serve a 4-year term. An individual is limited to serving two 4-year terms as president, which may or may not be consecutive (U.S. Const. amend. XXII, § 1).ᶜ To be eligible for election, candidates must be at least 35 years old, a natural-born citizen of the United States, and a resident of the country for at least 14 years.

Presidents have many roles. As the unofficial *Chief of State*, the president is seen as the symbol of the country and its citizens (H.R. Doc. No. 106-216, 2000, p. 40). As the official *Chief Executive Officer*, the president manages the cabinet and executive branch. The president also holds the position of *Commander in Chief of the Armed Forces*, and as such is the top-ranking military official in the country. The U.S. Constitution vests the president with other powers, such as the ability to appoint judges to the federal courts, sign treaties with foreign nations, and appoint ambassadors as liaisons to other countries. These powers are all subject to the advice and consent of the Senate (H.R. Doc. No. 106-216, 2000, p. 41).

Agenda Setting. A key tool of the presidency is the ability to put issues on the national agenda and offer a recommended course of action: "Framing agendas is what the presidency is all about" (Davidson, 1984, p. 371). Presidents help set the national agenda because of the role of the president as the country's leader and the amount of media attention given to presidential actions, decisions, and policy recommendations. Unlike many other politicians or interest groups, the president does not have to work hard to receive media coverage. Whether it is the annual State of the Union address, release of the president's budget proposal, a major speech, a press conference, a photo shoot with a foreign leader, or the release of a report, the president's message is continually publicized. In addition, the president's message can be delivered by the vice president, cabinet officers, and party leaders in Congress.

The notion of appealing directly to the country's citizens to focus on a particular issue and to influence legislative debates is referred to as "going public." In going public, presidents try to use support from the American people to gain the attention of Congress and sway votes on policy decisions. Because members of Congress are highly concerned about pleasing their constituency to improve their chance for reelection, "the president seeks the aid of a third party—the public—to force other politicians to accept his preferences" (Kernell, 1997, p. 3).

Sometimes it may be advantageous for the president to place an item on the policy agenda in a less public manner. For example, if a policy is controversial with the general public or if members of the president's party disagree with a proposal, it may be more effective to promote a policy behind the scenes. The president, either directly or through intermediaries, can carefully let members of Congress know which policies are favored. Using combinations of promises of favors and threats to members' interests, the president may be able to influence the outcome of policy debates in Congress even without going public.

In addition to deciding whether to approach Congress publicly or behind the scenes, the president must choose whether to present a preferred policy decision with more or less detail. A policy can be presented broadly through principles or general guidelines, or specifically through proposed legislation that is presented to Congress. Each method for conveying the president's goals has pros and cons. If a policy choice is presented in a broad manner, Congress may interpret the policy in a way that the president dislikes. However, if the president presents Congress with a specific proposal or draft legislation, congressional members may view such an act as an infringement on their role as the legislative body and resist working with the president.

Whether presidents are successful in placing policy issues on the national agenda and having them resolved in accordance with their preferences depends in part on how much "political capital" a president has available. Political capital is defined as the strength of the president's popularity and of the president's party, in Congress and in other contexts. Members of Congress are more likely to support a popular president who has the ability to mobilize the public's support, improve members' standing by association with the president and the president's party, and raise money for their campaigns.

Even the most popular president cannot always dictate what issues are on the national agenda, however. Events and decisions outside the president's control often influence what topics most concern the nation. The terrorist attacks of September 11, 2001, the subsequent anthrax scare, and the subway and bus bombings in London and Madrid all served to place combating terrorism at the top of the policy and political agenda during the George W. Bush administration. Concerns about an avian flu epidemic and numerous food recalls put public health and food safety issues on the national agenda. The devastation wrought by the BP oil spill in the Gulf of Mexico made improved responses to environmental disasters a high priority for a short time. Of course, the COVID-19 pandemic put public health in the spotlight. Thus, even the most popular presidents must be responsive to national and international events that may be beyond their control.

Presidential Powers. As noted earlier, the president has the power to veto legislation passed by Congress, thereby rejecting the bill. However, the president does not have to actually use the veto to shape policy. The president may be able to persuade Congress to change a piece of legislation simply by threatening to veto it, especially if it is a law that is expected to pass by only a slim majority. In general, vetoes are used infrequently, with presidents vetoing only 3% of all legislation since George Washington was president (H.R. Doc. No. 106-216, 2000, p. 43).

Presidents also have the power to issue executive orders. These are legally binding orders that the president gives to federal administrative agencies under the control of the Executive Office. In general, these orders are used to direct federal agencies and their officials in how they implement specific laws. Executive orders are controversial because under our system of government, Congress, not the executive, is tasked with making laws. In addition, significant policy decisions can be accomplished by using executive orders. For example, an executive order was used by President Truman to integrate the armed forces, by President Eisenhower to desegregate schools, by President Clinton to designate 1.7 million acres in southern Utah as a national monument, and by President George W. Bush to create the federal Office of Homeland Security (which subsequently became a cabinet-level department when Congress established it through legislation). President Trump issued several executive orders intended to alter the Patient Protection and Affordable Care Act (ACA) after Congress was unable to pass a bill to repeal and replace it (see Chapter 11, "Health Reform and the Patient Protection and Affordable Care Act" for a detailed discussion). President Biden signed 30 executive orders, presidential memoranda, and agency directives in his first three days in office (Sullivan et al., 2021).

If Congress believes an executive order is contrary to congressional intent, it has two avenues of recourse. It can amend the law at issue to clarify its intent and effectively stamp out the executive order that is now clearly contrary to the law. (Bear in mind that because the president may veto any bill, in effect it takes a two-thirds majority of Congress to override an executive order.) As an alternative, Congress may challenge the executive order in court, claiming that such actions exceed the president's constitutional powers.

Constituents of the Executive Branch.

From this description of the presidency, it is evident that presidents have several layers of constituents to consider when making policy choices. Certainly, the president represents every citizen and the country as a whole as the only nationally elected official (along with the vice president) in the nation. However, the president is also a representative of a particular political party and therefore must consider the views of that party when making policies. The party's views may be evident from the party platform, policies supported by party leadership in Congress, and voters who identify themselves as party members. In addition, the president must keep in mind the foreign policy duties of the office. Depending on the issue, it may be important for the president to take into account the views of other nations or international organizations, such as the United Nations or the World Health Organization.

How does the president decide which policies to pursue? Presidents are driven by multiple goals. They want "their policies to be adopted, they want the policies they put in place to last, and they want to feel they helped solve the problems facing the country" (Weissert & Weissert, 2002, p. 82). In addition, presidents often speak of wanting to leave a legacy or ensure their place in history when they leave office.

Given the vast array of constituents that presidents must consider, the president's policy decision-making process involves several layers. As shown in **Figure 2.2**, presidents consult their agency staff to identify problems, decide which problems are priorities, determine what solutions are available to address those problems, and choose the policy option that is the preferred course of action. In addition, the president's staff interacts with members of Congress and other political players to gauge their support for or opposition to various policies. Of course, how the media portrays both the problems and the potential solutions can be an important ingredient in whether politicians and the general public support the president's initiatives.

In addition, which policies presidents choose to promote may depend in part on when policy decisions are made. First-term presidents must satisfy their constituents if they hope to be reelected. Although all presidents want to see their favored policies implemented throughout their time in office, second-term presidents may be more willing to support more controversial goals because they cannot run for reelection. Yet, second-term presidents may also be constrained by the desire to keep their party in power, even though another individual will hold the presidential office.

Administrative Agencies

When studying the structure of our government, it is common to review Congress, the presidency, and the court system. Administrative agencies, however, are

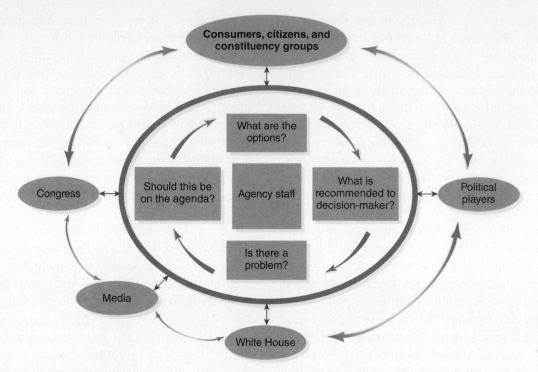

Figure 2.2 Executive Agency Policymaking
Courtesy of Jeff Levi, Professor of Health Policy, George Washington University

often overlooked despite the power they wield over the way our country is run.

Structurally, almost all administrative agencies are part of the executive branch and, thus, are under the power and control of the president. Practically, administrative agencies often work out of the public's eye to implement the laws passed by Congress and the executive orders signed by the president.

Federal agencies fall into two main categories: executive department agencies and independent agencies. Executive department agencies are under the direct control of the president, and department heads serve at the pleasure of the president. These departments include the 15 cabinet-level departments and their subunits; some of the more well-known executive departments are the Department of Health and Human Services, Department of Education, Treasury Department, Department of State, Department of Defense, and Department of Homeland Security. Independent agency heads are appointed by the president and confirmed by the Senate. They serve a fixed term and may be removed only "for cause," meaning there must be a legitimate reason to fire them. Examples of independent agencies include the Securities and Exchange Commission, U.S. Postal Service, and National Labor Relations Board.

Overall, the president fills approximately 4000 federal jobs (Yoder, 2016). In general, these political appointees have short tenures, lasting an average of

2 years (Weissert & Weissert, 2002, p. 161). When the administration changes hands after an election, new appointees are usually selected to run the agencies. The daily operations of agencies are run by career civil servants, public employees who do not necessarily come and go with each administration but who often remain at an agency for many years, gaining expertise and institutional knowledge about the agencies in which they work. Frequently, there may be tension between the goals of the political appointee and those of the career bureaucrat, who may have the advantage of familiarity with members of Congress and who knows that the political appointee is likely to be replaced in a few years.

Administrative agencies can be created by statute, internal department reorganization, or presidential directive (H.R. Doc. No. 106-216, 2000, p. 50). Regardless of how they are initially created, agencies must have statutory authority in order to receive appropriations from Congress and act with the force of law. This statutory authority, or enabling statute, outlines the agency's responsibilities and powers.

Agency Powers. By necessity, statutes are usually written broadly. Congress does not have the time or expertise to include every detail about how a new program should operate or how a new department will be structured. It is up to the executive branch agency to fill in the details, and it does so by issuing policy statements, developing rules, and promulgating regulations.

The ACA is a classic example. Although the statute itself is lengthy (over 2400 pages), the regulations needed to implement the law have been even more extensive—with some estimates putting the total page count at 20,000. To give just one example for now (a detailed discussion of the ACA occurs in Chapter 11, "Health Reform and the Patient Protection and Affordable Care Act"), the ACA includes a list of essential health benefits that must be provided by health insurance plans offered in state exchanges. The statute outlines numerous such services, including mental health services, maternity and newborn care services, prevention and wellness services, and chronic disease management services. Even with this level of detail, many unanswered questions remain regarding which services must be covered. Do mental health services include inpatient and outpatient services? Do prevention and wellness services include contraceptive coverage? Does chronic disease management include all chronic disease management models? These (and many other) questions must be answered through regulations. The ACA includes numerous provisions that require the relevant agencies to issue detailed regulations necessary for implementing the law.

In addition, agencies must follow the requirements set forth in the Administrative Procedure Act of 1946 (APA). The APA contains detailed requirements compelling agencies to issue a notice of their intent to issue a new rule or change an existing rule, and provide for and respond to public comments on the proposed rule. Some agencies are also required to hold hearings and develop rules based on the evidence presented in those hearings (Weissert & Weissert, 2002, p. 172). It is important to know that the APA creates procedural standards that require an agency to follow a particular *process* when promulgating regulations, but that the APA does not relate to the *substance* of the regulations. As long as an agency follows the necessary notice and comment requirements of the APA, it has wide latitude to issue rules within its scope of power, even if many of the public comments opposed the proposed rules. If an agency does not follow the APA requirements, interested parties may sue the agency in court to force compliance with the law.

Constituents of Agencies. Agency heads, because they are not elected, do not have constituents in the same way that the president and members of Congress do. In theory, as members of the executive branch, agency heads should be concerned only with the wishes of the president. In reality, however, that is not always the case. Some presidents have firmer control of their departments than others. If the president gives the departments and agencies broad discretion to make policy decisions, the agencies may have few policy constraints. Practically, however, agency heads want their operation to run smoothly, which includes having a good working relationship with the individuals or entities regulated by that agency. If an agency antagonizes the people or groups being regulated, they might reach out to their congressional representatives to try to change or limit the agency's personnel or authority. In addition, because Congress appropriates funds to and maintains oversight of many agencies, agency heads are well served by taking Congress's interests into account.

Table 2.3 summarizes the general public policymaking machinery. We next turn our attention to

Table 2.3 Summary of Public Policymaking Entities

	Congress	President	Administrative Agencies
Main function	Legislative body	Chief executive of the country	Implement statutes through rulemaking
Main tools/ powers	Support/oppose/pass legislation Appropriations Oversight	Agenda setting Persuasion Propose solutions Budget proposals Executive orders Sign legislation into law	Create regulations Provide information
Constituents	Voters in state or district Voters in nation if in leadership role or have national aspirations Party President	Nation (all voters) Public who voted for the president Party Other nations International organizations	President Congress Individuals and entities regulated or served by the agency

the specific parts of the government bureaucracy that operate in the health arena.

The Health Bureaucracy
The Federal Government

Although several federal agencies have healthcare-related responsibilities, three significant health agencies include HHS, the DoD, and the Department of Veterans Affairs (VA). HHS houses many of the major public health insurance programs and health services that provide care, information, and more to millions of U.S. residents; the DoD and VA operate health insurance programs specifically for military personnel and their families.

Department of Health and Human Services

HHS includes hundreds of programs that cover activities as varied as medical and social science research, preschool education services, substance abuse and prevention services, and health insurance programs, just to name a few. As shown in **Figure 2.3**, the department has 11 operating divisions. The main purpose of each agency is described in **Table 2.4**.

Each operating division has numerous bureaus or divisions that operate health programs. For example, the HIV/AIDS Bureau (HAB) is one of five bureaus in the Health Resources and Services Administration. The HAB implements the Ryan White CARE Act of 1990, which provides health care to individuals with HIV and AIDS. Similarly, the Food and Drug Administration has several offices or centers; the one whose job is perhaps best known to the general public is the Center for Drug Evaluation and Research, which is responsible for testing and approving new drugs before they can be sold to the public. These are just two examples of the many subagency units that perform vital functions in our federal healthcare bureaucracy.

HHS also includes numerous offices that assist the Secretary of HHS in running the department. The Office of the Assistant Secretary of Health (OASH) is the principal advisor to the HHS secretary on public health matters. Through the Office of the Surgeon General, OASH oversees the U.S. Public Health Service (PHS), the Commissioned Corps (health professionals used for both emergency responses and as health promoters), and the Office of Disease Prevention and Health Promotion. The PHS employs both commissioned corps members and civilians to run its public health programs.

Nine of the offices and agencies within HHS are part of the PHS. In addition, the PHS employees also work in the Bureau of Prisons, U.S. Coast Guard, National Oceanic and Atmospheric Administration, Environmental Protection Agency (EPA), Division of Immigration Health Services, and U.S. Marshal Services. HHS also has divisions concerned with planning and evaluation, legislation, administration and management, budget and finance, program support, public affairs, and global health affairs. Offices concerned with the legality and efficiency of the department's activities include those of the General Counsel and Inspector General, and the Office for Civil Rights.

The federal government includes a variety of offices and departments that focus on emergency preparedness (also see Chapter 13, "What Is Public Health Emergency Preparedness?" for more discussion of public health emergency preparedness). HHS includes an Assistant Secretary for Preparedness and Response. This individual is the principal advisor to the Secretary of HHS on matters relating to bioterrorism and other public health emergencies and helps coordinate efforts in these areas at all levels of government. HHS' Office of Global Affairs houses the Office of Pandemics and Emerging Threats, whose mission is to "prevent, detect, and respond to health threats" (Office of Global Affairs, 2019). The Department of Homeland Security (DHS), which includes the Federal Emergency Management Agency (FEMA), is tasked with preparing for and coordinating the federal response to emergencies, whether due to natural or human-made disasters. The CDC houses the Strategic National Stockpile of emergency pharmaceutical supplies. Other agencies, such as the EPA, DoD, and VA, play significant roles in emergency preparedness and response.

Department of Veterans Affairs and Department of Defense

Any veteran who does not receive a dishonorable discharge is potentially eligible for healthcare services through the Veterans Health Administration (VHA). The VHA is the largest healthcare delivery system in the country, with hundreds of medical centers, nursing homes, and outpatient clinics that serve over 9 million patients each year (Department of Veterans Affairs, n.d.).

VHA-sponsored health plans offer a wide array of preventive, ambulatory, and hospital services as well as medications and medical and surgical supplies. VHA providers are organized into integrated networks aimed at providing cost-effective services

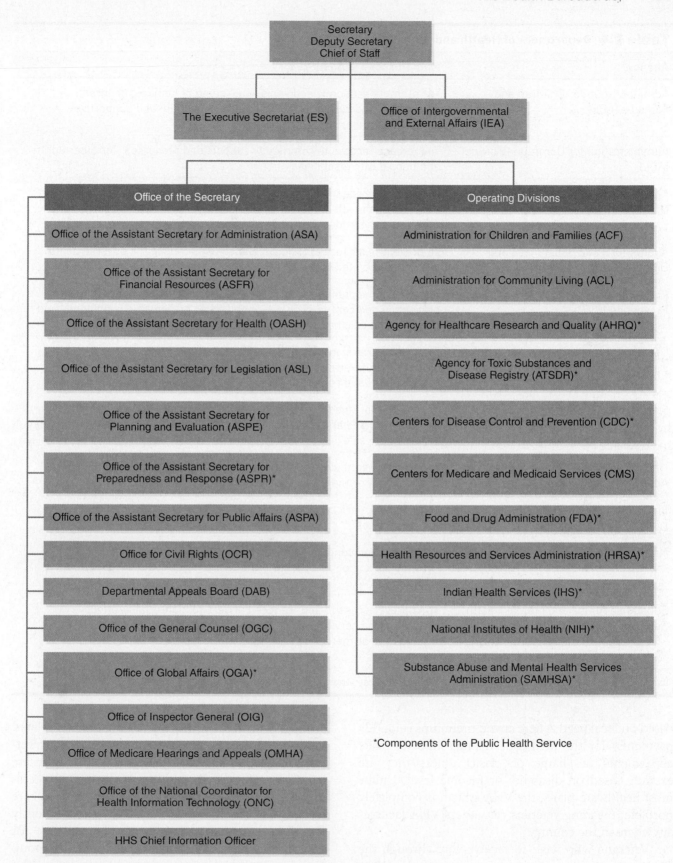

Figure 2.3 Department of Health and Human Services Organizational Chart

U.S. Department of Health and Human Services. (2021). *HHS organizational chart.* https://www.hhs.gov/about/agencies/orgchart/index.html

Table 2.4 Department of Health and Human Services Agencies

Agency	Main Purpose of Agency
Administration for Children and Families (ACF)	To "promote economic and social well-being of families, children, individuals, and communities" through educational and supportive programs
Administration for Community Living (ACL)	To increase "access to community support and resources" for older adults and people with disabilities
Agency for Healthcare Research and Quality (AHRQ)	To "produce evidence to make health care safer, high quality, more accessible, and affordable, and to work with HHS and other partners to make sure the evidence is understood and used"
Agency for Toxic Substances and Disease Registry (ATSDR)	To prevent "exposure to toxic substances and reduce the adverse health effects" associated with such exposure
Centers for Disease Control and Prevention (CDC)	To protect "the public health of the nation by providing leadership in the prevention and control of diseases and other preventable conditions" and to respond to public health emergencies
Centers for Medicare and Medicaid Services (CMS)	To provide "oversight of Medicare, the federal portions of the Medicaid and State Children's Health Insurance Program, the Health Insurance Marketplace, and related quality assurance activities"
Food and Drug Administration (FDA)	To ensure that "food is safe, pure, and wholesome," drugs and medical devices are "safe and effective," and that "electronic products that emit radiation are safe"
Health Resources and Services Administration (HRSA)	To provide "health care to people who are geographically isolated, or economically or medically vulnerable"
Indian Health Service (IHS)	To provide "American Indians and Alaska Natives with comprehensive health services"
National Institutes of Health (NIH)	To support and conduct "biomedical and behavioral research," to train "promising young researchers," and to promote "collecting and sharing knowledge"
Substance Abuse and Mental Health Services Administration (SAMHSA)	To improve access to and "reduce barriers to high-quality, effective programs and services for individuals who suffer from or are at risk for addictive or mental disorders, as well as for their families and communities"

Department of Health and Human Services. (2015). *HHS agencies and offices*. https://www.hhs.gov/about/agencies/hhs-agencies-and-offices/index.html

based on local need. There are no premiums (monthly payments) for the plan, but veterans have to make copayments (a charge per visit) unless they are exempt based on disability or income level. Unlike most healthcare plans, the VHA system is completely portable, meaning veterans can access VHA facilities anywhere in the country.

Veterans who wish to receive care through the VHA must enroll in the program. Because the VHA receives an annual appropriation from Congress, it may not have sufficient funds to pay for all of the care demanded by eligible veterans. For that reason, the VHA uses a priority system to ensure that veterans who are low income or have service-related disabilities can be enrolled into a plan. Other veterans may have to wait to be enrolled if there are insufficient funds. In addition, priority in accessing care is given to enrolled veterans who need care for service-related disabilities or have a sufficiently severe service-related disability and need care for any health concern. Veterans not in a priority group may have to wait to see an appropriate provider once they are enrolled.

Although veterans may receive care through the VHA, they are not required to do so. If eligible, they may choose to obtain services through other public or private healthcare programs or health insurance plans. They may also choose to receive some services through the VHA and others from non-VHA programs or plans. As a result of scandals pertaining to excessive wait times and falsified patient logs, Congress passed several bills to improve the medical care veterans receive. For example, the bipartisan VA Mission Act of 2018 is intended to streamline various VA programs that allow veterans to access care in the private sector and improve payment systems for providers (Rein, 2018).

The DoD provides coverage to current and retired military personnel and their families through its TRICARE program. TRICARE offers a variety of plans with various eligibility requirements and costs to the patient. If family members are not eligible through TRICARE, they may be able to receive benefits through VHA's Civilian Health and Medical Program.

State and Local Governments

As discussed earlier, the Constitution gives states primary responsibility for protecting the public's health. States have health-related agencies that deal with health financing, aging, behavioral health, environmental health, children and family services, veterans, facility licensing and standards, provider credentialing, and more. Although all states have agencies that generally cover the same functions, their structure, responsibilities, and lines of authority vary greatly.

With the variation among state agencies, it is not surprising that there are significant differences across the states in terms of their approach to public health and health services needs. All states have agencies to run their Medicaid and CHIP programs, as well as other state-specific health services programs. Local health departments (LHDs) carry out the public health functions of the state. Most commonly, LHDs are formed by, managed by, and report to a local government, such as a county commission or local board of health. This structure provides LHDs with significant latitude to interpret and implement state statutes. In some states, the state and local governments jointly oversee the LHD. LHDs may provide services directly or, as is increasingly common, may contract or provide support to others who perform the services. The services provided by LHDs vary considerably, although there is an emphasis on addressing communicable diseases, environmental health, and children's health issues. LHDs often provide services such as immunizations; infectious disease investigations, epidemiology, and surveillance; food safety and inspections; nutrition services; and environmental health

services. Some also provide diabetes care, glaucoma screening, substance abuse treatment, mental health services, and more (Turnock, 2016, pp. 235–239). (Chapter 5, "What Is Public Health?" provides a more detailed discussion of various public health agencies.)

Interest Groups

Before leaving the discussion of policy, the policy-making process, and the health bureaucracy, we must say a few words about interest groups. *Interest group* is a general term used for a wide variety of organizations that are created around a particular issue or population and have the goal of influencing policy and educating others about their views and concerns (Weissert & Weissert, 2002, p. 117). Interest groups are different from most of the other stakeholders that have been discussed because interest groups do not have the power to make policy. Although members of the executive and legislative branches of government have a key role in determining which policies are adopted, interest groups have the limited, but still significant, role of trying to influence the decisions of policymakers.

There are many types of interest groups, including trade associations, think tanks, advocacy groups, and lobbying firms. A few examples include the Pharmaceutical Research and Manufacturers of America (n.d.), whose mission is to "conduct effective advocacy for public policies that encourage discovery of important, new medicines for patients by biopharmaceutical research companies" (Our Mission section, para. 1); America's Essential Hospitals (n.d.), which "champions excellence in health care for all, regardless of social or economic circumstance, and advances the work of hospitals and health systems committed to ensuring access to care and optimal health for America's most vulnerable people" (Mission and Service section, para. 2); the Center on Budget and Policy Priorities (n.d.), which conducts nonpartisan research and pursues "federal and state policies designed both to reduce poverty and inequality and to restore fiscal responsibility in equitable and effective ways" (About the Center section, para. 1); and the Heritage Foundation (n.d.), which strives to "formulate and promote conservative public policies based on the principles of free enterprise, limited government, individual freedom, traditional American values, and a strong national defense" (About Heritage section, para. 1).

Just as members of Congress do not have the time or ability to become experts in every issue that comes before them, the same is true for the average citizen. Many people do not have the time and ability to learn about all of the issues that are important to them, develop proposals, rally public support for their positions, monitor current activity, lobby to add or remove issues from the agenda, and reach out to politicians who make policy decisions. Instead, interest groups take on those duties: "Their job is to make the case for their constituents before government, plying the halls of Congress, the executive branch, the courts, and the offices of other interest groups to provide a linkage between citizens and government" (Weissert & Weissert, 2002, p. 119).

Interest Group Powers

Interest groups do not have the power to pass laws. However, they can influence policy in a variety of ways throughout the policymaking process. For example, recall all of the steps it takes for a bill to become a law. Anywhere along that continuum is an opportunity for interest groups to make their case. The first step for interest groups is often to commission research that they use to support their position. This can be most important in the early stages of policy development, when politicians might have an open mind about various proposals (Weissert & Weissert, 2002, p. 131). However, it does not matter how much information a group has if it is not able to gain access to the decision makers. Even a few minutes with a politician may be a few more minutes than the opposition has to make its case directly to a decision maker (Weissert & Weissert, 2002, p. 131). Finally, interest groups need to develop a persuasive argument, a way to frame the issue that convinces politicians to agree with their view of a policy matter.

Interest groups have a variety of tools at their disposal when developing strategies for lobbying. They may initiate a *grassroots* campaign, asking their members to contact their representatives with a particular message. Because interest group members are the voters with the power to reelect public officials, strong grassroots campaigns can be quite effective. Or they

may try a *grasstops* strategy and harness the influence of community leaders and other prominent individuals (Weissert & Weissert, 2002, p. 1319), or they may join with other interest groups to create coalitions and strengthen their influence through numbers. Interest groups may start a media campaign to align public sentiment with their goals. Of course, providing candidates with money, often through political action committees, is a time-honored way to try to influence the outcome of policy debates.

Whatever methodology they use, interest groups are an important part of the policymaking process. According to Lindbloom (1980), interest groups are an "indispensable" (p. 85) part of making policy decisions. They provide a way to give a voice to their members, who may not otherwise feel able to participate effectively in the policymaking process.

Conclusion

This journey through the policymaking process in the United States was intended to provide you with an understanding of policy and a context for your discussions and analysis of health policy issues. It is vital that you become familiar with both the nature of policy and the institutions that make and influence policy. As you have seen, the definition of policy is subject to much debate, yet it is necessary to define what policy means before attempting to engage in policy analysis. We have also walked through the specific duties and powers of the executive and legislative branches of the federal government and included key points about state-level policymaking as well. Finally, all policy students must be aware of and understand the influence of interest groups. They have and use numerous opportunities to influence the policymaking process, and their strength and concerns must be accounted for when analyzing policy issues. As you move further into health policy study, use the information provided in this overview to help you think about and frame your own policy positions.

References

Administrative Procedure Act of 1946, 5 U.S.C. § 500 (2018).
America's Essential Hospitals. (n.d.). *Mission and service.* https://essentialhospitals.org/about-americas-essential-hospitals/mission-driven-and-ready-to-serve/
Center on Budget and Policy Priorities. (n.d.). *About the center.* https://www.cbpp.org/about

Center on Budget and Policy Priorities. (2018). *Policy basics: State supermajority rules to raise revenues.* https://www.cbpp.org/research/state-budget-and-tax/state-supermajority-rules-to-raise-revenues

Davidson, R. H. (1984). The presidency and the Congress. In M. Nelson (Ed.), *The presidency and the political system* (p. 371). Congressional Quarterly Press.

Department of Veterans Affairs. (n.d.). *Veterans Health Administration.* https://www.va.gov/ABOUT_VA/index.asp

Government Accountability Office. (2021). *Operation Warp Speed: Accelerated COVID-19 vaccine development status and efforts to address manufacturing challenges.* https://www.gao.gov/products/gao-21-319

Hanley, B. E. (1999). Policy development and analysis. In J. K. Leavitt, D. J. Mason, & M. W. Chaffee (Eds.), *Policy and politics in nursing and health care* (3rd ed., pp. 125–138). W. B. Saunders.

Heitshusen, V. (2018). *Introduction to the legislative process in the U.S. Congress* (CRS Report No. R24843). https://fas.org/sgp/crs/misc/R42843.pdf

Heritage Foundation. (n.d.). *About Heritage.* https://www.heritage.org/about-heritage/mission

House Committee on the Budget Majority Caucus. (2001). *Basics of the budget process.* U.S. Government Printing Office.

H.R. Doc. No. 106-216, at 40–50 (2000).

Kernell, S. (1997). *Going public: New strategies of presidential leadership* (3rd ed.). CQ Press.

Lindbloom, C. (1980). *The policy-making process.* Prentice-Hall.

Longest, B. B., Jr. (2016). *Health policymaking in the United States* (6th ed.). Health Administration Press.

Office of Global Affairs. (2019). *About the pandemic team.* https://www.hhs.gov/about/agencies/oga/about-oga/what-we-do/policy-and-program-coordination/pandemics-emerging-threats.html

Pharmaceutical Research and Manufacturers of America. (n.d.). *Our mission.* https://www.phrma.org/about/our-mission

Rakich, N., & Best, R. (2020). *There wasn't that much split-ticket voting in 2020.* https://fivethirtyeight.com/features/there-wasnt-that-much-split-ticket-voting-in-2020/

Rein, L. (2018, May 23). Congress sends massive veterans bill to Trump, opening door to more private care. *The Washington Post.* https://www.washingtonpost.com/politics/congress-sends-massive-veterans-bill-to-trump-opening-door-to-more-private-health-care/2018/05/23/48e91220-5ea8-11e8-a4a4-c070ef53f315_story.html

Rueben, K. S., & Randall, M. (2017). *Tax expenditure limits: How states restrict revenues and spending.* https://www.urban.org/research/publication/tax-and-expenditure-limits

Ryan White Comprehensive AIDS Resources Emergency Act of 1990, 42 U.S.C. § 300ff (2000).

Senate Committee on the Budget. (1998). *The congressional budget process: An explanation.* U.S. Government Printing Office.

Subcommittee on Health and Environment of the Committee on Interstate Commerce, U.S. House of Representatives. (1976). *A discursive dictionary of health care.* U.S. Government Printing Office.

Sullivan, K., Hickey, C., & O'Key, S. (2021, January 24). *Here are the 30 Executive Orders and actions Biden signed in his first three days.* https://www.cnn.com/2021/01/22/politics/joe-biden-executive-orders-first-week/index.html

Turnock, B. J. (2016). *Public health: What it is and how it works* (6th ed.). Jones & Bartlett Learning.

U.S. Const. amend. XXII, § 1.

U.S. Const. art. I, § 1.

U.S. Const. art. I, § 2.

U.S. Const. art. I, § 3.

U.S. Const. art. I, § 8.

U.S. Const. art. II, § 1.

Weissert, C. S., & Weissert, W. G. (2002). *Governing health: The politics of health policy* (2nd ed.). Johns Hopkins University Press.

Yoder, E. (2016, November 9). Trump and the federal workforce: Five key issues. *The Washington Post.* https://www.washingtonpost.com/news/powerpost/wp/2016/11/09/trump-and-the-federal-workforce-five-key-issues/

Endnotes

a. Under Article 1 of the Constitution, Congress has jurisdiction over the District of Columbia. Both the Senate and the House have committees that oversee some governmental functions of the District. The District elects two "shadow senators" who are allowed to lobby Congress on issues but who do not have voting rights. In terms of representation, this places the District in a position similar to other political bodies administered by the United States, such as Puerto Rico, the U.S. Virgin Islands, and American Samoa. The District's shadow senators (and a shadow representative in the House) were created by the citizens of the District in anticipation of the passage of the 1978 District of Columbia Voting Rights amendment to the U.S. Constitution, which would have granted the District the same voting rights as the states. The amendment never passed, but the District government has maintained the shadow positions nonetheless.

b. In addition to the 435 representatives, Puerto Rico has a resident commissioner, and the District of Columbia, Guam, the U.S. Virgin Islands, and American Samoa each has a delegate who is allowed to sponsor legislation and vote in committees, but may not vote on the House floor. The citizens of the District of Columbia also elect a nonvoting shadow representative.

c. In circumstances where the president serves 2 years or less of the term of another president, that president may hold office for 10 years.

CHAPTER 3

Law and the Legal System

LEARNING OBJECTIVES

By the end of this chapter you will be able to:

1. Describe the role of law in everyday life
2. Define the term *law*
3. Identify the various sources of law
4. Describe key features of the legal system

"It is perfectly proper to regard and study the law simply as a great anthropological document."

—Former U.S. Supreme Court Justice Oliver Wendell Holmes (1899, p. 444).

Introduction

The importance and complexity of law and the legal system in the United States cannot be overstated. Law's importance stems from its primary purpose: to function as the main tool with which we organize ourselves as an advanced, democratic society. The complexity of law and the legal process is a function of the multiple sources of law that may apply to any one of the millions of actions and interactions that occur daily in society, the division of legal authority between the federal and state governments and among the branches within them, the fact that the words used to create laws are constantly open to reinterpretation,[a] and more. For all its complexity, however, there is also an undeniable pervasiveness and openness when it comes to law. We are not left to wonder where it comes from or how it is made. Generally speaking, we are privy to lawmakers' rationales for the laws they write and to judges' reasoning for their legal opinions, just as we are generally privy to the process by which law is made, and once made, laws are not hidden from us; to the contrary, they are discussed in the media and catalogued in books and online services available for public consumption. (Indeed, one is *expected* to know what the law is, because its violation can have potentially severe consequences.) If you want to know more about law than the average person, you can study it formally in law and other schools, or you can consult with one of the million or so lawyers in practice today. In other words, although law is complicated, it is also accessible in a way that may not be clear at first blush.

Furthermore, as the quotation at the outset of this chapter implies, the study of law is in essence the study of human beings, particularly their evolving customs, beliefs, and value systems. Because law is the key tool with which we regulate social behavior, it stands to reason that it also reflects our foremost values and normative standards. Indeed, law "takes an understanding, a norm, an attitude, and hardens it into muscle and bone" (Friedman, 2002, p. 29); however, this is subject to change, for as our society evolves, so too does our law. A relevant example of legal evolution can be seen in the updating of state public health laws, which before the tragic events of September 11, 2001, and the subsequent anthrax scare had not been updated in most states for over a century. Soon after the 2001 attacks, however, many states, concerned about new risks to the public's health, reviewed and overhauled these laws (Ziskin & Harris, 2007).

This chapter begins by briefly considering the role law plays in everyday life, and then turns to defining law and describing its multiple sources. It then discusses several key features of the legal system, including the separation of powers among branches of government, federalism (i.e., the separate sovereignty and authority of the federal and state governments), the role of courts, due process, and more.

For some, reading this chapter may bring to mind a previously taken course on civics or government. In this case, the chapter should serve as a helpful refresher. For those of you who are new to the study of law, consider the following pages a condensed but important introduction to one of the most critical and influential aspects of the society in which you live. In either event, this chapter is designed to better position you to understand the law's application to the specific fields of health care and public health and to digest the health policy and legal concepts discussed throughout this textbook.

The Role of Law

The law reaches into nearly every corner of American life. Its impact is inescapable from the moment you wake up to the time you go to sleep at night (and perhaps beyond, if your community has a curfew or other means of controlling activity and noise after dark). Have you ever stopped to think about the regulations pertaining to the flammability of the mattress you sleep on, or the safety of the water you shower with, cook with, and drink? How about the consumer protection laws regulating the quality of the food you eat throughout the day, and the quality of the establishments that serve it? Then there are the laws pertaining to the safety of the cars, buses, and subways you travel in each day, and the traffic laws that control their movement. You encounter laws daily pertaining to the environment, property ownership, the workplace, civil rights, copyright, energy, banking, and much more. And these are just the laws implicated by the relatively mundane actions of day-to-day life. Steering into activities that are not as common—say,

international travel, or adoption, or being admitted to a hospital—you encounter the law swiftly and noticeably. If you need final proof of the ubiquitous nature of law, pick up today's newspaper and count how many stories have some sort of legal angle to them. Then do it tomorrow and the next day. What you will almost certainly find is that a great majority of the stories concern law or legal process.

The law's pervasive nature is no surprise, given the important societal role we assign to it—namely, to serve as the tool with which we govern our relationships with one another, our government, and society at large. A society as sprawling and complex as ours needs formal, enforceable rules of law to provide a measure of control (for example, the need to regulate entities or actions that are potentially dangerous or invidious—a polluting power plant, or acts of discrimination based on race or gender). Furthermore, many people believe that law should be used not just to organize and control the society in which we live, but to achieve a more just society; in other words, according to this view, the country's key organizing principle should not simply be grounded in law, but rather grounded in a legal system designed to affirmatively produce outcomes based on fairness, justice, and equality (Smith, 1991).

The main way the law governs societal relationships is to recognize and establish enforceable legal rights and responsibilities, and to create the institutions necessary to define and enforce them. Take constitutional law, for example. Constitutions are charters establishing governments and delineating certain individual and governmental rights and obligations. However, with the notable exception of the 13th Amendment's ban on slavery, constitutional provisions are triggered only when one party to a relationship works for or on behalf of the government, and when the governmental party played a significant role in the specific policy or action being challenged. Thus, constitutional law governs the relationship between individuals and their government—not the relationship between two private parties, even when one party's actions are clearly discriminatory or wrongful. Thus, although it would be a violation of a public school student's First Amendment right to be forced by his principal to pray in class, forced prayer in private schools passes constitutional muster.

A legal right (constitutional or otherwise) denotes a power or privilege that has been guaranteed to an individual under the law, not merely something that is claimed as an interest or something that is a matter of governmental discretion. Conceptually, legal rights derive from the fact that the government sometimes creates what are called individual "property rights"—a generic term referring to an entitlement to personal or real property—for specified groups of persons (Reich, 1964). Importantly, legal rights also presuppose that their enforcement can be achieved through public institutions, including state and federal courts, because a person's ability to secure a remedy when a legal right is denied, reduced, or terminated goes to the very heart of what it means to be "entitled" to something. Indeed, whether particular healthcare benefits rise to the level of being a legal "right" and whether the healthcare right can be enforced in court are two of the most fundamental legal questions in the area of healthcare law. For example, the federal Medicare program for the aged and disabled confers on eligible individuals not only the right to healthcare services, but also the ability to enforce their right to benefits when program violations occur.

The Definition and Sources of Law

Defining "Law"

Although many legal scholars agree on the general function of law in society, there is far less consensus on how to define "the law." As with many legal terms, there are several plausible interpretations of what is meant by the law, and thus there is no single way to correctly define it. For example, *Black's Law Dictionary* includes the following definitions in its primary entry:

> That which is laid down, ordained, or established. A rule or method according to which phenomena or actions co-exist or follow each other. Law, in its generic sense, is a body of rules of action or conduct prescribed by controlling authority, and having binding legal force. That which must be obeyed and followed by citizens subject to sanctions or legal consequences is a law. (Garner, 2014, p. 884)

However, even these commonly accepted definitions are not entirely satisfactory, because "a body of rules" that "must be obeyed" in the face of "sanctions or legal consequences" necessarily envisions a process by which the rules are created, disseminated, enforced, violated, disputed, interpreted, applied, revised, and so on. Considered in this way, "the law" essentially amounts to a "legal system"—and a system, by definition, entails regularly interacting or interdependent parts and subparts coming together to form a functional, unified whole. As you read this text, think of "the law" not just as words on a page (e.g., codified statutes or regulations), but as the many interacting parts that are involved in drafting those words in the first place, and in bringing them to life once they have been enacted as laws. Note that this broad conceptualization of law as a system squares nicely with the primary purpose of law described previously, because there must, by necessity, be a sizeable system in place if law is going to carry out its role as the primary organizing tool in society. This broad definition of law also encompasses key legal doctrines, like separation of powers and federalism, described later in this chapter.

Sources of Law

Regardless of the breadth of the definition attached to the term *law*, at the core of the nation's expansive legal system lies a body of written rules meant to maintain order, define the outer limits of our interactions with one another and with our governments, and delineate legal rights and responsibilities. These rules derive from several sources, which collectively are called *primary* sources of law. The sources of primary legal authority include constitutions, statutes, regulations, and common (i.e., judge-made) law. There are also *secondary* sources of law, which are not laws in the technical sense, but rather are a collection of treatises, law review articles, reports, legal encyclopedias, and more that analyze, interpret, and critique primary laws. This section discusses each of the four types of primary sources of law.

Constitutions

A constitution is a charter that both establishes a government and delineates fundamental rights and obligations of that government and of individuals who fall within the territory covered by the constitution. In this country, there is a federal constitution and separate constitutions in each of the 50 states. The Constitution of the United States, completed in 1787 and subsequently ratified in each of the original 13 states, took effect in 1789. It provided for a federal union of sovereign states, and a federal government divided into three branches (legislative, executive, and judicial) to operate the union. This governmental structure was not easily agreed upon. Prior to the creation of the federal Constitution, the colonies of the American War of Independence first adopted, in 1777, the Articles of Confederation, which represented the first formal governing document of the United States and which were ratified in 1781. However, a defining feature of the Articles was a weak national government; fairly quickly, a movement for a stronger central government took hold, the colonies elected to throw out their original plan, and the Constitutional Convention—and with it the Constitution—was born.

The federal Constitution is rather short and, for the most part, quite general. One explanation for this is that the framers of the Constitution viewed it as a "document for the ages" that needed to include enduring principles to serve a growing, evolving society that has certainly proved to be more complex than it was at the time of the Constitution's ratification. In the words of former U.S. Supreme Court Justice Robert Jackson, the Constitution is a compilation of "majestic generalities" that collect meaning over a span of many years (*Fay v. New York*, 1947).

But the fact that some of the most important constitutional provisions are written in broad terms leads to many thorny legal controversies, because there are many competing approaches and theories regarding how courts should interpret ambiguous constitutional phrases, and many different value systems and lived experiences among the people who ultimately enforce and interpret those provisions. Broadly speaking, the leading approaches to constitutional interpretation include the "living constitution," the "moral constitution," "originalism," and "strict constructionism." The living constitution model reflects a belief that the broadly written Constitution should be interpreted to reflect *current* moral, political, and cultural values in society, not the values that were predominant at the time of the Constitution's ratification. Under this view, the meaning of the Constitution is not fixed, but instead evolves along with society. Moral constitutionalists infuse their interpretation of constitutional law with principles of moral philosophy. Originalism, technically, is an umbrella term referring to a small group of constitutional interpretation theories, all of which share a common belief that constitutional provisions have a fixed and knowable meaning. For example, "original intent," one well-known theory under the originalism umbrella, adheres to the position that constitutional interpretation should be consistent with the intent of the Constitution's original drafters. Finally, strict constructionists limit their interpretation to the Constitution's actual words and phrases, and decline to consider contextual factors such as shifts in societal values or the commentaries or intent of the framers. The most well-known interpretational controversy in the area of health pertains to the breadth and reach of the due process clause of the federal Constitution's 14th Amendment, which prohibits states from depriving "any person of life, liberty, or property, without due process of law" (U.S. Const. amend. XIV, § 1). This provision rests at the heart of the Supreme Court's "right to privacy" jurisprudence, including the right to obtain an abortion. For readers interested in theories of constitutional interpretation, there is a vast body of literature at your disposal (Baker, 2004; Fallon, 1999).

One of the general principles underpinning the Constitution is that citizens should not be subjected to arbitrary and oppressive government. Given that the Constitution was drafted on the heels of the Revolutionary War, this is no surprise. But one consequence of the prevailing mood of the framers toward the reach of a national government is that they drafted the Constitution with an eye toward limiting federal government, as opposed to viewing the Constitution as a vehicle for extending benefits to the public—in other words, that "the men who wrote the Bill of Rights were not concerned that government might do too little for the people but that it might do too much to them" (*Jackson v. City of Joliet*, 1983). This logic helps explain why several key constitutional provisions were drafted in "negative" terms—the First Amendment prohibits government from abridging free speech, the Fourth Amendment makes unreasonable searches illegal—rather than as conferring positive rights, like a generalized right to receive healthcare services. At the same time, the First and Fourth Amendments, along with eight others, make up the Bill of Rights, a series of important, specifically guaranteed rights in the Constitution the framers believed to be inalienable.[b]

In addition to the federal Constitution, each state has its own constitution. All state constitutions are like the federal one in that they provide for the organizational structure of the particular state's government, and all contain some measure of a state bill of rights. Here the similarities can end, however. Although state constitutions cannot limit or take away rights conferred by the U.S. Constitution (or by federal statutes), some state constitutions go further than federal law in conferring rights or extending protections. For example, under current U.S. Supreme Court case law, the death penalty does not always violate the federal Constitution, but the Massachusetts Supreme Court has ruled that the death penalty is prohibited under the state's constitution in every instance. Maryland's constitution requires that a jury be unanimous in order to convict a person of a crime, a standard that differs from federal criminal law. Furthermore, state constitutions are amended much more easily and frequently than is their federal counterpart. While state constitutions have been amended, on average, 150 times per state (Dinan, 2018, p. 23), the language of the federal Constitution has not been dramatically altered since its inception; there have been just 27 amendments, and the 10 that make up the Bill of Rights were all added by 1791.

Statutes

Statutes are laws written by legislative bodies at all levels of government (federal, state, county, city) that, generally speaking, command or prohibit something. It is the fact of their being legislatively created that sets them apart from other sources of law, because legislatures are understood as creating laws that are forward-looking and apply to large numbers of people. Indeed, the two hallmarks of statutes are their prospectivity and generality. These hallmarks result mainly from the fact that legislatures are in the "regulation business" across an enormous array of issues, and as a result, legislators often lack both the time and the substantive expertise to regulate other than in broad fashion.

Because statutes tend to be written as broad policy statements (and because words on a page can never communicate intent with absolute accuracy), there are few statutes that are utterly unambiguous. This, coupled with the fact that our evolving society continuously presents situations that may not have been foreseeable at the time a statute was written, results in the need for courts to interpret and apply general statutes to millions of specific legal cases or controversies. This practice is called "statutory construction." Although it is a tenet of the separation of powers doctrine (discussed later under the section "Key Features of the Legal System") that legislatures represent the law-making branch of government and the judiciary's role is to interpret law, it is commonly understood that judges and courts "make" law as well through statutory construction, because the continual interpretation and application of broad policy statements (i.e., statutes) can put a "gloss" on the original product, potentially altering its meaning over time.

As discussed more fully later in the section, "Federalism: Allocation of Federal and State Legal Authority," state legislatures have greater ability than does Congress to use statutes to regulate across a broad range of issues, pursuant to states' plenary authority under the Constitution. For instance, the number of state statutes regarding population health and safety (e.g., disease control and prevention, the creation of public health agencies, the ability of governors to classify public health emergencies) far exceeds congressional output on the same topic. Notwithstanding states' broader regulatory power, however, federal statutes have primacy over state statutes.

Administrative Regulations

The fact that statutes are written in broad generalities has another consequence beyond their need to be interpreted and applied in vast numbers of unique instances: Specific regulations must be written to assist with the implementation of statutory directives and to promote statutes' underlying policy goals. This is where administrative agencies of the executive branch of government come in. Because these federal and state agencies—the U.S. Department of Health and Human Services, the U.S. Department of Labor, the California Department of Social Services, the Wisconsin Department of Commerce, and so on—are organized and created to deal with specific policy subject matters, they have more time and expertise than Congress or state legislatures have to enforce statutes and promulgate regulations, rules, and orders necessary to carry out statutory prerogatives. It is important to note that, assuming the process for creating the regulations was itself legal, and provided that the regulations do not stray beyond the intent of the enacted statute, regulations have the full force of law.

Administrative law is crucial in the area of health policy and law.[c] For example, consider the Medicaid program, which functions primarily as a health insurance program for low-income individuals. The Medicaid statute embodies Congress's intentions in passing the law, including standards pertaining to program eligibility, benefits, and payments to participating healthcare providers. Yet there are literally thousands of Medicaid administrative regulations and rules, which over the past 55 years have become the real battleground over the stability and scope of the program. In a very real sense, the Medicaid regulations passed by the federal Department of Health and Human Services and state-level agencies are what bring the program to life and give it vitality. This "operationalizing" function of administrative law can be seen across a wide spectrum of important health issues, including the reporting of infectious diseases, the development of sanitation standards, and the enforcement of environmental laws (Mensah et al., 2004).

In order to be lawful, regulations must be proposed and established in a way that conforms to the requirements of the federal Administrative Procedure Act of 1946 (APA), which provides procedural restrictions for agency rulemaking and adjudication. Compared to state administrative procedure acts, which tend to be technical and detailed, the APA is broad and sweeping; thus it is relatively more ambiguous and open to various interpretations by federal courts.[d] Once Congress delegates rulemaking authority to an executive branch agency via a statute (known as the "enabling statute"), the APA dictates how the agency must go about promulgating specific rules and regulations, unless the statute itself specifies the procedure an agency must follow. If the enabling statute dictates a formal rulemaking process, the APA requires the agency to follow cumbersome procedures, and it can adopt rules only after a trial-like hearing on the proposed rule. If Congress does not specify in an enabling statute how an agency must adopt rules, the APA permits the agency to follow a more informal rulemaking process. This generally requires the agency to publish a notice of proposed rulemaking, or NPRM, in what's called the *Federal Register*, the official daily publication for rules, proposed rules, and federal agency notices. The NPRM process is an important aspect of administrative law because it gives people likely affected by the proposed rule the ability to weigh in on it. Typically, the general public is given 60 days to share comments and concerns. Once that window closes, the authoring agency must take the comments under consideration (although it need not revise the proposed rule in response to them), and then publish a final rule in the *Code of Federal Regulations* (which houses permanent federal regulations under 50 separate titles representing broad areas subject to federal oversight).

In delegating authority to an agency through an enabling statute, Congress must provide an "intelligible principle" that the agency can (and must) follow. That said, the amount of direction and discretion given to agencies varies widely. For example, the enabling statute for the Occupational Health and Safety Administration provides broad discretion by delegating the authority to create and enforce workplace safety standards (Occupational Health and Safety Act of 1970). Contrast this with the Americans with Disabilities Act, which has very specific provisions and does not allow agencies much discretion when implementing and enforcing the statutory language.

In addition to the power of rulemaking, Congress may also delegate adjudicatory and enforcement powers to administrative agencies. Adjudicatory power refers to claims of public rights, which are claims that involve private persons as one party and the government as the other party (excluding criminal cases). Congress may set up a court, known as an administrative court, within an agency to adjudicate these claims. Because these courts are located in the executive, rather than judicial, branch of government, they are not subject to the same rules and procedures as traditional courts, although they still must provide for the rights and protections prescribed by the Bill of Rights (e.g., the right to legal counsel). Administrative hearings are often much less formal than judicial trials: There are no juries, and although some evidence may be gathered through witness testimony, the majority of evidence derives from written reports. Decisions by administrative law judges (known as ALJs) often do not represent the final word on the matter being adjudicated, as these decisions are subject to approval or rejection by the agency's lead official or by a traditional (judicial branch) federal court. At the same time, federal courts generally apply a deferential standard of review to administrative decisions, reviewing only to see whether an agency has acted in an "arbitrary and capricious" manner.

The third type of authority granted to agencies by Congress is that of enforcement. As this authority already inherently resides in the executive branch under the federal Constitution, Congress uses its power to specify which agencies have authority to enforce certain statutes and substantive areas of law.

Once Congress grants power to agencies to promulgate rules, adjudicate claims, and enforce statutes, its ability to constrain agency action is limited. Because agencies are located in the executive branch and thus are under the control of the president, Congress is limited to passing a new statute overturning the questioned agency action or investigating agency action for impropriety.

Common Law

In each of the prior discussions about constitutions, statutes, and administrative regulations, we pointed out the generality and ambiguity of those types of law, and the corresponding responsibility of courts to interpret and apply them to specific cases. It is via the common law—essay-like opinions written by appellate courts articulating the bases for their decisions in individual cases—that courts carry out this responsibility. Common law is also referred to as case law, judge-made law, or decisional law.

Common law is central to legal systems in many countries, particularly those that were territories or colonies of England, which is how the United States came to rely on common law as part of its legal system. Both historically and in modern times, case law is premised on the traditions and customs of society, the idea being that courts could continuously (and relatively efficiently, compared to the legislative process) interpret and apply law in such a way as to match the values of a society undergoing constant evolution. At the same time, the common law is heavily influenced by legal precedent and the doctrine of *stare decisis*, which refers to the legal principle that prior case law decisions should be accorded great deference and should not be frequently overturned. The importance and function of *stare decisis* in American law is discussed later in the section detailing the role courts play in maintaining stability in the law.

Although courts are expected to overturn their own prior decisions only in rare circumstances and lower courts can never overturn decisions by higher courts that have jurisdiction over them, legislatures can modify or even overturn common law decisions interpreting statutes and regulations. Imagine that the U.S. Supreme Court interpreted a federal civil rights statute as protecting individuals from intentional acts of race discrimination, but not from conduct that has the unintended effect of discriminating against racial minorities. If Congress disagreed with the court's interpretation of the statute, it could effectively overturn the court's decision by amending the statute to make it clear that the law was intended to prohibit intentional discrimination *and* presumably neutral acts that nonetheless resulted in unintended discrimination. However, because the judicial branch has final authority to determine whether statutes violate the federal Constitution, Congress would be powerless to overturn a federal court decision that ruled the same civil rights statute unconstitutional.

Notice the "checks and balances" at play in this example, with one branch of government acting as a restraint on another. In the next section, we discuss the separation of powers doctrine—including checks and balances—and other key features of the legal system. But first, see **Table 3.1**, which provides a summary of the sources of law.

Key Features of the Legal System

Recall the earlier description of the law as something more than just words on a page, something more than statutes and constitutional provisions. Although the laws themselves are obviously critical, they are just one component of a complex, interacting legal system that creates the laws in the first instance and brings them to life after they hit the pages of legal code books, texts, and treatises.

All legal systems rest on unique principles, traditions, and customs. This section describes a handful

Table 3.1 Summary of the Primary Sources of American Law

Source of Law	Key Points
Constitutions	■ Establish governments and delineate fundamental rights and obligations of government and individuals. ■ There is a federal constitution and separate constitutions in each state. ■ The federal constitution restrains government more than it confers individual rights; however, the Bill of Rights specifically guarantees several important individual rights. ■ The Supreme Court has the final word on the constitutionality of laws created by the political branches of government.
Statutes	■ Created by legislatures at all levels of government. ■ Two hallmarks: prospectivity and generality. ■ As broad policy statements, statutes are often ambiguous as applied to specific cases or controversies, requiring courts to interpret them through the practice of statutory construction. ■ State legislatures can use statutes to regulate across a broader range of issues than can Congress; however, federal statutes have primacy over conflicting state statutes.
Regulations	■ Created by executive branch administrative agencies to implement statutes and clarify their ambiguities. ■ Play a particularly critical role in health policy and law.
Common law	■ Court opinions interpreting and applying law to specific cases. ■ Also referred to as case law, judge-made law, or decisional law. ■ Based on the traditions and customs of society, yet heavily influenced by legal precedent and the doctrine of *stare decisis*.

of the most important features and principles of the U.S. legal system, including the separation of powers doctrine, federalism, the role and structure of federal and state courts, judicial review, due process, and constitutional standards of review.

Separation of Powers

This country's government, both federal and state, has an underpinning structure of three independent and equally powerful branches, a fact that sets it apart from parliamentary systems of government—such as those found in Canada, Germany, the United Kingdom, and many other countries—in which the legislature appoints the executive. The legal doctrine that supports the arrangement of shared governance among multiple branches is the *separation of powers* doctrine. This doctrine is considered one of the most important aspects of both federal and state constitutional design. The framers of the U.S. Constitution were well aware that nothing was more likely to foster tyrannical government than the concentration of governing powers in one person or political party. To guard against a concentration of political power, the framers did two related things: They divided governmental powers and responsibilities among separate, coequal branches, and they structured the elections of officials for the two political branches of government (legislative and executive) so that they would take place at different intervals and through different mechanisms (e.g., the president is elected through the electoral college system, whereas members of Congress are not).

Inherent in the separation of powers doctrine is the important concept of checks and balances. "Checks" refers to the ability and responsibility of one branch of government to closely monitor the actions of the other two, including when one branch grasps at an amount of power not envisioned by the Constitution. The "balance" at work in the separation of powers framework prevents one branch from exerting power in an area of responsibility that is the province of another branch.

The constitutional doctrine of separation of powers represents, in the words of one legal scholar, an "invitation to struggle for the privilege" of governing the country (Corwin, 1957, p. 171). Alexis de Tocqueville, a French philosopher and political theorist who studied American government in the 1830s, viewed the concept of checks and balances in much starker terms:

> The president, who exercises a limited power, may err without causing great mischief in the state. Congress may decide amiss without destroying the union, because the electoral

body in which the Congress originates may cause it to retract its decision by changing its members. But if the Supreme Court is ever composed of imprudent or bad men, the union may be plunged into anarchy or civil war. (de Tocqueville, 1835/1990, p. 152)

For example, a fairly common separation of powers debate between Congress and a president concerns the nation's soaring debt and the appropriateness of raising the debt ceiling. Some policymakers (and many presidents) maintain that the president can act unilaterally to raise the debt ceiling and allow the federal government to borrow more money, while others argue that such a move is solely within the purview of Congress and beyond the scope of presidential power.

Throughout this text, there are health policy and law questions that distinctly highlight our government's divided powers. For instance, how will the struggle between some members of Congress and leaders of the executive branch over implementation of the Patient Protection and Affordable Care Act (ACA) play out? And how has the Supreme Court applied its constitutional right to privacy jurisprudence to the matter of abortion in response to federal and state legislative enactments? As you consider these and other health policy and law questions from a separation of powers angle, consider the peculiar roles of each branch of government, taking into account their duties, powers, and limitations. Through this prism, continually reflect on which governmental body is best equipped to effectively respond to health policy problems.[e]

Federalism: Allocation of Federal and State Legal Authority

In the legal system, the powers to govern, make and apply law, and effect policy choices are not just apportioned among three governmental branches at both the federal and state levels; they are also divided *between* the federal government and the governments of the various states. This division of authority—which also plays a key role in the development of health policies and laws—is referred to as *federalism*. Like the separation of powers doctrine, federalism derives from the U.S. Constitution.

Under the Constitution, the federal government is one of limited powers, while the states more or less retain all powers not expressly given to the federal government. In essence, this was the deal consented to by the states at the time our federal republic was formed: They agreed to surrender certain enumerated powers (like foreign affairs) to the federal government in exchange for retaining many aspects of sovereignty.

The Constitution's 10th Amendment states that "the powers not delegated to the United States by the Constitution . . . are reserved to the States respectively." For example, because the Constitution does not explicitly define the protection and promotion of the public's health as a power of the federal government, public health powers are primarily held by the states. (In fact, compared to the federal government, the states handle the vast majority of *all* legal matters in this country. Consider just a sampling of typical legal affairs overseen by state government: marriages, divorces, and adoptions; law enforcement and criminal trials; schooling; driving, hunting, medical, and many other licenses; consumer protection; and much more [Adelson, 2003, pp. 481–488]. Furthermore, the vast majority of all litigation that takes place occurs in state, rather than federal, courts [Refo, 2004, p. 3].) As a result, all states regulate the area of public health through what are known as their "police powers," which allow state and local governments to (among other things) legislate to protect the common good. Examples of the kinds of laws passed under this authority include childhood immunization standards, infectious disease data collection mandates, and environmental hazard regulations. Moreover, under the 10th Amendment, states historically have had the power to regulate the practice of medicine and the licensing of hospitals and other healthcare institutions.

Recall, however, that the federal government also plays a role in regulating health care and public health. The national government's enumerated powers include the ability to tax, spend, and regulate interstate commerce, all of which have been utilized in ways to improve health care and promote public health. For example, Congress has used its taxing power to increase the cost of cigarettes (in the hopes of driving down the number of smokers) and to generate funds for programs such as Medicare, and congressional spending powers are the legal cornerstone for federal health programs like Medicaid. Furthermore, the sharing of power under the 10th Amendment notwithstanding, the Constitution's supremacy clause declares that federal laws—the Constitution, statutes, and treaties—are the "supreme" law of the land, and thus preempt state laws that conflict with them (U.S. Const. art. VI, para. 2).

Although federalism is built solidly into the nation's political branches through separate federal and state legislatures and executives, it is also on display in the structure of U.S. courts. There are both federal and state court systems, and each has unique authority and jurisdiction: Federal courts are limited to ruling only in certain kinds of cases, including those involving federal constitutional or statutory law, those in which the United States is a party to the lawsuit, and those specified by statutory law; state courts, by contrast, have jurisdiction to hear just about any case (unless explicitly precluded from doing so by federal statute), including those over which federal courts also have jurisdiction. State court jurisdiction includes cases implicating state statutory and regulatory law, the state constitution, and the U.S. Constitution.

Over the years, defining the boundaries of federalism (i.e., defining the federal government's sphere of authority and determining the scope of state sovereignty) has been a contentious legal and political issue. At the dawn of the country's independence, after the colonies scrapped the Articles of Confederation in favor of a stronger central government, the Supreme Court decided federalism cases with a nod toward expansive national powers (much to the dislike of some states). Two famous cases make the point. In the 1819 case of *McCulloch v. Maryland*, the Supreme Court enhanced the power of the U.S. government by establishing the principle that federal governmental powers are not strictly limited to those expressly provided for in the Constitution. At issue in the case was whether Congress had the power to charter a national bank to help the federal government shoulder wartime debt. In 1824, the court for the first time had the opportunity to review the Constitution's commerce clause (which grants Congress the authority to regulate interstate commerce) in the case of *Gibbons v. Ogden* (1824), which resulted from a decision by the state of New York to grant a monopoly to a steamboat operator for a ferry between New York and New Jersey. Again, the court ruled broadly in favor of the federal government, stating that the commerce clause reserved exclusively to Congress the power to regulate interstate navigation.

By the mid-1800s, however, this approach to defining the relative power of the federal and state governments gave way to one that was more deferential to states and more willing to balance their sovereign interests against the interests of the federal government. This approach, in turn, lost ground during the New Deal and civil rights eras, both of which were marked by an acceptance of federal authority to provide social services and regulate the economy. The arrival of Ronald Reagan's presidency in 1981 marked yet another turning point in the evolution of federalism. For 8 years, the Reagan administration acted to restrict national authority over the states, a process that took on even more force after the Republican Party took control of Congress in the mid-1990s. Indeed, since the early 1980s, a defining feature of federalism has been the purposeful devolution of authority and governance over social and economic policy from the federal government to state legislators and regulators.

The Role of Courts

Elsewhere, we have discussed the structure and powers of two of the political branches of government: the legislative and executive branches. The third branch is that of the judiciary, made up of justices, judges, magistrates, and other "adjudicators" in two separate court systems—one federal, one state. Although the federal and state court systems have critically distinctive authority, they do not look very different structurally. The federal court system has three tiers, with cases proceeding from the lowest-level court (a trial court) to two separate, higher-level courts (appellate courts). Federal trial courts are called district courts, and they exist in varying numbers in each state, with the size of the state determining the actual number of "districts," and thus the number of federal trial courts. In total, there are nearly 100 federal district courts. After a district court renders a decision, the losing party to a lawsuit is entitled to appeal the decision to a federal circuit court of appeals. There are 13 U.S. circuit courts of appeals—12 with jurisdiction over designated multistate geographic regions, or "circuits," and a court of appeals for the federal circuit (residing in Washington, DC), which has nationwide appellate jurisdiction over certain kinds of cases, such as patent and international trade disputes. For many individuals, losing a case in a federal circuit court represents the end of the line for their case, since litigants have no entitlement to have their case heard by the U.S. Supreme Court, the highest court in the country. Although parties have a right to *petition* the Supreme Court to hear their case, at least four of the nine justices on the court must agree to grant the petition. Although the Supreme Court is undeniably the most important court in the country in terms of its authority, it by no means renders the most decisions. Out of approximately 8000 petitions annually, the Supreme Court typically accepts only 70 to 80, whereas the 13 circuit courts collectively decide approximately 61,000 cases each year. This fact is more than trivial; it effectively means that in the huge majority of federal cases, lower appellate courts, and not the Supreme Court, have final say over the scope and meaning of federal law.

As mentioned, each state also has its own court system, most of which are organized like the federal system: one trial court, followed by two separate appellate courts (generally termed "[name of state] court of appeals" and "[name of state] supreme court"). However, some state systems provide for only one appellate court. State systems also tend to include courts that are "inferior" even to their general trial courts; these handle relatively minor disputes (think of the small claims courts frequently shown on daytime television). Furthermore, state trial courts are sometimes divided by specialty so that certain courts hear cases that involve only family matters, juvenile matters, and the like.

Within the federal and state court system hierarchy, appellate courts have two powers unavailable to trial courts: reviewing lower court decisions to determine whether there were errors of law made during the trial that necessitate a new one, and establishing legal precedents that lower courts are bound to follow. But appellate courts lack trial courts' powers to actually conduct trials, including empanelling juries, hearing testimony from witnesses, reviewing evidence, and the like. Instead, appellate reviews are generally limited to the written record created at trial by the lower court.

Adjudication refers to the legal process of resolving disputes. It is in the context of resolving specific legal disputes that the judiciary interprets and applies the law, and also indirectly "makes" law under its common law authority. The results of adjudication are the common law decisions described earlier. Because U.S. courts are generally not permitted to issue advisory opinions, courts in this country effectively only act in response to a specific "case or controversy" that is brought to them by parties to a lawsuit. (Where permitted, advisory opinions are released by courts not in response to a particular legal dispute, but in response to a request from another branch of government regarding the interpretation or permissibility of a particular law. Federal courts are bound from issuing advisory opinions because the Supreme Court has ruled that constitutional provisions establishing the federal courts prevent them from reviewing hypothetical or moot disputes. Although several exceptions exist, state courts are likewise prohibited from issuing advisory opinions.) This limitation essentially means that in order for a court to rule in a particular case, an individual initiating a lawsuit must assert an enforceable legal right, a measurable violation of that right, actual damage or harm, and a court-fashioned remedy that could appropriately respond to the lawsuit.

Courts play a vital role in the legal system. This role stems in large part from their responsibility to determine what, ultimately, the nation's various constitutions mean, permit, and prohibit. In discharging this responsibility, courts are asked to protect and enforce individual legal rights, determine whether the political branches of government have acted in a way that violates the law, and maintain stability in the law through the application of legal precedent. The judicial branch is viewed as uniquely able to fulfill these key responsibilities because it is the branch of government considered to be the most insulated from politics. At the state level, however, this alleged separation is now more or less a fiction, as most state judges are subject to popular election, either at the time of initial selection or subsequently, when it is determined whether they will be retained as judges (Brennan Center for Justice, 2015). At the federal level, judges are in fact not elected, but rather are nominated by the president and voted on by the Senate, and if approved for the bench they are granted life tenure under the Constitution. But whether these aspects of the federal appointment process result in an impartial, nonpolitical judiciary is an open, and important, question in today's partisan environment. Indeed, it is no longer uncommon for individuals to spend decades being "groomed" for certain federal appellate judgeships; for politicians to portray the federal courts as little more than a political prize to be "won" or "lost"; for Senate votes on judicial nominees to fall along partisan lines; and for Supreme Court law clerks to match the ideology of the president that appointed the justice for whom they work.

What is the problem with a politicized judiciary? In a nutshell, it puts the legitimacy of courts, and thus their decisions, at risk. Federal and state courts rely on the power of persuasion when it comes to the legitimacy of their decisions. Courts have no ability to actually enforce their rulings, nor do they have the power to allocate resources to fund their decisions. Instead, courts must persuade the American public and the policymaking branches of government that their decisions are just and reasoned, and based on law, rather than on politics. As people become convinced that politics plays an outsized role in judicial decision-making, the judicial branch's legitimacy erodes. And after enough erosion, the public may begin to question the need to abide judges' decisions, and policymakers may attempt to redraw the lines that delineate the branches of government. Essentially, as politics chip away at courts' perceived authority to make unpopular decisions and reign in legislative abuses, individual rights—say, the ability of historically disenfranchised populations to participate in elections devoid of unlawful barriers—stand to suffer.

Enforcing Legal Rights

As described earlier, two main functions of the legal system are to establish legal rights and to create institutions to enforce those rights. The primary enforcers of individual legal rights, and those in the best position to create remedies for their violation, are the courts. For example, the federal courts (and the Supreme Court in particular) were critical to the success of the civil rights movement, during which time federal judges expansively interpreted civil rights laws and maintained close oversight of the implementation of their rulings. At the same time, however, the Supreme Court has not often been at the forefront of advancing individual rights. Certainly, there have been times when the court has played an enormous role in advancing societal expectations with respect to individual equality—*Brown v. Board of Education* (1954) being the most obvious example—but this decision, and a few others, are actually quite anomalous, and the court has been more a follower of evolving attitudes and expectations.

Among the most important rights courts are expected to uphold and enforce is the constitutional right to *due process*, which protects individuals from arbitrary and unfair treatment at the hands of government. Both the 5th and 14th Amendments to the Constitution make clear that no person can be deprived of "life, liberty, or property, without due process of law," with the 5th Amendment applying to the federal government and the 14th Amendment applying to the states. An important component of due process is the principle that when government establishes a legal right or entitlement for individuals, it may not then decide to deny the right or entitlement unfairly.

When courts consider due process claims, they are often thought of as reviewing *how* laws operate and *why* laws have been established in the first place. This results from the fact that the due process clause has been interpreted by the Supreme Court as including *procedural* due process (the "how") and *substantive* due process (the "why"). Procedural due process requires that laws be enacted and applied fairly and equitably, including procedural fairness when individuals challenge government infringements on their life, liberty, or property. Thus, due process requirements might be triggered if a law is too vague or is applied unevenly, if government threatens to withdraw a previously granted license, or if an individual's public benefits are withheld. For example, before a physician can lose his state-granted license to practice medicine, the state must provide the physician advance notice of the termination and a formal hearing before an impartial examiner with all the usual legal trappings (right to legal representation, right to present evidence in one's defense, right to appeal the examiner's decision, etc.). Similarly, Medicaid beneficiaries must be given notice of, and an opportunity to challenge, benefit coverage denials made by a managed care company participating in the Medicaid program. And the courts' most well-known jurisprudence in the area of health-related due process rights concerns abortion, specifically whether federal and state laws impermissibly infringe on the right to terminate a pregnancy, which is part of the right to "liberty" under the due process clause.

However, that clause has been interpreted by courts to require more than just procedural fairness when a law deprives an individual of life, liberty, or property; it also requires that the government provide a sound reason for having invaded personal freedoms in the first place. This form of due process, which is termed *substantive due process*, serves as a proscription against arbitrary government activity. For instance, when states have been unable to adequately explain the reasoning behind statutes requiring involuntary confinement of mentally ill individuals who were not dangerous to themselves or others, courts ruled the laws unconstitutional on substantive due process grounds. Substantive due process is unquestionably more controversial than its procedural counterpart, because many critics argue that the former gives courts unrestrained power to invalidate, on constitutional grounds, government actions with which they simply disagree. In other words, some view this form of due process "as a potentially limitless warrant for judges to impose their personal values on the Constitution" (Lazarus, 1999, p. 474).

Reviewing the Actions of the Political Branches

An important piece of the separation of powers puzzle, and one that grants the courts wide authority to enforce individual legal rights in this country, is the doctrine of *judicial review*. Judicial review refers to the power of the courts to declare laws unconstitutional and to determine whether the actions of the legislative and executive branches of government are lawful. The theory behind judicial review is that, as the branch of government originally designed to be most independent of the political process, courts can pass judgment on the actions of the political branches free of partisanship.

Judicial review has its roots in the famous 1803 case of *Marbury v. Madison*, in which the Supreme Court ruled that it had the power to review acts of

Congress and determine their constitutionality. The facts of the case are fascinating. In 1800, Thomas Jefferson won the presidential election, besting incumbent John Adams. In the final days of President Adams's term, the Federalist-controlled Congress passed, and Adams signed into law, a statute called the Judiciary Act of 1801. Among other things, the law created several new judgeships, and the idea was to fill the new judicial posts with Federalists before Jefferson assumed the presidency. Among the new judicial appointments made by Adams and approved by the Senate before Jefferson took office were 42 justices of the peace, including one for William Marbury. Prior to Jefferson's taking office, Marbury's commission was signed by Adams and by John Marshall—who at the time was Secretary of State under Adams—but not delivered. After his inauguration, Jefferson ruled that Marbury's commission (and those of several other Adams-appointed justices of the peace) was invalid because it had not been delivered during the Adams presidency, and therefore directed his new Secretary of State, James Madison, to withhold delivery. Marbury sued to force delivery of his commission, petitioning the Supreme Court directly to issue a *writ of mandamus*, which is an order by a court compelling a government officer to perform his duties. Marbury was able to ask the court directly for the writ because the recently enacted Judiciary Act also authorized the Supreme Court to issue writs of mandamus.

The Supreme Court's decision in *Marbury v. Madison*[f] first established the important principle that for every violation of a legal right, there must be a corresponding legal remedy. With this principle in place, the court ruled that Marbury was in fact entitled to his commission and to a legal remedy for Jefferson's decision to withhold it,

> since [Marbury's] commission was signed by the President, and sealed by the secretary of state . . . and the law creating the office, gave the officer a right to hold for five years, independent of the executive, the appointment. . . . To withhold his commission, therefore, is an act deemed by the court not warranted by law, but violative of a vested legal right.

The *Marbury* court then did something monumental: It established and justified the power of judicial review. This outcome flowed from the fact that Marbury had filed his legal petition directly with the Supreme Court, and the court needed to determine whether Congress acted constitutionally in granting the court power under the Judiciary Act to issue writs of mandamus as a matter of "original jurisdiction." (Original jurisdiction refers to cases on which a court rules before any other court does so, contrasted with situations in which a court reviews a decision of a lower court, which is called "appellate jurisdiction.")

It was not apparent that the mandamus component of the new Judiciary Act was constitutional because Article III of the Constitution—which established the judicial branch of the federal government, including the Supreme Court—says,

> In all Cases affecting Ambassadors, other public Ministers and Consuls, and those in which a State shall be a Party, the Supreme Court shall have original Jurisdiction. In all the other Cases [subject to Supreme Court jurisdiction], the Supreme Court shall have appellate Jurisdiction, both as to Law and Fact, with such Exceptions, and under such Regulations as the Congress shall make. (U.S. Const. art. III, § 2, clause 2)

Interpreting this clause, Chief Justice Marshall determined the court could issue a writ of mandamus under the Constitution only as an exercise of appellate, but not original, jurisdiction and that Congress had no power to modify the court's original jurisdiction. As a result, the court held that the Judiciary Act of 1801 was in conflict with Article III, and thus unconstitutional.

Marbury represented the first time the Supreme Court exercised the power of judicial review and declared unconstitutional a law passed by Congress. Over the years, the court has exercised this power sparingly, explaining in 1867 that although it clearly had the authority to strike down congressional legislation repugnant to the Constitution, this "duty is one of great delicacy, and only to be performed where the repugnancy is clear, and the conflict unreconcilable" (*Mayor v. Cooper*, 1867).

For example, the Supreme Court invalidated few congressional acts in the first 50 years after *Marbury*, although the pace picked up somewhat after that, to an average of about one invalidation every 2 years. During William Rehnquist's term as chief justice (1986–2005), however, the court ruled unconstitutional more than 30 laws or statutory provisions, with most of these decisions occurring between 1995 and 2005. This uptick in the court's use of its most powerful judicial review tool has led to a discussion about the court's proper place in the separation of powers framework. As stated in one opinion piece,

> Declaring an act of Congress unconstitutional is the boldest thing a judge can do. That's because Congress, as an elected legislative body representing the entire nation, makes decisions that can be presumed to possess a high degree of democratic legitimacy. (Gewirtz & Golder, 2005, p. A19)

When determining whether a statute violates the Constitution, courts necessarily take into account the subject of the regulation and Congress's purpose in regulating. Certain kinds of laws—say, affirmative action laws, or a law that classifies people on the basis of their gender—require a greater level of governmental justification and thus are held to a higher constitutional *standard of review*. In other words, these laws are scrutinized more closely by the court and thus stand a greater chance of failing the constitutionality test.

By way of example, the Supreme Court has developed a tiered standard of review framework for equal protection jurisprudence. Under the Constitution's equal protection clause, states are prohibited from denying "to any person within its jurisdiction the equal protection of the laws" (U.S. Const. amend. XIV, § 1).

The Court employs one of three standards when it reviews whether a particular law satisfies this constitutional mandate. The first, termed *rational basis* or *rational relations* review, is applied to everyday legislation pertaining to things like public safety, tax rates, and consumer protection and thus is the review standard most frequently used. It is nearly impossible for a law to run afoul of this standard, because as long as the challenged statute is *rationally* related to *any* legitimate government purpose in passing the law, it will be upheld as constitutional.

The second standard is that of *intermediate* review. This is the court's choice when the measure under review classifies individuals or groups on, for example, the basis of gender. The assumption here—and the point of the heightened review standard—is that when politicians legislate with gender (or another potentially baseless characteristic) in mind, there is a greater likelihood they are doing so for nefarious reasons. In order to pass constitutional muster under intermediate review, a statute must serve an *important* government objective and be *substantially* related to that objective. A good deal of legislation reviewed under this standard is found to be unconstitutional.

Finally, the court has at its disposal in equal protection lawsuits a review standard known as *strict scrutiny*. The court reserves this standard for laws that tread on fundamental constitutional rights (defined in part as those that are firmly established in American tradition), including an individual's right to be free of governmental discrimination on the basis of race. In theory, otherwise discriminatory laws that are *necessary* to achieve a *compelling* government interest, meaning that the law in question is the least discriminatory way to meet the legislature's compelling objective, can survive this intense form of scrutiny. However, of all the equal protection claims measured against this standard, only one survivor emerged—when the Supreme Court permitted the federal government to intern individuals of Japanese descent during World War II (*Korematsu v. United States*, 1944)—and this almost universally vilified decision was finally condemned (if not formally overruled) by the Supreme Court in 2018 (*Trump v. Hawaii*, 2018).[g]

Maintaining Stability in the Law

In addition to enforcing legal rights and passing on the constitutionality of actions of the two political branches of government, courts are expected to maintain a measure of stability, continuity, and predictability in the law. This expectation derives from the idea that those subject to the law should not have to contend with continuous swings in the direction law takes. In theory, the relatively nonpolitical judicial branch of government is in the best position to bring this expectation to fruition.

The way courts implement their responsibility to maintain legal stability is through application of *stare decisis*, a Latin legal term meaning "let it stand." *Stare decisis* is a policy of the courts to stand by existing legal precedent; that is, where rules of law have been established in prior judicial decisions, these decisions should be adhered to in subsequent cases where the questions of law and fact are substantially similar to those in the original case. Stability in the law is considered so important that *stare decisis* is usually applied, and the original judicial decision given deference, *even when the original decision is subsequently determined to be wrongly decided or not legally sound*. This is especially true where the original decision is an old one on which society has come to rest, as opposed to a relatively young decision with few deep roots in terms of societal expectations. The role of legal precedent has been described in this way:

> Legal doctrines are shaped like family trees. Each generation of decisions is derived from ones that came before as, over time, each branch of the law grows and spreads or, occasionally, withers and dies away. The most recent decisions almost always draw their strength by tracing back through an ancestral

line, choosing among parents, uncles, and cousins according to the aptness of their bloodlines. Rarely, a branch of doctrine is disowned, repudiated, and left vestigial until perhaps revived in another legal era. (Lazarus, 1999, p. 77)

At the same time, legal precedent is not completely sacred, and prior decisions are sometimes reconsidered and, on occasion, overturned. For instance, changes in societal values might outweigh strict application of *stare decisis*, as was the case with the Supreme Court's 1954 decision in *Brown v. Board of Education* to overturn the invidious idea of "separate but equal" from the court's 1896 decision in *Plessy v. Ferguson*. *Stare decisis* is, however, generally understood to trump mere changes in a court's makeup. In other words, courts are expected to remain anchored to precedential rules of law even when current individual members may not be.[h] Indeed, in a well-known Supreme Court case, former Justice John Marshall Harlan II wrote:

> A basic change in the law upon a ground no firmer than a change in our membership invites the popular misconception that this institution is little different from the two political branches of the Government. No misconception could do more lasting injury to this Court and to the system which it is our abiding mission to serve. (*Mapp v. Ohio*, 1961)

Conclusion

This chapter led you on a short journey through the complex world of the legal system. Along the way, you visited several of its essential elements and doctrines: legal rights, the various types of law, separation of powers, federalism, judicial review, and more. To be sure, the trip was abbreviated and, in some cases, concepts were oversimplified in an effort to concisely cover a complex and expansive topic.

As you encounter myriad health policy and law topics and concepts that are complex in their own right, bearing in mind a few important details about law might help you achieve a greater measure of clarity. First, law's primary purpose is to organize and control an ever-changing, ever-expanding, ever-more-complex society, and it does this in part by regulating a variety of relationships among parties with often competing interests (e.g., individual citizen and government; patient and physician; beneficiary and public program or private insurance company; physician and managed care organization; individual and her family). This function of law helps explain why in the context of a specific relationship, one party has a legal right and the other party has a legal responsibility to refrain from acting in a way that infringes that legal right. It also helps explain why an individual can justifiably claim a particular legal right in the context of one specific relationship, but not in others (for example, a patient who believes that he has been treated negligently might have a legitimate legal claim against the physician who provided his care, but not against the hospital where the care was provided).

A second detail worth reflecting on periodically is that law is established, enforced, interpreted, and applied by human beings, and thus one must accept

that law and the legal process comprise a certain amount of imperfection. This characteristic of law helps explain why statutes and regulations are sometimes difficult to understand, why laws are sometimes enforced sporadically or not at all, why reasonable jurists can disagree about the intended meaning of statutory and constitutional provisions, and why law is too often applied unevenly or inequitably.

Finally, bear in mind the fact that laws and the broader legal system are reflective of the beliefs and values of the society from which they flow. This *fait accompli*, perhaps more than anything else, provides an object lesson in the role of law across a wide range of subjects, including matters related to health care and public health.

References

Adelson, R. G. (2003).The enumerated powers of states. *Nevada Law Journal, 3*, 469–494.

Administrative Procedure Act of 1946. 5 U.S.C. § 551 et seq.

Baker T. E. (2004). Constitutional theory in a nutshell. *William and Mary Bill of Rights Journal, 13*(1), 57–123.

Brennan Center for Justice. (2015). *Judicial selection: Significant figures*. https://www.brennancenter.org/rethinking-judicial-selection/significant-figures

Brown v. Board of Ed., 347 U.S. 483 (1954).

Corwin, E. S. (1957). *The president: Office and powers, 1787–1957*. New York University Press.

de Tocqueville, A. (1990). *Democracy in America* (H. Reeve, Trans.). Vintage Books. (Original work published 1835)

Dinan, J. (2018). *State constitutional policies: Governing by amendment in the United States*. University of Chicago Press.

Fallon, R. H., Jr. (1999). How to choose a constitutional theory. *California Law Review, 87*(3), 535–579.

Fay v. New York, 332 U.S. 261 (1947).

Friedman, L. M. (1964). Law and its language. *George Washington University Law Review, 33*, 563–579.

Friedman, L. M. (2002). *Law in America: A short history*. The Modern Library.

Garner, B. (2014). *Black's law dictionary* (10th ed.). Thomson West.

Gewirtz, P., & Golder, C. (2005, July 6). So who are the activists? *The New York Times*. https://www.nytimes.com/2005/07/06/opinion/so-who-are-the-activists.html

Gibbons v. Ogden, 25 U.S. (9 Wheat.) 1 (1824).

Holmes, O. W. (1899). Law in science and science in law. *Harvard Law Review, 12*(7), 443–463.

Jackson v. City of Joliet, 715 F.2d 1203 (7th Cir. 1983).

Korematsu v. United States, 323 U.S. 214 (1944).

Lazarus, E. (1999). *Closed chambers: The rise, fall, and future of the modern Supreme Court*. Penguin Books.

Mapp v. Ohio, 367 U.S. 643 (1961).

Marbury v. Madison, 1 Cranch (5 U.S.) 137 (1803).

Mayor v. Cooper, 73 U.S. 247 (1867).

McCulloch v. Maryland, 17 U.S. (4 Wheat.) 316 (1819).

Mensah, G. A., Goodman, R. A., Zaza, S., Moulton, A. D., Kocher, P. L., Dietz, W. H., Pechacek, T. F., & Marks, J. S. (2004). Law as a tool for preventing chronic diseases: Expanding the spectrum of effective public health strategies. *Preventing Chronic Disease: Public Health Research, Practice, and Policy, 1*(2), 1–6.

Occupational Health and Safety Act of 1970. 29 U.S.C. § 655.

Plessy v. Ferguson, 163 U.S. 537 (1896).

Refo, P. L. (2004). The vanishing trial. *Litigation Online, 30*(2), 1–4.

Reich, C. A. (1964). The new property. *The Yale Law Journal, 73*(5), 733–787.

Smith, S. D. (1991). Reductionism in legal thought. *Columbia Law Review, 91*(1), 68–109.

Trump v. Hawaii, 138 S. Ct. 923 (2018).

U.S. Const. amend. XIV, § 1.

U.S. Const. art. III, § 2, clause 2.

U.S. Const. art. VI, para. 2.

Ziskin, L. Z., & Harris, D. A. (2007). State health policy for terrorism preparedness. *American Journal of Public Health, 97*(9), 1583–1588.

Endnotes

a. Although the important role that language plays in law is not a topic we delve into in this chapter, it is, particularly for students new to the study of law, one worth thinking about. Words are the basic and most important tool of the law and of lawyers. Without them, how could one draft a law, legal brief, contract, or judicial opinion? Or engage in oral advocacy on behalf of a client, or conduct a negotiation? Or make one's wishes known with respect to personal matters near the end of life? As one renowned legal scholar puts it, "law is primarily a verbal art, its skills verbal skills" (Friedman, 1964, p. 567).

Of course, one problem with the language of law is that it is full of legal jargon, making it difficult sometimes for laypeople to understand and apply to their own particular situation. For example, if government regulation is to be effective, the language used to do the regulating must be understandable to those being regulated. Another problem relates to the interpretation of words and terms used in the law, because both ambiguity (where language is reasonably capable of being understood in two or more ways) and vagueness (where language is not fairly capable of being understood) are common to laws, leaving those subject to them and those responsible for applying them unsure about their true meaning. Furthermore, as the preface to *Black's Law Dictionary*, under the heading "A Final Word of Caution," states:

> The language of the law is ever-changing as the courts, Congress, state legislatures, and administrative agencies continue to define, redefine and expand legal words and terms. Furthermore, many legal terms are subject to variations from state to state and again can differ under federal laws. (Garner, 2014, p. iv)

b. For an overview of the Bill of Rights in a public health context, see Gostin, L. O. (2000). *Public health law: Power, duty, restraint* (pp. 62–65). Berkeley, CA: University of California Press.

c. For a full description of the intertwined nature of administrative and health law, see Jost, T. S. (2004). Health law and administrative law: A marriage most convenient. *Saint Louis University Law Journal, 49*, 1–34.

d. For an in-depth discussion of the relationship between the APA and state administrative procedures, see Bonfield, A. E. (1986). The federal APA and state administrative law. *Virginia Law Review, 72*(2), 297–336.

e. For a full discussion of each government branch's role in health policymaking, see Gostin, L. O. (1995). The formulation of health policy by the three branches of government. In R. E. Bulger, E. M. Bobby, & H. V. Fineberg (Eds.), *Society's choices: Social and ethical decision making in biomedicine* (pp. 335–357). Washington, DC: National Academy Press.

f. The decision was written, as it turned out, by Chief Justice John Marshall—the very same person who, as Secretary of State, signed Marbury's commission. Marshall was sworn in as Chief Justice of the United States just before Jefferson took office.

g. For a fuller discussion of how the equal protection standards of review operate, see Lazarus, 1999, pp. 293–294.

h. This understanding is often put to the test, however, as seen in the national discussion of the right to abortion that takes place each time a new U.S. Supreme Court nominee is announced whose political stripes seem to clash with the prevailing law that abortion is a constitutionally protected right.

CHAPTER 4

Overview of the Healthcare System

LEARNING OBJECTIVES

By the end of this chapter you will be able to:

1. Identify the key players who provide and finance health care in the United States
2. Identify common characteristics of the uninsured
3. Understand the effect of insurance on access to care and on health status
4. Identify barriers to accessing health care
5. Understand concerns regarding the quality of health care provided in the United States
6. Describe differences in how health care is delivered in various countries

Introduction

Coordinated. Efficient. Cost-effective. Goal oriented. These are words one might use to describe a well-functioning system. Unfortunately, they are not words that are often used when discussing how healthcare services are delivered in the United States. Unlike most other developed nations, the United States does not have a unified healthcare system. Even with the passage of the Patient Protection and Affordable Care Act of 2010 (ACA), the first major health reform law passed in this country in nearly 50 years, the United States will continue to provide healthcare services through a patchwork of public and private insurance plans; federal, state, and local governments; and institutions and individual providers who are often unconnected to one other.

The United States has never been accused of providing healthcare services in an efficient or cost-effective manner. On average, this country spends over twice as much on health care per person as other developed countries (Organization for Economic Cooperation and Development [OECD], 2019, p. 32). Although the U.S. healthcare system does some things well, it ranks at or near the bottom on important health outcome measures such as life expectancy, infant mortality, and adult obesity rates (OECD, 2019, pp. 34–96). The lack of a unified healthcare system makes it difficult to provide a straightforward overview of how healthcare services are delivered and financed. For example, the following are some of the various players in the provision and delivery of health care:

- Educational institutions such as medical, dental, nursing, and physician assistant programs
- Research organizations including private entities, public agencies, and nonprofit foundations
- Private suppliers of goods and services such as hospital equipment manufacturers, home health agencies, and uniform suppliers

- Private health insurance provided through employers, on the individual market, and through state health exchanges
- Public health insurance programs such as Medicaid, Medicare, and TRICARE (the Department of Defense healthcare program for members of the uniformed services and their families)
- Individual providers such as physicians, dentists, pharmacists, and physical therapists
- Institutional providers such as hospitals, community health centers, and skilled nursing facilities
- Private trade associations representing providers (e.g., the American Medical Association, which represents physicians), institutions (e.g., the National Association of Community Health Centers), and industries (e.g., PhRMA, which represents the pharmaceutical industry)
- Private accreditation agencies that provide quality certifications to healthcare institutions
- Consumers of healthcare goods and services
- Local, state, and federal government agencies that have roles in delivering care, financing care, setting health policy, developing laws and regulations, and conducting and funding research

In the absence of a unified system or single government program to describe, it is easiest to understand the provision of U.S. health care through the concepts of finance (How do individuals pay for health care, and how are providers reimbursed for their services?), access (How do individuals access healthcare services, and what barriers to access exist?), and quality (What is the quality of healthcare services that are provided, and what can be done to improve the quality of care?). It is also helpful to consider the health system choices made by this country against those made by other developed countries. This chapter begins with a discussion of the concepts of finance, access, and quality and then turns to a comparative overview of how other countries have designed their healthcare systems.

Healthcare Spending

In 2019, the United States spent $3.8 trillion on aggregate healthcare spending, the equivalent of $11,582 per person and 17.7% of the nation's gross domestic product (GDP) (**Figure 4.1**). This total represents a 4.6% increase over 2018 spending (Centers for Medicare and Medicaid Services [CMS], 2020c).

National health expenditures are expected to average 5.4% growth from 2019 to 2028 and reach 19.7% of the GDP by 2028 (CMS, 2020c). This growth is projected to be driven by an increase in prices for medical goods and services, higher Medicare and Medicaid enrollment and spending due to the aging baby boomer population and Medicaid expansion, and spending growth on prescription drugs and hospital services (CMS, 2020a). Over the next decade, the growth in intensity and use of services is expected to increase at a slower rate than the years right after when the ACA was implemented and millions gained insurance. At the same time, rapid growth is projected for personal healthcare spending due to rising input

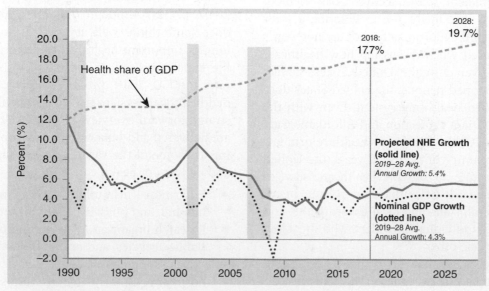

Note: Shaded areas for 1990–91, 2001, and 2007–09 represent recession periods.

Figure 4.1 National Health Expenditure, Gross Domestic Product (GDP) Growth, and Health Share of GDP, 1990–2028

Centers for Medicare and Medicaid Services, Office of the Actuary. (2020, March 24). *National health expenditure projections 2019–28.* https://www.cms.gov/files/document/national-health-expenditure-projections-2019-28.pdf

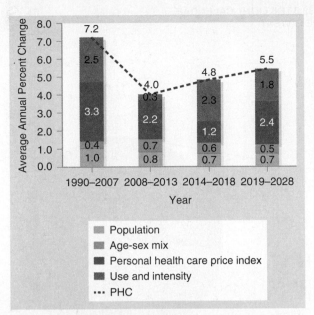

Notes: Growth in the total PHC (personal health care) price index is equal to the sum of economywide and relative PHC inflation and is a chain-weighted index of the price for all personal health care deflators."Use and intensity" includes quantity and mix of services. As a residual, this factor also includes any errors in measuring prices or total spending. "Age-sex mix" refers to that mix in the population.

Figure 4.2 Factors Accounting for Growth in per Capita National Health Expenditures, Selected Calendar Years, 1990–2028

Centers for Medicare and Medicaid Services, National Health Expenditure Projections 2019-28, March 24, 2020. https://www.cms.gov/files/document/national-health-expenditure-projections-2019-28.pdf

prices for medical providers that will be passed on to the consumer, as well as overall inflation (Keehan et al., 2020) (**Figure 4.2**). Put differently, come 2028, one-fifth of the nation's economy will be consumed by healthcare spending. This is nothing short of staggering. As shown in **Figure 4.3**, the largest portion of national healthcare spending in 2019 was on hospital services, followed by physician and clinical services.

Health Insurance

Having health insurance reduces the risk of financial ruin when expensive health services are needed and often provides coverage for preventive services at low or no cost. As discussed in the upcoming section on healthcare access, individuals without health insurance must pay for services themselves, find services provided at no cost, or go without care. Although most people in the United States have health insurance, one of the main goals of the ACA is to decrease the number of uninsured people.

The ACA includes a number of provisions designed to reduce the uninsured rate. These provisions, as well as the changes that have taken place since the ACA was signed into law, will be discussed in detail in Chapter 11, "Health Reform and the Patient Protection and Affordable Care Act"; however, a brief overview is useful here. The ACA attempts to reduce the number of uninsured through three main strategies. First, the law initially included a mandate on individuals to purchase insurance and still includes a mandate on (many) employers to provide insurance. Second, the law expands Medicaid, the federal–state program for the poor, to the poorest uninsured individuals across the country. Third, the ACA created state health insurance exchanges, which are aimed at individuals and small businesses that are not able to obtain affordable health insurance through other means.

When President Obama signed the ACA into law in 2010, the uninsured rate was 16.3%, or 49.9 million individuals (U.S. Census Bureau, 2011, pp. 22–23). The ACA was effective in reducing the uninsured rate; by 2019 it had dropped to 8%, or 26.1 million individuals (U.S. Census Bureau, 2020a). A number of legal and policy developments since the 2016 election have reduced the ACA's effectiveness. As a result, the Congressional Budget Office (CBO) estimates that the number of individuals younger than age 65 years without insurance will increase to 35 million (13%) by 2029 (CBO, 2019). According to the CBO, one reason for this increase is the 2018 repeal of the penalty associated with the individual mandate. The elimination of this penalty is projected to increase the uninsured rate by 7 million people in 2021, because without the penalty, some individuals will simply choose to go without coverage (as they might have done before the ACA was passed) to avoid the cost of carrying insurance. Furthermore, some individuals who applied for marketplace coverage in order to avoid the penalty discovered they were eligible for Medicaid; now, without the penalty, individuals who might otherwise have shopped for marketplace coverage may not, and thus may not realize they are eligible for Medicaid coverage (CBO, 2019).

As shown in **Figure 4.4**, most people in the United States are privately insured and obtain their health insurance through their employer. Employer-sponsored insurance plans may be self-funded (meaning employers set aside funds to pay for their employees' health insurance claims instead of paying a premium to a health insurance carrier) or fully insured (meaning employers pay a premium to a private health insurance company to administer employees' plans and pay the healthcare claims of the employees). Another significant portion of the population is publicly insured through Medicaid, the Children's Health

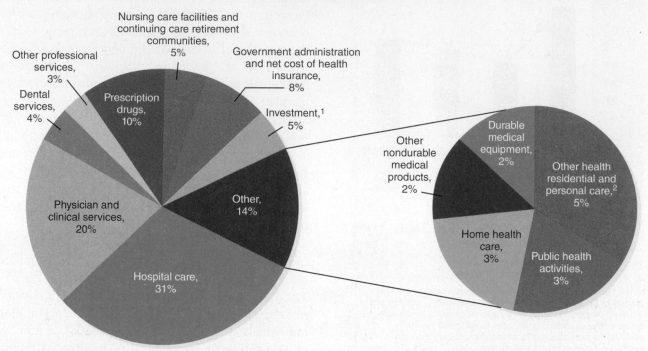

THE NATION'S HEALTH DOLLAR ($3.8 TRILLION), CALENDAR YEAR 2019 WHERE IT WENT

[1] Includes noncommercial research and structures and equipment.

[2] Includes expenditures for residential care facilities, ambulance providers, and medical care delivered in nontraditional settings (such as community centers, senior citizens centers, schools, and military field stations) and expenditures for home and community waiver programs under Medicaid.

Note: Sum of pieces may not equal 100% due to rounding.

Figure 4.3 The Nation's Health Dollar, Calendar Year 2019: Where It Went

Centers for Medicare and Medicaid Services, Office of the Actuary. (n.d.). *National health expenditures data.* https://www.cms.gov/files/document/nations-health-dollar-where-it-came-where-it-went.pdf

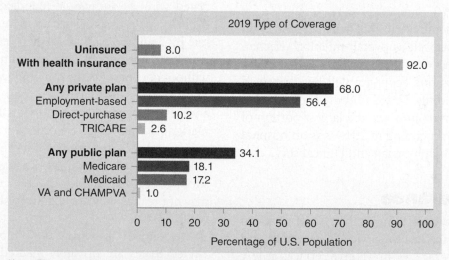

Notes: The estimates by type of coverage are not mutually exclusive; people can be covered by more than one type of health insurance during the year. For information on confidentiality protection, sampling error, nonsampling error, and definitions in the Current Population Survey, see https://www2.census.gov/programs-surveys/cps/techdocs/cpsmar20.pdf

Figure 4.4 Healthcare Coverage in the United States, 2019

Keisler-Starkey, K., & Bunch, L. N. (2020). *Health insurance coverage in the United States: 2019.* United States Census Bureau. https://www.census.gov/content/dam/Census/library/publications/2020/demo/p60-271.pdf

Insurance Program (CHIP), Medicare, the Veteran's Administration, and the Department of Defense. Public programs are funded and run by federal and/or state government agencies, depending on the program.

Figure 4.5 illustrates how health insurers act as an intermediary between consumers (sometimes referred to as "insureds") and providers (which refers to both individual providers, such as physicians or nurses,

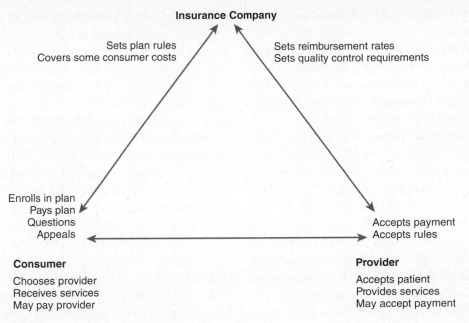

Figure 4.5 Insurance Company–Consumer–Provider Interaction

and institutions, such as hospitals and community health centers). The specifics regarding eligibility for a particular insurance plan, choice of plans, how much a plan costs to enroll in or use, what benefits are covered, and how much providers are reimbursed vary by plan or government program. In some circumstances, providers may accept insurance from only a single plan, but often providers will accept patients from a variety of plans.

Consumers interact with health insurance companies or government programs by enrolling into an insurance plan by which they are accepted (in the case of private plans) or for which they are eligible (in the case of public programs), providing payments to the insurance plan for being enrolled (either directly or through a payroll deduction), choosing which provider to see based on plan restrictions or incentives, and working with the plan if they have questions or complaints. Providers that agree to be part of a plan's "network" (i.e., the group of providers who will see patients insured by the plan) are reimbursed a contractually agreed-upon amount from the insurance company and/or the patient for providing services covered under the plan, may accept consumers who are enrolled in the plan, may be subject to plan quality control measures, and will participate as necessary in plan appeals processes.

Direct Services Programs

In addition to providing publicly funded health insurance to certain populations through programs such as Medicare and Medicaid, federal, state, and local governments also fund numerous programs that directly provide healthcare services to vulnerable populations. Many of these programs also receive private funding and donations to support their operations. Direct service programs generally exist to fill gaps in the private healthcare delivery system. Examples of these types of programs include the following:

- **Federally qualified health centers (FQHCs):** These centers are located in medically underserved areas and provide primary care services to individuals on a sliding fee scale (meaning that how much one pays for services depends on the individual's income level). While anyone may use an FQHC, the health center patient population is made up of mostly uninsured and publicly insured patients. Funding for health centers usually comes from the federal and state governments, and sometimes from local governments and private donations.

- **HIV/AIDS services:** The Ryan White HIV/AIDS Program works with states, cities, and local organizations to provide services to patients with human immunodeficiency virus (HIV) or acquired immunodeficiency syndrome (AIDS) who do not have health insurance coverage or the financial resources to pay for needed care. The program is federally funded and provides grants to state agencies that deliver care to patients. The Ryan White program includes the state AIDS Drug Assistance Program (ADAP), which provides medications to low-income individuals with HIV. A supplementary ADAP for high-need states includes federal funding and a state matching requirement. States often supplement federal funding with state-funded HIV prevention and treatment programs. Some local public health departments provide HIV testing and counseling services and help individuals access treatment. Many programs also accept private donations.

- **Family planning services:** Title X of the Public Health Service Act provides federal funding for family planning services offered to women who do not qualify for Medicaid, maintains family planning centers, and establishes standards for providing family planning services (although federal dollars may not be used to support abortion services except in the case of rape, incest, or danger to the life of the pregnant woman). In addition, states also fund family planning services. Services provided vary by state but may include contraception, cervical cancer screening, tubal sterilization, sexually transmitted disease screening, HIV testing, and abstinence counseling. State laws vary on the use of state funds for abortion services. Local health departments may also offer some of these services as well as help people access family planning services from private providers. Private donations provide revenue to many family planning clinics.

Healthcare Access

Access to care refers to the ability to obtain needed health services. A variety of factors can hinder access to care. Barriers may exist if individuals are underinsured and cannot afford the cost-sharing required by their health insurance policy, if needed services are not covered by health insurance, if providers will not take a particular insurance plan, or if providers are not available in certain geographical areas. Access problems are exacerbated by provider shortages, especially in primary care fields (e.g., internal medicine and pediatrics). Many areas of the country already experience workforce shortages, and the influx of newly insured individuals as a result of health reform will make this problem even more pronounced in the years to come.

Of course, one important factor relating to access is lack of health insurance. Individuals without health insurance have to pay more for comparable services because they do not have the advantage of sharing costs as part of a pool of consumers. Because many individuals without health insurance are low income, they may be unable to pay for the cost of needed care, and providers are often unwilling to accept uninsured patients because of the risk of not being paid for their services. Some providers, referred to as "safety

net" providers, focus on providing care to uninsured patients, but gaining access to needed care remains a significant issue for this population.

As noted previously, many changes that took place in 2014 as part of ACA implementation are intended to reduce the number of uninsured people. Even so, it is important to understand the healthcare problems faced by the uninsured due to the uncertainty surrounding the ACA's future. Furthermore, millions would remain uninsured even with a fully implemented ACA. The ACA did not help almost half the uninsured in 2017 because their state did not expand Medicaid, their income was too high to allow them to obtain subsidies, or they were ineligible for insurance or assistance due to immigration restrictions (Garfield et al., 2019). Many of those who could be assisted by the ACA's provisions also remain uninsured. A 2018 survey conducted by the Commonwealth Fund found that two-thirds of the uninsured did not look for coverage in a state marketplace, and more than one-third (36%) of uninsured adults who knew about state exchanges did not think they could find affordable coverage (Gunja & Collins, 2019).

The Uninsured
Characteristics of the Uninsured

There are many myths relating to the uninsured. It is often assumed that the uninsured do not work or simply choose not to purchase health insurance even though it is available and affordable. Although this assumption may be true in some cases, in most instances it is not. Furthermore, many people believe that all employers offer insurance or that those individuals without private insurance are always eligible for public programs. As you will see, these and other assumptions are also false.

Income Level. Although the poor saw significant gains in insurance coverage under the ACA, the primary reason people do not have health insurance is still financial—available coverage is simply too expensive (**Figure 4.6** and **Figure 4.7**). There was an increase of 18.3 million Medicaid and CHIP enrollees from September 2013 to January 2020, accounting for much of the decrease in the uninsured rate among the poor (Medicaid and CHIP, n.d.). Overall, the uninsured rate in states that did not expand Medicaid (15.8%) was almost twice as high as the rate in expansion states (8.3%) in 2019 (Garfield et al., 2021). In addition, most (86%) of the 10.5 million individuals enrolled in ACA marketplace coverage were eligible to receive premium subsidies and over 5 million also

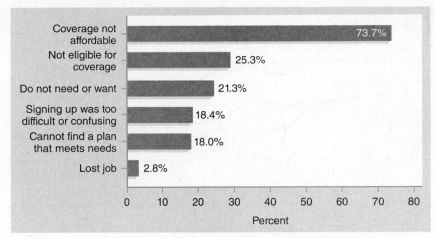

Note: Includes nonelderly individuals ages 18 to 64. Respondents can select multiple options.

Figure 4.6 Reasons for Being Uninsured Among Nonelderly Adults, 2019

Tolbert, J., Orgera, K., Singer, N., & Damico, A. (2020). *Key facts about the uninsured population.* https://www.kff.org/uninsured/issue-brief/key-facts-about-the-uninsured-population/

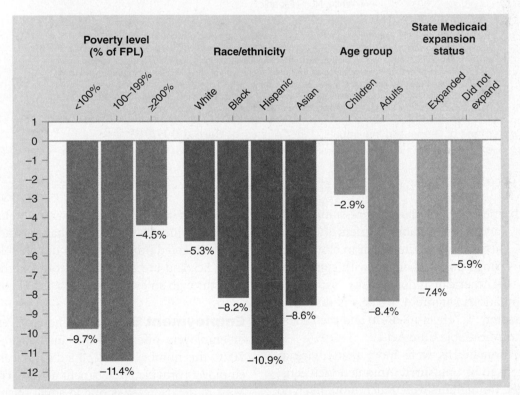

Note: FPL = federal poverty level. Includes nonelderly individuals ages 0 to 64. The U.S. Census Bureau's poverty threshold for a family with two adults and one child was $19,730 in 2017. Asian includes Native Hawaiians and Other Pacific Islanders (NHOPIs).

Figure 4.7   Change in Uninsured Rate Among the Nonelderly Population by Selected Characteristics, 2013–2016

Garfield, R., Orgera, K., & Damico, A. (2019). *The uninsured and the ACA: A primer—key facts about health insurance and the uninsured amidst changes to the Affordable Care Act.* https://files.kff.org/attachment/The-Uninsured-and-the-ACA-A-Primer-Key-Facts-about-Health-Insurance-and-the-Uninsured-amidst-Changes-to-the-Affordable-Care-Act

received cost-sharing subsidies (Norris, 2021). These subsidies were created to make health insurance more affordable for lower-income individuals.

Race, Ethnicity, and Immigrant Status.

Prior to the ACA, the uninsured rate was much higher for Hispanics (30.7%) and Blacks (20.8%) than for non-Hispanic Whites (11.7%) (U.S. Census Bureau, 2011, pp. 22–23). As shown in Figure 4.7 and **Figure 4.8**, minority populations experienced significant coverage gains in the early years of the ACA, although Whites continue to have one of the lowest uninsured rates (U.S. Census Bureau, 2020a). These differences are due to a variety of factors, such

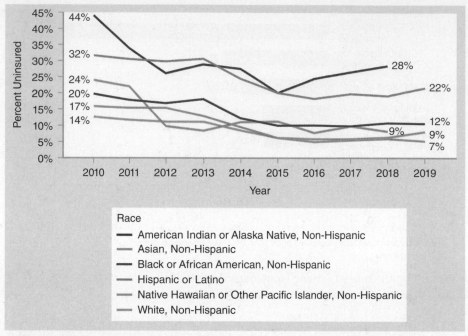

Figure 4.8 Percentage of Uninsured Individuals Under Age 65, by Race, 2010–2019

Finegold, K., Conmy, A., Chu, R.C., Bosworth, A., & Sommers, B. D. (2021). *Trends in the U.S. uninsured population, 2010–2020.* Assistant Secretary for Planning and Evaluation. https://aspe.hhs.gov/system/files/pdf/265041/trends-in-the-us-uninsured.pdf

as language barriers, income level, work status, state of residence, and immigration barriers (Garfield et al., 2019). The uninsured rate began to climb after 2016 due to various policy changes, with significant increases in the American Indian/Alaska Native and Hispanic populations (Figure 4.8). This is discussed further in Chapter 11, "Health Reform and the Patient Protection and Affordable Care Act."

In 2018, noncitizens were more than twice as likely as citizens to be uninsured. Among noncitizens, undocumented immigrants were much more likely to be uninsured (45%) than lawfully present immigrants (23%; Garfield et al., 2019; Kaiser Family Foundation [KFF], 2020a). Restrictive eligibility rules pertaining to immigrants in public programs make it difficult for non-natives to obtain public coverage. In addition, anti-immigration policies, such as the Trump administration's expansion of the public charge policy that helps determine whether immigrants can gain entry to the United States, deterred eligible immigrants from seeking coverage through Medicaid and other public programs. The Biden administration began reversing this expansion via executive order in February 2021 (Whitener, 2021). Although legal immigrants

may obtain subsidies to assist with purchasing health insurance through the state exchanges under the ACA, undocumented immigrants are not eligible for federal subsidies and are prohibited from purchasing insurance through an exchange, even at full cost.

Employment Status. Whereas over half (56%) of employers offered health insurance coverage in 2020, this number has declined significantly; 68% of employers provided this benefit in 2000 (KFF, 2020b). Most of the decrease is due to small businesses dropping coverage. As shown in **Figure 4.9**, premium costs nearly doubled while wages and inflation grew at a much slower pace, meaning coverage became less affordable even for those employees who were offered coverage (Garfield et al., 2019). Even though the ACA includes an employer mandate that requires medium and large employers (those with over 50 full-time-equivalent [FTE] employees) to provide coverage, the percentage of employers offering health insurance coverage, the number of employees eligible for coverage, and the take-up rate by employees choosing to purchase coverage did not change significantly after the ACA was implemented (KFF, 2020b). This is not

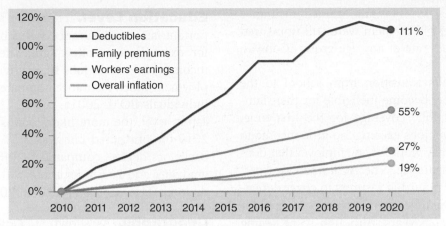

Note: Average general annual deductibles are for single coverage and are among all covered workers. Workers in plans without a general annual deductible for in-network services are assigned a value of zero.

Figure 4.9 Employer Premiums and Deductibles Have Risen Much Faster than Wages Since 2010

Kaiser Family Foundation, (2020, October 8). Average family premiums rose 4% to $21,342 in 2020, benchmark KFF Employer Health Benefit Survey finds. *KFF Health Affairs.* https://www.kff.org/health-costs/press-release/average-family-premiums-rose-4-to-21342-in-2020-benchmark-kff-employer-health-benefit-survey-finds/

surprising, because medium and large businesses were the most likely to offer coverage before the ACA, and concerns about affordability remain the primary obstacle for individuals obtaining insurance.

As shown in **Figure 4.10**, most of the uninsured work or are in families with at least one full-time worker, and many more have part-time workers in the family. In 2019, 72.5% of nonelderly uninsured workers were not offered health insurance by their employer (Tolbert et al., 2020). Most uninsured workers are low income and/or work in blue-collar fields

such as agriculture, construction, and the service industry (Alker, 2021; Boal et al., 2021).

Age. Because Medicaid and CHIP provide extensive coverage to low-income children and Medicare covers older adults, working-age adults between 19 and 64 years are the age group most likely to be uninsured. In 2019, 1.1% of adults older than 65 years and 5.2% of children younger than 19 years were uninsured, compared to 11.1% of working-age adults (U.S. Census Bureau, 2020a). Even though many

Note: FPL = federal poverty level. Includes nonelderly individuals ages 0 to 64. AI/AN refers to American Indian/Alaska native. NHOPI refers to native Hawaiians and other Pacific Islanders. Hispanic people may be of any race but are categorized as Hispanic; other groups are all non-Hispanic. The 2019 Census Bureau poverty threshold for a family of three was $20,578.

Figure 4.10 Characteristics of the Nonelderly Uninsured, 2019

Tolbert, J., Orgera, K, & Damico, A. (2020). *Key facts about the uninsured population.* Kaiser Family Foundation. https://www.kff.org/uninsured/issue-brief/key-facts-about-the-uninsured-population/

young adults (ages 19–34 years) gained insurance under the ACA, 15.6% of them were still uninsured in 2019, the highest rate of any age group (Conway, 2020).

As young adults transition from school to the workforce, they may become ineligible for their family's coverage or public coverage for the first time, may have entry-level jobs earning too little income to afford a policy, or may work for an employer that does not offer health insurance. The ACA addresses part of this problem by requiring insurers to cover dependents (someone who relies on the primary insured for support) until age 26 years. Although some young adults do not consider health insurance a priority expense because they are relatively healthy, studies have shown that cost is the primary determinant of whether people in this age bracket obtain coverage (Institute of Medicine [IOM], 2001a, pp. 73–74). Although adults ages 55 to 64 years are more likely to be insured than are younger adults, the uninsured who fall into this age group are a cause for concern because they are medically high risk and often have declining incomes (IOM, 2001a, p. 72). The disability provisions of Medicaid and Medicare and the availability of employer-based insurance keep the number of uninsured in this group relatively small, which is important because it is very expensive for individuals in this demographic to purchase individual insurance policies in the private market.

Education Level. Education level is also an important factor in insurance status because it is easier, for example, for college graduates to earn higher incomes and obtain jobs that provide affordable employment-based insurance compared to less-educated individuals (IOM, 2001a, p. 74). The higher the education level, the more likely one is to be insured. In 2019 the uninsured rate was 5.6% for adults with a bachelor's degree, compared to 14% for high school graduates and 26.8% for those without a high school diploma (U.S. Census Bureau, 2020a).

Geography. As shown in **Figure 4.11**, residents of the South and West are more likely to be uninsured than are residents of the North and Midwest. There are variations in the uninsured rate from state to state. These differences are based on numerous factors, including racial/ethnic composition, other population characteristics, public program eligibility, economic conditions, and employment rates and sectors (Tolbert et al., 2020). This trend is likely to continue, at least in the short run, with many states in the South opting not to expand Medicaid coverage under the ACA.

Uninsurance is a particular problem among the 52 million people (20% of the nonelderly population) who live in rural areas. These people are more likely to be poorer, less educated, unemployed, or employed in blue-collar jobs and are less likely to have access

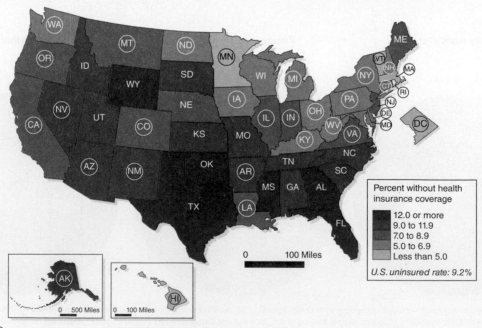

○ A state with a circle around its abbreviation expanded Medicaid eligibility on or before January 1, 2019.

Figure 4.11 Uninsured Rates by State, 2019

Keisler-Starkey, K., & Bunch, L. N. (2020). *Health insurance coverage in the United States: 2019.* United States Census Bureau. https://www.census.gov/content/dam/Census/library/publications/2020/demo/p60-271.pdf

to employer coverage than are their urban counterparts (Foutz et al., 2017). In addition, rural residents have relatively high healthcare needs—they tend to be older, poorer, and less healthy than urban residents—and there is often a provider shortage in these areas. The uninsured rate fell almost twice as much in rural states that expanded Medicaid than nonexpansion rural states (Foutz et al., 2017). Rural residents are clustered in Southern and Midwestern states. Almost all of the residents who live in nonexpansion states and have incomes that are too poor to qualify for ACA subsidies also live in the South, meaning insurance is likely to be more unaffordable for them (Garfield et al., 2021). (See **Boxes 4.1** and **4.2**.)

The Importance of Health Insurance Coverage to Health Status

Having health insurance provides tangible health benefits. For a variety of reasons discussed in this section, having health insurance increases access to care and positively affects health outcomes. Conversely, the uninsured, who do not enjoy the benefits of health insurance, are more likely to experience adverse health events and a diminished health-related quality of life and are less likely to receive care in appropriate settings or receive the professionally accepted standard of care (Tolbert et al., 2020).

Box 4.1 DISCUSSION QUESTIONS

From a policy perspective, are the characteristics just described interrelated, or should they be addressed separately? If you are trying to reduce the number of uninsured, do you believe the focus should be on altering insurance programs or changing the effect of having one or more of these characteristics? Whose responsibility is it to reduce the number of uninsured? Government? The private sector? Individuals?

Box 4.2 DISCUSSION QUESTIONS

The ACA made it a priority to reduce the number of uninsured. At what point, if any, should the government step in to provide individuals with assistance to purchase insurance coverage? Do you think such assistance should be a federal or a state responsibility?

Centers for Disease Control and Prevention. (1996). History of CDC. *MMWR 45*, 526–528.

Health insurance is an important factor in whether someone has a "medical home," or consistent source of care. Having a consistent source of care is positively associated with better and timelier access to care, better chronic disease management, fewer emergency department (ED) visits, fewer lawsuits against EDs, and increased cancer screenings for women (Garfield et al., 2019; Lambrew et al., 1996; Starfield & Shi, 2004). Unfortunately, the uninsured are much less likely to have a usual source of care than are insured individuals (**Figure 4.12**).

The uninsured are also less likely to follow treatment recommendations and more likely to forgo care due to concerns about cost (Garfield et al., 2019). In addition, the uninsured are less likely to receive preventive care and appropriate routine care for chronic conditions (Garfield et al., 2019). One result of these conditions is that children without insurance are more likely to have developmental delays, often leading to difficulties in education and employment. Also, quality of life may be lower for the uninsured due to their lower health status and anxiety about both monetary and medical problems.

Because the uninsured are less likely to obtain preventive care or treatment for specific conditions, they have a higher mortality rate overall, have a higher in-hospital mortality rate, and are more likely to be hospitalized for avoidable health problems (Garfield et al., 2019). Of course, without regular access to care, it is less likely that a disease will be detected early when treatment may be cheaper and more effective. For example, uninsured cancer patients are diagnosed at later stages of the disease and die earlier than insured cancer patients.

Ways to Assess the Cost of Being Uninsured

There are several ways to think about the costs of being uninsured. These costs include the health status costs to the uninsured individual, as discussed previously; financial cost to the uninsured individual; financial cost to state and federal governments and to private insurers; financial cost to providers; productivity costs from lost work time due to illness; costs to other public priorities that cannot be funded because of the resources spent on providing care to the uninsured; and costs to the health status and patient satisfaction of *insured* individuals.

The financial burden of being uninsured is significant. Although on average the uninsured spend fewer dollars on health care than the insured, those without insurance spend a greater proportion of their overall income on medical needs. Furthermore, when

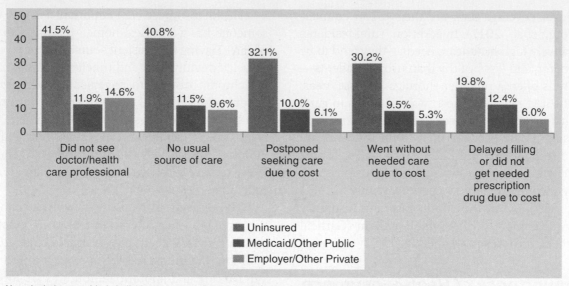

Note: Includes nonelderly individuals ages 18 to 64. Includes barriers experienced in the past 12 months. Respondents who said usual source of care was the emergency room were included among those not having a usual source of care. All Medicaid/Other public and Employer/Other private are statistically different from uninsured at the p<0.05 level.

Figure 4.12 Barriers to Health Care Among Nonelderly Adults by Insurance Status, 2019

Tolbert, J., Orgera, K., & Damico, A. (2020). *Key facts about the uninsured population.* Kaiser Family Foundation. https://www.kff.org/uninsured/issue-brief/key-facts-about-the-uninsured-population/

the uninsured receive care, it is often more expensive because the uninsured are not receiving care as part of an insurance pool with leverage to negotiate lower rates from providers. In fact, the uninsured are charged rates two to four times higher than the rates paid by insurance companies or public programs (Garfield et al., 2019). The uninsured are less likely to be able to pay for healthcare needs because the average uninsured household does not have savings or assets to fund their healthcare needs. In 2016, less than half of households with an uninsured person had more than $1000 in savings (Garfield et al., 2019). Not surprisingly, the uninsured are much more likely to be concerned about being able to pay their medical bills than are their insured counterparts (**Figure 4.13**).

Costs of medical care provided by, but not fully reimbursed to, health professionals are referred to as uncompensated care costs. In 2013, it was estimated that uncompensated care costs surpassed $85 billion in the United States, with federal, state, and local spending covering most of the tab, primarily through "disproportionate share" (DSH) payments to hospitals that serve many uninsured individuals and Medicaid beneficiaries (Garfield et al., 2019). Under the ACA, however, DSH payments are set to be reduced drastically, because it was projected that uncompensated care costs would fall as the uninsured rate fell (Congressional Research Service, 2021). As expected, uncompensated care shrank by about one-third between 2015 and 2017. Even so, providers

continue to incur substantial costs; between 2015 and 2017 uncompensated care reached $25.1 billion for hospitals, $13.4 billion for community-based providers, and $3.9 billion for prescription drugs (Karpman et al., 2021). Although hospitals provide about 60% of all uncompensated care services and receive significant government assistance, most of the uncompensated care provided by nonhospital physicians is not subsidized (Karpman et al., 2021). Every dollar spent by providers, governments, and communities to cover uncompensated care costs is a dollar that is not spent on another public need. There are a variety of high-cost public health needs, such as battling infectious diseases like tuberculosis, engaging in emergency preparedness planning, and promoting healthy behaviors. Public and private funds used to cover uncompensated care, especially when the care is more expensive than necessary because of the lack of preventive care or early interventions, are resources that are no longer available to meet the country's other health needs.

An additional cost associated with the uninsured is the cost of lower productivity. This cost refers to the reduced productivity in the workforce stemming from the lower health status associated with being uninsured. Productivity may be reduced when workers are absent or when they are not functioning at their highest level due to illness. In addition, several studies show that providing health insurance and other wellness benefits helps employers recruit better employees and that workers with health insurance are less likely

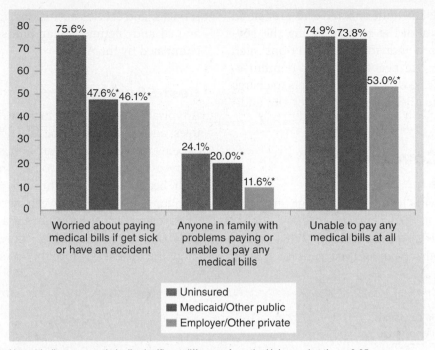

Note: * indicates a statistically significant difference from the Uninsured at the p<0.05 level. Includes nonelderly individuals ages 18 to 64.

Figure 4.13 Problems Paying Medical Bills by Insurance Status, 2019

Tolbert, J., Orgera, K., & Damico, A. (2020). *Key facts about the uninsured population.* Kaiser Family Foundation. https://www.kff.org/uninsured/issue-brief/key-facts-about-the-uninsured-population/

to change jobs, reducing the costs of hiring and training new employees (Centers for Disease Control and Prevention, 2015; Families USA, 2005; Wein, 2018).

Finally, there is a "spillover" effect of uninsurance for insured individuals. In communities with high rates of uninsured, even *insured* individuals are less likely to have a usual source of care, schedule an office visit, be satisfied with the quality of care they receive, and obtain needed care (Gresenz & Escarce, 2011; Pauly & Pagán, 2007). This spillover occurs because providers in communities with high uninsured rates may earn less revenue relative to costs. Insured individuals may suffer if subsidies are not available to providers to allow for higher revenue or if government spending on subsidies for the uninsured crowd out spending on services that might benefit the insured (Pauly & Pagán, 2007). In addition, physicians in communities with high uninsurance rates may choose to provide fewer types of services or fewer office hours due to profitability concerns. Finally, the insured may suffer if their provider treats them the same as uninsured patients, who may demand and receive fewer services or lower-quality services from their providers (Gresenz & Escarce, 2011).

The Underinsured

Although there are disagreements regarding how to measure the underinsured, in general, being underinsured means individuals do not have the financial means to cover the gap between what their insurance coverage pays for and the total cost of their medical bills. As a result, they spend a high proportion of their income on healthcare services. An August 2020 survey found that 21.3% of adults ages 19 to 64 years were underinsured (Collins et al., 2020). Not surprisingly, lower income individuals were much more likely to be underinsured than those with higher incomes. Having a private plan does not ensure adequate coverage; in fact, 42% of people who bought plans on the individual market and 26% who had employer coverage were also underinsured (Collins et al., 2020).

The underinsured problem is exacerbated during a recession when more individuals cannot afford to pay their deductibles and copayments. Insurance status is clearly linked to the decision to delay care due to cost. In the 2020 survey, 56% of uninsured individuals and 43% of underinsured respondents reported avoiding care due to cost, compared to 23% of insured individuals (Collins et al., 2020). In addition, 50% of underinsured adults indicated they had problems paying medical bills or were currently paying off medical debt, which is twice the rate of other insured adults who are not underinsured (Collins et al., 2020). As a result, everyone ends up paying for the underinsured. Providers attempt to shift the cost associated with the underinsured and uninsured to others who can afford to pay, including the government and insured individuals. Institutions such as hospitals may try to negotiate higher reimbursement for their services, which leads insurers to charge higher premiums to their clients to cover the additional costs.

Insurance Coverage Limitations

Even individuals with insurance coverage may face healthcare access problems due to coverage limitations. These limitations could include high levels of cost-sharing, reimbursement and visit caps for specific services, and service exclusions. (Another problem—annual and lifetime dollar limits on coverage—was eliminated by the ACA.)

Cost-Sharing

A typical insurance plan includes premiums, deductibles, and copayments (the latter can also be designed as coinsurance). A premium is an annual cost, typically charged monthly, for enrolling in a plan. For those with health insurance through their employer, the premium is often split between employer and employee. The average annual premium for a single coverage was $7470 in 2020 (KFF, 2020b). Figure 4.9 and **Figure 4.14** show the increase in monthly premiums over the last

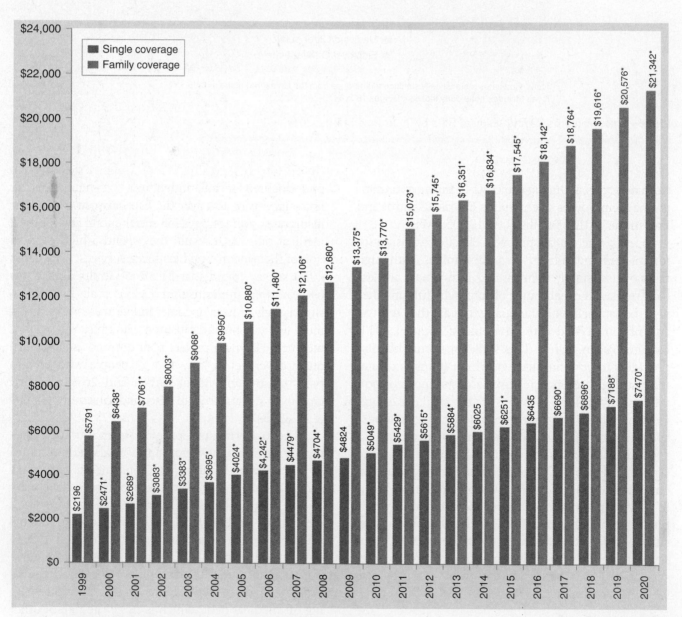

*Estimate is statistically different from estimate for the previous year shown (p<0.05).

Figure 4.14 Average Annual Premiums for Single and Family Coverage, 1999–2020

Kaiser Family Foundation. (2020). *Employer health benefits: 2020 Annual survey.* https://files.kff.org/attachment/Report-Employer-Health-Benefits-2020-Annual-Survey.pdf

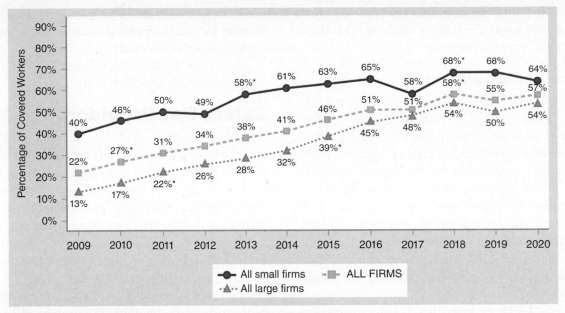

Figure 4.15 Percentage of Covered Workers Enrolled in a Plan with a General Annual Deductible of $1000 or More for Single Coverage, by Firm Size, 2009–2020

Kaiser Family Foundation. (2020). *Employer health benefits: 2020 Annual survey.* https://files.kff.org/attachment/Report-Employer-Health-Benefits-2020-Annual-Survey.pdf

decade and underscore how much faster premiums have risen relative to wages and inflation. A deductible is an amount the insured pays out-of-pocket before the insurance plan assists with the costs of healthcare services. There may be an annual deductible for the plan overall or separate deductibles for different types of services covered by the plan, such as inpatient care, outpatient care, and prescription drug coverage. Copayments refer to a specific dollar amount that patients pay when they receive services or drugs. For example, one might have a $15 copayment to see a primary care provider for an office visit. Coinsurance refers to a percentage of service cost that patients pay when they receive services or drugs. For example, an insured might have a 20% coinsurance requirement to see a primary care provider for an office visit. If the visit cost $150, a 20% coinsurance requirement would cost $30. Copayment and coinsurance amounts may vary depending on the service received.

Cost-sharing requirements can vary widely by plan and plan type. Some plans do not have general deductibles, and for those with general deductibles, the amount varies significantly. For example, in 2020 the average deductible for a single worker was $1644, although deductibles vary by plan type and employer size. Preferred provider organizations (PPOs) and health maintenance organizations (HMOs) had similar average deductibles in 2020 (approximately $1200) while high-deductible health plans averaged

$2303 for single workers. Coverage for single workers in small firms is much higher ($1888) than it is for those in large firms ($960) (KFF, 2020b). A significant number of plans have deductibles of $1000 or more (**Figure 4.15**).

Variation also exists for service-specific costs. It is rare for private plans to have separate deductibles for hospital admissions, outpatient surgery, or ED visits, but patients generally have cost-sharing arrangements for these services. For example, in 2020, the average copayment for a hospital admission in large private plans was $311 and the average copayment for outpatient surgery was $188 (KFF, 2020b). Medicare, on the other hand, charged a $1408 deductible for the first 60 days of hospitalization in 2020. Medicare beneficiaries do not pay a per diem for the first 60 days in a hospital, but they then pay $371 per day for the next 3 months. This fee increases for longer stays (CMS, 2020b).

Reimbursement and Visit Caps

Insurance plans may limit the amount they will reimburse for a specific service during the year, with patients responsible for costs that exceed dollar amount limits. In addition, plans may limit the number of times a patient may see a certain type of provider during the year. Visit caps vary by insurance plan. For example, a plan might limit a member to 90 physical therapy visits per year per injury or to 20 visits per calendar year for acupuncture. Once a patient reaches these limits, the insurance plan will not cover additional visits and the patient must pay the entire cost of a visit out-of-pocket.

Service Exclusions

Health insurance plans may also partially or fully exclude certain types of services from coverage altogether. For example, a plan might cover high-dose chemotherapy associated with bone marrow transplants for only specified organ and tissue transplants or home health services only if certain conditions are met. Examples of services not covered at all by a plan include nonrigid orthopedic or prosthetic devices, such as wigs or elastic stockings, eyeglasses, hearing aids, exercise programs, assisted reproductive technology, and physical exams for obtaining or continuing employment.

Coverage for abortion and family planning services is also limited in many instances. Federal funds may be used for abortion services only in cases of rape or incest or to save the life of the pregnant woman. The ACA does not include abortion services as part of its essential health benefits package, and any coverage of abortion services must be paid with private dollars, not with federal subsidies. As of June 2020, 11 states have enacted laws that restrict abortion coverage in all private plans in the state, 26 states restrict abortion coverage in private plans offered through their exchange, and 22 states restrict abortion coverage in public employee plans (Guttmacher Institute, 2021b, 2021c).

Regarding contraceptive coverage, the ACA requires most health insurance plans to cover all contraceptive methods approved by the Food and Drug Administration and related counseling services without cost-sharing. Federal regulations exempt religious organizations from having to provide contraceptive coverage and make an accommodation for certain other employers with religious objections to avoid paying for or arranging contraceptive coverage, while still allowing employees to obtain coverage through their health insurance plan (Guttmacher Institute, 2021a). This issue is discussed in more detail in Chapter 11, "Health Reform and the Patient Protection and Affordable Care Act." Due to concerns that federal guarantees for contraceptive coverage may be limited in the future, many states have passed laws protecting coverage. As of June 2020, 29 states require insurance plans to cover the full range of contraceptive drugs, 16 states prohibit cost-sharing for contraceptives, and 9 states prohibit other restrictions and delays by insurers. At the same time, 20 states exempt select employers and insurers from providing contraceptive coverage based on religious objections

(Guttmacher Institute, 2021a). Given the litigation relating to contraceptive coverage requirements and exemptions/accommodations, it is not yet clear what requirements, if any, plans will have to follow regarding contraceptive coverage in the future.

Safety Net Providers

Securing access to care can be difficult for those without comprehensive private insurance. For the uninsured, the high cost of care is often a deterrent to seeking care. For those with public coverage, it is often difficult to find a provider willing to accept their insurance due to the low reimbursement rates and administrative burdens associated with participating in these programs. For these patients and the underinsured, the "healthcare safety net" exists.

The healthcare safety net refers to providers who serve disproportionately high numbers of uninsured, underinsured, and publicly insured patients. Although there is no formal designation indicating that one is a safety net provider, the National Academy of Medicine (NAM; formerly the Institute of Medicine, or IOM) defines the healthcare safety net as "those providers that organize and deliver a significant level of health care and other related services to uninsured, Medicaid, and other vulnerable populations" (publishing as Institute of Medicine [IOM], 2000, p. 21). "Core" safety net providers are those who serve vulnerable populations and have a policy of providing services regardless of patients' ability to pay. Some safety net providers have a legal requirement to provide care to the underserved, while others do so as a matter of principle (IOM, 2000, p. 21).

Who are safety net providers? It is a difficult question to answer because there is no true safety net "system." Safety net providers can be anyone or any entity providing health care to the uninsured and other vulnerable populations, whether community or teaching hospitals, private health professionals, school-based health clinics, or others. Those providers that fit the narrower definition of "core" safety net providers include some public and private hospitals, community health centers, family planning clinics, and public health agencies that have a mission to provide access to care for vulnerable populations. Safety net provider patient loads are mostly composed of people who are poor, on Medicaid, or uninsured, and are members of racial and ethnic minority groups. For example, in 2018, 91% of federally qualified health center (FQHC) patients had incomes at or below 200% of the federal poverty level (FPL), 71% were on Medicaid or uninsured, 22% were African American, and 36% were Hispanic/Latino (National Association of Community Health Centers [NACHC], 2020). Of the America's Essential Hospitals (formerly National Association of Public Hospitals and Health Systems) member hospital inpatient discharges, in 2019, about 75% were covered by Medicaid, Medicare, or uninsured, and 51% were racial or ethnic minorities (America's Essential Hospitals, 2021).

FQHCs provide comprehensive primary medical care services, culturally sensitive care, and enabling services such as transportation, outreach, and translation that make it easier for patients to access services. Many health centers also provide dental, mental health, and pharmacy services. Because health centers are not focused on specialty care, public hospitals are often the sole source of specialty care for uninsured and underserved populations (Makaroun et al., 2017). In addition, public hospitals provide traditional healthcare services, diagnostic services, outpatient pharmacies, and highly specialized trauma care, burn care, and emergency services (America's Essential Hospitals, 2021). Although not all local government health departments provide direct care, many do. Local health departments often specialize in caring for specific populations, such as individuals with HIV or drug dependency, as compared to public hospitals and health centers, which provide a wider range of services (IOM, 2000, pp. 63–65).

Safety net providers receive funding from a variety of sources, but they often struggle financially. Medicaid is the single largest funding stream for health centers, accounting for 48% of their revenue (NACHC, 2021). Due to low Medicaid reimbursement, Medicaid revenue accounts for only 80% of the cost of providing care to Medicaid patients served by health centers (NACHC, n.d.). Federal grants to health centers are intended to cover the cost of caring for the uninsured; however, this grant funding has not kept pace with the cost of provided care. Due to low federal reimbursement, health centers incurred a $1.5 billion gap in the cost of care for treating the uninsured in 2018 (NACHC, 2020). In addition, payment from private insurance is unreliable due to the high-cost-sharing plans held by many privately insured, low-income individuals. Furthermore, Medicare payments to health centers are capped under federal law at an amount that does not match the growth in healthcare spending.

Public hospitals face a similarly difficult economic picture. Many public hospital services are not fully reimbursed because payments made by individuals or insurers do not match the cost of care. In 2019, America's Essential Hospitals members provided almost $6.9 billion in uncompensated care, which equals almost 16.5% of all the uncompensated care provided nationally (America's Essential Hospitals, 2021). Like health centers, public hospitals receive funds to cover low-income patients, including Medicaid DSH payments, state and local subsidies, and other revenues such as sales tax and tobacco settlement funds. In 2019, America's Essential Hospitals had an average aggregate operating margin of 2.9%, compared to 8.8% for all U.S. hospitals. Without DSH payments, America's Essential Hospitals' aggregate operating margin would dip to –1.5% (America's Essential Hospitals, 2021). Thus, the reduction in DSH payments that occurred as part of health reform is particularly concerning for safety net hospitals.

Despite all of the positive work accomplished by safety net providers, they cannot solve all healthcare problems for vulnerable populations. Safety net patients may lack continuity of care, whether because they cannot see the same provider at each visit or because they have to go to numerous sites or through various programs to receive the care they need. Even though safety net providers serve millions of patients every year, there are not enough providers in enough places to satisfy the need for their services. Although Medicaid expansion, the Community Health Center Fund in the ACA, and the coronavirus relief laws included an infusion of funds to safety net providers, these providers are also serving an influx of newly insured patients. For example, community health centers served 28 million patients in 2018, a 31% increase from 2013 (Shin et al., 2020). And, as noted earlier, many safety net providers are underfunded and constantly struggling to meet the complex needs of their patient population.

The problems facing the uninsured and the stressors on the healthcare safety net highlight the inadequacies of the current "system" of providing health care, and many of these problems will remain even after the ACA is implemented. Given the country's patchwork of programs and plans, decisions made in one area can significantly affect another. For example, if Medicaid reimbursement rates are cut or program eligibility is reduced, safety net providers will have a difficult time keeping their doors open. Simultaneously, more patients will become uninsured and seek care from safety net providers. If more people choose high-deductible private insurance plans that they cannot easily afford, individuals may go without needed services, or safety net providers will end up providing an increasing amount of uncompensated care. If employers decide to reduce or end coverage or increase employee cost-sharing previously insured people may fall into the ranks of the uninsured.

💡 **Box 4.3** DISCUSSION QUESTIONS

Safety net providers mostly serve uninsured and publicly insured low-income patients. Many of the safety net provider features you just read about are in place to assist these patients in accessing health care. Instead of pursuing universal coverage, would it be an equally good strategy to expand the number of safety net providers? Are there reasons for both safety net providers and health insurance to exist? How does having insurance relate to accessing care?

As a result, safety net providers and their patients are affected by many policies that are not directed at them, but greatly impact their ability to provide or access care nonetheless. (See **Box 4.3**.)

Workforce Issues

Problems accessing care may also occur due to provider shortages and an uneven distribution of providers throughout the country. This problem affects both the uninsured and the insured alike. If a provider is not available to take you as a patient, it matters little if you have an insurance plan that would cover the cost of your care. Of course, if a provider shortage is so great that those with insurance are turned away, the uninsured will have an even harder time accessing care.

There are a variety of estimates regarding a future healthcare workforce shortage. For example, the Association of American Medical Colleges estimates a physician shortfall between 54,100 and 139,000 by 2033 (Dall et al., 2020). On the other hand, if healthcare delivery approaches that rely heavily on nonphysician providers are used more often in the future, the estimates for physician shortages decline significantly (Kerns & Willis, 2020; Morgan, 2019). Two such models are the patient-centered medical home (PCMH), which relies on a team of providers to supply and coordinate care, and the nurse-managed health center (NMHC), which is a clinic with nurse practitioners (NPs) as the primary caregivers (Auerbach et al., 2013). One study estimated that increased use of PCMHs or NMHCs alone would reduce a primary care physician shortage from 45,000 to 35,000. Used together, the combination of approaches could cut the physician shortage in half (Auerbach et al., 2013).

One of the main concerns with the healthcare workforce is a shortage of primary care providers. It is expected that there will be between 21,400 and 55,200 fewer primary care physicians than are needed to meet demand by 2033 (Dall et al., 2020). More providers are choosing specialty care over primary care. About 33% of physicians practiced primary care in 2015, as opposed to 50% in 1961 (Dalen et al., 2017). Other provider career choices have followed a similar pattern. Both primary care and specialty practices hired more NPs and physician assistants (PAs) from 2008 to 2016 (Morr, 2018). Yet, from 1974 to 2018, the percentage of PAs working in primary care declined from 70% to 26% (Dunker et al., 2014; National Commission, 2019; Wolters Kluwer, 2020). Long work hours, increased demands (particularly administrative demands associated with insurance companies), lack of respect, and comparatively low pay for primary care providers are sending future practitioners to other fields (Castellucci, 2016; Dalen et al., 2017). For example, in 2020 the average annual salary for a plastic surgeon was $526,000, compared to $236,00 for a family medicine practitioner and $221,000 for a pediatrician (Wilcox, 2021).

While fewer graduates are turning to primary care, demand for primary care services is expected to increase in the next several years. Most of the increased demand will be due to population growth and aging, with the remaining uptick in demand based on the increase of insured individuals under the ACA (Dall et al., 2020). The U.S. population is aging, with individuals older than 65 years projected to increase from 15% in 2016 to 25% in 2060 (U.S. Census Bureau, 2020b). These older patients are heavy users of healthcare services. In 2016, older patients (65+) averaged 498 office visits per 100 patients, as compared to 302 for those aged 45 to 64 and 190 for 18- to 44-year-olds (Ashman et al., 2020). Furthermore, geriatric training is lacking among primary care providers. An NAM report on aging and the healthcare workforce concluded that medical school curricula on geriatric medicine were "inadequate" (publishing as IOM, 2008, p. 129). One study found that only 41% of medical schools had a "structured geriatrics curriculum" and less than 23% of medical schools required a clerkship in the field (Bardach & Rowles, 2012). Providers shy away from geriatrics: In 2018, only 25% of geriatric fellowship programs were filled, and in 2012 fewer than 1% of registered nurses (RNs) and 3% of advanced practice registered nurses (APRNs) were certified in geriatrics (Castellucci, 2018; Robert Wood Johnson Foundation, 2012).

In addition to provider shortages, access problems may exist because providers are not distributed as needed throughout the country (**Figure 4.16** through **Figure 4.18**). In 2013, 29 states had a primary care physician shortage, with Texas and Florida

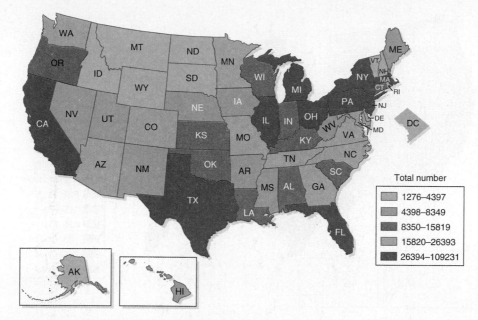

Figure 4.16 Number of Physicians, by State, 2011–2015

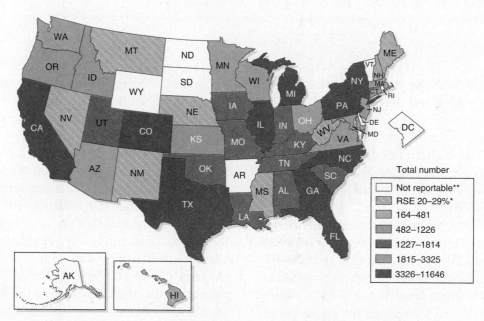

* Estimates in states with an RSE = 20%–29% should be considered with caution because of large sampling error.
**Data are not reported at the state level, because the RSE ≥ 30%; estimate does not meet standard of reliability.

Figure 4.17 Number of Physician Assistants, by State, 2011–2015

experiencing the greatest deficits (over 1000 FTE providers). By 2025, it is estimated that 37 states will have a primary care physician shortage, with 12 states experiencing a deficit of 1000 FTE providers or more (Health Resources Services Administration [HRSA], 2016). In contrast, Massachusetts has a primary care physician surplus that it expects to maintain through 2025. Similarly, primary care NP and PA shortages vary across the country. In 2013, 23 states had a primary care NP shortage, but no states are projected to have a shortfall by 2025 (HRSA, 2016). Regarding primary care PAs, 22 states had a shortage in 2013. In 2025, 9 states are expected to have a PA shortage, while 5 states (New York, North Carolina, Texas, California, and Colorado) are projected to have a surplus of more than 1000 FTE (HRSA, 2016).

Rural areas are particularly susceptible to provider shortages. This is an especially pressing problem

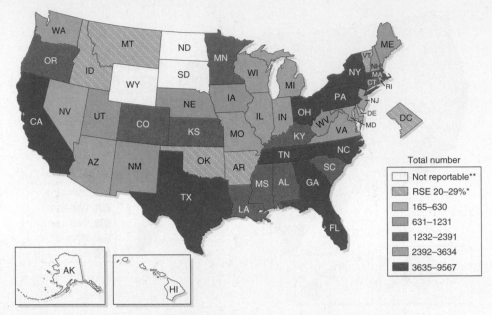

*Estimates in states with an RSE = 20%–29% should be considered with caution because of large sampling error.
**Data are not reported at the state level, because the RSE ≥ 30%; estimate does not meet standard of reliability.

Figure 4.18 Number of Nurse-Midwives and NPs, by State, 2011–2015

U.S. Department of Health and Human Services. (2018). *The U.S. health workforce chartbook*. https://bhw.hrsa.gov/sites/default/files/bureau-health-workforce/data-research/hrsa-us-health-workforce-chartbook-part-1-clinicians.pdf

because individuals who live in rural areas are more likely to be sicker, older, and poorer than their urban counterparts. Compared to urban dwellers, rural residents are more likely to lack access to a primary care physician, have higher rates of chronic diseases and teen pregnancies, and engage in more unhealthy behaviors such as smoking (National Conference of State Legislatures, 2017).

In 2017, 59% of designated Health Professional Shortage Areas were in rural areas (National Conference of State Legislatures, 2017). The number of specialists in rural areas is only 30 per 100,000 people, compared to 263 per 100,000 in urban areas (National Rural Health Association [NRHA], n.d.). Although the gap is not as prominent for primary care physicians, they also prefer urban locations. The patient–primary care physician ratio in rural areas is 39.8 per 100,000, compared to 53.3 per 100,000 in urban areas (NRHA, n.d.). Primary care providers are vital to the healthcare workforce in rural areas. Whereas family physicians comprise only 15% of outpatient physicians in the country, they provide 42% of services in rural areas (NRHA, n.d.).

Rural areas are more likely to attract NPs and PAs than physicians, suggesting that alternative care models that focus on nonphysician providers may be particularly useful in addressing access issues in rural areas (Graves et al., 2016). FQHCs have already embraced this model, hiring NPs, PAs, and nurse–midwives at a faster rate than physicians (Proser et al., 2015).

Shortages also exist within the public health workforce. The public health workforce has been defined to include anyone who is providing one of the essential public health functions (discussed in Chapter 5, "What Is Public Health?"), regardless of whether their employer is a government agency, not-for-profit organization, private for-profit entity, or some other type of organization (Center of Excellence, 2013). The public health workforce includes professions such as public health physicians and nurses, epidemiologists, health educators, and administrators. It is difficult to count everyone involved in the public health workforce, given the wide array of jobs and the numerous data sources needed to compile the information. After the 2008 recession, 19% of government public health workforce positions (approximately 50,000 jobs) were cut and never replaced (Wilson et al., 2020). Furthermore, a 2017 survey found that almost half of state and local public health employees plan to retire or leave their job within 5 years. Top reasons for leaving the public health workforce include low pay, few advancement opportunities, poor working environment, low job satisfaction, and lack of support (de Beaumont, 2019). Given the difficulties endured during the COVID-19 pandemic, it would not be surprising if even more public health workers choose to exit the field. In a 2021 survey, over half of responding public health workers indicated they experienced depression, anxiety, posttraumatic stress, and/or suicidal thoughts in the prior 2 weeks, with the severity of the condition directly connected to time spent on pandemic-related work (Smith-Schoenwalder, 2021).

The ACA and COVID-19 relief bills contain a number of provisions aimed at accomplishing the following goals (White House, 2021):

- Increase funding for community health centers.
- Increase funding for the National Health Service Corps, which provides scholarships and loan repayments to students who agree to become primary care providers and work in medically underserved communities.
- Increase funding for PA and NP training.
- Provide new funding to establish NP-led clinics.
- Provide new funding for states to plan and implement innovative strategies to boost their primary care workforce.
- Establish a National Health Care Workforce Commission to coordinate federal workforce efforts and bolster data collection and analysis.
- Establish teaching health centers.
- Provide payments for primary care residencies in community-based ambulatory care centers.
- Increase the number of Graduate Medical Education slots available to primary providers by redistributing unused slots.
- Promote residency training in outpatient settings.
- Provide grants to training institutions to promote careers in the healthcare sector.
- Increase reimbursement for primary care providers under Medicare and Medicaid.
- Provide new funding for state and local public health departments to add staff, increase training, support essential public health functions, and hire school nurses.
- Launch a Public Health AmeriCorps program to build a new public health workforce.
- Expand Centers for Disease Control and Prevention workforce programs, including the Epidemic Intelligence Service, which responds to local outbreaks.
- Build the public health laboratory workforce.

Given the uncertain political future of the ACA, it remains to be seen whether these provisions will be implemented or funded in the years to come.

Healthcare Quality

As noted earlier in this chapter, the United States spends more on health care than most other developed countries, yet frequently the care provided does not result in good health outcomes. Researchers and policymakers have highlighted the need to improve the quality of care provided in this country. A 2003 landmark study by McGlynn and colleagues raised many quality concerns, including findings that patients received the appropriate medical care only 55% of the time and that patients were much more likely not to receive appropriate services than to receive potentially harmful care (McGlynn et al., 2003). The lack of appropriate care was seen across medical conditions, affecting treatments relating to preventive care, acute care, and chronic diseases (McGlynn et al., 2003, p. 2641). The degree to which patients received appropriate care varied greatly. For example, only 10% of patients with alcohol dependence received the standard of care, as opposed to 78% of those with senile cataracts (McGlynn et al., 2003, p. 2641). A 2002–2013 review of 46 quality measures found mixed results in improving quality of care since the McGlynn research and a 2015 study found that only 8% of respondents ages 35 years and older reported receiving all of the recommended preventive measures, and only 20% reported receiving most (75%) of them (Borsky et al., 2018; Levine et al., 2016). Efforts to improve quality of care have occurred at all levels of government, and *Healthy People 2030*—a federal project laying out the nation's healthcare goals for the decade 2020 to 2030—includes a wide variety of quality objectives (Department of Health and Human Services [HHS], n.d.).

Key Areas of Quality Improvement

In 2001, the NAM released *Crossing the Quality Chasm: A New Health System for the 21st Century*, which represented nothing less than an urgent call to redesign the healthcare system to improve the quality of care provided (publishing as IOM, 2001b). The NAM attributes our inability to provide consistent, high-quality health care to a number of factors, including the growing complexity of health care, including quickly developing technological advancements; an inability to meet rapid changes; shortcomings in safely using new technology and applying new knowledge to practice; increased longevity among the population, which carries concerns relating to treating chronic conditions in a system better designed to address episodic, acute care needs; and a fragmented delivery system that lacks coordination, leading to poor use of information and gaps in care (IOM, 2001b, pp. 2–4). In its call to redesign the healthcare system to improve quality, the NAM focuses on six areas of improvement: safety, efficacy, patient-centeredness, timeliness, efficiency, and equity (IOM, 2001b, p. 43).

Safety

In a safe healthcare system, patients should not be endangered when receiving care that is intended to help them, and healthcare workers should not be harmed by their chosen profession (IOM, 2001b, p. 44). Medical errors may result in up to 3 million preventable adverse events and 100,000 deaths, and account for as much as $17 billion in excess health costs (Pronovost et al., 2018). A safe health-care system also means that standards of care should not decline at different times of the day or week or when a patient is transferred from one provider to another. In addition, safety requires that patients and their families are fully informed and participate in their care to the extent they wish to do so (IOM, 2001b, p. 45).

Efficacy

While scientific evidence regarding a particular treatment's effectiveness is not always available, an effective healthcare system should use evidence-based treatments whenever possible. This effort includes avoiding the underuse of effective care and the overuse of ineffective care (IOM, 2001b, p. 47). Evidence-based medicine is not limited to findings from randomized clinical trials, but may use results from a variety of research designs. To promote the use of evidence-based medicine, healthcare providers and institutions should improve their data collection and analysis capabilities so that it is possible to monitor results of care provided (IOM, 2001b, p. 48). (See **Box 4.4**.)

💡 Box 4.4 DISCUSSION QUESTIONS

Unfortunately, evidence is not available to support the effectiveness or cost–benefit of every procedure or drug. How should policymakers and providers make decisions when faced with a dearth of evidence? Do you prefer a more cautious approach that does not approve procedures or drugs until evidence is available or a more aggressive approach that encourages experimentation and use of treatments that appear to be effective? What about medical care for children, who are generally excluded from clinical and research trials for ethical reasons? When, if ever, is it appropriate for insurers to cover or the government to pay for treatments that are not proven effective?

Patient-Centeredness

A patient-centered healthcare system is sensitive to the needs, values, and preferences of each patient; includes smooth transitions and close coordination among providers; provides complete information and education at a level and in a language patients can understand; involves the patient's family and friends according to the patient's wishes; and, to the extent possible, reduces physical discomfort experienced by patients during care (IOM, 2001b, pp. 49–50). A language or cultural barrier may be a significant hurdle to receiving high-quality and patient-centered care. In 2018, 21.9% of Americans spoke a language other than English at home (Camarota & Zeigler, 2019). Individuals with language barriers are less likely to adhere to medication regimens, have a usual source of care, and understand their diagnosis and treatment, and are more likely to have lower patient satisfaction, use more healthcare services, have more adverse events, leave a hospital against a provider's advice, and miss follow-up appointments (Al Shamsi et al., 2020; Speaking Together, 2007). While use of interpreters can improve a patient's quality of care, when friends or family members serve as interpreters, there is greater risk that the interpreter will misunderstand or omit a provider's questions and that the patient will not disclose embarrassing symptoms (Speaking Together, 2007). Similarly, cultural differences between provider and patient can result in patients receiving less than optimal care. Cultural differences can define how healthcare information is received, whether a problem is perceived as a healthcare issue, how patients express symptoms and concerns, and what type of treatment is most appropriate. As a result, healthcare organizations should ensure that patients receive care that is both linguistically and culturally appropriate (Office of Minority Health, n.d.).

Timeliness

A high-quality healthcare system will provide care in a timely manner. Currently, U.S. patients experience long waits when making appointments, sitting in doctors' offices, standing in hallways before receiving procedures, waiting for test results, seeking care at EDs, and appealing billing errors (IOM, 2001b, p. 51). These delays can take an emotional as well as physical toll if medical problems would have been caught earlier with more timely care. Timeliness problems also affect providers because of difficulties in obtaining vital information and delays that result when consulting specialists. In addition, lengthy waits are the result of a system that is not efficient and does not respect the needs of its consumers (IOM, 2001b, p. 51).

Efficiency

An efficient healthcare system makes the best use of its resources and obtains the most value per dollar spent on healthcare goods and services. The uncoordinated and fragmented U.S. system is wasteful when it provides low-quality care and creates higher than necessary administrative and production costs (IOM, 2001b, p. 52). As indicated previously, the high level of spending and poor outcomes relating to preventable conditions, the number of patients who do not receive appropriate care, and the high number of medical errors make it clear that the quality of healthcare services provided can be improved.

In addition, significant geographical variations in the provision of healthcare services suggest a lack of efficiency in the system; however, this is a complicated issue to understand and solve. For example, the Dartmouth Atlas Project has studied regional variations in healthcare practices and spending for several decades. Even after controlling for level of illness and prices paid for services, researchers have found a twofold difference in Medicare spending in the country (Cubanski et al., 2015; "Health Policy," 2014).

Furthermore, higher spending areas are not associated with better quality of care, more patient satisfaction, better access to care, more effective care, or improved outcomes (Cassidy, 2014; Fisher et al., 2009). Instead, both health system capacity and local practice styles appear to be key factors in geographical variations in cost. An NAM report addressing this issue also found that health status, demographics, insurance plan coverage, and market factors did not explain the variation (publishing as IOM, 2013). The report highlighted the use of post-acute care and acute care services as a key concern and noted that other factors, such as patient preference and provider discretion, are not included in the data analyzed. In the end, the NAM concluded, "an overall explanation for geographic variation remains elusive" (IOM, 2013). As policymakers try to improve quality of care in the United States, they will have to continue to untangle difficult questions of why some parts of the country spend more on services than others.

The nation spends about one-quarter of its healthcare expenditures on administration, which is four times more per person than other comparable countries. More per-person resources are devoted to administrative costs in the United States than for long-term care, cancer care, or preventive care (Bodenheimer, 2005, p. 934; Cutler, 2018; Papanicolas et al.,

2018; Peter G. Peterson Foundation, 2020) (**Figure 4.19**). Extensive use of private insurers, which often have high administrative costs relative to public insurance programs, as well as the use of multiple insurers instead of a single-payer system, result in high administrative costs in the United States.

Equity

An equitable healthcare system provides essential health benefits to all people and includes universal access to care. Equity can be considered on an individual level and on a population level (IOM, 2001b, p. 53). While the ACA should improve individual access to services by reducing the number of uninsured, insurance alone is not sufficient to ensure access to care. The care itself still must be accessible (providers are willing to accept you as a patient), affordable, and available (sufficient providers are available).

Population-level equity refers to reducing healthcare disparities among subgroups. In the United States, racial and ethnic minority groups often receive lower-quality care and fewer routine preventive procedures than White people. A 2003 NAM report found that African Americans were less likely than Whites to receive appropriate cardiac medication, undergo necessary coronary artery bypass surgery, and use dialysis or receive a kidney transplant even when controlling for factors such as age, insurance status, income level, and comorbidities. Not surprisingly, African Americans also had higher mortality rates than their White counterparts (publishing as IOM, 2003, pp. 2–3).

These trends continue. Even before the disparities in healthcare access and outcomes made headlines during the COVID-19 pandemic (discussed more in Chapter 11, "Health Reform and the Patient Protection and Affordable Care Act"), numerous studies highlighted entrenched health disparities in our country. For example, Black, Indigenous, and People of Color (BIPOC) populations report lower health status and poorer outcomes relating to infant mortality, pregnancy-related deaths, chronic diseases, mental health status, overall health status, and life expectancy (Ndugga & Artiga, 2021).

Hispanics are more likely than Whites to have asthma, liver disease, tuberculosis, and diabetes, and to die from cervical cancer and HIV. (Families USA, 2018). In 2020, the Agency for Healthcare Quality and Research (AHQR) found access to care was worse for African Americans on 48% of their measures and for Hispanics on 65% of their measures (AHQR, 2020).

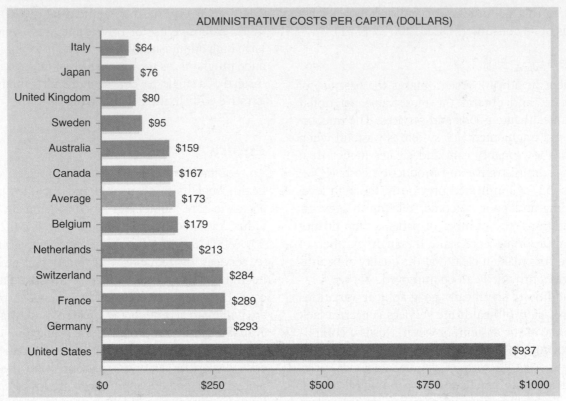

Notes: The five countries with the largest economies and those with both an above median GDP and GDP per capita, relative to all OECD countries, were included. Average does not include the U.S. Data are for 2019 or latest available. Chart uses purchasing power parties to convert data into U.S. dollars.

Figure 4.19 Administrative Costs Comprise a Larger Share of Healthcare Spending in the United States than in Other High-Income Countries, 2016

Reproduced from Peter G. Peterson Foundation. (2020). *How does the U.S. healthcare system compare to other countries?* https://www.pgpf.org/blog/2020/07/how-does-the-us-healthcare-system-compare-to-other-countries

Assessment of Efforts to Improve Quality

The NAM has called for sweeping changes to the healthcare system to address the numerous ways in which the quality of care could be improved. Although the ACA makes significant changes to the healthcare system, the law is focused more on improving access than improving quality or the delivery system. Many of the law's quality improvement provisions are pilot programs and demonstration projects that may eventually result in significant changes—or fall to the wayside once they expire.

None of the quality improvement tasks the NAM calls for will be simple to achieve, and, at times, they seem to have conflicting goals. For example, making the healthcare system patient-centered may not always result in enhanced efficiency. Furthermore, the NAM's proposed changes would require increased resources at a time when the United States is facing record deficits and unsustainable healthcare spending levels. Improving the quality of the healthcare system is an enormous challenge and one that is likely to remain on the nation's agenda for years to come.

Comparative Health Systems

A review of the U.S. healthcare system and a discussion of its flaws often lead one to ask, how do other countries deliver health care, and do they do a better job? Because the United States spends more overall and more per person on health care and yet often lags in many quality and outcome indicators, perhaps there are lessons to learn from other countries (**Figure 4.20**). Although there are many problems with healthcare delivery in the United States, it is also true that each type of healthcare system has its advantages and drawbacks.

Healthcare systems found in other countries typically fall into three general categories: (1) a national health insurance system that is publicly financed, but in which care is provided by private practitioners (e.g., Canada); (2) a national health system that is publicly financed and where care is provided by government employees or contractors (e.g., Great Britain); and (3) a socialized insurance system that is financed through mandatory contributions by employers and

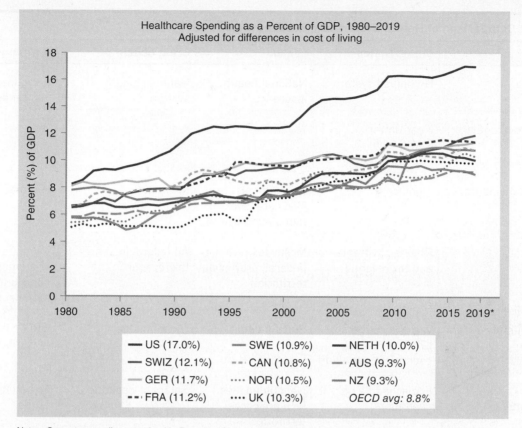

Healthcare Spending as a Percent of GDP, 1980–2019
Adjusted for differences in cost of living

Legend:
- US (17.0%)
- SWIZ (12.1%)
- GER (11.7%)
- FRA (11.2%)
- SWE (10.9%)
- CAN (10.8%)
- NOR (10.5%)
- UK (10.3%)
- NETH (10.0%)
- AUS (9.3%)
- NZ (9.3%)
- OECD avg: 8.8%

Notes: Current expenditures on health. Based on System of Health Accounts methodology, with some differences between country methodologies. OECD average reflects the average of 37 OECD member countries, including ones not shown here.

*2019 data are provisional or estimated.

Figure 4.20 Healthcare Spending as a Percentage of GDP, 1980–2019

Reproduced from Tikkanen, R., & Fields, K. (2020). *Multinational comparisons of health systems data, 2020.* The Commonwealth Fund. https://www.commonwealthfund.org/sites/default/files/2021-02/Tikkanen_Fields_2020_multinational_comparisons_chartpack.pdf

employees and in which care is delivered by private practitioners (e.g., Germany) (Shi & Singh, 2019, p. 22). Of course, variations exist within these types of systems in terms of the role of the central government, the presence of private insurance, the way the healthcare system is financed, and how care is administered by providers and accessed by patients. Although comparing the systems in the three countries used here as examples does not cover all possible permutations of how healthcare systems are designed, it provides an overview of the choices made by policymakers in different countries (**Table 4.1**).

A National Health Insurance System: Canada

Canada's healthcare system is called Medicare. Prior to establishing the Medicare program in 1966, Canada provided insurance in a manner that was similar to the U.S. method, with private plans offering coverage to many, even while millions remained uninsured. Incremental changes were made to the Canadian healthcare system until the Medical Care Act of 1966 established Medicare's framework; it was later modified through the Canadian Health Act of 1984. The Canadian Health Act established five principles for healthcare delivery: (1) public administration, (2) comprehensive coverage, (3) universality, (4) portability across Canada, and (5) uniform and reasonable access to care (Johnson et al., 2018).

Canada's healthcare system is largely decentralized, with Canada's provinces and territories each responsible for setting up its own delivery system. As such, Canada's Medicare system is a collection of single-payer systems governed by the provinces and territories, with the central government taking a more limited role. The provinces and territories set their own policies regarding many healthcare and other social issues, administer their own individual single-payer systems, reimburse hospitals directly or through regional health authorities, and negotiate physician fee schedules with provincial medical associations. Provinces and territories use regional health authorities as their primary payer of healthcare services.

Table 4.1 Comparison of Health Systems Across Four Countries

	United States	Canada	Great Britain	Germany
System type	No unified system	National health insurance	National health system	Socialized health insurance
Universal coverage	Near universal if ACA fully implemented	Yes	Yes	Yes
Role of private insurance	Significant	Supplemental to Medicare, two-thirds purchase	Minimal	Minimal
Financing	Private payments and tax revenue	Mostly tax revenue (federal, provincial, territorial)	All federal income tax revenue	Mandatory employer and employee contributions to national health fund
Hospital reimbursement	Varies by payer (DRG[a], FFS[b], capitation, per diem)	Global budget	Global budget	DRG[a]
Physician reimbursement	Fee schedule or capitation	Negotiated fees with provinces/territories	Salary or capitation	Negotiated fees with funds

[a]DRG = diagnostic-related group (payment based on bundle of services needed for diagnosis).
[b]FFS = fee for service (payment per service rendered).

Although funding methods vary by location, regional health authorities have the ability to tailor funds in a way that best serves the needs of their population. In addition to paying for care, regional health authorities also organize the delivery of care. They hire staff at most acute care facilities and contract for some ambulatory care services. General practitioners and specialists mostly work on a fee-for-service arrangement and in private practice (Allin et al., 2020). The federal government has responsibility for specific health areas such as prescription drugs, public health, and health research, as well as for providing care to certain populations (e.g., veterans, indigenous peoples; Allin et al., 2020).

Financing for health benefits varies by benefit type. Hospital services, physician services, and public health services are financed through public taxation. Hospitals mostly operate under global budgets that they negotiate with a ministry of health or regional health authority, although a few provinces are considering activity-based funding (Allin et al., 2020). Certain services, including prescription drugs, home care, and institutional care, are financed through a combination of public taxation and private insurance coverage. Other goods and services, such as dental

and vision care, over-the-counter drugs, and alternative medicines are covered only through private insurance. Approximately two-thirds of Canadians purchase private insurance, which is used to cover goods and services not provided by Medicare (Allin et al., 2020).

Tax revenue from the provincial, territorial, and federal governments pays for 70% of total Medicare expenditures, private insurance reimbursement accounts for 12% of costs, patient out-of-pocket payments cover 15%, and various sources account for the remaining amount (Allin et al., 2020). Healthcare spending is expected to reach C$265.5 billion in 2019 (Canadian Institute for Health Information [CIHI], 2021). Healthcare spending varies considerably across the country. For example, Alberta spends C$7855 per person, compared to Yukon's C$12,633 per-person costs (CIHI, 2021).

A National Health System: Great Britain

Great Britain's healthcare system was designed by Sir William Beveridge as part of a social reconstruction plan after World War II. The National Health

Services Act of 1946 created the National Health Service (NHS), a centrally run healthcare system that provides universal health care to all residents of Great Britain. It was designed based on the principle that the government is responsible for providing equal access to comprehensive health care that is generally free at the point of service (Johnson et al., 2018, pp. 174–176).

The Health and Social Care Act of 2012 introduced significant changes to the NHS system. In the prior system, health care was delivered through a variety of trusts that covered services such as primary care, mental health care, acute care, and ambulance services (Johnson et al., 2018, pp. 178–179). In the new system, Primary Care Trusts were replaced with Clinical Commissioning Groups (CCGs), which are led by clinicians. CCGs are bodies that consist of general practitioners in their service area, and they are responsible for providing urgent and emergency care, elective hospital care, community health services that go beyond general practitioner services, maternity and newborn services, and mental health and learning disability services. The 2012 legislation also created an independent organization called NHS England to focus on improving health outcomes and quality of care. NHS England provides national leadership, supervises CCGs, allocates resources to CCGs, and commissions primary care, certain specialty care, and offender care (Thorlby, 2020).

The NHS is the largest publicly financed national health system in the world. The 2020–2021 budget is £212.1 billion. The 2018 five-year funding included a £33.9 billion increase by 2023–2024, bringing its growth rate closer to the long-term average (King's Fund, 2021b). NHS is using a number of cost containment strategies to address its budgetary concerns, including freezing wages, increasing use of generic drugs, reducing hospital payments, lowering administrative costs, and improving hospital management (Thorlby, 2020).

The NHS is financed primarily through general tax revenues. It is NHS England's responsibility to identify necessary healthcare services and Monitor's (England's regulatory body for health care) role to set prices for those services. Although most residents receive their care through the NHS, private insurance is also available. Approximately 10.5% of residents have private health insurance, which provides the same benefits as the NHS but allows for reduced waiting times, more convenient care, and greater access to specialists (Johnson et al., 2018, p. 182; Thorlby, 2020).

NHS services are provided by provider organizations that are classified as NHS foundation trusts or NHS trusts. NHS foundation trusts are not directed by the government and are free to make financial decisions based on a framework established by law and regulation. NHS trusts are directed by the government and are financially accountable to the government (Johnson et al., 2018, p. 181; Thorlby, 2020). Most general practice physicians and nurses are private practitioners who work for the NHS as independent contractors, not salaried employees, while the NHS owns the hospitals and the hospital staff are salaried employees. Patients select a general practitioner in their service area, and this provider is the gateway to NHS services. Almost everyone has a registered general practitioner, and most patient contact is with this provider (Thorlby, 2020). Services are provided free of charge, except for specific services designated by law.

The Health and Social Care Act also renewed focus on public health needs. Public Health England was created in 2013 as an autonomous executive agency of the Department of Health. Its role is to protect the public's health, reduce health disparities, promote health knowledge and information, and support local government systems in their healthcare delivery. In addition, local Health and Wellbeing Boards were created to improve the public's health and reduce disparities through local government action (King's Fund, 2021a).

In 2019, NHS unveiled a 10-year Long-Term Plan that brought together a variety of 5-year plans that addressed challenges to the healthcare system, with a focus on improving early identification of high-risk patients and exploring new payment models. The models focused on "scaled up multidisciplinary primary care," long-term care, "vertically integrated hospital and community care," and emergency care (Thorlby, 2020). The 10-year plan also emphasized cardiovascular disease, respiratory disease, cancer, mental health, and improved primary care networks (Thorlby, 2020).

A Socialized Insurance System: Germany

In 1883, Germany's Otto von Bismarck created the first healthcare system in the world. He viewed a strong health and pension system as a way to build a superior nation, earn support from Germany's working class, and undermine any attempts by Germany's socialist party to gain power. The central government is responsible for setting health policy and regulating the Social

Health Insurance System (SHIS). German healthcare policy emphasizes solidarity, the idea that all should have equal access to health care regardless of ability to pay (Johnson et al., 2018, pp. 217–223). Germany's legislature passed several major health reform bills in recent years. These reforms include integration of inpatient and ambulatory care, premium payment changes, an insurance mandate, and revised long-term care policies (Johnson et al., 2018, pp. 230–231).

SHIS comprises a collection of nonprofit regional sickness funds with a standard benefit package that includes inpatient services, outpatient services, medications, rehabilitation therapy, and dental benefits. The funds are organized around industry or geography and are responsible for managing healthcare services. Germans must enroll in sickness funds or obtain coverage through private insurance (Blümel & Busse, 2020). Some populations are required to be under SHIS, including individuals who earn less than $60,750 per year. Funds may not refuse to cover these individuals, and physicians may not refuse to treat them. Germans who earn more than $68,000 per year or who are self-employed may choose to opt out of SHIS and purchase private coverage. Exempt citizens and individuals choosing to opt out of SHIS may purchase private substitutive private health insurance. Of those individuals with a choice between SHIS or private insurance, about 75% remain with the public plan. Overall, 88% of the population use sickness funds, 11% enroll in private insurance, and the remaining 1% have other plans (e.g., military) (Blümel & Busse, 2020).

Health care is provided in the public and private sectors. SHIS ambulatory care physicians generally work in private practice and are members of regional associations that negotiate a fee schedule with sickness funds. Fee schedules are also used by private insurers, but often at a higher rate than the SHIS fee schedule. Hospitals are split between public, private nonprofit, and private for-profit institutions, with the latter increasing its share of the market in recent years. Hospitals are staffed by salaried providers and reimbursed based on a diagnostic-related group methodology (Blümel & Busse, 2020; Johnson et al., 2018, p. 235).

Sickness funds are financed through employer and employee contributions. As of 2016, employer and employees split the 14.6% of gross wage contribution. In addition, there is a supplementary contribution based on income that is set by each sickness fund. The sickness fund contributions are pooled and then reallocated to individuals based on a risk-adjusted formula that accounts for age, sex, and morbidity (Blümel &

Busse, 2020). In 2014, Germany spent $492 billion in health expenditures, mostly through SHIS (Johnson et al., 2018, p. 234).

The Importance of Health Insurance Design

Reviewing the healthcare systems of four countries—the United States, Canada, Great Britain, and Germany—shows how varied healthcare systems are around the world. Differences exist regarding the role of government, the ability to purchase private insurance, cost-sharing requirements, and how the system is financed. Even countries that share the same general type of system have variations based on their specific culture, politics, and needs. How a system is designed matters in terms of access to care, financing, and patient satisfaction. (See **Box 4.5**.)

A 2021 survey in 11 countries asked residents about their experience with their country's healthcare system (Schneider et al., 2021). What issues were primary concerns and how different residents fared within a system varied by country. The United States ranked last on overall health system ranking and last in four of five categories (**Table 4.2** and **Figures 4.21** and **4.22**).

As shown in Table 4.2, the only category in which the United States shined was care process, which "includes measures of *preventive care, safe care, coordinated care*, and *engagement and patient preferences*" (Schneider et al., 2021). As part of the care process, the United States was a top performer for preventive care, safe care, patient preferences, and use of Internet healthcare portals. New Zealand, Switzerland, and the Netherlands excelled at coordinating care. Affordability is a key concern in the United States. The United States ranked last in affordability; individuals in England, the Netherlands, Norway, and Germany were the least likely to have difficulty paying bills or having a claim denied (Schneider et al., 2021). Australia, New Zealand, and England received high marks for administrative efficiency. Individuals

---

💡 Box 4.5 DISCUSSION QUESTIONS

Do you prefer one of these health systems to the others? Why or why not? Are there features that you think should be incorporated into the U.S. healthcare system? Are there reasons why certain features might be difficult to incorporate into the U.S. healthcare system?

Table 4.2 Healthcare System Performance Rankings

	Australia	Canada	France	Germany	The Netherlands	New Zealand	Norway	Sweden	Switzerland	United Kingdom	United States
OVERALL RANKING	3	10	8	5	2	6	1	7	9	4	11
Access to care	8	9	7	3	1	5	2	6	10	4	11
Care process	6	4	10	9	3	1	8	11	7	5	2
Administrative efficiency	2	7	6	9	8	3	1	5	10	4	11
Equity	1	10	7	2	5	9	8	6	3	4	11
Healthcare outcomes	1	10	6	7	4	8	2	5	3	9	11

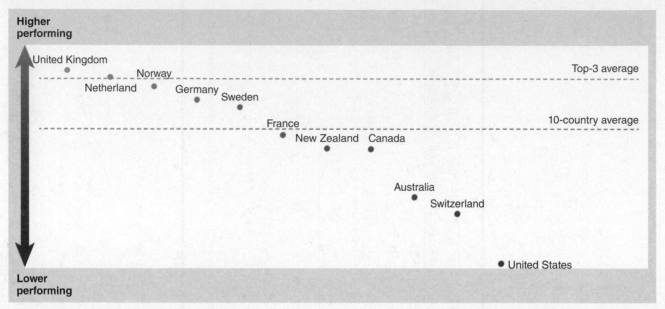

Note: To normalize performance scores across countries, each score is the calculated standard deviation from a 10-country average that excludes the United States.

Figure 4.21 Healthcare System Performance Scores: Affordability

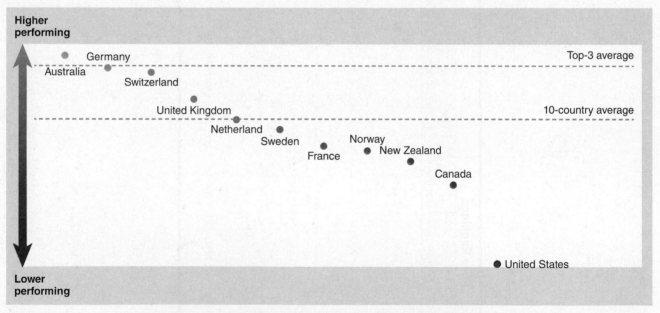

Note: To normalize performance scores across countries, each score is the calculated standard deviation from a 10-country average that excludes the United States.

Figure 4.22 Healthcare Systems Performance Scores: Equity

in the United States and Canada were more likely than residents of other countries to visit an emergency room for nonemergent care and to have higher income-related inequities. Overall, Australia, Germany, and Switzerland had the most equitable systems, while the United States was the least equitable by a noticeable margin (Schneider et al., 2021).

Conclusion

This wide-ranging review of the U.S. healthcare system was intended to provide readers with a general sense of how health care is accessed, financed, and administered in this country. Understanding the various players in the healthcare system, from providers to researchers to policymakers, is crucial to being able to participate in debates over current issues in health policy and law. While the U.S. system excels on many fronts, it falls short in many areas relating to access, quality, and efficiency. Perhaps policymakers in this country could learn lessons from successes abroad, but the United States

has a unique political environment and it is clear there is no silver bullet that will solve all of the problems we face. Specific health policy and law concerns will be described in much greater detail elsewhere, providing a foundation to tackle the many problems that will confront the country in the years ahead.

References

Agency for Healthcare Quality and Research. (2020, December). *2019 national healthcare quality and disparities report.* https://www.ahrq.gov/research/findings/nhqrdr/nhqdr19/index.html

Alker, J. (2021, April 28). *Low-wage uninsured workers: Who are they and where do they work?* https://ccf.georgetown.edu/2021/04/28/low-wage-uninsured-workers-who-are-they-and-where-do-they-work/

Allin, S., Marchildon, G., & Peckham, A. (2020, June 5). *International health care system profiles, Canada.* https://international.commonwealthfund.org/countries/canada/

Al Shamsi, H., Almutairi, A. G., Al Mashrafi, S., & Al Kalbani, T. (2020). *Implications of language barriers for healthcare: A systematic review.* https://www.ncbi.nlm.nih.gov/pmc/articles/PMC7201401/

America's Essential Hospitals. (2021, May). *Essential data: Our hospitals, our patients.* https://essentialhospitals.org/wp-content/uploads/2021/05/EssentialData2021_Web.pdf

Ashman, J., Schappert, S., & Santo, L. (2020, June). *Emergency department visits among adults aged 60 and over: United States, 2014–2017.* https://www.cdc.gov/nchs/products/databriefs/db367.htm

Auerbach, D. I., Chen, P. G., Friedberg, M. W., Reid, R., Lau, C., Buerhaus, P. I., & Mehrotra, A. (2013). Nurse-managed health centers and patient centered medical homes could mitigate expected primary care physician shortage. *Health Affairs, 32*(11), 1933–1941. https://doi.org/10.1377/hlthaff.2013.0596

Bardach, S. H., & Rowles, G. D. (2012). Geriatric education in the health professions: Are we making progress? *Gerontologist, 52*(5), 607–616. https://doi.org/10.1093/geront/gns006

Blümel, M., & Busse, R. (2020, June 5). *International health care system profiles, Germany.* https://www.commonwealthfund.org/international-health-policy-center/countries/germany

Boal, W., Li, J., & Silver, S. (2021, March 9). *Health care access among essential critical infrastructure workers, 31 states, 2017–2018.* https://journals.sagepub.com/doi/full/10.1177/0033354921996688

Bodenheimer, T. (2005). High and rising health care costs, part 2: Technological innovation. *Annals of Internal Medicine, 142*(11), 932–937. https://doi.org/10.7326/0003-4819-142-11-200506070-00012

Borsky, A., Zhan, C., Miller, T., Ngo-Metzger, Q., Bierman, A. S., & Myers, D. (2018). Few Americans receive all high-priority, appropriate clinical preventive services. *Health Affairs, 37*(6), 925–928. https://doi.org/10.1377/hlthaff.2017.1248

Camarota, S. A., & Zeigler, K. (2019, October 29). *Some 67 million people in the United States spoke a foreign language at home.* https://cis.org/Report/673-Million-United-States-Spoke-Foreign-Language-Home-2018

Canadian Institute for Health Information. (2021). *National health expenditures trends, 2020.* https://www.cihi.ca/sites/default/files/document/nhex-trends-2020-narrative-report-en.pdf

Cassidy, A. (2014, March 6). *Geographic variation in Medicare spending.* https://www.healthaffairs.org/do/10.1377/hpb20140306.633790/full/

Castellucci, M. (2016, November 5). Medical schools tackle primary-care shortages. *Modern Healthcare.* https://www.modernhealthcare.com/article/20161105/MAGAZINE/311059982/medical-schools-tackle-primary-care-shortages

Castellucci, M. (2018, February 27). Geriatrics still failing to attract new doctors. *Modern Healthcare.* https://www.modernhealthcare.com/article/20180227/NEWS/180229926/geriatrics-still-failing-to-attract-new-doctors

Center of Excellence in Public Health Workforce Studies. (2013). *Public health workforce enumeration, 2012.* http://www.phf.org/resourcestools/Documents/UM_CEPHS_Enumeration2012_Revised_July_2013.pdf

Centers for Disease Control and Prevention. (2015, December 5). *Increase productivity.* https://www.cdc.gov/workplacehealthpromotion/model/control-costs/benefits/productivity.html

Centers for Medicare and Medicaid Services. (n.d.). *National health expenditure projections 2018–2027.* https://www.cms.gov/Research-Statistics-Data-and-Systems/Statistics-Trends-and-Reports/NationalHealthExpendData/Downloads/ForecastSummary.pdf

Centers for Medicare and Medicaid Services. (2020a, April 15). *NHE projections 2019–2028—Forecast summary.* https://www.cms.gov/files/document/nhe-projections-2019-2028-forecast-summary.pdf

Centers for Medicare and Medicaid Services. (2020b, November 6). *2021 Medicare parts A & B premiums and deductibles.* https://www.cms.gov/newsroom/fact-sheets/2021-medicare-parts-b-premiums-and-deductibles

Centers for Medicare and Medicaid Services. (2020c, December 16). *NHE fact sheet* https://www.cms.gov/Research-Statistics-Data-and-Systems/Statistics-Trends-and-Reports/NationalHealthExpendData/NHE-Fact-Sheet

Collins, S. R., Gunja, M. Z., & Aboulafia G. N. (2020, August 19). *U.S. health insurance coverage in 2020: A looming crisis in affordability.* https://www.commonwealthfund.org/publications/issue-briefs/2020/aug/looming-crisis-health-coverage-2020-biennial

Congressional Budget Office. (2019). *Federal subsidies for health insurance coverage for people under age 65: 2019 to 2029*. https://www.cbo.gov/system/files/2019-05/55085-Health CoverageSubsidies_0.pdf

Congressional Research Service. (2021, February 9). *Medicaid disproportionate share hospital (DSH) reductions*. https://crsreports.congress.gov/product/pdf/IF/IF10422

Conway, D. (2020, October 26). *Adults age 26 had highest uninsured rate among all ages, followed by 27-year-olds*. https://www.census.gov/library/stories/2020/10/uninsured-rates-highest-for-young-adults-aged-19-to-34.html

Cubanski, J., Neuman, T., & White, C. (2015). *The latest on geographic variation in Medicare spending: A demographic divide persists but variation has narrowed. Kaiser Family Foundation*. https://www.kff.org/report-section/the-latest-on-geographic-variation-in-medicare-spending-findings/

Cutler, D. (2018). What is the US health spending problem? *Health Affairs, 37*(3), 1838–1847. https://doi.org/10.1377/hlthaff.2017.1626

Dalen, J., Ryan, K., & Alpert, J. (2017, February 16). *Where have the generalists gone? They became specialists, then subspecialists*. https://www.amjmed.com/article/s0002-9343(17)30134-1/fulltext

Dall, T., Reynolds R., Chakrabarti, R., Jones, K., & Iacobucci, W. (2020, June). *The complexities of physician supply and demand: Projections from 2018 to 2033*. https://www.aamc.org/media/45976/download

de Beaumont. (2019, January 14). *New workforce survey: Public health turnover could pose threat to community health*. https://debeaumont.org/news/2019/new-workforce-survey-public-health-turnover-could-pose-threat-to-community-health/

Department of Health and Human Services. (n.d.). *Healthy people 2030*. https://health.gov/healthypeople

Dunker, A., Krofah, E., & Isasi, F. (2014, September 22). *The role of physician assistants in health care delivery*. https://www.nga.org/files/live/sites/NGA/files/pdf/2014/1409TheRoleOfPhysicianAssistants.pdf

Families USA. (2005). *Paying a premium: The added cost of care for the uninsured*. http://www.policyarchive.org/handle/10207/6261

Families USA. (2018, September 25). *Latino health inequities compared to non-Hispanic Whites*. https://familiesusa.org/resources/latino-health-inequities-compared-to-non-hispanic-whites/

Finegold K, Conmy, A., Chu, R. C., Bosworth, A., & Sommers, B. D. (2021). *Trends in the U.S. uninsured population, 2010–2020*. Assistant Secretary for Planning and Evaluation. https://aspe.hhs.gov/system/files/pdf/265041/trends-in-the-us-uninsured.pdf; Figure 4.

Fisher, E., Goodman, D., Skinner, J., & Bronner, K. (2009). *Health care spending, quality, and outcomes: More isn't always better*. http://www.dartmouthatlas.org/downloads/reports/Spending_Brief_022709.pdf

Foutz, J., Artiga, S., & Garfield, R. (2017). *The role of Medicaid in rural America*. https://www.kff.org/medicaid/issue-brief/the-role-of-medicaid-in-rural-america/

Garfield, R., Orgera, K., & Damico, A. (2019, January 25). *The uninsured and the ACA: A primer—key facts about health insurance and the uninsured amidst changes to the Affordable Care Act*. https://www.kff.org/uninsured/report/the-uninsured-and-the-aca-a-primer-key-facts-about-health-insurance-and-the-uninsured-amidst-changes-to-the-affordable-care-act/

Garfield, R., Orgera, K., & Damico, A. (2021, January 21). *The coverage gap: Uninsured poor adults in states that do not expand Medicaid*. https://www.kff.org/medicaid/issue-brief/the-coverage-gap-uninsured-poor-adults-in-states-that-do-not-expand-medicaid/

Graves, J. A., Pranita, M., Dittus, R. S., Parikh, R., Perloff, J., Buerhaus, P. I. (2016). Role of geography and nurse-practitioner scope of practice in efforts to expand primary care system capacity: Health reform and the primary care workforce. *Medical Care, 54*(1), 81–89. https://doi.org/10.1097/MLR.0000000000000454

Gresenz, C. R., & Escarce, J. J. (2011). Spillover effects of community uninsurance on working age adults and seniors: An instrumental variable analysis. *Medical Care, 49*(9), e14–e21. https://doi.org/10.1097/MLR.0b013e31822dc7f4

Gunja, M., & Collins, S. (2019, August 28). *Who are the remaining uninsured and why do they lack coverage?* https://www.commonwealthfund.org/publications/issue-briefs/2019/aug/who-are-remaining-uninsured-and-why-do-they-lack-coverage

Guttmacher Institute. (2021a, June 1). *Insurance coverage of contraceptives*. https://www.guttmacher.org/state-policy/explore/insurance-coverage-contraceptives

Guttmacher Institute. (2021b, June 1). *An overview of abortion laws*. https://www.guttmacher.org/state-policy/explore/overview-abortion-laws#

Guttmacher Institute. (2021c, June 1). *Regulating insurance coverage of abortion*. https://www.guttmacher.org/state-policy/explore/regulating-insurance-coverage-abortion

Health policy brief: Geographic variation in Medicare spending." (March 6, 2014). *Health Affairs*. https://www.healthaffairs.org/do/10.1377/hpb20140306.633790/full/healthpolicybrief_109.pdf

Health Resources Services Administration. (2016). *State-level projections of supply and demand for primary care practitioners: 2013–2025*. https://bhw.hrsa.gov/sites/default/files/bureau-health-workforce/data-research/primary-care-state-projections2013-2025.pdf

Institute of Medicine. (2000). *America's health care safety net: Intact but endangered*. National Academy Press.

Institute of Medicine. (2001a). *Coverage matters: Insurance and health care*. National Academy Press.

Institute of Medicine. (2001b). *Crossing the quality chasm: A new health system for the 21st century*. National Academy Press.

Institute of Medicine. (2003). *Unequal treatment: Confronting racial and ethnic disparities in health care*. National Academy Press.

Institute of Medicine. (2008). *Retooling for an aging America: Building the health care workforce*. National Academy Press.

Institute of Medicine. (2013). *Variation in health care spending: Target decision making, not geography*. National Academy Press.

Johnson, J., Stoskopf, C., & Shi, L. (2018). *Comparative health systems: A global perspective* (2nd ed.). Jones & Bartlett Learning.

Kaiser Family Foundation. (2020a). *Health coverage of immigrants*. https://www.kff.org/racial-equity-and-health-policy/fact-sheet/health-coverage-of-immigrants/

Kaiser Family Foundation. (2020b). *2020 Employer health benefits survey*. https://files.kff.org/attachment/Report-Employer-Health-Benefits-2020-Annual-Survey.pdf

Karpman, M., Coughlin, T., & Garfield, R. (2021, April 6). *Declines in uncompensated care costs for the uninsured under the ACA and implications of recent growth in the uninsured rate*. https://www.kff.org/uninsured/issue-brief/declines-in-uncompensated

-care-costs-for-the-uninsured-under-the-aca-and
-implications-of-recent-growth-in-the-uninsured-rate/

Keehan, S., Cuckler, G., Poisal, J., Sisko, A., Smith, S., Madison, A., Rennie, K., Fiore, J., & Hardesty, J. (2020, March 24). *National health expenditure projections, 2019–28: Expected rebound in prices drives rising spending growth.* https://www.healthaffairs.org/doi/full/10.1377/hlthaff.2020.00094

Kerns, C., & Willis, D. (2020, March 16). *The problem with U.S. health care isn't a shortage of doctors.* https://hbr.org/2020/03/the-problem-with-u-s-health-care-isnt-a-shortage-of-doctors

King's Fund. (2021a). *The new NHS: Health and wellness boards.* https://www.kingsfund.org.uk/projects/new-nhs/health-and-wellbeing-boards

King's Fund. (2021b). *The NHS budget and how it has changed.* https://www.kingsfund.org.uk/projects/nhs-in-a-nutshell/nhs-budget

Lambrew, J. M., DeFriese, G. H., Carey, T. S., Ricketts, T. C., & Biddle, A. K. (1996). The effects of having a regular doctor on access to primary care. *Medical Care, 34*(2), 138–151.

Levine, D. M., Linder, J. A., & Landon, B. E. (2016). The quality of outpatient care delivered to adults in the United States, 2002–2013. *JAMA, 176*(12), 1778–1790. https://doi.org/10.1001/jamainternmed.2016.6217

Makaroun, L. K., Bowman, C., Duan, K., Handley, N., Wheeler, D. J., Pierluissi, E., & Chen, A. H. (2017). Specialty care access in the safety net—The role of public hospitals and health systems. *Journal of Health Care for the Poor and Underserved, 28*(1), 566–681. https://doi.org/10.1353/hpu.2017.0040

McGlynn, E. A., Asch, S. M., & Adams, J. (2003). The quality of health care delivered to adults in the United States. *New England Journal of Medicine, 348*, 2635–2645.

Medicaid and CHIP Payment and Access Commission. (n.d.). *Medicaid enrollment changes following the ACA.* https://www.macpac.gov/subtopic/medicaid-enrollment-changes-following-the-aca/

Morgan, P. (2019, October). *Predicted shortages of physicians might even disappear if we fully account for PAs and NPs.* https://journals.lww.com/jaapa/Fulltext/2019/10000/Predicted_shortages_of_physicians_might_even.12.aspx

Morr, M. (2018, May 3). *NP, PA employment increasing in primary care and specialty practices.* https://www.clinicaladvisor.com/home/topics/practice-management-information-center/np-pa-employment-increasing-in-primary-care-and-specialty-practices/

National Association of Community Health Centers. (n.d.). *The facts about Medicaid's FQHC Prospective Payment System (PPS).* https://www.nachc.org/wp-content/uploads/2018/06/PPS-One-Pager-Update.pdf

National Association of Community Health Centers. (2020, January). *Community health center chartbook.* https://www.nachc.org/wp-content/uploads/2020/01/Chartbook-2020-Final.pdf

National Association of Community Health Centers. (2021, April). *Health centers and Medicaid.* https://www.nachc.org/wp-content/uploads/2021/03/Medicaid-Factsheet-2021-1.pdf

National Commission on Certification of Physician Assistants, Inc. (2019, September). *2018 Statistical profile of recently certified physician assistants: An annual report of the National Commission on Certification of Physician Assistants.* https://prodcmsstoragesa.blob.core.windows.net/uploads/files/2018StatisticalProfileofRecentlyCertifiedPAs.pdf

National Conference of State Legislatures. (2017). *Improving access to care in rural and underserved communities: State workforce strategies.* http://www.ncsl.org/research/health/improving-access-to-care-in-rural-and-underserved-communities-state-workforce-strategies.aspx

National Rural Health Association. (n.d.). *About rural health care.* https://www.ruralhealthweb.org/about-nrha/about-rural-health-care

Ndugga, N., & Artiga, S. (2021, May 11). *Disparities in health and health care: 5 key questions and answers.* https://www.kff.org/racial-equity-and-health-policy/issue-brief/disparities-in-health-and-health-care-5-key-question-and-answers/

Norris, L. (2021, March 26). *The ACA's cost-sharing subsidies.* https://www.healthinsurance.org/obamacare/the-acas-cost-sharing-subsidies/

Office of Minority Health. (n.d.). *The national CLAS standards.* https://minorityhealth.hhs.gov/omh/browse.aspx?lvl=2&lvlid=53

Organization for Economic Cooperation and Development. (2019). *Health at a glance 2019: OECD indicators.* https://www.oecd-ilibrary.org/social-issues-migration-health/health-at-a-glance-2019_4dd50c09-en

Papanicolas, I., Woskie, L. R., & Jha, A. K. (2018). Health care spending in the United States and other high-income countries. *New England Journal of Medicine, 319*(10), 1024–1039. https://doi.org/10.1001/jama.2018.1150

Patient Protection and Affordable Care Act of 2010, 42 U.S.C. § 18001 (2010).

Pauly, M. V., & Pagán, J. A. (2007). Spillovers and vulnerability: The case of community uninsurance. *Health Affairs, 5*, 1304–1314. https://doi.org/10.1377/hlthaff.26.5.1304

Peter G. Peterson Foundation. (2020, July 14). *How does the U.S. healthcare system compare to other countries?* https://www.pgpf.org/blog/2020/07/how-does-the-us-healthcare-system-compare-to-other-countries

Pronovost, P., Johns, M. M. E., Palmer, S., Bono, R. C., Fridsma, D. B., Gettinger, A., Goldman, J., Johnson, W., Karney, M., Samitt, C., Sriram, R. D., Zenooz, A., & Wang, Y. C. (Eds.). (2018). *Procuring interoperability: Achieving high-quality, connected, and person-centered care.* https://nam.edu/wp-content/uploads/2019/08/Interop_508.pdf

Proser, M., Byshhe, T., Weaver, D., & Yee, R. (2015). Community health centers at the crossroads: Growth and staffing needs. *Journal of the American Academy of PAs, 28*(4), 49–53. https://doi.org/10.1097/01.JAA.0000460929.99918.e6

Robert Wood Johnson Foundation. (2012, February 27). *United States in search of nurses with geriatrics training.* https://www.rwjf.org/en/library/articles-and-news/2012/02/united-states-in-search-of-nurses-with-geriatrics-training.html

Schneider, E. C., Shah, A. Doty, M. M., Tikkanen, R., Fields, K., William II, R. D. II. (2021). *Mirror, mirror 2021: Reflecting poorly—health care in the U.S. compared to other high-income countries.* https://www.commonwealthfund.org/publications/fund-reports/2021/aug/mirror-mirror-2021-reflecting-poorly

Shi, L., & Singh, D. A. (2019). *Delivering health care in America: A systems approach* (7th ed.). Jones & Bartlett Learning.

Shin, P., Morris, R., Casoni, M., Rosenbaum, S., & Somodevilla, A. (2020, April 10). *Keeping community health centers strong during the coronavirus pandemic is essential to public health*. https://www.healthaffairs.org/do/10.1377/hblog20200409.175784/full/

Smith-Schoenwalder, C. (2021, June 25). *Survey: Over half of public health workers experienced mental health problems during COVID-19 pandemic*. https://www.usnews.com/news/health-news/articles/2021-06-25/survey-over-half-of-public-health-workers-experienced-mental-health-problems-during-coronavirus-pandemic

Speaking Together. (2007). *Addressing language barriers in health care: What's at stake*. https://www.rwjf.org/content/dam/farm/reports/issue_briefs/2007/rwjf30140

Starfield, B., & Shi, L. (2004). The medical home, access to care, and insurance: A review of evidence. *Pediatrics, 113*, 1493–1498.

Thorlby, R. (2020, June 5). *International health care system profiles, England*. https://international.commonwealthfund.org/countries/england/

Tolbert, J., Orgera, K., & Damico, A. (2020, November 6). *Key facts about the uninsured population*. https://www.kff.org/uninsured/issue-brief/key-facts-about-the-uninsured-population/

U.S. Census Bureau. (2011). *Income, poverty, and health insurance coverage in the United States: 2010*. [Current Population Reports, P60-239]. U.S. Government Printing Office.

U.S. Census Bureau. (2020a). *Health insurance coverage in the United States: 2019*. [Current Population Reports]. U.S. Government Printing Office. https://www.census.gov/content/dam/Census/library/publications/2020/demo/p60-271.pdf

U.S. Census Bureau. (2020b). *Demographic turning points for the United States: Population projections from 2020 to 2060*. [Current Population Reports, P25-1144]. U.S. Government Printing Office. https://www.census.gov/content/dam/Census/library/publications/2020/demo/p25-1144.pdf

Wein, D. (2018, August 27). Win with wellness—Attract and retain talent. *Forbes*. https://www.forbes.com/sites/forbesbusinessdevelopmentcouncil/2018/08/27/win-with-wellness-attract-and-retain-talent/?sh=1b27ea431648

White House.gov. (2021, May 13). *Fact sheet: Biden-Harris administration to invest $7 billion from American rescue plan to hire and train public health workers in response to COVID-19*. https://www.whitehouse.gov/briefing-room/statements-releases/2021/05/13/fact-sheet-biden-harris-administration-to-invest-7-billion-from-american-rescue-plan-to-hire-and-train-public-health-workers-in-response-to-covid-19/

Whitener, K. (2021, February 8). *President Biden's executive order on public charge*. https://ccf.georgetown.edu/2021/02/08/president-bidens-executive-order-on-public-charge/

Wilcox, L. (2021, May 26). *Physician salary report 2021: Compensation steady despite COVID-19*. https://weatherbyhealthcare.com/blog/annual-physician-salary-report

Wilson, R., Troisi, C., & Gary-Webb, T. (2020, April 5). *A deficit of more than 250,000 public health workers is no way to fight COVID-19*. https://www.statnews.com/2020/04/05/deficit-public-health-workers-no-way-to-fight-covid-19/

Wolters Kluwer. (2020). *NPs and PAs by the numbers: The data behind America's frontline healthcare providers*. https://www.wolterskluwer.com/en/expert-insights/nps-and-pas-by-the-numbers-the-data-behind-americas-frontline-healthcare-providers

CHAPTER 5

What Is Public Health?

Guthrie S. Birkhead
Cynthia B. Morrow
Sylvia Pirani

LEARNING OBJECTIVES

By the end of this chapter you will be able to:

- Formulate a working definition and describe the functions of public health in the 21st century; key aspects of this objective include being able to:

  1. Articulate several different definitions of public health
  2. Describe the origins and evolutionary themes of public health in the United States
  3. Trace the development of the public health system in the United States
  4. Broadly characterize the contributions and value of the public health field
  5. Identify three or more distinguishing features of public health approaches
  6. Describe public health as a system, emphasizing the role of the three core functions and 10 Essential Public Health Services
  7. Identify five or more Internet websites that provide useful information on the public health system in the United States

Introduction

The passing of one century and the early decades of the next afford a rare opportunity to look back at where public health has been and to look forward toward the challenges that lie ahead. Imagine a world 100 years from now where life expectancy is 30 years more and infant mortality rates are 95% lower than they are today. The average human life span would be greater than 107 years, and fewer than 1 of every 2000 infants would die before their first birthday. These seem like unrealistic expectations and unlikely achievements; yet, they are no greater than the gains realized during the 20th century in the United States. In 1900, few envisioned the century of progress in public health that lay ahead. Yet by 1925, public health leaders such as C.-E.A. Winslow (1877–1957), the founder of what is now the Yale School of Public Health, were noting a nearly 50% increase in life expectancy (from 36 years to 53 years) for residents of New York City between the years 1880 and 1920 (Winslow, 1926). Accomplishments such as these caused Winslow to speculate what might be possible through widespread application of scientific knowledge. Based on the even more spectacular achievements over the rest of the 20th century, we all should wonder what is possible in the 21st century.

Authors' note: This chapter was completed in September 2021. The COVID-19 pandemic continues to evolve.

In any given year, it may be difficult to point to a particular public health discovery, innovation, or triumph. Yet on closer examination, perhaps public health gains are like the grains of wheat in the story of the wise man who invented the game of chess for his king. The wise man asked for payment by having the king place one grain of wheat on the first square of the chessboard, two on the second, four on the third, eight on the fourth, and so on. Similarly, the small victories of public health over the past 120 years have resulted in cumulative gains so vast in scope that they are difficult to comprehend.

Today, there are nearly 895,000 fewer cases of measles reported per year than in 1941, over 200,000 fewer cases of diphtheria reported per year than in 1921, more than 250,000 fewer cases of whooping cough reported per year than in 1934, and 21,000 fewer cases of polio reported per year than in 1951, the peak year for reported cases for each disease, respectively (Hinman, 1999). The first two decades of the 21st century have seen 50 million fewer smokers than would have been expected, given trends in tobacco use through 1965. More than 2 million Americans are alive who otherwise would have died from heart disease and stroke, and almost 100,000 Americans are alive as a result of automobile seat belt use. Protection of the U.S. blood supply has prevented millions of hepatitis B, hepatitis C, and human immunodeficiency virus (HIV) infections, as well as billions of dollars in medical costs associated with these three diseases (U.S. Public Health Service, 1994). Today,

average blood lead levels in children are less than one-third of what they were just a quarter century ago. This catalog of accomplishments could be expanded many times over. **Figure 5.1** summarizes this progress, including two of the most widely followed measures of a population's health status—life expectancy and infant mortality.

These results did not occur by themselves. They came about through decisions and actions that represent the essence of what public health is. With this impressive litany of accomplishments, it would seem that public health's story would be easily told. For many reasons, however, it is not. As a result, public health remains poorly understood by its prime beneficiary—the public—as well as many of its dedicated practitioners. Although public health's results—as measured in terms of improved health status, diseases prevented, scarce resources saved, and improved quality of life—are more apparent today than ever before, society seldom links the activities of the public health enterprise with its results. This suggests that the public health community must communicate more effectively what public health is and what it does, so that its results can be readily traced to their source.

In 2020, the world faced an unprecedented global crisis that put a spotlight on public health—a novel virus, severe acute respiratory syndrome coronavirus 2 (SARS-CoV-2). This virus sparked a worldwide epidemic, or pandemic, of coronavirus disease 2019 (COVID-19). Reminiscent of the great influenza

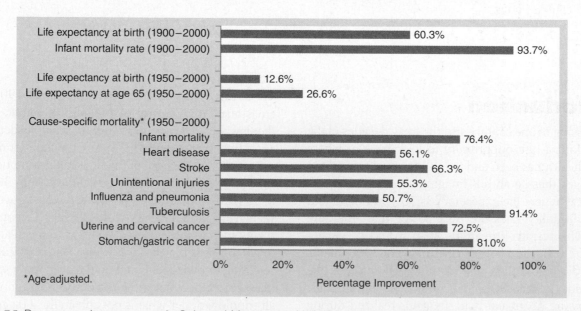

Figure 5.1 Percentage Improvement in Selected Measures of Life Expectancy and Age-Adjusted, Cause-Specific Mortality for the Time Periods 1900–2000 and 1950–2000, United States

Data from Centers for Disease Control and Prevention, National Center for Health Statistics. (2009). *Health, United States 2009.* NCHS; and Rust, G., Satcher, D., Fryer, G. E., Levine, R. S., & Blumenthal, D. S. (2010). Triangulating on success: Innovation, public health, medical care, and cause-specific US mortality over a half century (1950–2000). *American Journal of Public Health, 100,* S95–S104.

pandemic of 1918–1919, the COVID-19 pandemic has killed millions of people and disrupted societies worldwide. While public health measures have been essential in decreasing the impact of the pandemic, they have been inconsistently implemented, and in many places, applied without full political and societal support. Furthermore, the public health workforce has been greatly stressed and under-resourced to carry out its functions to fight the pandemic. However, the pandemic has also highlighted the importance of public health and the need to support it. As a result of the pandemic, many more people have a better idea of what public health does than ever before.

This chapter provides an introduction to public health that links basic concepts to practice. It considers three questions:

- What is public health?
- Where did it come from?
- Why is it important in the United States today?

To address these questions, this chapter begins with a short history of public health in the United States. It then examines several definitions and characterizations of what public health is and explores some of its distinguishing features. Finally, it offers insight into the value of public health in protecting and improving health, as well as presenting the subject in economic and human terms. Taken together, these topics provide a foundation for understanding what public health is and why it is important.

A Brief History of Public Health in the United States

Early Influences of Epidemics on the Development of Public Health

Although the complete history of public health is a fascinating saga in its own right, this section presents only selected highlights. When ancient cultures perceived illness as the manifestation of supernatural forces, they felt that little in the way of either personal or collective action to respond to or prevent illness was possible, except to appeal to those same supernatural forces. For many centuries, disease was synonymous with epidemic. Diseases, including horrific epidemics of infectious diseases such as the Black Death (plague), smallpox, and cholera, were phenomena to be accepted. It was not until the so-called Age of Reason and the Enlightenment that scholarly inquiry began to challenge the "givens" or accepted realities of the time. Eventually, expansion of the science and knowledge base would reap substantial rewards.

With the advent of industrialism and imperialism, the stage was set for epidemic diseases to increase their terrible toll. As populations shifted to urban centers for the purpose of commerce and industry, public health conditions worsened. The mixing of dense populations living in unsanitary conditions and working long hours in unsafe and exploitative industries was a formula for disaster and resulted in wave after wave of cholera, smallpox, typhoid, tuberculosis, yellow fever, and other diseases. Such disasters struck again and again across the globe, but most seriously and most often at the industrialized seaport cities that provided the portal of entry for diseases transported by people, rats, fleas, and other stowaways alongside commercial cargo. The lack of previous exposure to these diseases and the subsequent susceptibility to severe disease complications of different cultures partly explains how relatively small bands of Europeans were able to overcome and subjugate vast Native American cultures. Seeing the Europeans unaffected by scourges such as smallpox served to reinforce beliefs that these light-skinned visitors were supernatural figures, unaffected by natural forces (McNeil, 1977).

The Beginnings of Public Health in the Americas

The British colonies in North America and the new American republic bore their share of these burdens. American diaries of the 17th and 18th centuries chronicle one infectious disease onslaught after another. These epidemics left their mark on families, communities, and even history. For example, the national capital had to be moved out of Philadelphia because of a devastating yellow fever epidemic in 1793. This epidemic also prompted the city to develop its first board of health in that same year.

The formation of local boards of distinguished citizens, the first boards of health, was one of the earliest organized responses to epidemics. This response was important in that it represented an attempt to confront disease collectively, a forerunner of the organized efforts by society to protect and improve the health of the public that are the hallmark of public health today (Holsinger & Scutchfield, 2013). Because science had not yet determined that specific microorganisms were the causes of epidemics, later dubbed the germ theory, avoidance of diseased individuals had long been the primary tactic used.

Boards of health began to exercise what today are called the "police powers" of public health—the government's ability to limit the actions of individuals to protect the health of the public. These police power actions included evacuating the general location of the epidemic until disease activity subsided or isolating diseased individuals and quarantining those recently exposed to diseases. At this time, many people subscribed to the miasma theory, which blamed disease outbreaks on the malodorous accumulations of garbage and general filth prevalent in enlarging cities. As a result, many early boards of health also required removing garbage and keeping the streets clean. Although initially based on a mix of fear, tradition, and scientific speculation, these actions formed the basis of public health into the 20th century, and some continue to be part of public health's armamentarium today. The effectiveness of many of these actions was unclear at the time; however, several scientific and social developments in the mid-1800s were swinging the pendulum ever closer to more scientifically based and effective public health interventions.

Scientific and Social Developments in England

The work of public health pioneers in England such as Edward Jenner, John Snow, and Edwin Chadwick illustrates the value of public health, even when its methods are applied amid scientific uncertainty. Well before Louis Pasteur (1822–1895) conducted experiments in France to help establish the germ theory (the proposition that diseases can be caused by microorganisms) and before Robert Koch (1843–1910) developed his four postulates in Germany that established the scientific methods for proving that a specific bacterium caused a specific disease, both Jenner and Snow used deductive logic and common sense to do battle with smallpox and cholera, respectively. In 1796, Jenner (1749–1823), an English physician, successfully used vaccination to prevent smallpox, a disease that ran rampant through communities across the globe. This was the innovation that was eventually employed in the long and arduous public health campaign that, by the year 1977, had totally eradicated smallpox from the earth, the first time human collective action had resulted in the elimination of an infectious disease. (The potential for smallpox's possible reemergence through the actions of bioterrorists is now part of public health emergency preparedness planning to detect and respond to natural and man-made infectious disease threats and disasters.)

Snow (1813–1858), also an English physician, further advanced the art and science of public health. In 1854, Snow used basic descriptive epidemiological methods to analyze the pattern of deaths in a cholera outbreak and traced the source of the outbreak to the well water drawn from the community pump at Broad Street in a neighborhood of London. Based on this information, Snow persuaded the community leaders to remove the pump handle (Johnson, 2006). Although the outbreak was already waning and the number of additional cases this action prevented is debatable, this episode is one of the foundational stories of epidemiology and public health. The metaphor of "removing the pump handle" is used throughout public health to describe the actions taken to prevent further disease based on the results of an investigation by public health workers.

Snow later demonstrated that another large cholera outbreak in London could be traced to one particular water company that drew its drinking water from the Thames River from a location that was downstream of London's drainage. He demonstrated that people supplied by that company developed cholera while people supplied by another water company that drew its water from the Thames River upstream from London did not, thus implicating the source of contamination. In both efforts, Snow's ability to collect and analyze data allowed him to determine causation, which, in turn, allowed him to recommend corrective actions that prevented additional cases. All of this occurred without benefit of the knowledge of the germ theory of disease—that an odd-shaped bacterium in the water was the cause of the disease.

England's General Board of Health conducted its own investigations of these outbreaks and concluded that air, rather than contaminated water, was the cause (Paneth et al., 1998). However, its approach was one of collecting a vast amount of information and accepting only that which supported its view of disease causation. Snow, on the other hand, systematically tested his hypothesis by exploring evidence, even when it ran contrary to his initial expectations.

Chadwick (1800–1890) was a leader of what has become known as the sanitary movement of the mid- and latter half of the 19th century. In a variety of official capacities, he played a major part in structuring the government's role and responsibilities for protecting the public's health. Because of the growing concern over the social and sanitary conditions in England, Chadwick's *Report on an Inquiry into the Sanitary Conditions of the Laboring Population of Great Britain* articulated a framework for broad public actions that served as a blueprint for the growing sanitary movement. (One result was the establishment in 1848 of a General Board of Health, which examined Snow's analysis a decade later.) Interestingly, Chadwick's interest in public health had its roots in the utilitarian movement founded by Jeremy Bentham (1748–1832), a philosopher and social reformer in England. For Chadwick, disease was viewed as causing poverty, and poverty was responsible for the great social ills of the time, including societal disorder and high taxation to provide for the general welfare (Hamlin, 1995). Public health efforts were necessary to reduce poverty and its wider social effects. This utilitarian view recognizes a link between poverty and health, although this is in an opposite direction to current thinking about the role of social determinants of health in causing poor health. Today, it is more common to consider poor health as a result of poverty, rather than as its cause, although poor health certainly also can lead to impoverishment.

Chadwick was also a key participant in the partly scientific, partly political debate that took place in British government regarding whether deaths should be attributed to pathological conditions or to their underlying factors, such as hunger and poverty. It was Chadwick's view that medical and pathological, rather than less proximal, more "upstream" (in the causal chain of disease) social and behavioral factors should be the basis for classifying deaths (Hamlin, 1995). Chadwick's arguments prevailed then, although aspects of this debate continue to the present day. William Farr (1807–1883), sometimes called the father of modern vital statistics because he established, in England and Wales, a system of collecting death certificates detailing the cause of death that is utilized to guide public health efforts around the world today, championed the opposing view.

In the latter half of the 19th century, sanitation and environmental engineering methods improved, which allowed effective interventions to prevent epidemic diseases, particularly in assuring safe drinking water and disposal of human sewage, as well as the development of new vaccines. Furthermore, the scientific advances of this period paved the way for modern disease control efforts targeting specific microorganisms.

Growth of Local and State Public Health in the United States

Lemuel Shattuck (1793–1859), a legislator in Massachusetts and a founder of the American Statistical Association, was the author of the *Report of the Sanitary Commission of Massachusetts* in 1850. The report outlined existing and future public health needs for that state and became the roadmap for development of a public health system in the United States. Shattuck called for the establishment of state and local governmental health departments in Massachusetts to organize public efforts aimed at sanitary inspections, communicable disease control, and food sanitation (employing the police functions of public health), as well as vital statistics (recording of births, deaths, fetal deaths, marriages, and divorces), and medical services for infants and children. Winslow called the report "the most outstanding single 'Book of Prophecy' in the history of public health" (Winslow, 1949).

Although Shattuck's report closely paralleled Chadwick's efforts in Great Britain, acceptance of his recommendations did not occur for several decades. In the latter part of the century, his far-reaching recommendations came to be widely implemented in many states. With greater understanding of the value of environmental controls for clean drinking water and disposal of human sewage and of the role of specific control measures for specific diseases (quarantine, isolation, and vaccination), the creation of local health departments to carry out these activities supplemented and, in some cases, supplanted the local boards of health. These local health departments developed rapidly in major seaports and other industrial urban centers where epidemics including smallpox, typhoid fever, plague, and yellow fever were reaching unacceptable levels. It was during this period that a common pattern, which has repeated to this day, was also established: During epidemic periods or periods of public health crisis there is a tremendous outcry and support for public health activities, but when the epidemic subsides, that support evaporates and objections to stringent public health measures become more strident.

Because infectious and environmental hazards do not respect local jurisdictional boundaries, states began to develop their own health boards and health departments after 1870. These agencies often had very broad powers, including police powers, to protect the health and lives of state residents, although the clear intent at the time was to use these powers to battle epidemics of infectious diseases. These powers and duties serve as both a stimulus and a limitation for what can be done to address many contemporary public health issues and problems, including, and extending beyond, infectious diseases.

Throughout the late 1800s and early 1900s, state and local health departments' main roles continued to be the application of police powers to control infectious diseases; the institution of environmental protections, particularly drinking water and sewage disposal;

Box 5.1 DISCUSSION QUESTIONS

Pick a major historical public health figure mentioned in this chapter or of whom you are aware. What was the most important contribution of this individual to the evolution of public health? Why was it important? What is this individual's enduring legacy to public health?

and the provision of services for infants and children, which were closely tied to the control of infectious diseases, prevention of infant and child mortality, and improvement of maternal and child health.

By the 1920s, public health figures such as C.-E.A. Winslow, recognized that as infectious diseases were better controlled, chronic diseases such as heart disease, stroke, and cancer were emerging as public health problems (see **Box 5.1**). Additionally, occupational diseases due to industrialization and injuries from motor vehicles and other advances of the industrial age were first recognized. This presaged a vast increase in the scope of public health activities in the 20th century to encompass all threats to health facing the population.

Federal Role in Public Health in the United States

This sketch of the development of public health in the United States would be incomplete without a brief introduction to the roles and powers of the federal government. Federal health powers, at least as enumerated in the U.S. Constitution, are minimal. It is surprising to some to learn that the word "health" does not even appear in the Constitution. As a result of not being a power explicitly granted to the federal government (such as defense, foreign diplomacy, international and interstate commerce, or printing money), health is a power that is exercised by states or reserved to the people themselves.

Two sections of the Constitution have been interpreted over time to allow for federal roles in health. These are the ability to tax in order to provide for the "general welfare" (a phrase appearing in both the preamble and body of the Constitution) and the specific power to regulate commerce, both international and interstate. These provisions allowed the federal government to establish a beachhead in health, initially through the Marine Hospital Service, which was established in 1798 (it would eventually become the U.S. Public Health Service). After the 1913 ratification of the 16th Amendment authorized a national income tax, the federal government acquired the ability to raise

substantial sums of money that could then be directed toward promoting the general welfare. The specific means to this end were a variety of grants-in-aid to state and local governments. Beginning in the 1950s and 1960s, federal grant-in-aid programs designed to fill gaps in the medical care system nudged state and local governments further and further into the business of medical service provision for people without access to health care. Federal grant programs for other social, substance abuse, mental health, nutrition, and community prevention services soon followed. The expansion of federal involvement into these areas, however, was not accomplished by these means alone.

Before the Great Depression during the 1930s, most Americans did not believe that the federal government should intervene in their social circumstances. Social values shifted dramatically during the Depression, a period of such great social insecurity and need that the federal government was now permitted—indeed, expected—to intercede. One result was the Social Security program, which began providing monetary benefits for persons age 65 years and older in 1935, for spouses and children of retired or deceased persons in 1939, and for disabled persons in 1954. The program provided economic resources to those in need and had a direct impact on their health. The federal role was also evident in the Hospital Services and Construction (Hill-Burton) Act of 1946, which provided support for local healthcare systems across the county. In 1965, the federal Medicare (health insurance for the elderly and disabled) and Medicaid (health insurance for the poor, administered by the states) programs were established with a great ability to impact health, but interestingly, were kept separate from the U.S. Public Health Service and organized public health activities.

Following World War II and into the 1980s, federal funding enabled state and local health departments to expand public health efforts beyond infectious diseases and maternal, infant, and child health. However, these efforts were subject to unpredictable swings in funding support as congressional interest in specific diseases or at-risk populations waxed and waned, or as funding across multiple program areas was combined to generate budget savings. The federal government also encouraged state and local health departments to get involved in the delivery of gap-filling clinical medical services for people without health insurance and for those Medicaid recipients to whom the private medical sector declined service. Up to three-quarters of federal funding for state and local health departments was devoted to such care (Holsinger & Scutchfield, 2013).

The terrorist attacks of September 11, 2001, serve as an example of federal funding swings. Following the attacks, federal resources flowed to state and local health departments for public health and healthcare system emergency preparedness activities. Yet those funds have, in turn, been reduced by more than half over time. The 2010 Patient Protection and Affordable Care Act (ACA) includes public health provisions and provided significant additional public health funding, although these provisions and related funding are generally in flux as national elections continue to influence the interest of policymakers in public health.

The Public Health System in Crisis and the 1988 Institute of Medicine Report

By the mid-1980s, despite the achievements of recent decades, public health's mission had become diffuse and underfunded, public health departments were not prepared to face the increasing burden of chronic diseases and emerging diseases such as acquired immunodeficiency syndrome (AIDS), the capabilities of health departments varied widely, and public health's ability to lead was questioned. At this juncture, the National Academy of Medicine (NAM; formerly the Institute of Medicine)—part of the National Academies of Sciences, Engineering, and Medicine—issued its groundbreaking report *The Future of Public Health*. In the report, the NAM stated bluntly, "this nation has lost sight of its public health goals and has allowed the system of public health to fall into 'disarray'" (publishing as Institute of Medicine [IOM], 1988).

The report highlighted the problems facing public health, summarized as follows (IOM, 1988):

- There is a lack of agreement regarding the mission of public health.
- Tension between professional expertise and politics is present throughout the nation's public health system.
- Public health professionals appear to have been slow to develop strategies that demonstrate to legislators and the public the worth of their efforts.
- The relationship between private medicine and public health has been uneasy.
- Public health research has not been adequately supported.
- The linkage between academia and public health practice needs to be strengthened.

To address these issues, the report spelled out the mission and three core functions of public health, and led to the formulation of the 10 Essential Public Health Services (discussed later). The recommendations of the 1988 and subsequent NAM reports form the basis for the definition of public health, its mission, and its functions.

Public Health 1.0, 2.0, and 3.0

In order to provide some structure to the historical development of public health, described previously, and to lay down the challenges of the next era of public health, in 2016 Karen DeSalvo, then the acting Assistant Secretary for Health in the U.S. Department of Health and Human Services, and colleagues (2016) proposed the evolution of public health in the United States as occurring in three phases, which they dubbed Public Health 1.0, 2.0, and 3.0. Public Health 1.0 encompassed the development of public health from the mid-19th century up to the time of the 1988 NAM report (**Figure 5.2**). As noted, this

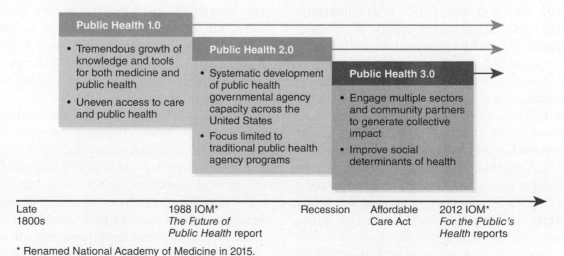

Figure 5.2 Evolution of Public Health in the United States

DeSalvo, K. B., Wang, Y. C., Harris, A., Auerbach, J., Koo, D., & O'Carroll, P. (2017). Public Health 3.0: A call to action for public health to meet the challenges of the 21st century. *Preventing Chronic Disease, 14*, 170017.

was an era of incredible growth of scientific knowledge about medicine and health, including the development of the scientific disciplines of epidemiology, engineering, and vaccinology. Public health programs were aimed primarily at combating infectious diseases, providing gap-filling medical services, and addressing health issues in specific populations such as maternal and child health. However, the growing demands to broaden the role of public health, combined with the lack of adequate resources and uneven access to public health services around the country, led to the crisis that the NAM report sought to address.

The 1988 NAM report ushered in the era of Public Health 2.0. This era saw the systematic development of the capacity of state and local public health departments. This included categorical funding for immunizations, specific infectious diseases, and chronic diseases, which were traditional public health program areas. There was also an increased focus on developing state and local public health agency capacity through funding, for example, to encourage strategic planning and quality improvement activities. A system for national accreditation of state and local health departments was established in 2007 in an effort to improve public health practices and the organization of public health services.

Despite these efforts, funding remained inadequate to scale up evidence-based programs to serve all populations in all states. The categorically funded programs were almost totally reliant on federal funding, an approach that lacked flexibility to respond to local priorities. Many funding streams followed a familiar pattern of funding reductions when the perception of a crisis in a particular area had faded. Additionally, state and local public health programs lost funding and staff during the economic recession of 2007–2009, from which they had difficulty recovering. It is estimated that local health departments alone lost over 50,000 staff as a result of the recession (Newman et al., 2016).

These and other factors prompted the need to move beyond Public Health 2.0, which DeSalvo and coauthors show lasting roughly 20 years (Figure 5.2). First, the ACA resulted in dramatic increases of people with health insurance, which reduced the need for gap-filling medical services provided by public health agencies. There was also increased attention focused on the social determinants of health (a discussion in one form or another dating back to Chadwick), the leading role that behaviors played in the risk of poor health, and the vast disparities in

health status among different populations (e.g., by race, ethnicity, or socioeconomic status). Finally, the NAM issued additional reports, including the 2003 *The Future of the Public's Health in the 21st Century* (publishing as IOM, 2002), further developing the ideas presented in *The Future of Public Health* that highlighted the need for public health to engage more sectors of society and for the health departments to lead their communities in an understanding of the importance of public health principles and approaches.

The need to move beyond Public Health 2.0 was eloquently summarized by DeSalvo et al. (2016) as follows: "Despite nearly $3.0 trillion in annual healthcare spending, the United States ranks 27th in the world in life expectancy, and relatively low in many other measures of health and well-being. Worse yet, for the poor in this country, life expectancy is actually decreasing. Given these trends, and persistent gaps in health status, it's time for a major upgrade to Public Health 3.0."

The definition of Public Health 3.0 in a nutshell is "cross sector collaboration and environmental, policy, and systems-level actions that directly affect the social determinants of Health" (DeSalvo et al., 2016). The main recommendations of the Public Health 3.0 report (**Table 5.1**) include enhancing state and local public health departments' leadership and workforce to take on the mantle of the community's "chief health strategist"; engaging new partners in support of public health in sectors such as employers and business, the media, academia, the healthcare delivery system, and community organizations and communities themselves; encouraging state and local health departments to seek formal national accreditation; developing adequate data and metrics to measure success; and encouraging state and local health departments to seek additional funding for these efforts. It is important to recognize that Public Health 3.0 did not abandon the principles developed in Public Health 2.0; rather it expanded upon them.

The COVID-19 pandemic has challenged the public health community even further to view health as a global issue, and it has highlighted the ongoing need to better address health disparities and to engage and coordinate public health partners more efficiently. The next phases of public health's development, with an ongoing goal to build stronger and more supported public health systems, will undoubtedly be influenced by the gaps identified in Public Health 2.0 and 3.0 that were further magnified by the pandemic.

Table 5.1 Final Recommendations from the Public Health 3.0 Report

- Public health leaders should embrace the role of **Chief Health Strategist for their communities**—working with all relevant partners so that they can drive initiatives, including those that explicitly address "upstream" social determinants of health. Specialized Public Health 3.0 training should be available for those preparing to enter or already within the public health workforce.
- Public health departments should engage with community stakeholders—from both the public and private sectors—to form vibrant, **structured, cross-sector partnerships** designed to develop and guide Public Health 3.0–style initiatives and to foster shared funding, services, governance, and collective action.
- Public Health Accreditation Board (PHAB) criteria and processes for department **accreditation should be enhanced** and supported so as to best foster Public Health 3.0 principles, as we strive to ensure that every person in the United States is served by nationally accredited health departments.
- Timely, reliable, granular (i.e., subcounty), and **actionable data** should be made accessible to communities throughout the country, and **clear metrics** to document success in public health practice should be developed in order to guide, focus, and assess the impact of prevention initiatives, including those targeting the social determinants of health and enhancing equity.
- **Funding for public health should be enhanced and substantially modified**, and innovative funding models should be explored to expand financial support for Public Health 3.0–style leadership and prevention initiatives. Blending and braiding of funds from multiple sources should be encouraged and allowed, including the recapturing and reinvesting of generated revenue. Funding should be identified to support core infrastructure as well as community-level work to address the social determinants of health.

Office of the Assistant Secretary for Health, U.S. Department of Health and Human Services. *Public Health 3.0: A call to action to create a 21st century public health infrastructure.* https://www.healthypeople.gov/sites/default/files/Public-Health-3.0-White-Paper.pdf

Definitions of Public Health

Early 20th Century Definitions

Having now briefly reviewed the history of the development of public health in the United States and understanding the broad context of and challenges with public health, it is appropriate to pause and formally define public health more precisely. A century ago, in 1920, C.-E.A. Winslow delivered an address at the second annual meeting of the American Association for the Advancement of Science titled "The Untilled the Fields of Public Health," in which he provided a definition of public health that describes both what public health does and how it gets it done. It is a comprehensive definition that has stood the test of time, and forms the basis against which to compare all subsequent definitions. Winslow (1920) characterized public health as

. . . the science and art of preventing disease, prolonging life, and promoting health and efficiency through organized community effort for the sanitation of the environment, the control of communicable infections, the education of the individual in personal hygiene, the organization of medical and nursing services for the early diagnosis and preventive treatment of disease, and for the development of the social machinery to insure everyone a standard of living adequate for the maintenance

of health, so organizing these benefits as to enable every citizen to realize his birthright of health and longevity.

To this he added

Public health conceived in these terms will be something vastly different from the exercise of the purely police power which has been its principal manifestation in the past. (Winslow, 1920)

There is much to consider in Winslow's definition. The phrases, "science and art," "organized community effort," and "birthright of health and longevity" capture the substance and aims of public health and foreshadow the 1988 NAM report. Winslow's catalog of methods illuminates the scope of the endeavor, embracing public health's initial targeting of infectious and environmental risks, as well as current activities related to the organization, financing, and accountability of medical care services. His allusion to the "social machinery to insure everyone a standard of living adequate for the maintenance of health" speaks to the relationship between social conditions and health in all societies.

The 1988 National Academy of Medicine Definition of Public Health

The 1988 NAM report, *The Future of Public Health*, provides a useful definition of public health. The NAM report characterized public health's mission as "fulfilling society's interest in assuring conditions in which people can be healthy" (IOM, 1988). The definition directs attention to the many conditions that influence health and wellness, underscoring the broad scope of public health and legitimizing its interest in social, environmental, economic, political, and medical care factors that affect health and illness. The definition's premise that society has an interest in the health of all its members implies that everyone benefits when the conditions and health status of the population improve. This is a core value of public health. The NAM report's characterization of public health stands as a bold philosophical statement of mission and purpose. Importantly, NAM does not see this definition as applying only to government, but to all sectors of society, including the public itself.

The NAM report also sought to further define the scope of public health by identifying the three core functions of governmental public health agencies: assessment, policy development, and assurance. There is a temporal order in the core functions, similar to the sequence in clinical medicine of diagnosis, treatment and treatment monitoring and modification, if necessary (this last step brings the process back to the beginning of re-diagnosis). Assessment identifies health problems, policy development devises policies and programs to address them, and assurance monitors the application and success of these policies and programs. The process cycles back around to reassessing the health status and leading to further development and application of policies. The NAM core public health functions are defined more formally as follows (IOM, 1988):

1. **Assessment** is the analogue of diagnosis, except that the diagnosis is made for a group or population of individuals. It calls for public health to regularly and systematically collect, assemble, analyze, and make available information on the health of the community, including statistics on health status, community health needs, and epidemiological and other studies of health problems. Not every agency is large enough to conduct these activities directly; intergovernmental and interagency cooperation is essential. Nevertheless, each agency bears the responsibility for seeing that the assessment function is fulfilled. This basic function of public health cannot be delegated. (p. 7)

2. **Policy development** is a responsibility of every public health agency. The NAM calls for public health to serve the public interest in the development of comprehensive public health policies by promoting the use of the scientific knowledge base in decision-making about public health and by leading in developing public health policy. Policymakers in health departments and elsewhere in government should use the technical knowledge and professional expertise of public health agency staffs in developing new policies. However, they must also take a strategic approach, developed on the basis of a positive appreciation for the democratic political process, in order for this expertise to have the most impact in developing well-founded policies that will receive political support. (p. 8)

3. **Assurance** calls for public health to ensure their constituents that services necessary to achieve agreed-upon goals are provided, either by encouraging actions by other entities (private or public), by requiring such action through regulation or by providing services directly. Each public health agency should involve key policymakers and the general public in determining a set of high-priority personal and community-wide health services that government will guarantee to every member of the community. This guarantee should include subsidization or direct provision of high-priority personal health services for those unable to afford them. (p. 8)

The 10 Essential Public Health Services

In response to the 1988 NAM report, a national Working Group of the Core Public Health Functions Steering Committee was assembled by the U.S. Public Health Service in 1994. The working group developed a consensus statement of what public health is and does in language that is understandable to those both inside and outside the field of public health and which describes in greater detail that the mission of public health is to "promote physical and mental health and prevent disease, injury and disability." The working group also further operationalized the three core functions by developing 10 corresponding essential public health services. The statement was published in a document titled "Public Health in America" (Centers for Disease Control and Prevention [CDC], 2021). (For a comparison of different definitions of public health, see **Table 5.2**.) In 2020, the Public Health National Center for Innovations and the de Beaumont Foundation collaborated to convene a task force to review and revise this framework.

Table 5.3 and **Figure 5.3** present the results of the efforts of the working groups (CDC, 2021). The table and figure demonstrate how the 10 Essential Public Health Services relate to the three core public health

Table 5.2 Selected Definitions of Public Health

"The science and art of preventing disease, prolonging life, and promoting health and efficiency through organized community effort."

"Fulfilling society's interest in assuring conditions in which people can be healthy."

"Promote physical and mental health and prevent disease, injury and disability."

Data from Winslow, C.-E. A. (1920). The untilled field of public health. *Modern Medicine, 2*, 183–191; Institute of Medicine. (1988). *The future of public health.* National Academy Press; and Public Health Functions Steering Committee. (1995). *Public health in America.* U.S. Public Health Service.

Table 5.3 Public Health in America

Vision: *Healthy People in Healthy Communities*

Mission: *Promote Physical and Mental Health and Prevent Disease, Injury, and Disability*

Purposes of Public Health

Prevents epidemics and the spread of disease
Protects against environmental hazards
Prevents injuries
Promotes and encourages healthy behaviors
Responds to disasters and assists communities in recovery
Assures the quality and accessibility of services

10 Essential Public Health Services

Assessment Core Function
Monitor health status to identify and solve community health problems.
Diagnose and investigate health problems and health hazards in the community.

Policy Development Core Function
Inform, educate, and empower people about health issues.
Mobilize community partnerships to identify and solve health problems.
Develop policies and plans that support individual and community health efforts.

Assurance Core Function
Enforce laws and regulations that protect health and ensure safety.
Link people with needed personal health services and assure the provision of health care when otherwise unavailable.
Assure a competent public health and personal healthcare workforce.
Evaluate effectiveness, accessibility, and quality of personal and population-based health services.

Cross Cutting
Research for new insights and innovative solutions to health problems.

Data from Essential Public Health Services Working Group of the Core Public Health Functions Steering Committee, U.S. Public Health Service. (1994). *10 Essential Public Health Services.* https://www.cdc.gov/publichealthgateway/publichealthservices/essentialhealthservices.html

functions identified in the 1988 NAM report. Figure 5.3 also illustrates the temporal relationship between the core functions and their corresponding essential services. Assessment identifies problems, which then leads to the development of policy solutions, which then leads to the implementation of public health measures, and finally, to the assurance that they are being carried out. However, the job of public health is never done. As the pinwheel figure indicates, the process cycles back to assessment to see if the problem has been solved, and to be ever vigilant to arising new problems. The placement of health equity (the idea that all people should have an equal chance to live healthy lives) at the center of the pinwheel emphasizes the importance of working to improve the health of all community members. The extensive disparities in a wide range of health outcomes associated with the COVID-19 pandemic illustrate the importance of this change.

The Understanding of "Public Health" by the Public

The term *public health* evokes different images among the general public, professionals in other fields, and even

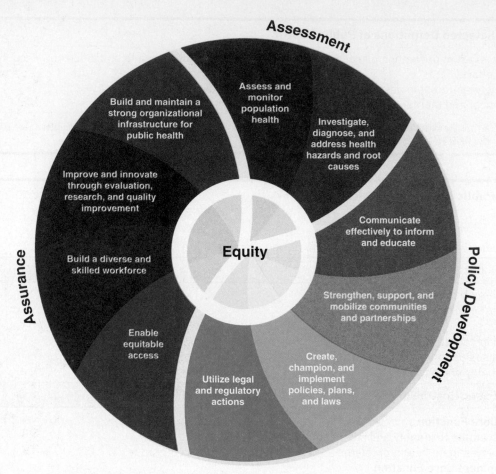

Figure 5.3 Public Health Core Functions and 10 Essential Public Health Services

Centers for Disease Control and Prevention. (2021). *Public health professionals gateway: 10 Essential Public Health Services.* https://www.cdc.gov/publichealthgateway/publichealthservices/essentialhealthservices.html

among some who work in public health. It is important, therefore, when talking or writing about public health, to understand how others may be using the term and to define your own use of it in order to avoid confusion.

To some, the term describes the workforce of professionals whose job it is to solve certain important health problems. When they use the term *public health*, they are referring to the people who respond to the disease outbreak or other health issue of concern to their community at the moment. This definition is sometimes limiting because it does not acknowledge the broad array of what constitutes public health, nor does it appreciate that all segments of the community play a part in protecting and improving health.

Another image of public health is that of a body of knowledge and techniques that can be applied to health-related problems. Here, public health is seen as what public health does.

Similarly, many people perceive public health primarily as the activities ascribed to governmental public health agencies, sometimes with the common view that public health primarily involves the provision of medical care to indigent populations.

In recent years, however, public health's mission has been much broader. Since 2001, for example, it has emerged as a frontline defense against bioterrorism and other threats to personal security, thus taking on a public safety role.

To many, public health may be described as the activities that the government takes to address health threats. While the government at all levels is the central player in public health, as described earlier in this chapter, this image of public health is also too narrow to fully capture what public health encompasses.

Another understanding of public health is that of its intended outcomes—literally, the health of the public, as measured in terms of health and illness in a population. The term *population health* has been frequently used in recent years, but it, too, has different meanings to different people. Its meaning may be similar to public health if it is meant to be addressing the health of the entire population in an area (Kindig, 2007). However, population health may also be used to refer to the population for which a particular employer or healthcare provider is responsible. This may not be the entire population in an area in need of public health services and is not synonymous with public health (Sharfstein, 2014).

Finally, public health can mean the broader system of organizations, agencies, and people who may impact the health of the population in any way, ranging from providing individual medical care at one end of the spectrum to addressing the broad social determinants of health on a population level at the other. To only a relative few outside the field of public health, the term describes a broad social enterprise or system, an understanding of public health that will be discussed in detail. As summarized in **Table 5.4**, the profession, the methods, the governmental agencies and health services, the ultimate

Table 5.4 Understandings of the Term *Public Health*

- Public health: the profession
- Public health: the methods, knowledge, and techniques
- Public health: governmental agencies and health services
- Public health: the health of the public
- Public health: the system and social enterprise

health outcomes, and even the broad social enterprise itself are all commonly encountered understandings of what public health is today. This chapter focuses primarily on public health as a social enterprise or system.

Public Health as a System

The Public Health System Players and Their Roles

The Future of Public Health report defined the public health system as encompassing "activities undertaken within the formal structure of government and the associated efforts of private and voluntary organizations and individuals" (IOM, 1988). Subsequent NAM reports provided more detail on who the nongovernmental players in the public health system should be. **Figure 5.4** provides a depiction of many of the key sectors in the system. At the center of the system diagram is the governmental public health infrastructure, the combination of local, state, and federal health

Figure 5.4 The Public Health System

agencies, the programs they collectively operate, and the body of laws and regulations that define their powers and responsibilities. They also serve to coordinate the efforts of the broader public health system, provide data on the health of the population and on evidence-based interventions to protect and improve health, and finally, serve as the "chief health strategist" for their communities (Public Health Leadership Forum, 2014). Their central location in the figure indicates the critical function that these governmental public health agencies have.

Around this center in Figure 5.4 are arrayed the other sectors of society that play a role in protecting and improving health. These include governmental agencies other than public health departments, including agencies that protect the environment or promote safe and affordable housing. There are also members of the healthcare delivery system that play a key role not only in providing curative medical care but also mental health and preventive medical services. There are other partners that at first glance might not appear to have a direct role but that actually do, for example, employers, businesses, and unions that provide or advocate providing health insurance, safe working environments for employees, or improved living conditions. The media and academia play a role in bringing attention to health issues, determining effective interventions (academia), and educating the public (see **Box 5.2**). Philanthropy may fund innovative pilot programs that demonstrate how to deliver new and more effective public health measures. Community organizations may provide supportive services to populations at risk and advocacy on behalf of needed public health programs. Policymakers and elected officials play a key role in assuring that laws and funding streams are adequate to support public health activities, and highlight the very political nature of public health. Last but not least, the community itself is part of the public health system, representing individuals and groups whose health is the ultimate goal. Without their support and understanding, and without an appreciation of what they view the issues impacting their health to be, no governmental programs can succeed.

💡 Box 5.2 DISCUSSION QUESTIONS

Review the news headlines for the last week. How many stories are related to health? Are these predominantly stories about health care or about public health, or both? To what extent is prevention of disease highlighted in the news? Is health equity mentioned? What other themes are mentioned?

One Health

An example of where disparate parts of the broad public health system described here need to work together is in addressing zoonoses (animal diseases that affect humans). The One Health initiative involves the interdisciplinary collaboration of professionals involved with human, animal, and environmental health (CDC, n.d.c). For example, this collaboration involves biosurveillance to track pathogens and diseases in people, animals, and the environment and to link them to their source and identify means of transmission. An area of focus for One Health is the problem of antimicrobial resistance, which can arise through use of antibiotics in food animals, be spread to humans in food products, and be present in the environment if farm animal waste is not properly disposed of or if people improperly dispose of unused antibiotics. At the federal level, One Health collaboration involves the Centers for Disease Control and Prevention (CDC), the Food and Drug Administration, the Department of Agriculture, and the Environmental Protection Agency. These agencies in turn engage their state and local counterparts. While each agency is concerned with the health of those entities under its jurisdiction, there is recognition that the problem must also be addressed globally for it to be controlled locally. Therefore, collaboration is not only helpful, but is also necessary to fully address the problem.

The Social-Ecological Model of the Determinants of Health

Why do the particular sectors in the public health system just described, play such an important role in assuring the public's health? The answer comes from a consideration of the many factors that help to determine health and health status, and how the sectors making up the public health system can impact these factors. A useful way of thinking about these determinants of health can be found in the social-ecological model shown in **Figure 5.5**.

At the center of the social-ecological model are the individual human beings whose health is at stake. Their biological makeup, genetic profile, age, sex, and other individual constitutional factors play a role determining their health now and in the future. These individual characteristics are often not modifiable, although their impacts on health may be ameliorated, for example, through following dietary and exercise recommendations for persons with a genetic risk for heart disease. Moving outward in the figure, the impact of individuals' behaviors and lifestyle factors on their

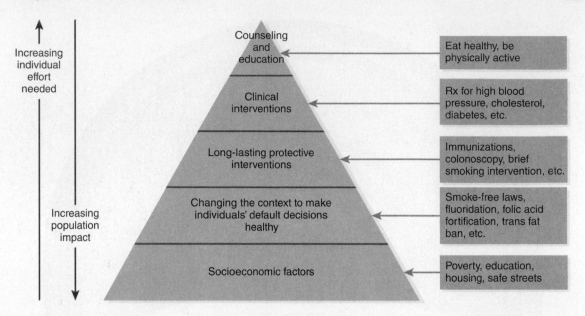

Figure 5.6 A Framework for Public Health Action: The Health Impact Pyramid with Examples of Public Health Interventions at Each Level

Data from Frieden, T. R. (2010). A framework for public health action: The health impact pyramid. *American Journal of Public Health, 100*(4), 590–595.

(2010), the former director of the CDC (**Figure 5.6**). The framework for action is displayed as a pyramid with its base encompassing the broad socioeconomic determinants of health such as poverty, education, and housing. Actions taken at this level are often outside the direct purview of governmental public health agencies but may have the greatest potential impact on the health of the population over time and require the least effort directed one-on-one at individuals. Other partners in the public health system, including elected officials, need to act to impact this level of the pyramid, although public health departments can still play a key role in providing the health data that highlight the problems and in tracking the impact of any actions taken. Nevertheless, interventions that impact socioeconomic status may take many years to bear fruit in terms of improved health.

The next level up in the pyramid addresses steps that can be taken to change health behaviors or to otherwise incentivize healthy behaviors so that the default behavior becomes the healthy one. Examples include smoke-free indoor air laws to prevent second-hand smoke exposure, fluoridation of drinking water to prevent dental caries, folic acid fortification of flour to prevent neural tube defects in newborns, and a ban on trans fats in foods to prevent cardiovascular disease. Benefiting from these public health interventions requires no conscious decision or learned behavior on the part of individuals; they obtain health benefits simply by accepting the default choice. Again, the public health system partners involved in making these changes to the living environment extend beyond the

health department, although the health department should inform and encourage these actions.

The upper levels of the pyramid move more into the provision of health care with preventive screenings and treatment of risk factors, such as high cholesterol, to prevent cardiovascular disease. Many of these actions will take place within healthcare delivery, but public health can play an important role by, for example, educating the public about the importance of such interventions, assuring that they have insurance coverage and access to health services, and monitoring the outcomes in the whole population.

As actions move up the pyramid, they become more directed at individuals, meaning more effort is needed to carry them out. The peak of the pyramid calls for individual counseling and education. Actions taken at all levels of the pyramid are important, but those taken at the base of the pyramid may be more impactful, for more people, in the long run by preventing disease so that actions at the top of the pyramid are less needed. CDC has launched the "Health Impact in 5 Years" (HI-5) initiative, which promotes evidence-based interventions in the first two levels of the pyramid (CDC, n.d.b).

Characteristics of a Public Health Approach

From the foregoing discussion of the public health system, the social-ecological model of determinants of health, and the framework for public health action, several characteristic features of a public approach to protecting and improving health are apparent. These are highlighted in **Table 5.5** and each is discussed in detail next. The first four characteristic features in the table represent the values of public health. The remaining five characteristics reflect the practical realities of working in public health.

Grounded in Science

A fundamental characteristic of public health is that it is grounded in science. This relationship is clear for science that governs our understanding of the biologic aspects of human beings, microorganisms, and disease vectors, as well as the risks present in our physical environments. However, it is also true for the social sciences of anthropology, sociology, psychology, and economics that affect our understanding of human culture and behaviors influencing health and illness. The quantitative sciences of epidemiology and biostatistics remain essential tools and methods of public health practice.

As we have seen, the history of public health began based on the so-called hard sciences underlying environmental sanitation and communicable disease control. This was supplemented in the 20th century by the rapid growth of biomedical science, which led to antibiotics, vaccines, and other equally significant advances. Epidemiology and biostatistics have also matured and advanced to become, with the assistance of computers, powerful tools to help determine what the true risk factors for disease are and whether interventions to improve health are indeed working. These "harder" sciences have been further supplemented by the social, behavioral, and economic sciences, which have become important tools for addressing the behavioral and social determinants of health. Although this latter group has been viewed in the past as the "soft" sciences, in fact they employ the same scientific and statistical approaches as epidemiology and clinical medicine.

These sciences have in common the scientific method and the appreciation for the replication of findings to lend strength to scientific arguments, although this can be difficult in the often-uncontrolled settings in which public health practice occurs. These sciences also share the important vehicle of peer-reviewed scientific publications to share their findings and to ultimately advance knowledge in each discipline. The journals that are important for public health are as diverse as the field itself, but focus on biomedical journals (e.g., *New England Journal of Medicine, Journal of the American Medical Association*) and general public health journals (e.g., *American Journal of Public Health, Morbidity and Mortality Weekly Report, Journal of Public Health Management and Practice, Public Health Reports*), as well as specialty journals in all of the fields just mentioned.

The publication of one article, even with eye-opening findings, usually does not change medical or public health practice overnight. Often there is a range of findings in published papers that may not all agree on any given topic. This is the nature of science. How, then, is the evidence base for public health established and agreed upon? An important part of advancing evidence-based public health practice is a series of governmental and professional advisory bodies that sift through the medical and public health literature and develop recommendations based on the best data available, often applying strict scoring systems to grade the strength of the evidence in peer-reviewed publications (Ahmeda et al., 2011; Guyatt et al., 2008). Some important public health advisory groups include the U.S. Preventive Services Task Force (for prevention recommendations related to clinical medical practice, such as disease screening recommendations), the Community Preventive Services Task Force (for recommendations related to community-based public health programs), the Advisory Committee on Immunization Practices (ACIP), and the Healthcare Infection Control Practices Advisory Committee; the latter three are based at CDC. These committees may

Table 5.5 **Selected Characteristics of a Public Health Approach**

Public health is . . .
Grounded in science
Focused on prevention as a primary strategy
Founded on social justice and health equity philosophies
Dedicated to ethical principles
Linked with government
Based on an inherently political nature
Reliant on the broader public health system/health in all policies approaches
Engaged as a multidisciplinary culture with common bonds
Dynamic, with an ever-expanding agenda

have strong, statutory-based influence over the public health system. For example, clinical screening recommendations from the U.S. Preventive Services Task Force with Grade A or B evidence, and all ACIP recommendations, have to be covered without a copay by health insurance plans covered by the Affordable Care Act (Office of Disease Prevention and Health Promotion, n.d). Also, ACIP indicates which vaccines are eligible for coverage under the national Vaccines for Children Program, a program that provides vaccines free of charge to physicians to administer to children who do not have health insurance coverage for vaccinations, who are covered by Medicaid, or who are Native American or Alaskan Native.

CDC maintains a list of evidence-based practices for public health and additional sites for specific advisory committees, as listed in **Table 5.6**. In addition, CDC maintains lists of "best" or "promising" practices (see Table 5.6, last two items), which appear to be beneficial but do not yet have high-level evidence to support them. Work is ongoing to validate these as evidence-based practices.

Focused on Prevention

If public health professionals were pressed to provide a one-word synonym for public health, the most frequent response would probably be prevention. Generally, prevention characterizes actions that are taken to reduce the possibility that something will happen or in hopes of minimizing the damage that may occur if it does happen. Although prevention is considered by many to be the purpose of public health, the specific intentions of prevention can vary greatly. Prevention can target deaths, hospital admissions, days lost from school, consumption of human and fiscal resources, and many other ends. There are as many targets for

prevention as there are various health outcomes and effects to be avoided.

It is often hard to marshal support for prevention efforts because their success results in outcomes that are often unseen: if prevention works, disease does not happen. Because these consequences are unseen, people are less likely to develop an attachment for or support the efforts preventing them. In arguing for more programmatic resources, advocates for such causes as mental health services, care for individuals with developmental disabilities, and organ transplants, for example, can point to the direct needs of people who would receive program services, and indeed, these are worthy and important causes. In contrast, it is difficult to rally the millions of people who did not get measles because of successful vaccination programs—they are part of an invisible constituency. Additionally, the long lag time before many preventive interventions bear fruit can be a barrier to marshaling support. For example, programs to improve diet and increase opportunities for physical activity may take decades to show results in terms of reducing cardiovascular disease. From this perspective, the undervaluation of public health is understandable; the majority of the beneficiaries of recent and current public health prevention efforts have not yet been born! Despite its lack of recognition, prevention as a strategy has been remarkably successful. Its success is exemplified in many of the 10 great public health achievements of the 20th century, discussed later in this chapter.

Primary, Secondary, and Tertiary Prevention

Public health and medical professionals speak of three different types of prevention, each of which utilizes different strategies and is carried out by different parts

---

Table 5.6 Resources for Evidence-Based Public Health Practice

- Evidence-Based Practices in Public Health
  www.cdc.gov/publichealthgateway/program/resources/evidence.html
- Guide to Community Preventive Services
  www.thecommunityguide.org/about/about-community-guide
- Advisory Committee on Immunization Practices
  www.cdc.gov/vaccines/acip/index.html
- Healthcare Infection Control Practices Advisory Committee
  www.cdc.gov/hicpac/index.html
- U.S. Preventive Services Task Force
  www.uspreventiveservicestaskforce.org/Page/Name/home
- CDC Best Practices for Cardiovascular Disease Prevention Programs
  www.cdc.gov/dhdsp/pubs/guides/best-practices/index.htm
- CDC Best Practices for Comprehensive Tobacco Control Programs
  www.cdc.gov/tobacco/stateandcommunity/best_practices/index.htm

of the public health system. Primary prevention, such as vaccinations to prevent communicable diseases or dietary and exercise measures to prevent heart disease, involves preventing disease from occurring at all. Secondary prevention involves identifying disease that is present before it causes symptoms; examples include screening for high blood pressure or breast cancer. In these cases, early identification of disease can result in treatment to prevent disease from progressing (e.g., treating high blood pressure) or curing it outright (surgery to remove early cancer). When a disease is already present and causing symptoms, tertiary prevention involves steps aimed at preventing further disease progression and disability. An example is the treatment of heart attack patients to reduce their cholesterol and blood pressure to prevent further heart damage.

Three Buckets of Prevention

Prevention has also been the focus of recent efforts to encourage more collaboration between the public health and healthcare systems. CDC has proposed a framework of three prevention domains, or "buckets," that span the spectrum between purely clinical prevention and community-based prevention (**Figure 5.7**; Auerbach, 2016). This approach is intended to impress upon the healthcare system, clinicians, health insurers, and public health professionals the importance of not only applying current clinical recommendations in the office setting, but also thinking outside the office to the broader community. The first bucket is in the

clinical setting and calls for full implementation of evidence-based preventive measures, such as cancer screenings. The second bucket involves increased services delivered outside the clinical setting, such as home visits to asthma patients to assure their adherence with prescribed asthma medications and to check their home environment to remove asthma triggers. The third bucket involves measures aimed at engaging the whole population in the community, not just the patients of a given healthcare practice, with preventive interventions. These include things like advocating for safe spaces in the community to exercise and making sure that healthy foods are available and accessible in local grocery stores so that peoples' food choices are not limited to fast food. Additional examples are at CDC's Community Health Improvement Navigator site (CDC, n.d.a).

Return on Investment in Prevention

In addition to the human aspect of improving health, there is an economic argument to be made for prevention. In the business world, the concept of "return on investment" (ROI) is an important one in determining where to invest new resources: It is easier to put money up front into a project that will return the initial investment and then more in the future. The same principle holds in public health. An analysis by Trust for America's Health showed that strategic investment in proven community-based prevention programs to increase physical activity, improve nutrition, and prevent smoking and other tobacco use could yield an

Figure 5.7 Three Buckets of Prevention
Centers for Disease Control and Prevention. *Evidence-based community-wide interventions slides* [HI-5 14]. https://www.cdc.gov/policy/hst/hi5/slides/index.html

ROI of 1.4-to-1 in 1 year and 7-to-1 in 5 years (Trust for America's Health, 2008).

Public health professionals should take every opportunity to educate the public and policymakers about the strength of prevention as an approach. Often a hard business case can be made for prevention, albeit with a sometimes-long time horizon to realize monetary returns. However, prevention is the right course, even if it is not cost neutral, if the definition of public health is to be honored.

National Prevention Strategy

Prevention plays such a central role in public health that the Surgeon General released the National Prevention Strategy (NPS) in 2011 with the goal to increase the number of Americans who are healthy at each stage of life (Office of the U.S. Surgeon General, 2011). The NPS has seven priority areas: tobacco-free living, preventing drug abuse and excessive alcohol use, healthy eating, active living, injury- and violence-free living, reproductive and sexual health, and mental and emotional well-being. These priorities are addressed through acting on the recommendations of four strategic domains: healthy and safe community environments, clinical and community preventive services, empowered people, and elimination of health disparities.

Founded on Social Justice and Health Equity Philosophies

Social justice—the idea that all members of a society should be treated fairly and justly—is the foundation of public health. Social justice argues that public health is properly a public matter and that its results, in terms of death, disease, health, and well-being, reflect the decisions and actions that a society takes, for good or for ill (Krieger & Brin, 1998). It is vital to recognize the social justice orientation as a fundamental characteristic of a public health approach, and it is critical to understand the potential for conflict and confrontation that it generates.

The World Health Organization (2002) Constitution recognizes health as a human right. Achieving health equity, as defined earlier, means addressing the social and other determinants of health, not just access to health care. The recognition of a widespread lack of health equity in the population, resulting in dramatic disparities in health status between people with different racial, ethnic, socioeconomic, and geographical backgrounds, and other characteristics, is a main driver of the social justice approach in public health practice today. Health inequity equals social injustice.

The concept of social justice first emerged around 1848, a time that might be considered the birth of modern public health. It has been an important element of public health practice ever since. For example, in 1911, Hermann Biggs, who revolutionized public health practice in New York City and later became the third New York State Health Commissioner, succinctly stated that "[p]ublic health is purchasable. Within natural limitations a community can determine its own death-rate" (Winslow, 1929). He further explained

> Disease is largely a removable evil. It continues to afflict humanity, not only because of incomplete knowledge of its causes and lack of adequate individual and public hygiene, but also because it is extensively fostered by harsh economic and industrial conditions and by wretched housing in congested communities. These conditions and consequently the diseases which spring from them can be removed by better social organization. No duty of society, acting through its governmental agencies, is paramount to this obligation to attack the removable causes of disease. (Winslow, 1929)

The potential for conflict and confrontation about the "duty of society" to address "removable causes of disease" arises from disagreements over responsibility. The concept of "market justice" emphasizes personal responsibility of the individual as the basis for distributing burdens and benefits. In terms of health, individuals assume primary responsibility for their own health. According to this view, there is little expectation that society should act to protect or promote the health of its members beyond addressing risks that cannot be controlled through individual action.

In contrast, "social justice" argues that there are significant factors outside of individuals' control that can impede the fair distribution of benefits and burdens (Beauchamp, 1976). Thus, there are times when collective action is needed to address these impediments. When the necessary collective actions are not taken, even the most important public policy problems remain unsolved, despite periodically becoming highly visible (Beauchamp, 1976). This explains our inadequate responses to such intractable American problems as inadequate housing, poor public education systems, racial discrimination, and poverty. This is also true for public health problems such as tobacco-related illnesses, infant mortality, substance abuse, lack of mental health and long-term care services, and environmental pollution. The bitter political conflict accompanying the enactment of the Affordable Care Act of 2010, and the subsequent pulling back from the law's commitments, reflect these same themes.

These and other examples suggest that a critical challenge for public health as a social enterprise lies in overcoming the social and ethical barriers that prevent us from doing more with the knowledge and tools already available to us (Beauchamp, 1976). Extending the frontiers of science and knowledge may not be as effective for improving public health as shifting the collective values of our society to act on what we already know. Recent public health successes, such as public attitudes toward smoking in both public and private locations and operating motor vehicles after alcohol consumption, provide evidence in support of this assertion. These advances came through changes in social norms, rather than through bigger and better science. Even more important for achieving equity in health status are concerted efforts to improve health status in population groups with the greatest disadvantage, mechanisms to monitor health status and contributing factors across all population groups, and participation of disadvantaged population groups in the key political decision-making processes within society (Susser, 1993).

Dedicated to Ethical Principles

From the previous discussion of social justice, it should be clear that public health has strong moral underpinnings. Given that public health has strong principles to live up to and has, in the case of governmental public health departments, strong police and other legal powers, it is imperative that public health has a strong code of ethics to assure that it is serving the best interests of the communities it is responsible for and to avoid potential abuses of power. A code of ethics for public health, targeting primarily traditional public health institutions such as health departments and schools of public health, was developed in 2000–2001 with extensive input from the public health community (Thomas et al., 2002). The 12 principles are shown in **Table 5.7**.

Linked with Government

A fifth characteristic of public health is its close link with government, which should be clear from reviewing the history and the definition of public health, the 10 Essential Public Health Services, and the central role of government in the public health system, discussed earlier. Although public health is far more than the aggregate activities of federal, state, and local health agencies, many people think only of governmental public health agencies when they think of public health. Government does play a unique role in seeing that the key elements are in place and that public health's mission is carried out. Only government can exercise the enforcement provisions of the public laws, regulations, and policies that limit the personal and property rights of individuals and corporations in areas such as retail food establishments, sewage and water systems, occupational health and safety, consumer product safety, infectious disease control, and drug efficacy and safety.

Government also can play the convener and facilitator role for identifying and prioritizing health

Table 5.7 Principles of the Ethical Practice of Public Health

Public health and its institutions and employees should . . .
- Address the fundamental causes of disease and requirements for health.
- Respect the rights of members of the community.
- Develop and evaluate policies, programs, and priorities providing opportunities for input from community members.
- Advocate and strive for the empowerment of disenfranchised communities and ensure that the conditions necessary for health are accessible to all.
- Seek the information needed to implement effective policies and programs.
- Provide communities with the information needed to develop policies or programs and should implement them only with the community's consent.
- Act in a timely manner on the available information within their resources and mandates.
- Develop programs and policies informed by and respecting the diverse values, beliefs, and cultures in the community.
- Implement programs and policies in ways that most enhance the physical and social environment.
- Protect the confidentiality of individuals or the community unless there is a high likelihood of significant harm to an individual or the community.
- Ensure the professional competence of their employees.
- Collaborate in ways that build the public's trust and their effectiveness.

Data from Thomas, J. C., Sage, M., Dillenberg, J., & Guillory, V. J. (2002). A code of ethics for public health. *American Journal of Public Health, 92*(7), 1057–1059.

problems that might be addressed through public resources and actions. This is a primary role of government in the broader public health system, as previously discussed, and is critical for the identification of public health problems and the implementation of public health program solutions that meet the community's needs and have the support of communities, public health partners, and other interested parties. Government also has a role as part of the political process of determining the budget for public health programs and developing new public health laws. Additionally, government has a strong role in developing evidence-based and best practice recommendations for public health programs to follow, and in providing and marshaling the scientific expertise in the community to make the evidence base the best possible. Advisory body recommendations are strengthened by being developed in as unbiased and transparent a process as possible, which government is in a position to achieve. Because government is a major funder of public health activities, it can also require the implementation of evidence-based practices with the funding it provides. This, in turn, can help their dissemination and adoption and can decrease the implementation of non–evidence-based programs. Health departments can also engage their sister governmental agencies to take a HiAP approach, as discussed earlier.

As noted previously, the link between government and public health can make for a particularly precarious funding situation for governmental public health agencies. The conflicting value systems of public health and the wider community, and the difficulty in making the argument for prevention, may translate into public health agencies having to document their failures in terms of poorer health, increased disease, and disease outbreaks in order to make progress. It is said that only the squeaky wheel gets the grease; in public health, it often takes an outbreak, disaster, or other tragedy to demonstrate the value of public health. Following the terrorist attacks of September 11, 2001, and the subsequent anthrax attacks, a massive infusion of federal funding occurred. However, that funding shrank by more than half in the succeeding decade.

A more recent example of a public health crisis is the epidemic of opioid use and overdose deaths. The epidemic has superseded the AIDS epidemic in terms of number of deaths per year, has resulted in a decline in life expectancy in some groups, and has been associated with outbreaks of HIV and hepatitis C among injection drug users. This comes despite years of warnings from public health agencies about the growing risk and the failure to adequately control opioid prescriptions, fund drug treatment programs, or adopt policies like syringe exchange to reduce infectious diseases. Whether adequate funding to address this issue will be made available, and how long it will last, are open questions.

Based on an Inherently Political Nature

The social justice underpinnings of public health serve to stimulate political conflict. Public health is both publicly visible and political in nature. It serves populations, which are composites of many different communities, cultures, and values. Politics allow for issues to be considered, negotiated, and finally determined within societies. At the core of political processes are differing values and perspectives regarding both the ends to be achieved and the means for achieving those ends. Advocating for certain causes and agitating various segments of society to identify and address unacceptable conditions that adversely affect health status often lead to increased expectations and demands on society, generally through government. As a result, public health advocates at times appear as antigovernment and anti-institutional. Governmental public health agencies seeking to serve the interests of both government and public health are frequently caught in the middle. This creates tensions and conflict that can put these public health professionals at odds with governmental leaders on the one hand, and external public health advocates on the other. The political nature of public health has been highlighted during the COVID-19 pandemic in the United States. Political leaders in different states have taken drastically different approaches to controlling the pandemic, in some cases even acting in direct opposition to public health recommendations such as mask requirements.

Reliant on the Broader Public Health System/Health in All Policies Approaches

As discussed earlier, public health can only work when all members of the broader public health system are collaboratively engaged. Individual agencies, community organizations, and even the public itself may engage in activities that promote the public health, whether they recognize that as the goal or not. Only working together, however, can the public's health be optimized. It is important for the members of the broader system to take a HiAP approach in their work.

Engaged with a Multidisciplinary Professional Culture with Common Bonds

The multidisciplinary nature of public health and its need to engage a wide range of partners in the public health system appear to be both a strength and weakness. The ties that bind public health professionals are neither a common preparation through education and training, nor a common set of work experiences and work settings. Public health is unique in that the common links are a set of intended outcomes and characteristics, as outlined in this section, toward which many different sciences, arts, and methods can contribute. As a result, public health professionals include anthropologists, sociologists, psychologists, physicians, nurses, nutritionists, lawyers, economists, political scientists, social workers, laboratory workers, managers, sanitarians, engineers, epidemiologists, biostatisticians, gerontologists, disability specialists, and dozens of other professions and disciplines. All are bound to common ends and all employ somewhat different perspectives from their diverse education, training, and work experiences. "Whatever it takes to get the job done" is the theme, suggesting that the basic task is one of problem solving around health issues. This aspect of public health is the foundation for strategies and methods that of necessity must rely heavily on collaborations and partnerships.

This multidisciplinary and interdisciplinary approach is unique among professions, calling into question whether public health is really a unified profession at all. An argument can be made that public health is not a profession. There is no minimum credential or training that distinguishes public health professionals from either other professionals or nonprofessionals. Only a tiny proportion of those who work in organizations dedicated to improving the health of the public possess one of the academic public health degrees (while the Master of Public Health degree may be the most commonly recognized one, there are several other undergraduate, master, and doctoral degrees granted by schools of public health and other institutions). With the vast majority of public health workers not formally trained in public health, it is difficult to characterize its workforce as a profession.

Indeed, until only recently, public health has lacked key characteristics that distinguish professions from occupations. However, significant progress has been made such that public health now meets several of the defining criteria of a profession, including (1) a distinct body of knowledge, (2) an educational credential offered by schools and programs accredited by a specialized accrediting body, (3) career paths that include autonomous practice, and (4) an independent national credential, Certified in Public Health (CPH), indicative of self-regulation based on the examination of the National Board of Public Health Examiners (Evashwick et al., 2013).

Nonetheless, several obstacles will continue to challenge an independent professional status for public health, including the viability of the credential and variability in the content of graduate training programs. The educational requirements of the Council on Education for Public Health (n.d.) for accreditation of schools and programs in public health go a long way to address this latter concern. The impact of complete professionalization could be considerable in terms of recruitment into the field, autonomy of practice, ultimate strengthening of the public health infrastructure, and impact on public health policy and outcomes.

Dynamic, with an Ever-Expanding Agenda

One inevitable characteristic of public health is its broad and ever-increasing scope. Traditional domains of public health interest include biology, environment, behavior, and health services organizations. Within each of these domains are many factors that affect health status. In recent decades, many new public policy problems have been moved onto the public health agenda as their predisposing factors have been identified and found to fall into one or more of these domains. Additionally, in response to several NAM reports, public health has expanded its work to encompass the broader public health system and all the components of the social-ecological model (see **Box 5.3**).

Box 5.3 DISCUSSION QUESTION

How does each of the characteristic features of a public health approach described in this chapter distinguish it from other fields, or not?

The assuming of new challenges onto the public health agenda is an ever-evolving phenomenon. For example, before 1900, the primary problems addressed by public health were infectious diseases and related environmental risks. After 1900, the focus expanded to include the problems and needs of children and mothers as public sentiment over the health and safety of children increased. In the middle of the century, chronic disease prevention and medical care fell into public health's realm as an epidemiological revolution began to identify causative agents for chronic diseases and links between use of health services and health outcomes. Later, substance abuse, mental illness, teen pregnancy, long-term care, chronic diseases, and injuries fell to public health, as did several emerging problems, most notably the epidemics of violence and HIV infections. The public health agenda expanded even further as a result of the recent national dialogue over health reform and how health services should be organized and managed.

Bioterrorism preparedness is an even more recent addition to this agenda amidst heightened concerns and expectations after the events of September 11, 2001, and the anthrax attacks the following month. Infectious diseases, thought to be controllable by antimicrobials and good medical care, are now recognized to be constantly changing, with new diseases emerging or being recognized. These emerging and reemerging diseases include pandemic influenza, antimicrobial-resistant organisms, and the Zika and Ebola virus infections, among many other potential threats. Noncommunicable diseases have emerged as well. The epidemic of opioid use is only the latest crisis to engage public health. The history of public health is the continual emergence and recognition of disease threats that demand a response, as evidenced by the COVID-19 pandemic. Given the scope of the pandemic, it has required the public health community to vastly expand the use of all of its tools, such as disease surveillance, providing access to laboratory testing, coordinating the public health system including acute and long-term care facilities, encouraging behavior change around social distancing and mask use, and encouraging and providing access to vaccinations, to name a few. Although pandemic planning has been going on for decades, the roles and responsibilities of public health in the actual COVID-19 response have expanded well beyond what was anticipated in the planning phases.

The Value of Public Health

How can we measure the contributions of public health and use them to engender among policymakers and the public an appreciation of the value of public health efforts? This question is addressed both directly and indirectly throughout this text. Some initial information presented here will set the stage for greater detail later on.

10 Great Public Health Achievements of the 20th Century

The 20th century was a time of dramatic improvements in the public's health in the United States. At the end of the century, CDC (1999) compiled a list of the 10 great public health achievements of the past 100 years (**Table 5.8**). This list gives an idea of the breadth of public health as a field and underscores how much improvement is possible through public health actions over time.

While these may appear to be distant and sterile accomplishments, each also tells the story of public health in human terms. A good example is the achievement of reductions in communicable diseases due to vaccination programs. In the 1950s, the United States was in the midst of a terrorizing polio epidemic. Public fear was so great that public libraries, community swimming pools, and other group activities were closed during the summers when the disease was most prevalent. Biomedical research had discovered a possible weapon against epidemic polio in the form of the Salk killed polio virus vaccine, which was

Table 5.8 10 Great Public Health Achievements— United States, 1900–1999

Vaccination
Motor-vehicle safety
Safer workplaces
Control of infectious diseases
Decline in deaths from coronary heart disease and stroke
Safer and healthier foods
Healthier mothers and babies
Family planning
Fluoridation of drinking water
Recognition of tobacco use as a health hazard

Centers for Disease Control and Prevention. (1999). Ten great public health achievements—United States, 1900–1999. *Morbidity and Mortality Weekly Report, 48*(12), 241–243.

developed in 1954 and licensed for use 1 year later. A massive and unprecedented campaign to immunize the public was quickly begun, setting the stage for a triumph of public health. Almost seven decades later, wild poliovirus has been eradicated from the western hemisphere and much of the rest of the world. However, public health always has its challenges and vaccinations are not an exception. Unless a disease is eliminated, vaccination efforts need to continue even when disease rates are low. The elimination or near elimination of diseases like polio and measles has led to antivaccination concerns by parents for whom vaccination seems like a bigger threat than diseases they have never experienced. The resulting undervaccination has led to recurring outbreaks of vaccine-preventable diseases in recent years. Similar stories accompany many of other the top 10 achievements.

Reduced Mortality and Increased Life Expectancy

The accomplishments in reducing communicable diseases, heart disease, and stroke point to a second way to appreciate the value of public health: looking at broad measures of the public's health as shown in mortality and life expectancy data. The dramatic reduction in deaths due to infectious diseases, particularly in the first half of the 20th century, is seen in **Figure 5.8**. This serves as a reminder that new and unexpected diseases, such as pandemic influenza, can emerge and have devastating consequences, underscoring the need to be prepared.

Studies have concluded that public health's prevention efforts are responsible for 25 years of the nearly 30-year improvement in life expectancy at birth in the United States since 1900, with only 5 years of the improvement resulting from better medical care (Bunker et al., 1994). Even within these 5 years, medical treatment accounted for approximately 3.5 years, while clinical preventive services (such as immunizations and screening tests) accounted for 1.5 years. The remaining 25 years of improvement have resulted largely from prevention efforts in the form of improved sanitation, better living conditions, social policies, community actions, and personal behavior change. Similarly, a study of life years gained from modern health disease treatments and changes in population risk factors in England and Wales from 1981 to 2000 concluded that 79% of the increase in life years gained was attributed to reductions in major risk factors. Only 21% of the life years gained could be attributed to medical and surgical treatments of coronary heart disease (Unal et al., 2005).

As with recent challenges with vaccination programs, as described earlier, declines in mortality and gains in life expectancy have reversed in selected populations since 2015 (Xu et al., 2018). These changes bring attention to the opioid epidemic and increases in suicide, and the need for public health to respond.

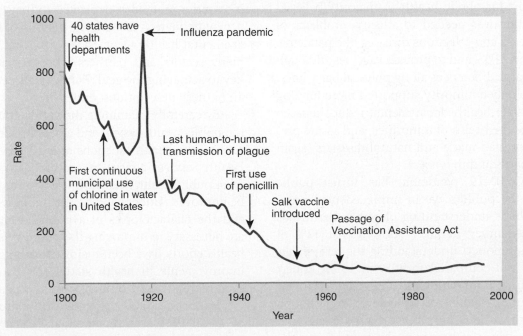

Figure 5.8 Crude Death Rate (per 100,000) for Infectious Diseases, United States, 1900–1996

Centers for Disease Control and Prevention. (1999). Public health achievements, United States, 1900–1999: Control of infectious diseases. *Morbidity and Mortality Weekly Report, 48,* 621–629.

The Value of Public Health to the Public

Perhaps the most important group to gain an understanding and appreciate the value of public health is the public itself, given that they elect the political leadership at all levels of government and that their cooperation and support are critical to the success of public health programs. Public opinion polls suggest that public health is already highly valued in the United States (Harris Polls, 1999). Public opinion surveys suggest that the overwhelming majority of the public rate a variety of key public health services as "very important." Substantially more Americans believe that "public health/protecting populations from disease" is more important than "medicine/treating people who are sick." Public opinion surveys such as these suggest that public health's contributions to health and quality of life have not gone unnoticed.

More recent assessments of the public's view of the value of public health support this contention. A summary of public opinion surveys on public health published in 2010 found that only 42% of respondents rated the nation's system for protecting the public from health threats and preventing illness as excellent/good, and 75% of respondents—a higher proportion than any other area except education—said the federal government expenditures for improving and protecting the nation's health were too low (Blendon et al., 2010). This indicates a level of concern on the part of the public that might be leveraged to help marshal more support for public health. A majority believed more spending was needed to address problems of chronic disease and infectious diseases like pandemic influenza and AIDS, and to provide vaccines, although there were large differences along political party lines. Of concern, only a minority supported more funding to support state health departments, reduce tobacco use, improve the health of minorities, and assure preparedness for man-made and natural disasters (again with wide partisan differences).

The COVID-19 pandemic has thrust public health into the public's eye in unprecedented ways, and the public's understanding of public health has improved. A survey in 2021 showed that 42% of respondents reported understanding the term *public health* very well compared to 25% in 1995 (Robert Wood Johnson Foundation & T.H. Chan Harvard School of Public Health, n.d.). However, even though public health workers have been praised along with healthcare workers as heroes in the fight against the pandemic, the political polarization of the country has resulted in vehement criticism of public health

officials and their recommendations in some areas (Pew Research Center, n.d.). As evidence of this polarization, in 2021, 59% of Democrats but only 22% of Republicans had a great deal/quite a bit of trust in their state health department; 85% of Democrats favored substantially increasing federal funding for public health compared to 40% of Republicans (Robert Wood Johnson Foundation & T.H. Chan Harvard School of Public Health, n.d.).

These data indicate that the public is concerned about health and that it values public health efforts to improve health, although support is divided. Much more needs to be done to impress on the public the value of public health.

Conclusion

Public health evokes different images for different people and, even to the same people, it can mean different things in different contexts. The intent of this chapter has been to define public health and to describe the characteristics of a public health approach to improving health. In defining and describing public health, we have tried to address the common perceptions of public health in the United States, which may in part be the cause of the uncertain valuing of public health by the public. Public health should be thought of as a complex, dynamic, social enterprise, akin to a movement. Public health can also mean a goal of improved health outcomes and health status. Or, it can be the collection of activities and a profession dedicated to that goal. Finally, it may be viewed as both the actions of official governmental health agencies and a system made up of many sectors and partners whose collaboration is key to achieving the goal. Public health encompasses all of these descriptions, and more.

By carefully examining the various dimensions of the public health system and assessing what the three core public health functions and 10 Essential Public Health Services consist of, we can gain insight into what public health does, how it works, and how it can be improved. Understanding the public health system and the characteristics of a public health approach are necessary to improving the public's health. Public health efforts have been major contributors to recent improvements in health status and can contribute even more in a new century with new challenges.

Prior to 2020, the great influenza pandemic of 1918–1919 was the seminal health catastrophe about which all students of public health learned. Similarly, the COVID-19 pandemic is a (hopefully) once-in-a-century event that will provide a touchpoint for public health practice for decades to come. Its impact on public health has been profound, including renewed attention to public health governance, the exercise of police powers, public health functions (surveillance, communications, policy development, and community relations), public health funding, federal-state-local public health relations, and how to address systemic health inequities (NAM, 2021).

If there is any silver lining in the COVID-19 pandemic, it may be the increased recognition of the role that public health and health departments play in protecting their communities and the support they require to do that. Across the country, collaborations that were strengthened between health departments and the healthcare delivery systems, local governments, and so many other community partners will serve to improve the community's health long after the pandemic subsides. It is not possible to return to the "old normal," but it is hoped that the "new normal" will find public health better able to fulfill its roles, and that society will be better able to seriously address the underlying causes of poor health and premature morbidity and mortality with guidance from their health departments.

References

Ahmeda, F., Temte, J. L., Campos-Outcalt, D., & Schünemann, H. J., for the ACIP Evidence Based Recommendations Work Group (EBRWG). (2011). Methods for developing evidence-based recommendations by the Advisory Committee on Immunization Practices (ACIP) of the U.S. Centers for Disease Control and Prevention (CDC). *Vaccine, 29*, 9171–9176.

Auerbach, J. (2016). The 3 buckets of prevention. *Journal of Public Health Management and Practice, 22*(3), 215–218.

Beauchamp, D. E. (1976). Public health as social justice. *Inquiry, 13*, 3–14.

Blendon, R. J., Benson, J. M., Steel-Fisher, G. K., & Connolly, J. M. (2010). Americans' conflicting views about the public health system, and how to shore up support. *Health Affairs (Millwood), 29*(11), 2033–2040.

Bunker, J. P., Frazier, H. S., & Mosteller, F. (1994). Improving health: Measuring effects of medical care. *Milbank Quarterly, 72*, 225–258.

Centers for Disease Control and Prevention. (n.d.a). *Community Health Improvement Navigator.* https://www.cdc.gov/CHInav/

Centers for Disease Control and Prevention. (n.d.b). *Health impact in 5 years initiative.* https://www.cdc.gov/policy/hst/hi5/index.html

Centers for Disease Control and Prevention. (n.d.c). *One Health Initiative.* https://www.cdc.gov/onehealth/index.html

Centers for Disease Control and Prevention. (1999). Ten great public health achievements—United States, 1900–1999. *Morbidity and Mortality Weekly Report, 48*(12), 241–243.

Centers for Disease Control and Prevention. (2021). 10 Essential public health services. https://www.cdc.gov/publichealthgateway/publichealthservices/essentialhealthservices.html

Council on Education for Public Health. (n.d.). https://ceph.org/

DeSalvo, K. B., O'Carroll, P. W., Koo, D., Auerbach, J. M., & Monroe, J. A. (2016). Public Health 3.0: Time for an upgrade. *American Journal of Public Health, 106*, 621–622.

Evashwick, C. J., Begun, J. W., & Finnegan, J. R. (2013). Public health as a distinct profession: Has it arrived? *Journal of Public Health Management and Practice, 19*(5), 412–419.

Frieden, T. R. (2010). A framework for public health action: The health impact pyramid. *American Journal of Public Health, 100*(4), 590–595.

Guyatt, G. H., Oxman, A. D., Vist, G. E., Kunz, R., Falck-Ytter, Y., Alonso-Coello, P., Schünemann, H. J., & GRADE Working Group. (2008). GRADE: An emerging consensus on rating quality of evidence and strength of recommendations. *BMJ, 336*(7650), 924–926.

Hamlin, C. (1995). Could you starve to death in England in 1839? The Chadwick-Farr controversy and the loss of the "social" in public health. *American Journal of Public Health, 85*, 856–866.

Harris Polls. (1999). *Public opinion about public health,* United States.

Hinman, A. (1999). Eradication of vaccine-preventable diseases. *Annual Review of Public Health, 20*, 211–229.

Holsinger, J. W., Jr., & Scutchfield, F. D. (2013). History and context of public health care. In J. W. Holsinger, Jr. (Ed.). *Contemporary public health: Principles, practice, and policy* (pp. 1–5). University Press of Kentucky.

Institute of Medicine. (1988). *The future of public health.* National Academy Press.

Institute of Medicine. (2002). *The future of the public's health in the 21st century.* National Academies Press.

Johnson, S. (2006). *The ghost map: The story of London's most terrifying epidemic – and how it changed science, cities and the modern world.* Riverhead Books.

Kindig, D. A. (2007). Understanding population health terminology. *Milbank Quarterly, 85*, 139–161.

Krieger, N., & Brin, A. E. (1998). A vision of social justice as the foundation of public health: Commemorating 150 years of the spirit of 1848. *American Journal of Public Health, 88*, 1603–1606.

McNeil, W. H. (1977). *Plagues and peoples.* Doubleday.

National Academy of Medicine, National Academies of Sciences, Engineering, and Medicine. (2021). *Public health COVID-19 impact assessment: Lessons learned and compelling needs.* https://nam.edu/public-health-covid-19-impact-assessment-lessons-learned-and-compelling-needs/

Newman, S. J., Ye, J., Leep, C. J., Hasbrouck, L., & Zometa, C. (2016). Assessment of staffing, services, and partnerships of local health departments – United States, 2015. *Morbidity and Mortality Weekly Report, 65*(25), 646–649.

Office of Disease Prevention and Health Promotion, Department of Health and Human Services. (n.d.). Healthfinder.gov. https://healthfinder.gov/myhealthfinder/

Office of the U.S. Surgeon General, Department of Health and Human Services. (2011, June). *National Prevention Strategy*. https://www.hhs.gov/sites/default/files/disease-prevention-wellness-report.pdf

Paneth, N., Vinten-Johansen, P., Brody, H., & Rip, M. (1998). A rivalry of foulness: Official and unofficial investigations of the London cholera epidemic of 1854. *American Journal of Public Health*, 88, 1545–1553.

Pew Research Center. (n.d.). *A year of U.S. public opinion on the coronavirus pandemic*. https://www.pewresearch.org/2021/03/05/a-year-of-u-s-public-opinion-on-the-coronavirus-pandemic/

Public Health Institute. (2013). *Health in all policies: A guide for state and local government*. http://www.phi.org/resources/?resource=hiapguide

Public Health Leadership Forum. (2014, May). The high achieving governmental health department in 2020 as the community chief health strategist. https://www.resolve.ngo/site-healthleadershipforum/hd2020.htm

Robert Wood Johnson Foundation, & T.H. Chan Harvard School of Public Health. (n.d.). *The public's perspective on the United States public health system*. https://www.rwjf.org/en/library/research/2021/05/the-publics-perspective-on-the-united-states-public-health-system.html

Sharfstein, J. M. (2014). The strange journey of population health. *Milbank Quarterly*, 92(4), 640–643.

Susser, M. (1993). Health as a human right: An epidemiologist's perspective on the public health. *American Journal of Public Health*, 83, 418–426.

Thomas, J. C., Sage, M., Dillenberg, J., & Guillory, V. J. (2002). A code of ethics for public health. *American Journal of Public Health*, 92(7), 1057–1059.

Trust for America's Health. (2008, July). *Prevention for a healthier America: Investments in disease prevention yield significant savings, stronger communities*. https://www.rwjf.org/content/dam/farm/reports/reports/2008/rwjf29920

Unal, B., Critchley, J. A., Fidan, D., & Capewell, S. (2005). Life-years gained from modern cardiological treatments and population risk factor changes in England and Wales, 1981–2000. *American Journal of Public Health*, 95, 103–108.

U.S. Public Health Service. (1994). For a healthy nation: Returns on investment in public health. Author.

Winslow, C.-E. A. (1920). The untilled fields of public health. *Science*, 51(1306), 23–33.

Winslow, C.-E. A. (1926). Public health at the crossroads. *American Journal of Public Health*, 16, 1075–1085 (reprinted in 1999 in *American Journal of Public Health*, 89, 1645–1647).

Winslow, C.-E. A. (1929). *The Life of Hermann M. Biggs*. Lea and Febiger.

Winslow, C.-E. A. (1949). Lemuel Shattuck – still a prophet: The message of Lemuel Shattuck for 1948. *American Journal of Public Health*, 39, 156–162.

World Health Organization. (2002). Constitution of the World Health Organization. *Bulletin of the World Health Organization*, 80(12), 983–984.

Xu, J., Murphy, S. L., Kochanek, K. D., Bastian, B., & Arias, E. (2018, July 26). Deaths: Final data for 2016. *National Vital Statistics Reports*, 67(5), 1–76.

PART II

Essential Issues in Health Policy and Law

Part I of this book introduced frameworks for conceptualizing health policy and law and described basic aspects of policy, the policymaking process, law, the legal system, and the healthcare and public health systems. Part II covers many of the essential issues in health policy and law. Chapter 6 addresses individual rights in health care and public health, Chapter 7 describes how law itself is a driver of health and how it relates to other structural and social determinants of health, and Chapters 8 and 9 cover the fundamentals of health insurance and health economics, respectively. Chapter 10 reviews key public insurance programs, while Chapter 11 provides an overview of health reform efforts and the Patient Protection and Affordable Care Act (ACA). Chapters 12 and 13 cover healthcare quality and public health emergency preparedness, respectively. After completing Part II, you will understand, among other things, how structural and social factors influence individual and population health, how health insurance functions, why private employer–based coverage dominates the health insurance market, why gaps in health insurance coverage remain, the importance of health economics to health policymaking, key provisions in the ACA, various policy and legal dimensions to healthcare quality, and the role of public health in preparing for and responding to national emergencies.

CHAPTER 6

Individual Rights in Health Care and Public Health

LEARNING OBJECTIVES

By the end of this chapter you will be able to:

1. Describe the meaning and importance of the "no-duty-to-treat" principle
2. Explain generally how the U.S. approach to health rights differs from that of other high-income countries
3. Describe the types and limitations of individual legal rights associated with health care
4. Describe the balancing approach taken when weighing individual rights against the public's health

Introduction

The real-life scenarios in **Box 6.1** touch upon the key issues you will confront in this chapter: namely, the ways in which the law creates, protects, and restricts individual rights in the contexts of health care and public health. Individuals are deeply impacted by law on a daily basis, and this fact is no less true when they navigate the healthcare system, or when an individual's actions are measured against the broader interests of the public's health. Over many decades, legal principles have been rejected, developed, and refined as the law continually struggles to define the appropriate relationship between individuals and the clinicians, hospitals, managed care companies, and others they encounter in the healthcare delivery system, and between individuals and government agencies charged with protecting public health and welfare. These balancing acts are made all the more difficult as the legal system bumps up against the quick pace of technological advancements

in medicine and against amorphous, potentially deadly risks to the public's health, such as bioterrorism and fast-spreading influenzas.

After a background section, this chapter considers individual legal rights in health care, beginning with a brief overview of health rights under international and foreign law. This sets up a much lengthier discussion of healthcare rights in the United States, which for purposes of this chapter are classified according to an important distinction: legal rights *to* health care and rights that individuals can claim only *within* the context of the healthcare system—that is, only once they have found a way to access needed care.[a] Examples of the latter type of rights include the right to refuse unwanted treatment, the right to autonomy in making personal healthcare decisions, and the right to be free from wrongful discrimination when receiving care. Finally, the chapter turns to a discussion of individual rights in the context of government-initiated public health efforts. This topic

Box 6.1 VIGNETTES At the turn of the 20th century, an Indiana physician named George Eddingfield repeatedly refused to come to the aid of Charlotte Burk, who was in labor, even though he was Mrs. Burk's family physician. Doctor Eddingfield conceded at trial that he made this decision for no particular reason and despite the facts that he had been offered monetary compensation in advance of his performing any medical services and that he was aware that no other physician was available to provide care to Mrs. Burk. Unattended by any medical providers, Mrs. Burk eventually fell gravely ill, and both she and her unborn child died. It was determined upon trial and subsequent appeals that Dr. Eddingfield did not wrongfully cause either death.

Around the same time as the scenario just described, the Cambridge, Massachusetts, Board of Health ordered everyone within city limits to be vaccinated against the smallpox disease under a state law granting local boards of health the power, under certain circumstances, to require the vaccination of individuals. After refusing to abide by the Cambridge Board's order, Henning Jacobson was convicted by a state trial court and sentenced to pay a $5 fine. Remarkably, Mr. Jacobson's case not only made its way to the U.S. Supreme Court, but it also resulted in one of the court's most important public health rulings and a sweeping statement about limitations to fundamental individual rights in the face of threats to the public's health.

The [state licensing] act is preventive, not a compulsive, measure. In obtaining the state's license (permission) to practice medicine, the state does not require, and the licensee does not engage, that he will practice at all or on other terms than he may choose to accept. (*Hurley v. Eddingfield*, 1901)

In other words, obtaining a license to practice medicine does not obligate an individual to actually practice, or to practice in a particular fashion or with a particular clientele; the licensure requirement exists instead to filter out individuals who may not have the requisite knowledge or skills to practice medicine. The same can be said for obtaining a law license, or even a driver's license: The former does not obligate a lawyer to practice, or to choose certain types of clients or cases; the latter does not require that a person actually drive, or drive a certain make of car. As with a medical license, the point of a law or driver's license is to guarantee that should the licensee *choose* to practice law or operate a motor vehicle, they are qualified to do so. Furthermore, you will recall from the facts provided in the vignette that Dr. Eddingfield was Mrs. Burk's family physician, and many students believe that this fact is enough to establish a sufficient legal relationship between the two to hold Dr. Eddingfield accountable for the death of Mrs. Burk. However, the general legal rule is that physician–patient relationships are specific to "spells of illness" and that past treatment is not tantamount to an *existing* physician–patient relationship. Put another way, under the law a physician–patient relationship does not exist as a general, continuous matter—even with one's family physician, internist, primary care physician, and so on—but rather it exists for a specific period of time and must be established (or renewed) accordingly.

Note that this basic premise—that there is no fundamental right to healthcare services in the United States—was not altered by the passage in 2010 of the Patient Protection and Affordable Care Act (ACA). Although it is arguable that the ACA moves the country in a direction that makes a legal right to health care more plausible down the road (Friedman & Adashi, 2010) and there can be no arguing that it makes health care more accessible to millions of people by virtue of its health insurance reforms (as discussed later in this chapter and in greater detail elsewhere), the ACA does not create a right to care.

As you begin to think through the significance and implications of the no-duty principle, it is important to understand that there are many other legal principles and health laws that define the relationship

is dominated by the role and scope of government "police powers," which permit governments, when acting to promote or protect public health, to curtail individual freedoms and liberties.

Background

Lurking behind any discussion of individual rights in a health context is one of the most basic principles in U.S. health law: Generally speaking, individuals have no legal right to healthcare services (or to public health insurance), and, correspondingly, there exists on the part of healthcare providers no general legal duty to provide care. This is referred to as the "no-duty" or "no-duty-to-treat" principle, which is aptly described by the Indiana Supreme Court in the well-known 1901 case of *Hurley v. Eddingfield*, the facts of which were referred to in the first vignette in Box 6.1. In its decision, the court wrote that the state law permitting the granting of a medical license

provides for . . . standards of qualification . . . and penalties for practicing without a license.

between an individual and another health system stakeholder (e.g., a physician, hospital, or government program). In fact, there are several federal and state laws that narrow the scope of the no-duty principle. For example, a federal law called the Examination and Treatment for Emergency Medical Conditions and Women in Labor Act enables all individuals to access some hospital care in medical emergencies, irrespective of the individual's ability to pay for that care or a hospital's willingness to treat the individual. Also, both federal and state laws that generally prohibit certain forms of discrimination (say, based on race or disability) apply in the context of health care and might thus result in access to health services that otherwise would not be forthcoming. Furthermore, some public health insurance programs—Medicaid and Medicare, most prominently—create entitlements (a legal concept denoting a legal claim to something) to services for individuals who meet the programs' eligibility criteria (Jost, 2003), and some health insurance products obligate physicians participating in the plan's networks to extend care to plan members. Finally, some states implemented universal healthcare coverage programs, such as Maine's Dirigo Health Reform Act, which was designed to provide access to health coverage to every person in Maine (and which ended at the end of 2014 as residents of the state were transitioned into the health insurance exchanges created by the ACA).

When thinking about the law's no-duty principle, you must also take into account the role of medical ethics, which might require more of a healthcare professional than does the law. For example, no law mandates that licensed physicians aid a stranger in medical distress, but many believe an ethical obligation exists in this instance. And although legally the no-duty principle would dictate otherwise, many healthcare providers consider themselves ethically obligated to furnish at least some level of care to those who cannot pay for it. In short, although there is no universal legal right to health care in the United States, certain situations give rise to healthcare rights, and specific populations may be entitled to health care or receive it purely through the magnanimity of ethics-conscious providers.

Perhaps because of the federal and state laws that chip away at the no-duty-to-treat principle, many students new to the study of health law erroneously assume that the principle is a legal anomaly, born solely of the incredible historical power and autonomy of the medical profession and without modern precedent. In this case, it is instructive to place the principle in a broader "welfare rights" context. During the 1960s, public-interest lawyers, social reform activists, and others pressed for an interpretation of the federal Constitution that would have created an individual right to welfare. Under this view, the government must provide individuals with minimally adequate levels of education, food, housing, health care, and so on (Davis, 1993). But in a series of cases, the Supreme Court rejected the notion of a constitutional right to welfare.

Consider the right to education. Even though every state provides free public schools and makes education for minors compulsory, there is no national, generalized legal right to education. In the case of *San Antonio Independent School District v. Rodriguez* (1973), the Supreme Court ruled that education is not a fundamental right under the federal Constitution's Equal Protection Clause. The plaintiffs in the *Rodriguez* case were Mexican-American parents whose children attended elementary and secondary schools in an urban San Antonio school district. They had attacked as unconstitutional Texas's system of financing public education and filed the suit on behalf of school children throughout the state who were members of minority groups or who resided in relatively poor school districts. But the court turned the plaintiffs' argument away, noting that although education is one of the most important services states perform,

> it is not among the rights afforded explicit protection under our Federal Constitution. Nor do we find any basis for saying it is implicitly so protected. . . . [T]he undisputed importance of education will not alone cause this Court to depart from the usual standard for reviewing a State's social and economic legislation. (*San Antonio Indep. School Dist. v. Rodriguez*, 1973)

In the wake of the *Rodriguez* decision, several states interpreted their own constitutions as prohibiting inequitable methods of financing public education, thereby recognizing on some level a right to a minimally "meaningful" education. Subsequently, lawyers and social activists seeking to promote equal access to all manner of critical services seized on these state determinations, arguing that an egalitarian approach to constitutional interpretation should not be limited to education (Stacy, 1993). Note, for example, how one author's writings about the right to education could just as well have been written with respect to health care:

> Requiring an adequate education will help to fulfill our nation's promise, articulated in

Brown [v. *Board of Education*], that an individual be free to achieve her full potential. Ensuring educational adequacy will promote children's emotional and intellectual development, their career path and earning potential and thus their success throughout life. A meaningful education offers the hope that children can escape the degradation of poverty and its lack of opportunity, and attain pride, participation in this country's economic and political life, and financial and emotional success. (Smith, 1997, p. 825)

However, efforts around ensuring adequate education have not been emulated in other social policy areas, such as health care. In fact, health care is treated not as a right, but as a commodity (like televisions or vacuum cleaners) subject to private market forces and socioeconomic status. During the public debate in 1993 over President Bill Clinton's failed attempt at national health reform, U.S. Representative Dick Armey (R-TX) stated that "health care is just a commodity, just like bread, and just like housing and everything else" (Reinhardt, 1996, p. 102). But why should this be the case, particularly when the private health insurance market has presumably found equilibrium at a point that continually leaves tens of millions of Americans uninsured, and particularly because health care (like education) is different from vacuum cleaners and other everyday goods in that it has "a fundamental bearing on the range of one's opportunities to realize one's life plans"? (Stacy, 1993, p. 80).

There is no single answer to the question of why health care is generally treated in this country as something less than an individual legal right. Many factors beyond the scope of this chapter are implicated: the nature and interpretation of the federal Constitution, politics, a weak labor movement, powerful interest groups, the nation's free market philosophies, the public's often negative view of the government, and more (Blum et al., 2003; Rich, 2000; Vladeck, 2003). In this chapter, we limit the discussion to describing the kinds of health rights that do exist and how they operate in the context of the healthcare delivery system and when considered against government-initiated public health efforts. Before we explore in depth the scope of individual health-related rights under U.S. law, however, we briefly describe these same types of rights under international law and under the law of other countries. Through this examination, we provide a backdrop for understanding this country's approach to legal rights in the context of health.

Individual Rights and Health Care: A Global Perspective

Despite being the world leader in terms of the development of medical technologies and the quantity of medical services, the United States is one of the only high-income nations that does not guarantee health care as a fundamental right, and it is the only high-income nation that has not implemented a system for insuring at least all but the wealthiest segment of its population against healthcare costs (Jost, 2003, p. 3). In essence, other high-income nations with social democracies treat the provision of health care as a social good[b] (i.e., something that could be supported through private enterprise but is instead supported by the government and financed from public funds). Furthermore, it is worth noting that nations that provide universal healthcare entitlements have not been bankrupted as a result. In fact, according to Professor Timothy Jost, "all of the other developed nations spend less on health care than does the U.S., in terms of both dollars per capita and proportion of gross domestic product" (Jost, 2003, p. 3).

A foreign nation's universal healthcare rights—whether an unlimited right to health, a right to medical care generally or to a basic package of services, a right to healthcare insurance, or something else—exist as the result of either a commitment to human rights principles generally, or as fidelity to the particular country's own constitution. When recognized by governments, human rights accrue to all individuals because the rights are based on the dignity and worth of the human being; thus, technically, a human right exists regardless of whether positive law (a constitution or statute) has given it expression (Barnes & McChrystal, 1998). Examples of positive expressions of health as a human right include Article 25 of the 1948 Universal Declaration of Human Rights, which states that "everyone has the right to a standard of living adequate for the health and well-being of himself and of his family, including . . . medical care . . . and the right to security in the event of. . . sickness [or] disability" (Claiming Human Rights, 2010), and the Constitution of the World Health Organization, which says that "the enjoyment of the highest attainable standard of health is one of the fundamental rights of every human being without distinction of race, religion, political belief, economic or social condition" (World Health Organization, 2006).

In terms of national constitutions, some two-thirds of constitutions worldwide specifically address health or health care, and almost all of them do so in universal terms, rather than being limited to certain populations (Kinney & Clark, 2004). For example, consider the health-related aspects of the constitutions of four politically and culturally diverse countries—Italy, the Netherlands, South Africa, and Poland—that have some type of "right to health": Italy's Constitution guarantees a right to health; under the Dutch Constitution, the government is mandated "to promote the health of the population"; the Constitution of South Africa imposes on government the obligation to provide access to health services; and under Polish constitutional law, citizens are guaranteed "the right to health protection" and access to publicly financed healthcare services (Littell, 2002). (See **Box 6.2**.)

💡 Box 6.2 DISCUSSION QUESTION

Depending on one's personal experience in obtaining health care, or one's view of the role of physicians in society, of law as a tool for social change, of the scope of medical ethics, or of the United States' place in the broader global community, the no-duty principle might seem appropriate, irresponsible, or downright wrong. Imagine you are traveling in a country where socialized medicine is the legal norm, and your discussion with a citizen of that country turns to the topic of your countries' respective health systems. When asked, how will you account for the fact that health care is far from being a fundamental right rooted in American law?

Of course, including language respecting health rights in a legal document—even one as profound as a national constitution—does not guarantee that the right will be recognized or enforced. As in the United States, multiple factors might lead a foreign court or other tribunal to construe rights-creating language narrowly or to refuse to force implementation of what is properly considered a right. Examples of these factors include the relative strength of a country's judicial branch vis-à-vis other branches in its national governance structure and a foreign court's view of its country's ability to provide services and benefits inherent in the health right.

Individual Rights and the Healthcare System

The "global perspective" you just read was brief for two reasons. First, a full treatment of international

and foreign health rights is well beyond the scope of this chapter, and second, historically speaking, international law has played a limited role in influencing this nation's domestic legal principles. As one author commented, "historically the United States has been uniquely averse to accepting international human rights standards and conforming national laws to meet them" (Yamin, 2005, p. 1156). This fact is no less true in the area of health rights than in any other major area of law. As described earlier in this chapter, universal rights to health care are virtually nonexistent in this country, even though this stance renders it almost solitary among the world's developed nations.

This is not to say that the United States has not contemplated health care as a universal, basic right. For instance, in 1952, a presidential commission stated that "access to the means for attainment and preservation of health is a basic human right" (President's Commission, 1983, p. 4). Medicaid and Medicare were the fruits of a nationwide debate about universal healthcare coverage. And during the 1960s and 1970s, the claim that health care was not a matter of privilege, but rather of right, was "so widely acknowledged as almost to be uncontroversial" (Starr, 1982, p. 389). Nor is it to say that certain populations do not enjoy healthcare rights beyond those of the general public. Prisoners and others under the control of state governments have a right to minimal health care (Wing, 1993), some state constitutions expressly recognize a right to health or healthcare benefits (e.g., Montana includes an affirmative right to health in its constitution's section on inalienable rights), and individuals covered by Medicaid have unique legal entitlements. Finally, it would be inaccurate in describing healthcare rights to cover only rights to obtain health care in the first instance, because many important healthcare rights attach to individuals once they manage to access needed healthcare services.

The remainder of this section more fully describes the various types of individual rights associated with the healthcare system. We categorize these rights as follows:

1. Rights related to receiving services explicitly provided under healthcare, health financing, or health insurance laws—for example, the Examination and Treatment for Emergency Medical Conditions and Women in Labor Act, Medicaid, and the ACA
2. Rights concerning freedom of choice and freedom from government interference when making healthcare decisions—for example, choosing to have an abortion

3. The right to be free from unlawful discrimination when accessing or receiving health care—for example, Title VI of the federal Civil Rights Act of 1964, which prohibits discrimination on the basis of race, color, or national origin by entities that receive federal funding (Annas, 2004; Barnes & McChrystal, 1998, p. 12)

Rights Under Healthcare and Health Financing Laws

We begin this discussion of rights-creating health laws with the Examination and Treatment for Emergency Medical Conditions and Women in Labor Act (also referred to as EMTALA, which is the acronym for the law's original name—the Emergency Medical Treatment and Active Labor Act—or, for reasons soon to become clear, the "patient anti-dumping statute"). We then briefly discuss the federal Medicaid program in a rights-creating context and wrap up this section with a brief discussion of the ACA.

Rights Under Healthcare Laws: EMTALA

Because EMTALA represents the only truly universal legal right to health care in this country—the right to access emergency hospital services—it is often described as one of the building blocks of health rights. EMTALA was enacted by Congress in 1986 to prevent the practice of "patient dumping"—that is, the turning away of poor or uninsured persons in need of hospital care. Patient dumping was a common strategy among private hospitals aiming to shield themselves from the potentially uncompensated costs associated with treating poor and/or uninsured patients. By refusing to treat these individuals and instead "dumping" them on public hospitals, private institutions were effectively limiting their patients to those whose treatment costs would likely be covered out-of-pocket or by insurers. Note that the no-duty principle made this type of strategy possible.

EMTALA was a conscious effort on the part of elected federal officials to chip away at the no-duty principle: By creating legally enforceable rights to emergency hospital care for all individuals regardless of their income or health insurance status, Congress created a corresponding legal *duty* of care on the part of hospitals. At its core, EMTALA includes two related duties, which technically attach only to hospitals that participate in the Medicare program (but then again, nearly every hospital in the country participates). The first duty requires covered hospitals to provide an "appropriate" screening examination to all individuals who present at a hospital's emergency department seeking care for an "emergency medical condition." Under the law, an appropriate medical screening is one that is nondiscriminatory and that adheres to a hospital's established emergency care guidelines. EMTALA defines an emergency medical condition as a

medical condition manifesting itself by acute symptoms of sufficient severity (including severe pain) such that the absence of immediate medical attention could reasonably be expected to result in (i) placing the health of the individual (or, with respect to a pregnant woman, the health of the woman or her unborn child) in serious jeopardy, (ii) serious impairment to bodily functions, or (iii) serious dysfunction of any bodily organ or part; or with respect to a pregnant woman who is having contractions, that there is inadequate time to effect a safe transfer to another hospital before delivery, or that transfer may pose a threat to the health or safety of the woman or the unborn child. (Examination and Treatment, 2011)

The second key duty required of hospitals under EMTALA is to either stabilize any condition that meets the preceding definition or, in the case of a hospital without the capability to treat the emergency condition, undertake to transfer the patient to another facility in a medically appropriate fashion. A proper transfer is effected when, among other things, the transferring hospital minimizes the risks to the patient's health by providing as much treatment as is within its capability, a receiving medical facility has agreed to accept the transferred patient, and the transferring hospital provides the receiving facility all relevant medical records.

The legal rights established under EMTALA are accompanied by heavy penalties for their violation. The federal government, individual patients, and "dumped-on" hospitals can all initiate actions against a hospital alleged to have violated EMTALA, and the federal government can also file a claim for civil money penalties against individual physicians who negligently violate an EMTALA requirement.

Rights Under Healthcare Financing Laws: Medicaid

Many laws fund programs that aim to expand access to health care, such as state laws authorizing the establishment of public hospitals or health agencies, and the federal law establishing the vast network of community health clinics that serve medically under-served communities and populations. However, the legal obligations created by these financing laws are generally enforceable only by public agencies, not by individuals.

The Medicaid program is different in this respect. (Medicaid is covered elsewhere in greater depth, but because of its importance in the area of individual healthcare rights, we mention it also in this context.) Although most certainly a law concerning health-care financing, Medicaid is unlike most other health financing laws in that it confers the right to indi-vidually enforce program obligations through the courts (Rosenblatt et al., 1997, pp. 419–424). This right of individual enforcement is one of the reasons why Medicaid, 50 years after its creation, remains a hotly debated public program. This is because the legal entitlements to benefits under Medicaid are viewed as a key contributor to the program's high cost. Yet whether Medicaid's legal entitlements are any more of a factor in the program's overall costs than, say, the generally high cost of health care, is not clearly established.

Rights Under Health Insurance Laws: The Affordable Care Act

The ACA is far more than a law that concerns only health insurance; it is a sweeping set of reforms that touch on healthcare quality, public health prac-tice, health disparities, community health centers, healthcare fraud and abuse, comparative effective-ness research, the health workforce, health informa-tion technology, long-term care, and more. You will learn more about the details of the ACA in subsequent chapters. However, for purposes of this chapter, we mention it briefly in terms of its impact on the rights of individuals to access health insurance and to equi-table treatment by their insurer. Details concerning the ACA's effect on the public and private insurance markets are discussed elsewhere.

Through a series of major reforms to existing poli-cies, the ACA reshapes the private health insurance market, transforming private health insurance from a commodity that regularly classified (and rejected) individuals based on their health status, age, disabil-ity status, and more into a social good whose avail-ability is essential to individual and population health (Rosenbaum, 2011). The key elements of this shift include a ban on exclusion and discrimination based on health status or preexisting health conditions; new protections that ensure that, once covered by insur-ance, individuals will have access to necessary care

without regard to artificial annual or lifetime expen-diture caps; a guarantee that once insurance coverage is in place, it cannot be rescinded except in cases of applicant fraud; a ban on additional fees for out-of-network emergency services; the provision of financial subsidies to help low- and moderate-income individ-uals and small businesses purchase insurance cover-age; the inclusion, in the individual and small group insurance markets, of a package of "essential health benefits" that must be covered; and the creation of state health insurance "exchanges" through which individuals and small employer groups can purchase high-quality health insurance in a virtual marketplace that is substantially regulated and that simplifies the job of learning about, selecting, and enrolling in insurance plans.

The ACA also reforms the public health insurance market, primarily through an expansion of Medicaid eligibility to cover all nonelderly low-income persons who are legal residents or citizens (this expansion is now voluntary on the part of states, as the result of a Supreme Court decision described in a subsequent chapter). If fully implemented, this reform would substantially close one of Medicaid's last remaining coverage gaps for the poor—namely, the program's historical denial of coverage for nonpregnant, work-ing-age adults without minor children—and in so doing would provide insurance coverage (and the resulting access to health care that often follows cov-erage) to many millions of people.

Rights Related to Freedom of Choice and Freedom from Government Interference

EMTALA and Medicaid are remarkable in terms of the rights *to* health care that they each provide, although as mentioned earlier in this chapter, individual rights that attach *within* the context of healthcare provision can be equally important. Important individual rights within health care include the right to make informed healthcare decisions and the right to personal privacy and autonomy.

The Right to Make Informed Healthcare Decisions

One of the most important healthcare rights is the right of individual patients to make informed deci-sions about the scope and course of their own care. This includes the right to *refuse* treatment, regard-less of the treatment's nature or urgency. That is, the right to refuse treatment exists whether the patient is considering ingesting prescribed medication for minor pain, undergoing a minimally invasive test or procedure, or consenting to a major, potentially life-sustaining operation like the removal of a brain tumor. However, the right pertaining to informed decision-making does not come without qualifiers and exceptions, as described here.

Modern notions of informed consent have their roots in the Nuremberg Code, which derived from the Nuremberg trials in the late 1940s of German physicians who performed horrendous experiments on prisoners in Nazi concentration camps during the Second World War. The code spells out principles of research ethics, including the need to secure in advance the voluntary consent of the research subject. These principles have been codified and expanded in American federal statutory and regulatory law concerning federally funded biomedical research (Protection of Human Subjects, 2009). But if the Nuremberg Code can be thought of as the roots of U.S. informed consent law, then the decision in *Canterbury v. Spence* (1972) can be thought of as the trunk.

In 1959, Jerry Canterbury was a 19-year-old suffering from severe back pain. His neurosurgeon, Dr. William Spence, informed him that he would need a laminectomy—a surgical procedure in which the roofs of spinal vertebrae are removed or trimmed to relieve pressure on the spinal cord—to correct what the doctor believed was a herniated disk. However, Dr. Spence did not inform Canterbury of any risks associated with the surgery. The day after the operation, while appearing to recuperate normally, Canterbury fell from his hospital bed while no attendant was on hand and a few hours later began suffering paralysis from the waist down. This led to a second spinal surgery, but Canterbury never fully recovered; years later, he needed crutches to walk and he suffered from paralysis of the bowels.

Canterbury sued Dr. Spence, alleging negligence in both the performance of the laminectomy and the doctor's failure to disclose risks inherent in the operation. The federal trial judge ruled in Dr. Spence's favor and Canterbury appealed, setting the stage for the now-famous decision in 1972 by the federal Court of Appeals for the District of Columbia Circuit (considered second in national importance to the Supreme Court).[c] The decision includes two important determinations pertinent to this chapter. The first is that "as a part of the physician's overall obligation to the patient, [there exists a] duty of reasonable disclosure of the choices with respect to proposed therapy and the dangers inherently and potentially involved." The court viewed this duty as a logical and modest extension of a physician's existing general duty to his patients. Importantly, the court discarded the notion that "the patient should ask for information before the physician is required to disclose." In other words, the duty to disclose requires more than just answering patient questions; it demands voluntary disclosure on the part of the physician of pertinent medical information.

The *Canterbury* court's second key determination concerns the actual scope of the disclosure required—in other words, once the physician's duty to disclose is triggered, what information satisfies the legal requirement? On this matter the court made several observations: that the patient's right of "self-decision" is paramount, that the right to consent can be properly exercised only if the patient has sufficient information to make an "intelligent choice," that the sufficiency test is met when all information "material to the decision" is disclosed, and that the disclosure's legality should be measured objectively, not subjectively from the perspective of a particular physician or patient. From these observations, the court settled on three required pieces of disclosed information: a proposed treatment's inherent and potential risks, any alternatives to a proposed treatment, and the likely outcome of not being treated at all. Applying these criteria, the court ruled that Dr. Spence's failure to disclose even the tiniest risk of paralysis resulting from the laminectomy entitled Canterbury to a new trial.

As mentioned earlier, the right to make informed healthcare decisions is not boundless. For example, the court in *Canterbury* wrote that where disclosure of a treatment's risks would pose a threat of harm to the patient (e.g., because it would severely complicate treatment or psychologically damage the patient) as to become "unfeasible or contraindicated from a medical point of view," the physician's duty to disclose could be set aside. Furthermore, a patient's competency from a legal vantage point plays a major role in their ability to consent to treatment.

The *Canterbury* decision and its progeny have over the years been interpreted expansively, and today the right to make informed healthcare decisions has many facets beyond a clear explanation of proposed treatments, potential risks and complications, and the like. For example, patients have the right to know whether outside factors, such as research interests or financial considerations, are coloring a physician's thinking about a proposed course of treatment; patients whose first language is not English have the right to an interpreter; and patients have the right to designate in advance their treatment wishes, whether through written advance directives or another individual. (See **Box 6.3**.)

💡 Box 6.3 DISCUSSION QUESTIONS

Go back to the first legal principle drawn from the *Canterbury* decision: namely, that physicians have a duty of reasonable disclosure to include therapy options and the dangers potentially involved with each. Do you agree with the court that this duty is both a logical and modest extension of physicians' "traditional" obligation to their patients? Why or why not? Depending on your answer, are you surprised to learn that some states have opted not to follow the *Canterbury* court's patient-oriented standard of informed consent, relying instead on the more conventional approach of measuring the legality of physician disclosure based on what a reasonable physician would have disclosed?

The Right to Personal Privacy

Another right related to freedom of choice and freedom from government interference is the constitutional right to personal privacy. Although the federal Constitution makes no explicit mention of the right to privacy, the Supreme Court has recognized some form of it since the 1890s.[d] The court has taken a more or less two-pronged approach to the right. The first approach defines the protected personal interest as "informational privacy," meaning the limiting of others' access to and use of an individual's private information.[e] The second approach—the focus of this section—is concerned with individual autonomy and freedom from governmental interference in making basic personal decisions. This right is one of the most debated in law, both because of its implicit nature (constitutionally speaking) and because it has served as the legal underpinning of several divisive social issues, including abortion, intimate associations, and the decisions as to whether, when, and how to end one's life.

The right to privacy achieved prominence beginning with the Supreme Court's landmark 1965 decision in *Griswold v. Connecticut* (1965), in which the court considered the constitutionality of a state law criminalizing the provision of contraception to married couples. In the early 1960s, Estelle Griswold, the executive director of the Planned Parenthood League of Connecticut, and one of her colleagues were convicted of aiding and abetting "the use of a drug, medicinal article, or instrument for the purpose of preventing conception" by providing contraceptives to a married couple in violation of Connecticut law. The court determined that although the Constitution does not explicitly protect a general right to privacy, certain provisions in the Bill of Rights create "penumbras," or zones, of guaranteed privacy, and that Connecticut's law constituted an undue intrusion into one of these zones (i.e., marriage).

After the *Griswold* decision, advocates of the constitutional right to privacy flooded the federal courts with cases designed to expand the scope of the right. Quickly, laws banning interracial marriage were struck down (*Loving v. Virginia*, 1967), as were laws prohibiting unmarried individuals from using contraception (*Eisenstadt v. Baird*, 1972). At the same time, federal courts were confronted with cases asking them to determine how the right to privacy applied in the context of abortion. The remainder of this section analyzes the courts' response to this particular issue. We selected the constitutional right to abortion as the focal point of the right to privacy discussion because it is not only one of the most contested rights in a health context, but also one of the most contested areas of public policy generally.

The *Roe v. Wade* Decision. Few judicial decisions have affected this country's legal, political, and social landscape as much as *Roe v. Wade* (1973).[f] In 1970, an unmarried pregnant woman filed a lawsuit under the pseudonym "Roe" challenging the constitutionality of a Texas criminal law that prohibited procuring or attempting an abortion at any stage of pregnancy, except for the purpose of saving the pregnant woman's life. Roe was joined in the lawsuit by a doctor who performed abortions in violation of the law. They argued that the constitutional right to privacy articulated in *Griswold* and its progeny included a woman's right to choose to obtain an abortion. Texas, through district attorney Henry Wade, claimed that the law was permissible because the state had a compelling interest in protecting women from an unsafe medical procedure and in protecting prenatal life. The federal trial court agreed with Roe and declared the law unconstitutional, and Texas immediately appealed to the U.S. Supreme Court, which agreed to hear the case (in rare circumstances, the Supreme Court will hear a case without an intermediate appellate court ruling).

At the Supreme Court, the work of drafting the majority opinion in *Roe v. Wade* fell to Justice Harry Blackmun, who earlier in his legal career had been counsel to a well-known and highly regarded medical clinic. By a 7–2 margin, the court ruled that the constitutional right to privacy, which in its view most strongly emanates from the 14th Amendment's due process protections, is broad enough to encompass a woman's decision to terminate her pregnancy.

Once the court established that a woman has a constitutional right to obtain an abortion, it went on to discuss the limits of that right. Roe had argued that the right to obtain an abortion is absolute and that no state or federal law abridging the right could be enacted. The court did not agree. Justice Blackmun wrote that states have both an interest in protecting the welfare of its citizens and a duty to protect them and that the duty extends to the unborn. According to the court, "a State may properly assert important interests in safeguarding health, in maintaining medical standards, and in protecting potential life. At some point in pregnancy, these respective interests become sufficiently compelling to sustain regulation of the factors that govern the abortion decision" (*Roe v. Wade*, 1973). The court then linked both a woman's "right to choose" and states' interest in protecting potential life to the viability of the fetus, setting forth the following "trimester framework" that enhances state power to regulate the abortion decision and restricts a pregnant woman's right as the fetus grows older:

a. For the stage prior to approximately the end of the first trimester, the abortion decision and its effectuation must be left to the medical judgment of the pregnant woman's attending physician.

b. For the stage subsequent to approximately the end of the first trimester, the State, in promoting its interest in the health of the mother, may, if it chooses, regulate the abortion procedure in ways that are reasonably related to maternal health.

c. For the stage subsequent to viability, the State, in promoting its interest in the potentiality of human life may, if it chooses, regulate, and even proscribe, abortion except where it is necessary, in appropriate medical judgment, for the preservation of the life or health of the mother. (*Roe v. Wade*, 1973)

As a matter of both policy and law, the Roe decision has been vigorously criticized (Barzelay & Heymann, 1973; Bopp & Coleson, 1989; Ely, 1979; Regan, 1979). For example, detractors claim that the court improperly made social policy by "finding" an expansive constitutional right to privacy (one broad enough to include the right to terminate a pregnancy) where one did not expressly exist. As a legal matter, many have argued that the decision relied too heavily on medical concepts that would be rendered obsolete as medical technology advanced and that would, in turn, result in a narrowing of the constitutional right advanced in the decision.[g]

Regardless of these and other criticisms, the *Roe* decision was monumental beyond its legal implications. It galvanized political forces opposed to abortion and prompted a movement to create ways to discourage the practice through state policies designed to regulate the factors involved in the abortion decision. For example, as described next, Pennsylvania enacted a law that imposed a series of requirements on women seeking abortion services, and it was this law that nearly 20 years after *Roe* set the stage for another battle at the Supreme Court over abortion and the right to privacy.

The *Planned Parenthood of Southeastern Pennsylvania v. Casey* Decision.

At issue in the 1992 case of *Planned Parenthood of Southeastern Pennsylvania v. Casey* were several amendments to Pennsylvania's Abortion Control Act that made it more difficult for a pregnant woman to obtain an abortion: One provision required that a woman seeking an abortion be provided with certain information at least 24 hours in advance of the abortion; a second stated that a minor seeking an abortion had to secure the informed consent of one of her parents, but included a "judicial bypass" option if the minor did not wish to or could not obtain parental consent; a third amendment required that a married woman seeking an abortion had to submit a signed statement indicating that she had notified her husband of her intent to have an abortion, although certain exceptions were included; and a final provision imposed new reporting requirements on facilities that offered abortion services. The revised law exempted compliance with these requirements in the event of a "medical emergency."

Before any of the new provisions took effect, they were challenged by five Pennsylvania abortion clinics and a group of physicians who performed abortions. The federal trial court struck down all of the provisions as unconstitutional violations under *Roe*. On appeal, the Third Circuit Court of Appeals reversed and upheld all of the provisions, except for the husband notification requirement, as constitutional. The plaintiffs appealed to the Supreme Court, which agreed to hear the case.

The court's 5–4 decision in favor of the plaintiffs in *Casey* expressly acknowledged the widespread confusion over the meaning and reach of *Roe*, and it used its opinion in *Casey* to provide better guidance to legislatures seeking to regulate abortion as a constitutionally protected right. Specifically, the court in *Casey* sought to define more precisely both the constitutional rights of pregnant women and the legitimate authority of states to regulate some aspects of the abortion decision. The deeply divided court wrote the following:

> It must be stated at the outset and with clarity that *Roe*'s essential holding, the holding we reaffirm, has three parts. First is a recognition of the right of the woman to choose to have an abortion before viability and to obtain it without undue interference from the State. Before viability, the State's interests are not strong enough to support a prohibition of abortion or the imposition of a substantial obstacle to the woman's effective right to elect the procedure. Second is a confirmation of the State's power to restrict abortions after fetal viability, if the law contains exceptions for pregnancies which endanger the woman's life or health. And third is the principle that the State has legitimate interests from the outset of the pregnancy in protecting the health of the woman and the life of the fetus that may become a child. These principles do not contradict one another; and we adhere to each. (*Planned Parenthood of Southeastern Pennsylvania v. Casey*, 1992)

Notice how, in interpreting *Roe*, the court in *Casey* makes some remarkable alterations to the contours of the right to choose to have an abortion. First, trimesters were replaced by fetal viability as the regulatory touchstone. Second, the pregnant woman, not her attending physician, makes the abortion decision. Third, a state's interest in protecting pregnant women and fetuses now attaches "from the outset of the pregnancy," not at the beginning of the second trimester. Fourth, and perhaps most important, the court's invalidation of the trimester framework enabled the establishment of a new "undue burden" standard for assessing the constitutionality of state abortion regulations. Under this new standard, a state may not prohibit abortion prior to fetal viability, but it may promulgate abortion regulations as long as they do not pose a "substantial obstacle" to a woman seeking to terminate a pregnancy. The court did not, however, alter its decision in *Roe* that, post-viability, a state may proscribe abortion except when pregnancies endanger a woman's life or health. Taken together, these alterations both maintain a pregnant woman's basic constitutional right to obtain an abortion pre-viability and enhance state interest in protecting the potentiality for human life.

Once the court established the undue burden standard for assessing the constitutionality of state abortion regulations, it applied the standard to each constitutionally questionable amendment to Pennsylvania's Abortion Control Act. In the end, only the spousal notification provision was struck down as an unconstitutional burden; the court determined that some pregnant women may have sound reasons for not wishing to inform their husbands of their decision to obtain an abortion, including fear of abuse, threats of future violence, and withdrawal of financial support. As a result, the court equated the spousal notification requirement to a substantial obstacle because it was likely to prevent women from obtaining abortions.

The court majority in *Casey* provided a new template for lower courts to use in deciding the constitutionality of state abortion regulations. Likewise, the opinion offered guidance to state legislatures regarding what kinds of abortion restrictions were likely to withstand a constitutional attack. Nonetheless, some state legislatures have tested the boundaries of *Casey* by enacting bans on a procedure known as "partial birth" abortion, an issue to which we now turn.

The *Stenberg v. Carhart* Decision.

The undue burden standard articulated in *Casey* for assessing the constitutionality of abortion regulations was put to the test in *Stenberg v. Carhart* (2000). At issue in the case was a Nebraska criminal law banning "an abortion procedure in which the person performing the abortion partially delivers vaginally a living unborn child before killing the unborn child and completing the delivery." It further defined "partially delivers vaginally a living unborn child before killing the unborn child" to mean "deliberately and intentionally delivering into the vagina a living unborn child, or a substantial portion thereof, for the purpose of performing a procedure that the person performing such procedure knows will kill the unborn child and does kill the unborn child." The Nebraska law penalized physicians who performed a banned abortion procedure with a prison term of up to 20 years, a fine of up to $25,000, and the automatic revocation of the doctor's license to practice medicine in Nebraska.

Dr. Leroy Carhart, a Nebraska physician who performed abortions, filed a lawsuit seeking a declaration that the Nebraska law violated the constitutional principles set forth in *Roe* and *Casey*. After a lengthy trial, a federal district court agreed with Dr. Carhart and declared the Nebraska law unconstitutional. The Court of Appeals for the Eighth Circuit agreed, concluding that Nebraska's statute violated the Constitution as interpreted by the Supreme Court in *Casey*. The Supreme Court then granted review.

The court was unequivocal in its opinion in *Stenberg* that the case was not a forum for a discussion on the propriety of *Roe* and *Casey*, but rather an application of the rules stated in those cases. In applying the undue burden standard to pre-viability abortions, the court considered trial court testimony from expert witnesses regarding several different abortion procedures that were then current in medical practice to flesh out the procedures' technical distinctions and to determine whether the procedures fell within Nebraska's definition of "partial birth" abortion. The court determined that two distinct abortion procedures were relevant—dilation and evacuation (D&E), and dilation and extraction (D&X)—and that the Nebraska law's vague definition of "partial birth" abortion effectively banned both procedures.

Again by a 5–4 majority, the Supreme Court struck down the Nebraska law as unconstitutional on two separate grounds. First, the court concluded that the statute created an undue burden on women seeking pre-viability abortions. The court reasoned that banning the most commonly used method for pre-viability second trimester abortions—the D&E procedure—unconstitutionally burdened a woman's ability to choose to have an abortion. Second, the court invalidated the state law because it lacked an exception for the preservation of the health of the pregnant woman. The court rejected Nebraska's claim that the banned procedures were never necessary to maintain the health of the pregnant woman and held that "significant medical authority" indicated that the D&X procedure is in some cases the safest abortion procedure available.

At the time *Stenberg* was decided, nearly 30 states had laws restricting D&E- and D&X-type abortions in some manner. Attempts to enact bans on these abortion procedures, however, have not been made only by state legislatures. Congress has tried numerous times to promulgate a federal ban, and after *Stenberg* was handed down, congressional opponents to abortion vowed to craft a ban that would pass constitutional muster. This effort culminated in the Partial Birth Abortion Ban Act of 2003 (PBABA).

Partial Birth Abortion Ban Act of 2003.
PBABA represented Congress's third attempt since 1996 to ban "partial birth" abortions. Previous bills were vetoed by President Bill Clinton in 1996 and 1997, but in late 2003, PBABA easily passed both houses of Congress and was signed into law by President George W. Bush. Immediately, the constitutionality of PBABA was challenged in federal court, and the Supreme Court ultimately decided the law's fate in 2007, as described here.

PBABA establishes criminal penalties for "any physician who . . . knowingly performs a partial birth abortion and thereby kills a human fetus." Attempting to avoid the definitional vagueness that affected the Nebraska law's constitutionality, the drafters of the federal law used more precise language in an effort to ban only D&X procedures, although PBABA does not specifically refer to any medical procedure by name. Instead, the law defines a "partial birth" abortion as

> an abortion in which the person performing the abortion deliberately and intentionally vaginally delivers a living fetus until, in the case of a headfirst presentation, the entire fetal head is outside the body of the mother, or, in the case of a breech presentation, any part of the fetal trunk past the navel is outside the body of the mother, for the purpose of performing an overt act that the person knows will kill the partially delivered living fetus. (PBABA, 2003)

PBABA contains an exception allowing for these otherwise illegal abortions when necessary to protect a pregnant woman's life, but not health. The law's authors claim that the banned procedure is never necessary to protect the health of a pregnant woman and thus that an exception is not required.

Separate lawsuits challenging PBABA were filed in federal courts in California, Nebraska, and New York. All three federal trial courts concluded that the lack of a health exception necessarily rendered the law unconstitutional under Supreme Court precedent. With enforcement of PBABA halted, the federal government appealed all three cases. The appellate courts that examined PBABA all found that substantial medical authority exists supporting the necessity of the banned procedure and declared PBABA unconstitutional because of its lack of a health exception. As noted, the fate of PBABA was then decided by the Supreme Court.

The *Gonzales v. Carhart* Decision.
The Supreme Court upheld the constitutionality of the PBABA in *Gonzales v. Carhart*, another 5–4 decision. The court rejected the reasoning of the appellate courts and found that PBABA was not on its face "void for vagueness" (a doctrine that permits courts to reject statutes under which a layperson could not generally understand who is being regulated or what is being prohibited) and did not pose an undue burden on the right to receive an abortion under *Casey*. Although the court reaffirmed again the various basic principles of *Roe* and *Casey*—that women have an unfettered right

to an abortion pre-viability, that the government has the power to restrict abortions post-viability, and that the government has an interest from the outset of pregnancy in protecting the health of the woman and the fetus—the court in *Carhart* focused on the latter and held that the government's legitimate interest in promoting fetal life would be hindered if the act was invalidated.

The court first ruled that PBABA was not void for vagueness simply because the law prohibits performing intact D&Es. According to the court, the law puts doctors on notice of the prohibited conduct by adequately describing the intact D&E procedure and requiring that the doctors have knowledge that they are performing the intact D&E for the purpose of destroying the fetus. The court also found that PBABA did not impose an undue burden for being overly broad. To distinguish it from the Nebraska law in *Stenberg*, the court majority stated that PBABA targets extraction of the entire fetus, as opposed to the removal of fetal pieces beyond a specific anatomic point in the pregnant woman.

The court then held that PBABA did not pose a "substantial obstacle" to obtaining an abortion under *Casey*'s undue burden test. According to the court, the ban on partial birth abortions furthers the government's interest in protecting fetal life and the government has the ability to prohibit practices ending fetal life that are similar to condemned practices. Finally, in a major shift that received relatively little attention by the court majority, the court ruled that the fact that PBABA did not contain language protecting the health of the woman did not render the law unconstitutional. Deferring to Congress because there are other safe procedures besides intact D&E that a doctor may use to perform an abortion and because according to the court PBABA promotes fetal life, the court simply declared the law constitutional notwithstanding the missing language. (See **Box 6.4**.)

The Right to Be Free from Wrongful Discrimination

We now transition to the final topic in the discussion of individual legal rights to and

within health care—namely, the topic of healthcare discrimination.[h] Like discrimination generally, healthcare discrimination has a lurid and lengthy history in this country. Prior to the *Brown v. Board of Education* decision in 1954 and the civil rights movement of the 1960s, healthcare injustice and exclusion based on race and other factors were commonplace, dating to slavery times and plantation-based racially segregated health care. After the end of the First Reconstruction, states passed so-called Jim Crow laws, cementing in place legally segregated health care. As a result, hospitals, physician practices, medical/nursing/dental schools, and professional medical societies were all separated based on race. In places where Jim Crow laws had not been passed, corporate bylaws and contracts between private parties often had the same discriminatory effect, and these "Jim Crow substitutes" were generally honored and enforced by the courts that interpreted them.

Federal law also played a role in perpetuating racially segregated health care. For example, the Hospital Survey and Construction Act of 1946 (more commonly known as the Hill–Burton Act, after the key congressional sponsors of the measure) provided federal money to states to build and refurbish hospitals after World War II, but explicitly sanctioned the construction of segregated facilities:

> A hospital will be made available to all persons residing in [its] territorial area . . . without discrimination on account of race, creed, or color, but an exception shall be made in cases where separate hospital facilities are provided for separate population groups, if the plan makes equitable provision on the basis of need for facilities and services of like quality for each such group. (Hospital Survey and Construction Act, 1946)

This provision was not ruled unconstitutional until the 1963 case of *Simkins v. Moses H. Cone Memorial Hospital*, which has been referred to as the "*Brown v. Board of Education* of health care" (Smith, 1999). *Simkins* also helped fuel the passage of the Civil Rights Act of 1964, this country's most important civil rights legislation of the 20th century. For purposes of health care, Title VI of the 1964 Act was of specific importance. Title VI is discussed in more depth later in this chapter; in sum, this portion of the Civil Rights Act makes it illegal for programs and activities that receive federal funding to discriminate on the basis of race, color, or national origin.

Box 6.4 DISCUSSION QUESTION

If you were asked to distill, down to their most essential parts, the constitutional right to privacy and the right to privacy as it applies to abortion, what elements would you include?

Notwithstanding the healthcare rewards brought about by the civil rights movement—Title VI, the passage of Medicaid and Medicare, the establishment of federally financed community health centers—the focus on healthcare civil rights was waning as early as 1968. Several factors led to this decline, but what is most striking is that compared to the progress made by public and private civil rights efforts over the past 45 years in education, employment, and housing, civil rights enforcement in the healthcare field has been anything but sustained.

Of course, even an enduring and well-funded enforcement effort is no guarantee of wiping out discrimination, regardless of its social context. There are, unfortunately, vestiges of discrimination in many important aspects of American society, including the healthcare system. Moreover, although historically healthcare discrimination on the basis of race and ethnicity has received the most attention, the existence of discrimination in health care on the basis of socioeconomic status, disability, age, and gender also raises troubling questions. The remainder of this section touches briefly on each of these areas, describing laws (where applicable) or legal theories used to combat the particular healthcare discrimination at issue.

Race/Ethnicity Discrimination

The fact that healthcare discrimination premised on race or ethnicity has dominated the healthcare civil rights landscape should not be surprising, because racist beliefs and customs have infected health care no less so than other areas of life, such as education, employment, and housing. This fact is chronicled to a staggering degree by W. Michael Byrd and Linda A. Clayton, two physician-researchers at the Harvard School of Public Health (2000, 2002). Byrd and Clayton paint a complex and disturbing picture of a healthcare system that itself perpetuates racism in health care in three distinct ways: by not destroying the myth that minority Americans should be expected to experience poorer health relative to Caucasians; by organizing itself as a private, for-profit system that marginalizes the indigent and minorities; and by refusing to acknowledge the historical and ongoing problem of racial exclusion in health care.

One key problem that in part results from the design of the healthcare system is that of racial and ethnic health disparities—differences in healthcare access, treatment, and outcomes between populations of color and Caucasians. In 2003, the National Academy of Medicine (then known as the Institute of Medicine) released an influential report that included overwhelming evidence of racial and ethnic health disparities and documented that these disparities could not be explained solely by the relative amount of health care needed by populations of color and nonminority populations (Smedley et al., 2003). For example, the report concluded that African Americans are relatively less likely to receive treatment for early-stage lung cancer, publicly insured Latinos and African Americans do not receive coronary artery bypass surgery at rates comparable to publicly insured nonminorities, and Latino and African American children on Medicaid experience relatively higher rates of hospitalization.

Furthermore, the study revealed that even when relevant patient characteristics are controlled for, racial and ethnic differences arise not only in terms of accessing care initially, but also after individuals have entered the healthcare system, a finding that supports the notion that both the system itself and physician practice style contribute to disparities. This notion is, of course, quite controversial, because it suggests that physician decision-making and clinical practice can increase the likelihood of racially disparate outcomes.

The key federal law used to combat race and ethnicity discrimination in health care is Title VI of the 1964 Civil Rights Act, which states that "no person in the United States shall, on the ground of race, color, or national origin, be excluded from participation in, be denied the benefits of, or be subjected to discrimination under any program or activity receiving federal financial assistance." Because it attaches only to recipients of federal funding, Title VI does not reach, for example, health professionals who do not directly participate in government-sponsored health programs; nor does it reach physicians whose only participation in federal assistance programs is under Medicare Part B (the basis for this exemption is historical and purely political, and the exemption is not codified in Title VI statutory or regulatory law [Smith, 1999, pp. 115–128]). Nonetheless, Title VI has long had the potential to greatly impact the field of health care, because an enormous amount of federal funding has been poured into the healthcare enterprise over the past 50 years.

The concept of "discrimination" under Title VI applies both to *intentional* acts and to actions or policies that unintentionally have the *effect* of discriminating against racial and ethnic minorities. This is so because federal regulations implementing the Title VI statute (which explicitly prohibits only intentional discrimination) reach actions that, even if neutral on their face, have a disproportionate adverse impact (or effect) on members of minority groups. In the case of healthcare access and delivery, you can imagine several types of conduct that might potentially violate the Title VI disproportionate impact regulations. For example, were a hospital to segregate patients by source of payment—say, by maintaining a ward or floor that treated only patients covered under Medicaid—racial and ethnic minorities may be adversely impacted, given the overall makeup of the Medicaid population. Similarly, the Title VI regulations could be violated if a managed care organization enrolled both privately and publicly insured persons but allowed participating providers to refuse to accept as patients those individuals covered by Medicaid.

The disproportionate impact regulations are crucial to realizing Title VI's full force, because much of the racism in post-1954 America does not take the form of overt, intentional acts. However, as a result of the 2001 Supreme Court decision in *Alexander v. Sandoval*, these regulations were severely undercut. Under *Alexander*, private individuals were barred from bringing a lawsuit under the disparate impact regulations, leaving the federal government as the sole enforcer when racial or ethnic minorities allege a violation of the regulations.[i]

Physical and Mental Disability Discrimination

Like discrimination based on race or ethnicity, healthcare discrimination premised on disability has a long, sad history in this country and, as with race, the health system itself is partly to blame for its perpetuation. For instance, historically, persons with mental disabilities were viewed from a medical standpoint as having little to offer to society, and they were, as a matter of practice, shipped to mental asylums isolated from communities. Those with physical disabilities were not spared discriminatory practices, either; because individuals with Down syndrome were viewed by medical practitioners as "Mongoloid idiots" and children with cerebral palsy or other serious physical limitations were regularly viewed as unable to contribute to society, they were all simply institutionalized. These historical practices and perspectives resonate even in the modern healthcare system, in which treatment opportunities for the disabled are skewed toward institutional, rather than community, settings, and disease-specific limitations in health insurance are commonplace.

However, passage of the Americans with Disabilities Act (ADA) in 1990 alleviated at least some of the problems associated with disability discrimination in health care. Like Title VI, the ADA is not specifically a "health law"; its intent is to extend to the disabled the maximum opportunity for community integration in many sectors of society, including employment, public services, public accommodations (i.e., privately owned entities open to the public), telecommunications, and more. For this reason, it prohibits discrimination generally against disabled individuals who satisfy the essential requirements of a particular job, or who meet the qualification standards for a program, service, or benefit.

But the ADA's impact on health care for disabled individuals is notable, in large part because the law defines "places of public accommodation" to include private hospitals and other private healthcare providers. So, for example, a dentist in private practice who does not receive any federal funds for his services is nonetheless prohibited from discriminating against a person who is HIV-positive, as the well-known case of *Bragdon v. Abbott* (1998) makes clear. This represents an important expansion of federal disability law because prior to the ADA, only recipients of federal funds were proscribed from discriminating on the basis of disability. Note also how this expanded concept of public accommodations differs from Title VI of the Civil Rights Act, which still requires the receipt of federal money on the part of the offending entity to trigger protections for racial and ethnic minorities.

Although the ADA has dramatically altered the disability law landscape, it is not without limitations. For example, the regulations implementing the ADA's statutory text require entities that implement public programs and services to make only "reasonable modifications"—but not "fundamental alterations"—to those programs and services. Under the ADA, a fundamental alteration is one that would change the essential nature of a public program or service. Whether a requested change to a public program or service by a disabled individual amounts to a "reasonable" or a "fundamental" one is potentially determinative to the outcome of the request. Why? Because if a court determines that the request would alter the essential nature of the program or service at issue, it is powerless under the ADA to order the change. Another way of understanding this reasonable modification/fundamental alteration dichotomy is to recognize that fundamental alterations to public services—alterations that might actually be necessary to achieve at least the spirit of the ADA's loftiest goals and meet the expectations of a modern, enlightened society—could be made only by the political branches of government, not by the courts.

Another important limitation of the ADA (at least as it has been interpreted by most courts) is that it does not prohibit arbitrary insurance coverage limits attached to certain medical conditions. A stark example of this is found in the case of *Doe v. Mutual of Omaha Insurance Company* (1999), in which a federal appellate court ruled that a lifetime benefit limitation in a health insurance policy of $25,000 for AIDS or AIDS-related conditions did not violate the ADA, even though the very same policy set a $1 million lifetime limit for other conditions.

Socioeconomic Status Discrimination

Compared to race or disability discrimination in healthcare access and treatment, healthcare discrimination based on class gains little attention—even though socioeconomic status is independently associated with health status, and the negative effects of poverty on health and healthcare access are incontrovertible. Class-related healthcare discrimination can take many forms. For example, healthcare providers might refuse to accept as patients individuals who are covered under Medicaid, or low-income individuals might fall victim to the practice of redlining, which refers to discrimination based on geographical location when companies offer goods and services to consumers. (Although insufficient data exist to know the extent of redlining in healthcare-related goods and services, industries such as home health care, pharmaceuticals, and managed care have come under particular scrutiny [Perez, 2003].) Another example stems from the fact that healthcare providers (e.g., physician and dental practices, hospitals) sometimes elect to not operate in relatively poor communities, leaving residents of these communities at heightened risk for experiencing a shortage of adequate healthcare resources.

Gender Discrimination

Discrimination against women is also a problem in health care. This bias appears to be of particular concern in the area of coronary heart disease (Bess, 1995), in which delayed or disparate care could have severe consequences. While it may seem that gender discrimination in health care could be remedied under the Equal Protection Clause of the federal Constitution, Equal Protection claims are difficult to win because they require proof of both state action (a sufficient government connection to the discriminatory acts) and proximate causation (a cause-and-effect link between the discrimination and the harm suffered). Also, consider the fact that healthcare practitioners who receive federal funds cannot face suit under Title VI for even obvious gender discrimination, because Title VI's prohibitions relate only to race, color, and national origin discrimination.

Age Discrimination

Finally, the medical care system also seems to be biased against older adults. Just one of several disturbing facts on the treatment front is that older adults sometimes do not receive needed surgical care because health professionals wrongfully assume that the chances of recovery are not good (Smith, 1996). Another concern pertains to insurance coverage, in that many employers are attempting to rescind lifetime health coverage benefits to retired workers, even where the benefits had been promised as part of negotiated labor contracts. At first blush, this may not seem like a critical issue, because many retirees are at or beyond the age required for Medicare eligibility. However, some retirees are not yet 65 years old, a retiree's employer-sponsored benefits might provide more or different coverage than Medicare, and employer benefits might cover a retiree's dependents, which Medicare does not do.

ACA Section 1557

One final aspect of antidiscrimination law deserves mention. The ACA includes its own nondiscrimination provision, best known as Section 1557 (for its location in the ACA statute). Section 1557 prohibits discrimination on the basis of race, color, national origin, sex, age, or disability in specified health programs or activities. While it largely builds on existing federal civil rights laws by expanding their reach via the ACA, Section 1557 does represent the first time that federal law has broadly prohibited sex discrimination in health care. Specifically, Section 1557 extends its several nondiscrimination protections to (1) individuals participating in any health program or activity, *any part of which* receives funding from the federal government (an important declaration because it effectively bars private entities that participate in public programs from limiting their compliance only to certain areas or services); (2) individuals participating in any program or activity that is administered by the U.S. Department of Health and Human Services under Title I of the ACA, including the ACA's federally facilitated insurance marketplace (discussed in detail in a later chapter); and (3) individuals who purchase health insurance products through state-level ACA marketplaces (also discussed in more detail elsewhere). Importantly, Section 1557 makes clear that federal funding (or "federal financial assistance," as it is technically called) includes health insurance policies purchased with federal subsidies, meaning that Section 1557 applies, for example, to insurers that participate in Medicaid, Medicare, and the Children's Health Insurance Program.

Individual Rights in a Public Health Context

The discussion thus far has focused on healthcare legal rights that individuals can claim in the context of access, receipt of services, freedom of choice, and antidiscrimination. In each of these areas, however, the right claimed is not absolute. For example, EMTALA does not make illegal all transfers of indigent patients from private hospitals to public ones; rather, it requires that patients be medically stabilized before a transfer can occur. Even eminent civil rights laws do not provide blanket protections, because they might be triggered only where federal funding is present, or where the assistance requested would not fundamentally alter a government health program.

In this section, we consider restrictions on individual rights and liberties of a different sort: those that derive not from the limitations of specific laws, but rather from governmental police powers used to protect the general public's health and welfare. One simple way to think about individual rights in a public health context is to use a balancing approach; that is, what might the appropriate legal trade-offs be between private rights and public welfare? Public discussion of this trade-off intensified after the terrorist attacks of September 11, 2001, because many government actions taken in their wake—the passage of new laws, the tightening of existing regulations, the detainment of alleged terrorists—starkly raised the question of where to draw the line between individual autonomy and government authority to restrain that autonomy in the name of public welfare and national security. The attacks raised new questions relating to public health law as well, including whether the potential for a bioterrorist attack using smallpox should compel the federal government to vaccinate individuals—even against their will—against the virus in order to protect the public at large in the event of an attack.

Similarly, fierce debates about whether and how to restrict private rights at the expense of public benefit have continuously roiled the United States (and many other countries) since the emergence of the COVID-19 pandemic. The same questions—should government (whether local, state, tribal, or federal) restrain the liberty of private entities (whether individuals, businesses, religious institutions, etc.) in order to protect the broader public and, if so, does the government have the legal authority to do so?—have been debated at every stage of the pandemic. Stay-at-home orders, workplace requirements for essential workers, mandatory business closures, capacity limits, face coverings, vaccine mandates, and more have all been wrangled over with these questions in mind. More broadly, and not unlike what the nation experienced in the wake of the attacks on U.S. soil in 2001, the COVID-19 pandemic is raising questions about the solidity of long-standing American public health and public health law principles. More and more, state and federal courts appear willing to question public health powers; some governors and legislatures seem inclined to weaken the ability of their own health officials to combat COVID-19 and its ilk; in many communities, public sentiment turned against local public health leaders charged with enforcing COVID-19 restrictions, leading to unprecedented numbers of resignations and retirements from the public health workforce. While an in-depth exploration of COVID-19 regulations is beyond the scope of this textbook, and while it is unknowable at this time whether the COVID-19 pandemic will force a shift in the tectonic plates that have underpinned public health practice for the past 100 years, there is little doubt that these topics will animate classrooms across the country for years to come.

Overview of Police Powers

Police powers represent state and local government authority to require individual conformance with established standards of conduct. These standards are designed to promote and protect the public's health, safety, and welfare, and to permit government control of personal, corporate, and other private interests. The government's police powers are broad and take many forms. Healthcare professionals are required to obtain licenses from government agencies. Healthcare facilities face accreditation standards. Food establishments are heavily regulated. Employers are bound by numerous occupational health and safety rules. Businesses are constrained by pollution control measures. Tobacco products can be marketed in only certain ways. The purchase of guns is controlled, buildings have to abide by certain codes, motorcyclists must wear helmets. The list goes on and on.

The government's police powers are often invasive, a result that stems in part from the fact that the American colonies were battling multiple communicable diseases during the time of the writing of the Constitution, and its drafters were thus well aware of the need for pervasive governmental public health powers. At the same time, the government may not overreach when restricting private autonomy in the name of public health promotion and protection. For example, police powers cannot be used as a form of punishment, they cannot be used arbitrarily and capriciously, and they cannot be used for purposes unrelated to public health and welfare.

A key principle inherent to the use of police powers is that of coercion. This is so because, in a country founded upon the twin ideals of individualism and a limited government, many individuals and businesses do not respond kindly to being told to conform with public health regulations that limit their actions. For example, sometimes a public health concern (e.g., pollution) requires a response (enhanced governmental regulation) that may not be in the best economic interests of an implicated party (a refinery). This is not to say that individuals and businesses do not voluntarily assume responsibilities and measures that are in the public's interest. For instance, one effect of poor exercise habits—obesity—has enormous implications for the public's health and for national healthcare costs. As a result, the government would prefer that all individuals exercise for a minimum amount of time each week, but there is of course no law requiring this; rather, voluntarism is the guiding principle when it comes to personal exercise. Nonetheless, personal coercion and industrial regulation have long been adopted (and accepted) practices of public health officials, and all of the major communicable disease outbreaks have been combated with some combination of compulsory screening, examination, treatment, isolation, and quarantine programs.

The *Jacobson v. Massachusetts* Decision

The fact that government coercion can be justified by important public health goals does not answer the question of where to draw the line between personal/economic freedom on the one hand, and the public welfare on the other. This question was taken up by the Supreme Court in *Jacobson v. Massachusetts* (1905), perhaps the most famous public health law decision in the court's history and the one to which we alluded in the second factual scenario in Box 6.1 at the opening of this chapter.

The facts in *Jacobson* are straightforward enough. At the turn of the 20th century, the state of Massachusetts enacted a law granting local health boards the power to require vaccination when necessary to protect the public's health or safety. In 1902, the Cambridge Board of Health, in the throes of attempting to contain a smallpox outbreak, took the state up on its offer and issued an order requiring all adults in the city to be vaccinated against the disease. Henning Jacobson refused vaccination on the ground that he previously

suffered negative reactions to vaccinations. Jacobson was fined $5 for his refusal, a penalty upheld by the state's highest court. Jacobson appealed to the U.S. Supreme Court, setting the stage for a decision that, more than 100 years later, remains both controversial and at least symbolically forceful (Gostin, 2005).

Like the enduring tension between private interests and public welfare underpinning public health law generally, the *Jacobson* decision amounts to "a classic case of reconciling individual interests in bodily integrity with collective interests in health and safety" (Mariner et al., 2005). The 7–2 decision went the state's way, with the Supreme Court recognizing that police powers were generally broad enough to encompass forced vaccination. Responding to Jacobson's argument that the Massachusetts law impermissibly infringed on his constitutional right to liberty, the court wrote the following:

> The liberty secured by the Constitution of the United States to every person within its jurisdiction does not import an absolute right in each person to be, at all times and in all circumstances, wholly freed from restraint. There are manifold restraints to which every person is necessarily subject for the common good. On any other basis organized society could not exist with safety to its members. Society based on the rule that each one is a law unto himself would soon be confronted with disorder and anarchy. (*Jacobson v. Massachusetts*, 1905)

Due to this and other language used by the court in the decision, *Jacobson* is often described as sweepingly deferential to public health officials and their use of police powers. And without question, social compact theory (the idea that citizens have duties to one another and to society as a whole) animates the court's decision. However, the *Jacobson* decision also recognizes the individual liberties protected by the Constitution, and in fact requires a deliberative governmental process to safeguard these interests.

According to the *Jacobson* court, public health powers must be exercised in conformity with four standards in order to pass constitutional muster:

- The first standard, that of "public health necessity," requires that government use its police powers only in the face of a demonstrable public health threat.
- The second standard, termed "reasonable means," dictates that the methods used when exercising police powers must be designed in such a way as

to prevent or ameliorate the public health threat found to exist under the first standard.

- "Proportionality" is the third *Jacobson* standard; it is violated when a particular public health measure imposes a burden on individuals that is totally disproportionate to the benefit to be expected from the measure.

- Finally, and axiomatically, the public health regulation itself should not pose a significant health risk to individuals subject to it. This is the standard of "harm avoidance."

These standards have never been explicitly overturned, but it can be argued that they have at the very least been implicitly replaced, given that in the 100 plus years since *Jacobson* was decided, the Supreme Court has developed a much more complex approach to applying constitutional provisions to cases implicating individual autonomy and liberty. (See **Box 6.5**.)

💡 Box 6.5 DISCUSSION QUESTION

Jacobson v. Massachusetts is a product of the early 20th century, and the public health law principles supporting it are vestiges of an even earlier time. This, coupled with more than a century of subsequent civil liberties jurisprudence and societal and political shifts, has led some commentators to question whether *Jacobson* should retain its paradigmatic role in terms of the scope of government police powers. At the same time, other public health law experts call for *Jacobson*'s continued vitality, arguing that it is settled doctrine and a still-appropriate answer to the private interest/collective good question. What do you think?

The "Negative Constitution"

The discussion of police powers up to this point might reasonably lead you to believe that the Constitution *obligates* the government to protect the public's health and welfare through affirmative use of its powers. This view, however, has never been adopted by the Supreme Court. Instead, the prevailing view is that the Constitution *empowers* government to act in the name of public health, but does not require it to do so. This interpretation of the Constitution refers to what is known as the "negative constitution"—that is, the idea that the Constitution does not require government to provide any services, public health or otherwise. This approach to constitutional law derives from the fact that the Constitution is phrased mainly in negative terms (e.g., the First Amendment prohibits

government abridgment of free speech). Professor Wendy Parmet describes the "negative constitution" this way:

> In the century that has witnessed Auschwitz and Chernobyl, it is easy to see the dangers posed by state power. This recognition tempers enthusiasm for public authority and leads us to use law as a limiting device. In our legal tradition, this view of law is integral to constitutional structure, with its emphasis on separation of powers, checks and balances, procedural protections, and individual rights. We rely on the Constitution to limit the power of the government to restrain our freedoms and cause us harm. In this sense, law is a negative force that prevents the state from intruding upon the individual. This negative conception of law, which sees legal rights as a restraint upon the state, has played a dominant role in the formulation of contemporary American public health law. It explains the central pillars of constitutional public health law: the search for limits on governmental authority to restrain individual freedoms in the name of public health, and the concomitant assumption that government has no obligation to promote public health. (Parmet, 1993, pp. 267, 271)

In two important decisions, *DeShaney v. Winnebago County Department of Social Services* (1989) and *Town of Castle Rock, Colorado v. Gonzales* (2005), the Supreme Court has advanced this view of the negative constitution. In the former case, 1-year-old Joshua DeShaney was placed in his father's custody after his parents divorced. Two years later, the father's second wife complained to county officials in Wisconsin that the father had been abusing Joshua physically. Social service workers opened a file on the case and interviewed Joshua's father, but the county did not pursue the matter further after the father denied the charges. One year after that, an emergency department physician treating Joshua alerted social services of his suspicion that Joshua's injuries were the result of abuse. The county again investigated but decided that insufficient evidence of child abuse existed to remove Joshua from his father's custody. This emergency department scenario played out two additional times over the next several months, but Joshua's caseworkers still believed that they had no basis on which to place Joshua in court custody. Some months later, when Joshua was 4 years old, he suffered a beating so severe that he fell into a life-threatening coma. He survived but was left with permanent, severe brain damage, and he was expected to live his life in an institution for the profoundly mentally disabled. Joshua's father was subsequently convicted of child abuse.

Joshua's mother filed a civil rights claim on Joshua's behalf against the county officials who failed to take the boy into their custody. The lawsuit was based on the Due Process Clause of the federal Constitution, which prohibits states from depriving any person of property without due process of law. However, the Supreme Court in *DeShaney* concluded that the "substantive" component of the Due Process Clause—which focuses on challenges to government conduct—could not be read to provide Joshua with a property interest in having state child welfare officials protect him from beatings by his father. For a 6–3 majority, Chief Justice Rehnquist held that state officials had no affirmative constitutional duty to protect Joshua:

> Nothing in the language of the Due Process Clause itself requires the State to protect the life, liberty, and property of its citizens against invasion by private actors. The Clause is phrased as a limitation on the State's power to act, not as a guarantee of certain minimal levels of safety and security. It forbids the State itself to deprive individuals of life, liberty, or property without "due process of law," but its language cannot fairly be extended to impose an affirmative obligation on the State to ensure that those interests do not come to harm through other means. (*DeShaney*, 1989)

The majority further rejected the argument that the state's knowledge of the danger Joshua faced, and its expression of willingness to protect him against that danger, established a "special relationship" that gave rise to an affirmative constitutional duty to protect.

In dissent, three justices in *DeShaney* argued that through the establishment of its child protection program, the state of Wisconsin undertook a vital duty and effectively intervened in Joshua's life, and its failure to live up to its child protection duty amounted to a constitutional violation. According to the dissenters, the majority opinion "construes the Due Process Clause to permit a State to displace private sources of protection and then, at the critical moment, to shrug its shoulders and turn away from the harm that it has promised to try to prevent" (*DeShaney*, 1989).

Sixteen years after *DeShaney*, the Supreme Court in *Castle Rock v. Gonzales* had an opportunity to again consider whether the government has a duty to affirmatively protect its citizens. This time, however, the court was concerned not with substantive due process, but rather with procedural due process, which mandates that when a state establishes a benefit or right for its citizens, it is not entitled to deny individuals the benefit or right in an arbitrary or unfair way.

Unfortunately, the facts in *Gonzales* are as tragic as those in *DeShaney*. In May 1999, Jessica Gonzales received a court order protecting her and her three young daughters from her husband, who was also the girls' father. On June 22, all three girls disappeared in the late afternoon from in front of the Gonzales home, and Jessica suspected that her husband had taken them in violation of the restraining order. This suspicion was confirmed in a phone conversation she had with her husband. In two initial phone conversations with the Castle Rock Police Department, she was told there was nothing the police could do and to wait until 10:00 P.M. to see if her husband brought the girls home.

Shortly after 10:00 P.M., Jessica called the police to report that her children were still missing, but this time she was told to wait until midnight to see what transpired. She called the police again at midnight, reported that her children were still missing, and left her home to go to her husband's apartment. Finding nobody there, she called the police again at 12:10 A.M. and was told to wait for an officer to arrive. Thirty minutes later, after no officer showed up, she went to the police station to submit a report. According to the Supreme Court decision, the officer who wrote up the report "made no reasonable effort to enforce the [restraining order] or locate the three children. Instead, he went to dinner." A couple of hours later, Jessica's husband pulled his truck up to, and began shooting at, the Castle Rock Police Department. After he was killed by police during the gunfight, the three Gonzales daughters were found dead in the back of the truck; they had been murdered by their father hours earlier.

Jessica sued the police department, claiming that her constitutional right to procedural due process was violated by the department's inaction. She argued that the restraining order she received was her "property" under the Constitution's Due Process Clause and that it was effectively "taken" from her without due process. Overturning the federal appellate court that ruled in her favor, the Supreme Court decided by a 7–2 margin that Jessica did not have a property interest in police enforcement of the restraining order against her husband.

The court said it was not clear that *even if* it had found an individual entitlement to enforcement of a restraining order under a Colorado state statute requiring officers to use every reasonable means to enforce restraining orders, that this entitlement would constitute a protected "property" interest that triggers due process protections under the federal Constitution. Justice Antonin Scalia wrote that the Due Process Clause does not protect all government "benefits," including those things that government officials have discretion to grant or deny. Applying this standard, the court ruled that Colorado's protection order law did not create an individual entitlement to police enforcement of restraining orders, explaining that police have discretion to act or not act under many circumstances, including when to enforce a restraining order (e.g., police officers have discretion to consider whether a violation of a protection order is too "technical" or minor to justify enforcement). Furthermore, the court noted that if the Colorado legislature included statutory language making police enforcement of a restraining order "mandatory," even that would not necessarily mean that Mrs. Gonzales had a personal entitlement to its enforcement, given that the statute makes no mention of an individual's power to demand—or even request—enforcement.

In dissent, two justices in *Gonzales* argued that restraining orders amount to a personal, enforceable property interest. They asserted that the majority opinion wrongly ruled that a citizen's interest in government-provided police protection does not resemble a "traditional conception" of property. Looking to the legislative history and text of Colorado's own protection order law and to the purpose of the state's domestic violence legislation, the dissent concluded that a particular class of individuals were indeed entitled beneficiaries of domestic restraining orders. (See **Box 6.6**.)

Conclusion

This chapter offered a snapshot of the current state of health-related legal rights. But, as alluded to early on in the chapter, there were times in its relatively short history that this country was closer to recognizing broader individual healthcare rights than is currently the case, just as there have been times (as the aftermath of September 11, 2001, proved) when concerns for the public's health and safety have eclipsed the nation's more natural inclinations toward individualism and a deregulated marketplace. That this is so is of no surprise: Legal rights are, by nature, subject to

> **Box 6.6** DISCUSSION QUESTIONS

The "negative constitution" is a concept over which reasonable people can easily disagree. Notwithstanding the "defensive" manner of some of the Constitution's key provisions, there are several arguments in support of more affirmative action on the part of government health and welfare officials than current Supreme Court jurisprudence requires. For example, the dissent in *DeShaney* argues persuasively that Wisconsin's implementation of a child protection program effectively created a constitutional duty to actually protect children from seemingly obvious danger. As one leading scholar put it,

> If an agency represents itself to the public as a defender of health, and citizens justifiably rely on that protection, is government "responsible" when it knows that a substantial risk exists, fails to inform citizens so they might initiate action, and passively avoids a state response to that risk? (Gostin, 2000)

What do you think of this argument? Can you think of other arguments that call into question the soundness of the negative theory of constitutional law?

shifts in the political and social terrain. For example, the Aid for Families with Dependent Children program (commonly known as AFDC), the federal welfare entitlement program for low-income populations, was dismantled in 1996 after more than 60 years in existence. Originally enacted under a slightly different name as part of the New Deal in 1935, the AFDC was replaced with the Temporary Assistance for Needy Families (TANF) program by a moderate Democrat (President Bill Clinton) and a conservative, Republican-controlled Congress. Compared to the AFDC, TANF dramatically limited the receipt of individual benefits and focused much more heavily on creating work opportunities for needy families. Like legal rights generally, health-related legal rights are similarly subject to changing political currents. For example, many state legislatures approved bills in recent years that protect health professionals from providing care that conflicts with their personal beliefs, reflecting the current political power of social conservatives.[j]

Of course, changes to legal rights are not always represented by restrictions of those rights. The enactment of Medicaid and Medicare, which created new health-related rights, is an obvious example. Other major examples include EMTALA and expanded state consumer rights for persons in managed care. On a less noticed scale, legal rights for persons with HIV/AIDS have expanded since the 1980s (Halpern, 2004), and federal courts now review the constitutionality of the treatment provided in, and conditions of, psychiatric hospitals (*Wyatt v. Stickney*, 1972). These are just a few of many examples.

Nonetheless, vast challenges remain. After all, many scholars, politicians, and consumers point to the millions of uninsured Americans as just one example of not only a failing healthcare financing and delivery system, but also a failing of the legal system. To reduce this nation's huge uninsured population takes not just political will, but also an enormous undertaking to change the law, as witnessed with the ACA. A "rights revolution" in a health context, like other major legal upheavals, requires something else too—a substantial amount of general economic and social unrest (Friedman, 1971). As historian Brooks Adams once noted, "Law is merely the expression of the will of the strongest for the time being, and therefore laws have no fixity, but shift from generation to generation" (Nash & Zullo, 1995).

References

Alexander v. Sandoval, 532 U.S. 275 (2001).

Americans with Disabilities Act of 1990, 42 U.S.C. §§ 12101 *et seq.* (1990).

Annas, G. J. (2004). *The rights of patients* (3rd ed.). Southern Illinois University Press.

Barnes, A., & McChrystal, M. (1998). The various human rights in health care. *Human Rights*, 25, 12–14.

Barzelay, D. E., & Heymann, P. B. (1973). The forest and the trees: *Roe v. Wade* and its critics. *Boston University Law Review*, 53, 765–784.

Bess, C. J. (1995). Gender bias in health care: A life or death issue for women with coronary heart disease. *Hastings Women's Law Journal*, 6(1), 41–65.

Blum, J. D., Talib, N., Carstens, P., Nasser, M., Tomkin, D., & McAuley, A. (2003). Rights of patients: Comparative perspectives from five countries. *Medical Law Review*, 22(3), 451–471.

Bopp, J., & Coleson, R. (1989). The right to abortion: Anomalous, absolute, and ripe for reversal. *Brigham Young University Journal of Public Law*, 3(2), 181–355.

Bragdon v. Abbott, 524 U.S. 624 (1998).

Byrd, W. M., & Clayton, L. A. (2000). *An American health dilemma: A medical history of African Americans and the problem of race, beginnings to 1900.* Routledge.

Byrd, W. M., & Clayton, L. A. (2002). *An American health dilemma: Race, medicine, and health care in the United States, 1900–2000.* Routledge.

Canterbury v. Spence, 464 F.2d 772 (D.C. Cir. 1972).

Civil Rights Act of 1964, 42 U.S.C. §§ 2000d (1964).

Claiming Human Rights. (2010). *The Universal Declaration of human rights: Article 25.* http://www.claiminghumanrights.org/udhr_article_25.html

Davis, M. F. (1993). *Brutal need: Lawyers and the welfare rights movement, 1960–1973.* Yale University Press.

DeShaney v. Winnebago Cnty., 489 U.S. 189 (1989).

Doe v. Mutual of Omaha Insur. Co., 179 F.3d 557 (7th Cir. 1999), cert. denied, 528 U.S. 1106 (2000).

Eisenstadt v. Baird, 405 U.S. 438 (1972).

Ely, J. H. (1979). The wages of crying wolf: A comment on *Roe v. Wade*. *Yale Law Journal*, 82, 920–949.

Examination and Treatment for Emergency Medical Conditions and Women in Labor, 42 U.S.C. § 1395dd (2011).

Friedman, E. A., & Adashi, E. Y. (2010). The right to health as the unheralded narrative of health care reform. *Journal of the American Medical Association*, 304(23), 2639–2640.

Friedman, L. M. (1971). The idea of right as a social and legal concept. *Journal of Social Issues*, 27(2), 189–198.

Garrow, D. J. (1994). *Liberty and sexuality: The right to privacy and the making of* Roe v. Wade. University of California Press.

Gonzales v. Carhart, 550 U.S. 124 (2007).

Gostin, L. O. (2000). *Public health law: Power, duty, restraint.* University of California Press.

Gostin, L. O. (2005). *Jacobson v. Massachusetts* at 100 years: Police powers and civil liberties in tension. *American Journal of Public Health*, 95(4), 576–581.

Griswold v. Connecticut, 381 U.S. 479 (1965).

Halpern, S. A. (2004). Medical authority and the culture of rights. *Journal of Health Politics, Policy and Law*, 29(4–5), 835–852.

Hospital Survey and Construction Act of 1946, 42 U.S.C. § 291e(f) (1946).

Hurley v. Eddingfield, 59 N.E. 1058 (Ind. 1901).

Jacobson v. Massachusetts, 197 U.S. 11 (1905).

Jost, T. S. (2003). *Disentitlement? The threats facing our public health-care programs and a rights-based response.* Oxford University Press.

Kinney, E. D., & Clark, B. A. (2004). Provisions for health and health care in the constitutions of the countries of the world. *Cornell International Law Journal*, 37(2), 285–355.

Littell, A. (2002). Can a constitutional right to health guarantee universal health care coverage or improved health outcomes? A survey of selected states. *Connecticut Law Review*, 35(1), 289–318.

Loving v. Virginia, 388 U.S. 1 (1967).

Mariner, W. K., Annas, G. J., & Glantz, L. H. (2005). *Jacobson v. Massachusetts*: It's not your great-great-grandfather's public health law. *American Journal of Public Health*, 95(4), 581–590.

Nash, B., & Zullo, A. (Eds.). (1995). *Lawyer's wit and wisdom: Quotations on the legal profession, in brief.* Running Press.

Navarro, V., & Shi, L. (2003). The political context of social inequalities and health. In R. Hofrichter (Ed.), *Health and social justice: Politics, ideology, and inequity in the distribution of disease.* Jossey-Bass.

Parmet, W. (1993). Health care and the constitution: Public health and the role of the state in the framing era. *Hastings Constitutional Law Quarterly, 20*(2), 267–335.

Partial Birth Abortion Ban Act, 18 U.S.C. §§ 1531 (a)-(b) (2003).

Perez, T. E. (2003). The civil rights dimension of racial and ethnic disparities in health status. In B. D. Smedley, A. Y. Stith, & A. R. Nelson. (Eds.), *Unequal treatment: Confronting racial and ethnic disparities in health care* (pp. 626–663). The National Academies Press.

Planned Parenthood of Southeastern Pa. v. Casey, 505 U.S. 833 (1992).

President's Commission for the Study of Ethical Problems in Medicine and Biomedical and Behavioral Research. (1983). *Securing access to health care: A report on the ethical implications of differences in the availability of health services.* The National Academies Press.

Protection of Human Subjects, 45 C.F.R. Part 46 (2009).

Regan, D. H. (1979). Rewriting *Roe v. Wade. Michigan Law Review, 77,* 1569–1646.

Reinhardt, U. (1996). The debate that wasn't: The public and the Clinton health care plan. In H. Aaron (Ed.), *The problem that won't go away: Reforming U.S. health care financing* (pp. 70–109). Brookings Institution.

Rich, R. F. (2000). Health policy, health insurance and the social contract. *Comparative Labor Law Policy Journal, 21,* 397–421.

Roe v. Wade, 410 U.S. 113 (1973).

Rosenbaum, S. (2011). Realigning the social order: The Patient Protection and Affordable Care Act and the U.S. health insurance system. *Suffolk Journal of Health and Biomedical Law, 7,* 1–31.

Rosenbaum, S., & Teitelbaum, J. (2003). Civil rights enforcement in the modern healthcare system: Reinvigorating the role of the federal government in the aftermath of *Alexander v. Sandoval. Yale Journal of Health Policy, Law, and Ethics, 3*(2), 215–252.

Rosenblatt, R. E., Law, S. A., & Rosenbaum, S. (1997). *Law and the American health care system.* Foundation Press.

San Antonio Indep. School Dist. v. Rodriguez, 411 U.S. 1 (1973).

Simkins v. Moses H. Cone Memorial Hospital, 323 F.2d 959 (4th Cir. 1963).

Smedley, B. D., Stith, A. Y., & Nelson, A. R. (Eds.). (2003). *Unequal treatment: Confronting racial and ethnic disparities in health care.* The National Academies Press.

Smith, D. B. (1999). *Health care divided: Race and healing a nation.* University of Michigan Press.

Smith, G. P. (1996). Our hearts were once young and gay: Health care rationing and the elderly. *University of Florida Journal of Law and Public Policy, 8*(1), 1–23.

Smith, P. S. (1997). Addressing the plight of inner-city schools: The federal right to education after *Kadrmas v. Dickinson Public Schools. Whittier Law Review, 18,* 825–835.

Stacy, T. (1993). The courts, the Constitution, and a just distribution of health care. *Kansas Journal of Law and Public Policy, 3,* 77–94.

Starr, P. (1982). *The social transformation of American medicine: The rise of a sovereign profession and the making of a vast industry.* Basic Books.

Stein, R. (2006, January 30). Health workers' choice debated: Proposals back right not to treat. *Washington Post.* http://www.washingtonpost.com/wp-dyn/content/article/2006/01/29/AR2006012900869.html

Stenberg v. Carhart, 530 U.S. 914 (2000).

Teitelbaum, J. B. (2005). Health care and civil rights: An introduction. *Ethnicity and Disease, 15*(2 Suppl. 2), 27–30.

Town of Castle Rock, Colorado v. Gonzales, 545 U.S. 748 (2005).

Vladeck, B. (2003). Universal health insurance in the United States: Reflections on the past, the present, and the future. *American Journal of Public Health, 93*(1), 9–16.

Wailoo, K., & Schlesinger, M. (2004). Transforming American medicine: A twenty-year retrospective on *The Social Transformation of American Medicine. Journal of Health Politics, Policy, and Law, 29*(4–5), 1005–1019.

Wing, K. R. (1993). The right to health care in the United States. *Annals of Health Law, 2,* 161–193.

World Health Organization. (2006). *Constitution of the World Health Organization.* http://www.who.int/governance/eb/who_constitution_en.pdf

Wyatt v. Stickney, 344 F. Supp. 373 (M.D. Ala. 1972).

Yamin, A. E. (2005). The right to health under international law and its relevance to the United States. *American Journal of Public Health, 95*(7), 1156–1161.

Endnotes

a. These competing concepts were given life in Paul Starr's influential 1982 book, *The Social Transformation of American Medicine: The Rise of a Sovereign Profession and the Making of a Vast Industry.* Incidentally, *The Social Transformation of American Medicine* should be read by all students with an interest in the history of medicine; the book's significance across a range of disciplines is hard to overstate. See Wailoo and Schlesinger, 2004.

b. For an interesting article describing the importance of political structures in determining the level of equalities/inequalities in a society, including the level of government-provided healthcare coverage, see Navarro and Shi, 2003.

c. Incidentally, the *Canterbury* decision was authored by Spottswood Robinson III, who, prior to becoming a highly regarded federal judge, was instrumental in the fight for civil rights, in part as one of the National Association for the Advancement of Colored People (NAACP) lawyers who initially brought suit in one of the cases that eventually morphed into *Brown v. Board of Education.*

d. A now-famous 1890 *Harvard Law Review* article titled "The Right to Privacy," written by Samuel Warren and Louis Brandeis, is often credited with introducing the constitutional "right to be let alone."

e. In a health context, this type of privacy is embodied by the Health Insurance Portability and Accountability Act (HIPAA) of 1996, found in large part at 29 U.S.C. §§ 1181–1187, 42 U.S.C. §§ 300gg *et seq.* and 42 U.S.C. §§ 1320a *et seq.*, which creates a federal right to maintain the confidentiality of one's personal health information.

f.   For a compelling look at what the case has meant to society, see Garrow, 1994.

g.   For example, notice how the Supreme Court linked states' power to ban abortions (with certain exceptions) to fetal viability, even though the progression of medical knowledge and technology could push back the point of viability earlier into pregnancy. Also, who appears to hold the power, under "(a)," to decide whether an abortion should occur? The *physician*, a fact often overlooked by those who hail *Roe* as a seminal women's rights case and one that calls into question how the pregnant

woman's constitutional right to privacy could be effectuated by her treating physician.

h.   This section was adapted from Teitelbaum, 2005.

i.   For a discussion of the implications of the *Alexander* decision in a healthcare context, see Rosenbaum and Teitelbaum, 2003.

j.   These bills represent a

> surge of legislation that reflects the intensifying tension between asserting individual religious values and defending patients' rights. . . . The flurry of political activity is being welcomed by conservative groups that consider it crucial to prevent health workers from being coerced into participating in care they find morally repugnant—protecting their "right of conscience" or "right of refusal." (Stein, 2006)

CHAPTER 7

Structural and Social Drivers of Health and the Role of Law in Optimizing Health

LEARNING OBJECTIVES

By the end of this chapter you will be able to:

1. Describe the significance of structural and social drivers on individual and population health
2. Describe how law can create or perpetuate health-harming social, economic, and environmental conditions
3. Explain how law can be used to ameliorate health-harming social, economic, and environmental conditions
4. Understand how innovative interventions to improve health, such as medical–legal partnership, can help address health-harming social, economic, and environmental conditions at the individual and population levels

> ### 📝 Box 7.1 VIGNETTE
>
> Living through brief periods without heat or electricity is a fact of life for most of us, perhaps as a result of a powerful weather system or a blown generator. But have you experienced or considered what it would be like to be without heat or electricity more chronically, due to homelessness, inadequate housing, or an unscrupulous landlord who neglects a property without concern for tenants? Even for the healthiest among us, a persistent utility concern would be incredibly challenging; for those with chronic illness, it can mean increased asthma attacks, severe pain associated with sickle cell disease, an inability to refrigerate needed medicine, and much more, including death. Indeed, factors such as homelessness, dilapidated homes, slum landlords—and many others—have nothing to do with biology, genetics, personal choice, or access to healthcare services, but they have a great deal to do with individual and population health.

Introduction

Disparities in health and health care are a systemic and deeply challenging problem in the United States (Smedley et al., 2003). While related, the two terms have different meanings. A *health* disparity exists when one population group experiences a higher burden of disability or illness relative to another group; a *healthcare* disparity, by contrast, tends to denote differences in access to healthcare services or health insurance, or in the quality of care actually received (Kaiser Family Foundation, 2012). What makes both types of disparities so invidious—and a major social justice concern—is that they can exist even when patient needs or treatment recommendations do not differ across populations (Hoffman et al., 2016). Furthermore, health and healthcare disparities appear through many different lenses; researchers have documented disparities based on race, ethnicity, socio-economic status, age, geography, language, gender, disability status, citizenship status, sexual identity and orientation, and more. As long as these disparities exist, a society cannot achieve what is known as *health equity*—a situation in which everyone has the opportunity to attain their full health potential.

Many different drivers contribute to health and healthcare disparities. For example, individual behaviors, healthcare provider bias, cultural expectations and differences, the location and financing of healthcare systems, local/state/national politics, and more can all be contributors. So, too, are public policies. For instance, the United States spends less than 3% of its overall health spending on public health and disease prevention, and it spends far less on nonmedical social services (e.g., housing and food programs, support services for older adults, disability and sickness benefits, employment programs, unemployment benefits, homeless shelters, utility assistance programs) than do other high-income countries. On average, nations that are members of the Organisation for Economic Cooperation and Development (OECD, a multinational organization that strives to fight poverty and achieve economic growth and employment in member countries) spend about $1.70 on social services for every $1 spent on health services; the United States spends just $0.56 in comparison. As it turns out, the former ratio is significantly associated with better population health outcomes, including less infant mortality, less premature death, longer life expectancy, fewer low-birth-weight babies, and more (Bradley et al., 2011). At the same time, despite spending two to three times more per capita on direct healthcare services than nearly all of our European counterparts, the United

States has significantly worse health outcomes in many respects, particularly among the poorest individuals and families (Tobin-Tyler, 2012).

In fact, a robust collection of evidence both globally and nationally shows that public policies targeting social, economic, and environmental factors can account for sizable reductions in morbidity and mortality (Gostin et al., 2011). Similarly, a generous body of evidence indicates that these types of drivers—factors not directly tied to individual behaviors, healthcare access, healthcare provider regulation, or the like—are far more influential on individual and population health than are things most people generally consider to be health related. These bodies of evidence reflect a simple truth: More than anything else, the *context* of people's lives determines their health and well-being. This truism is described in more detail next, with a distinction drawn between "structural" drivers of health (root causes) and "social" drivers of health (the social conditions that result from root causes). Before turning to that distinction, consider the discussion questions in **Box 7.2**.

Structural Drivers of Health

According to the federal Centers for Disease Control and Prevention (CDC; 2013), there are various drivers of health that combine to create a person's current state of health. Included within this broad definition are biological factors (e.g., carrying a genetic mutation that could increase one's chances of developing a particular disease, such as sickle cell anemia), psychosocial factors (e.g., conflicts within one's family that may lead to stress, anger, and/or depression), behavioral factors (e.g., alcohol/drug use, smoking, unprotected sex), and structural and social factors. Structural drivers of health are interchangeably referred to as "root," "upstream," or "top-level" causes of population-level health inequities because they include things like the nation's system of governance, laws and other public policies (in areas such as housing, education, working

> **Box 7.2** DISCUSSION QUESTIONS
>
> Do you think trying to achieve wide-scale health equity is a laudable goal? Why or why not? If yes, what do you think are the keys to achieving it? And what about people who are given the opportunity to achieve optimal health but do not take advantage of it; should they face consequences of some sort?

conditions, the minimum wage, etc.), the manner in which public institutions and systems operate, and cultural norms and practices.

There are a few important aspects of structural drivers that must be called out (examples of each aspect are provided in **Box 7.3**). First, of all the various drivers of health, structural ones should be thought of as those that actually design how society operates. As a result, structural drivers—and the individuals, groups, and political parties that control them—shape the distribution of power, health-promoting resources, and health-promoting opportunities across the American population. Put simply, structural drivers determine whether power, resources, and opportunities are equally distributed, or whether they are unjustly distributed based on characteristics such as race, ethnicity, gender, social class, geography, or sexual identity or orientation. Second, and relatedly, structural drivers are generally outside the direct control of individuals. This essentially means that at the individual level, there may be no amount of political engagement, knowledge, or health-promoting behavior that will actually make someone physically, mentally, or emotionally healthier—the structural barriers to good health and well-being may simply be impossible to overcome.

A third crucial aspect of structural drivers is that some of the nation's laws, policies, institutions, systems, norms, and practices date back to the founding of the country, which is to say that some current structural drivers of health remain rooted in a time marked by overt, legally sanctioned racism and discrimination. Indeed, America's earliest social mores, economic systems, and laws were conceived during an era of genocide, enslavement, and legalized racial oppression, as North America colonizers tortured Native Americans and African Americans alike. As barbaric as this treatment was, its long-term consequences have been equally damaging: centuries of race-based prejudice, discrimination, and injustice that flow from laws, policies, and societal practices that perpetuate and operationalize the myth that People of Color are inferior to White people. This is called *structural racism*, and it remains a devastating driver of health even today, as racialized laws, policies, and practices are carried through generations, perpetually relegating People of Color—Black people, in particular—to a lower social, financial, educational, and health status relative to White people. Structural racism refers, quite literally, to discrimination that is woven into the fabric of society, and it has left an indelible mark on the health of People of Color who have been systematically excluded from the health-promoting resources and opportunities necessary for maximal health outcomes (Tobin-Tyler & Teitelbaum, 2019).

Social Drivers of Health

If structural drivers of health are the methods and tools utilized by those in power to shape society and distribute resources and opportunities, then social drivers of health are the *actual conditions and material*

Box 7.3 Three Important Aspects of Structural Drivers of Health: Examples

1. Structural drivers help determine how society operates. For example, at the time of this writing—just 6 months after the 2020 election cycle—lawmakers in 47 states have introduced nearly 400 bills aiming to restrict voting rights (primarily in the areas of absentee voting, ID requirements, voter registration, the power of local election officials, and early voting). Where these bills are enacted into law, they will likely disproportionately burden People of Color and people with disabilities—groups of voters who historically have been suppressed from having their voices heard on important health and other matters.
2. Structural drivers are generally outside the direct control of individuals. For example, few individuals can control public policies concerning how robustly to subsidize health insurance premiums or education services, or officials' decisions about where to store and release toxic substances, or rules about working conditions at private companies.
3. The effects of structural drivers conceived during a time when race discrimination was legally sanctioned can still be felt today. For example, long-standing structural racism in the U.S. housing system has contributed to racial wealth (and thus health) disparities, especially between Black and White households. One form of structural racism in housing was "redlining," a commonplace practice from the 1930s through the 1960s in which federal agencies would draw red lines around portions of a map to indicate areas or neighborhoods considered to be poor financial risks. In turn, mortgage lenders and insurers would simply refuse to provide a loan or insurance product to anyone living within the red boundary. The practice effectively blocked African Americans from obtaining homes, home loans, and home repairs, and it remains a major factor today in the wealth gap between Black and White families given how important homeownership is to building and passing down wealth across generations.

circumstances that result from the use of those methods and tools. In other words, social drivers of health are the conditions in which people are born, grow, live, learn, work, and age (World Health Organization, 2018), and which are shaped by a set of forces generally beyond the control of the individual. Commonly, these types of drivers are referred to as the "social determinants of health" (although there appears to be a shift in some health policy circles away from "determinants" and toward "drivers" as better describing the relationship between structural and social factors and individual/population health).

Resources and opportunities that enhance the quality of one's life—such as the availability of healthy foods, access to education, and an environment free of toxins—all shape individual and population health. These and many other social factors are transient across the life cycle, with some becoming more pertinent depending on one's stage of life. For example, proximity to a high-quality school would be more meaningful for a child, while one's actual education level would be more significant to an adult who is either seeking work or aiming to increase their income. Social drivers may obviously include factors that could lead to an individual's disadvantaged state

to begin with—institutionalized racism, exposure to crime and violence, a lack of available community-based resources, and many other factors can all be harmful to health and well-being.

As you have likely gleaned already, social drivers that influence health cover a wide swath of topics and life events. As a result, it is not always easy to define exactly what role these social drivers—whether one standing alone, or many at once—play in shaping health. Researchers have for decades explored such questions as: Why are some populations more predisposed than others to develop and suffer from certain ailments? Why do differences persist in healthcare quality among racial and ethnic groups? Why do people in low-income families sometimes experience lower-quality care compared to high-income families? Why do studies show incremental improvements in health as one rises in social status? In some capacity, it is likely that social drivers are at play in all of these situations, but defining their role is a challenge. Before delving into some of the more specific research findings concerning the health effects of certain social factors, let us take a more detailed look at some different types of social drivers of health (**Figure 7.1**).

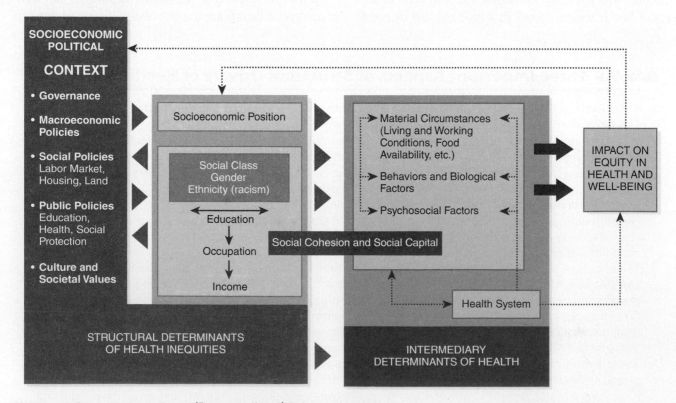

Figure 7.1 Structural and Social ("Intermediary") Drivers of Health

Sullivan, K., Thakur, N. (2020). Structural and social determinants of health in asthma in developed economies: A scoping review of literature published between 2014 and 2019. *Current Allergy and Asthma Reports, 20*(5). https://doi.org/10.1007/s11882-020-0899-6

Types of Social Drivers of Health

The *Healthy People 2030* initiative lists many different examples of social drivers of health (U.S. Department of Health and Human Services, 2021). We summarize several of them here to provide context for the discussion that follows.

- **Access to high-quality educational opportunities:** Individuals with access to consistent, high-quality educational opportunities are more likely to obtain higher-income jobs, and completion of undergraduate and graduate studies affords access to a greater number of these higher-paying opportunities. Many middle and high schools in low-income areas, however, have high dropout rates or do not adequately prepare students for higher education, and many of these areas do not have adequate access to job training resources for those seeking training in a vocation, which can provide a path to a well-paying career in the absence of a 4-year college degree. Furthermore, many low-paying positions do not offer health insurance as a job benefit, making it all the more difficult for individuals in these positions to access routine and specialty physician services. Overall, educational attainment and corresponding income levels tend to be strong predictors of individual and population health. From an early age, educational attainment and income provide valuable resources that protect individuals against stressors that tend to lead to health complications later in life.

- **Access to medical care services:** Individuals who do not live close to medical care providers (e.g., primary care doctors, clinics, hospitals) are less likely to see a physician regularly and will often seek care only in emergencies, eschewing preventive care. Access is also not just about geography—it entails affordability as well. People who do not receive health insurance coverage as a job-related benefit and cannot purchase it on their own can forgo seeing a doctor for several years before presenting to the emergency department for an acute problem, which can possibly lead to a lengthy hospitalization and/or decreased quality of life.

- **Access to social media and other technologies (e.g., Internet, cell phones):** The Internet and cell phones are becoming increasingly useful in individual and population health, from appointment time reminders, to learning more about one's symptoms and diagnoses, to buying insurance through state exchanges established under the Patient Protection and Affordable Care Act (ACA), to finding providers who are accepting new patients. In addition, many people connect to support groups or other valuable health-related resources through the Internet, and providers are increasingly making health records available via Internet portals.

- **Availability of community-based resources and opportunities for recreational activities:** Community-based resources can connect residents to local health providers and recreational/physical activities, both of which increase the likelihood that people will lead healthier lives overall. The absence of leisure activities in one's life can lead to increased stress, which in turn is associated with poorer overall health outcomes.

- **Availability of resources to meet daily needs (e.g., access to local food markets):** The farther an individual lives from a grocery store that offers healthy food options, like fresh fruits and vegetables, the more likely it is that the individual will consume fast foods or other relatively unhealthy options. Geographical areas that have no or few healthy food options are referred to as "food deserts." Food deserts tend to be identified based on their shortages of whole food providers and their abundance of "quick marts" and fast food establishments that stock processed, sugar-heavy, and fat-laden foods that contribute to a poor diet and can lead to higher levels of obesity and other diet-related diseases, such as diabetes and heart disease. Due to the enormous individual and public health effects of food deserts, the U.S. Department of Agriculture (2017) has developed a map of the nation's food deserts and many resources aimed at reducing their number.

- **Culture:** By way of example, some cultures rely heavily on time-honored approaches to illness, such as teas and other homemade remedies. While these can be effective, some commonly ingested herbals can in fact be quite dangerous when taken in conjunction with other regularly prescribed medications; for example, St. John's wort—a plant that is used for medicinal purposes in this country and many others—can have drastic effects when taken alongside certain antidepressant medications. So, while traditions can have important positive effects in treating illness, cultural norms can also impact health in unseen ways.

- **Language/literacy:** If adequate translation and interpretation services are not in place in healthcare facilities, foreign language–speaking patients may be discouraged from seeking care. Even when they do, many patients struggle to understand clinicians and medication or other treatment protocols.

- **Public safety:** Individuals who live in dangerous neighborhoods tend to remain indoors, which can close off opportunities for exercise and social interaction. People who must pass through a dangerous neighborhood in order to reach public transportation often have to make a choice between their own safety and attending work or a doctor's appointment. Furthermore, alcohol, drugs, violence, and the adverse health outcomes associated with them tend to be more prevalent in relatively unsafe neighborhoods.

- **Residential segregation:** Physicians may preferentially set up their practices in locations dominated by certain demographics. As a result, some patient populations—often minority and low-income populations—suffer from a lack of healthcare facilities and resources in their neighborhoods, a particularly strident problem in rural areas.

- **Social norms and attitudes (e.g., discrimination, racism, distrust of government):** Discriminatory attitudes remain a cause of health disparities (Tobin-Tyler & Teitelbaum, 2019). Multiple studies have shown that physicians are more likely to recommend medical best practices based on race, gender, and age (Schulman et al., 1999; van Ryn et al., 2006). These studies demonstrate that bias (unconscious or otherwise) in physicians and other health professionals still plays a significant role in how patients of certain races, ethnicities, social statuses, and education levels are treated. Patient attitudes about the medical professions can also affect health. The most infamous example of discriminatory practice creating negative patient attitudes toward the medical community stems from the Tuskegee syphilis experiment. In this experiment, hundreds of syphilis-infected, African American men in rural Alabama were used as unwitting research subjects by the U.S. Public Health Service, which wanted to study untreated syphilis in humans. The men were given free medical care but were never told they had the disease, nor were any of them treated with penicillin once it became the accepted course of treatment for syphilis. The study lasted a stunning 40 years, from 1932–1972, and has affected the attitudes and healthcare decisions of many African Americans ever since. In 1997, President Bill Clinton issued a formal apology for the Tuskegee Study, but government healthcare programs have been hard-pressed to earn back the trust of millions of patients that was shattered once the study was revealed.[a]

- **Socioeconomic conditions (e.g., concentrated poverty and the stressful conditions that accompany it):** While the link between poverty and poor health is discussed later, suffice it to say here that the connection between the two is well documented and undeniable, and the health effects of extreme financial hardship in childhood can be lifelong even in the event that people eventually escape poverty. A similar phenomenon, although with far different health effects, can be seen at the other end of the socioeconomic spectrum—greater wealth correlates with lower rates of morbidity and longer life spans.

- **Transportation options:** Many individuals miss medical appointments because they cannot afford private transportation and live long distances from reliable public transportation. It is common for patients without their own cars to spend hours on buses in an effort to reach medical appointments.

See **Box 7.4** for a group activity about which social drivers might play a more significant role in health than others.

The Link Between Social Drivers and Health Outcomes

While it is well beyond the scope of this chapter to provide a full discussion of the myriad ways in which social factors play important roles in individual and population health, we provide in this section a flavor of the types of links that researchers have drawn in this respect. We note at the outset that these links are not usually linear and directly causative—social drivers do not usually act alone or in "simple additive fashion," but rather in concert with one another in complex, interdependent, bidirectional relationships" (McGovern et al., 2014, p. 3). Indeed, "most diseases and injuries have multiple potential causes

---

Box 7.4 Group Activity

Each student should begin by rank-ordering a list of the half-dozen social drivers (from those listed in this chapter or otherwise; broad or specific) that they believe most significantly affect individual health. Then get together in groups of three or four people to compare lists, discussing disagreements and making the case for some drivers over others.

and several factors and conditions may contribute to a single death. Therefore, it is a challenge to estimate the contribution of each factor to mortality" (Mokdad et al., 2004, p. 1238). That said, "the overwhelming weight of evidence demonstrates the powerful effects of socioeconomic and related social factors on health, even when definitive knowledge of specific mechanisms and effective interventions is limited" (Braveman & Gottlieb, 2014, p. 22).

Links can be drawn between social drivers and both physical and mental health. Among many examples on the physical health front, research indicates that while half of all deaths in the United States involve behavioral causes (McGinnis & Foege, 1993), evidence shows that health-related behaviors are strongly shaped by three important social factors: income, education level, and employment (Braveman et al., 2011; Stringhini et al., 2010). Another study concluded that the number of U.S. deaths in 2000 attributable to low education, racial segregation, and low social support was comparable with the number of deaths attributable to heart attack, cerebrovascular disease, and lung cancer, respectively (Galea et al., 2011). The CDC has regularly found that individuals among the lowest levels of income and education suffered the greatest age-adjusted prevalence and incidence rate of diagnosed diabetes (CDC, 2013). Similarly, associations have been demonstrated between lower socioeconomic status and increased prevalence of disease, morbidity, and mortality in persons with arthritis and rheumatic conditions (Callahan et al., 2011).

Access to safe, quality, affordable housing represents one of the most influential social drivers of health. Indeed, for individuals and families trapped in a cycle of housing instability, this driver can almost completely dictate their ability to achieve and maintain a healthful state (Corporation for Supportive Housing, 2014). Several studies demonstrate that linking healthcare management to supportive housing—an evidence-based practice that combines permanent affordable housing with relevant support services—leads to improved health outcomes. For example, a study out of Denver, Colorado, found that 50% of supportive housing residents experienced improved health status, 43% had better mental health outcomes, and 15% reduced substance use (Perlman & Parvensky, 2006).

Regardless of income or housing cost, living in a predominately minority neighborhood increases the likelihood of having poor access to healthy food choices (Jack et al., 2012). For example, one study found that African American urban neighborhoods have only 41% of the chain supermarkets found in comparable White neighborhoods (Powell et al., 2007), and minority neighborhoods have an overabundance of fast food restaurants known for relatively inexpensive but unhealthful food options (Fleischhacker et al., 2011).

As noted, social drivers play a significant role in mental health outcomes as well. Emotional stressors—such as neighborhood violence, poverty, or familial abuse—during key developmental years in childhood can lead to severe consequences later in life. For example, several studies have been conducted regarding the mental health outcomes of children who have been subject to abuse, including one showing that survivors of childhood sexual abuse have higher levels of both general distress and major psychological disturbances, including personality disorders (Schneiderman et al., 2005). One particularly fascinating but worrisome study demonstrated that the brains of children in low-income families actually had less surface area than did the brains of children from families who were wealthier—specifically, 6% less surface area in children whose families made less than $25,000 a year compared with children whose families made more than $150,000 (Layton, 2015). One theory behind this finding was that children from poor families tend to be malnourished and have less access to high-quality education than their richer peers. Another theory proposed that poorer families tend to lead more chaotic lives, which can inhibit brain development in children.

Law as a Driver of Health

In the previous section, we provided a general description of various types of social drivers of health and some correlations between those drivers and the health of people who live in communities in which social factors may be relatively more compromised. We turn now to a discussion of one very influential *structural* driver of health: the law. Throughout the nation's history, law has played an integral role in causing, exacerbating, and alleviating health-harming social conditions, from the legally sanctioned, racially segregated—and horribly unequal—medical care systems used during slavery time, to the expansion of building codes in the 1920s, to the War on Poverty legislation of the 1960s, to the ACA's focus on health equity. Because the law's reach in this regard is so expansive, we provide only an overview for purposes of this chapter (for a far more in-depth discussion, see Tobin-Tyler & Teitelbaum, 2019).

Whether embodied in constitutions, statutes, regulations, executive orders, administrative agency decisions, or court decisions, the law plays a profound role in shaping life circumstances and, in turn, health. Indeed, law is the primary tool used by those in power to mold society, distribute resources and opportunities, and shape economic interactions. As a result, it is fair to say that the law exerts a powerful force on nearly *all* social drivers of health. The ways in which this occurs can be broken down into five categories.

1. **The law can be used to design and perpetuate social conditions that can have terrible physical, mental, and emotional effects on individuals and populations.** One obvious example in this category is the "separate but equal" constitutional doctrine that allowed racial segregation in housing, health care, education, employment, transportation, and more. Indeed, injustices in healthcare access and quality were commonplace in the United States prior to the civil rights movement. Racially segregated health care dates to slavery times, when plantations had on-site facilities to care for slave laborers. After the slaves were freed but also after the First Reconstruction ended in the late 1870s, Jim Crow laws ushered in a new era of discriminatory healthcare access and delivery through separate hospitals and physician practices; separate medical, nursing, and dental schools; and separate professional medical societies. For example, Alabama once had a law that stated: "No person or corporation shall require any White female nurse to nurse in wards or rooms in hospitals, either public or private, in which Negro men are placed" (Ferris State University, 2012).

2. **The law can be used as a mechanism through which behaviors and prejudices are transformed into distributions of well-being among populations.** By way of example, although Black and White people use illicit drugs at approximately the same rate, drug crime incarceration rates are far higher for Black people. Thus, who is chosen for surveillance and arrest, and how the arrested are selected for either punishment or treatment, turns out to be an important driver of how a supposedly neutral law (the federal Controlled Substances Act) differentially impacts people and communities, and in turn their health (Burris, 2011). Healthcare provider discrimination and bias reside in this category as well. Healthcare discrimination and bias can take many forms: It can be based on race, ethnicity, disability, age, gender, class (or socioeconomic status), or other classifications. Class-related healthcare discrimination alone can take multiple forms. For example,

some healthcare providers might refuse to accept as patients individuals who are covered under Medicaid (because the Medicaid population tends to be disproportionately poor and of color), or low-income individuals might fall victim to the practice of redlining, which results when healthcare entities relocate from poor neighborhoods to wealthier ones (Yearby, 2013). Finally, laws limiting the ability of transgender youths to receive certain medical treatments fall into this category too. In early 2021, Arkansas became the first state in the United States to ban some medical treatments (e.g., gender-conforming hormone therapy, puberty blockers, gender-confirmation surgeries) for transgender minors, and more than a dozen states are considering a range of similar restrictions.

3. **Laws can be determinative of health through their under-enforcement.** For example, a perfectly good set of housing regulations aimed at keeping housing units safe, clean, and quiet are of little value to individual and group health if there is neither the will, nor the resources, to enforce them. Substandard housing conditions, including the presence of rodents, mold, peeling lead paint, exposed wires, and insufficient heat—all of which are common among low-income housing units—can cause or exacerbate asthma, skin rashes, lead poisoning, fires, and common illnesses, yet none of these housing problems can be "cured" by a clinical encounter. While their consequences can be treated medically, the causes require robust enforcement of existing laws (Tobin-Tyler et al., 2011).

4. **Laws can be determinative of health through their interpretation.** In 2012, the U.S. Supreme Court was asked by half the states in the country to rule on whether the Medicaid expansion in the ACA was unlawfully coercive (*National Federation of Independent Business v. Sebelius*, 2012; note that this decision is discussed in more detail in Chapter 11, "Health Reform and the Patient Protection and Affordable Care Act). As originally passed into law, the ACA permitted the secretary of the U.S. Department of Health and Human Services to terminate *all* of a state's Medicaid funding if the state failed to implement the Medicaid expansion—even those Medicaid funds that a state would receive that were unconnected to the expansion. While determining that the Medicaid expansion itself was perfectly legitimate, the court ruled that Congress unconstitutionally forced states to

potentially have to choose between the Medicaid expansion and a total loss of Medicaid funding. This ruling had the effect of making the ACA's Medicaid expansion optional, rather than mandatory, and states have been deciding individually whether to implement the expansion ever since. At the time of this writing, 38 states and the District of Columbia have adopted the ACA's Medicaid expansion, while 12 states have not; thus, the court's interpretation of a statute has contributed to the fact that otherwise eligible individuals in "non-expansion states" do not have access to Medicaid benefits in the same way that individuals in "expansion states" do. Another example of how the interpretation of law can correlate with health concerns prisoners' well-being during the COVID-19 pandemic. In March 2020, residents at the District of Columbia Jail filed a lawsuit against the D.C. Department of Corrections, accusing the agency of failing to prevent the spread of COVID-19. A federal judge agreed and ordered the agency to devise precautionary safety measures. In response, the Department of Corrections implemented a 23-hour-per-day lockdown, relegating approximately 1500 prisoners to, effectively, prolonged solitary confinement. The lockdown lasted for more than a year (in May of 2021 prisoners were granted 2 hours outside their cells, and 1 month later they were granted more than 5 hours outside their cells each day, in a return to prepandemic levels). District of Columbia officials claimed the universal lockdown was the "only" way to adhere to the judge's order; however, other correctional officials, physicians, and civil liberties groups called the policy ineffective, health-harming, and a human rights abuse.

5. **Finally, the law can be used to structure direct responses to health-harming social needs that result from factors like impoverishment, illness, market failure, and individual behavior that harms others.** For example, the Emergency Medical Treatment and Active Labor Act (EMTALA) requires Medicare-participating hospitals to provide needed stabilization services to individuals who have an emergent condition. Notably, EMTALA's requirements are universal—meaning they have to be fulfilled by hospitals irrespective of the presenting patient's socioeconomic or insurance status—and were written into law because many private hospitals had long turned away emergent patients who were uninsured and could not pay out-of-pocket for their care.

Many financing laws that subsidize healthcare services for vulnerable populations also fit into this category. Medicaid is an obvious example, and the Public Health Service Act includes funding for community health centers, people with HIV/AIDS, people with mental illness or substance abuse disorders, and project grants to provide preventive and immunization services, and breast and cervical cancer screening and detection. Title VI of the 1964 Civil Rights Act prohibits discrimination on the basis of race, color, or national origin by any recipient of federal financing, including healthcare providers and facilities. Finally, public health departments funded under state and local legal authority provide primary and preventive healthcare services, such as childhood immunizations, to underserved populations. Programs such as the National Health Service Corps (NHSC) and the Indian Health Service (IHS) were established under federal law to address the lack of providers in rural and other underserved areas. The NHSC was founded in order to incentivize graduates of medical school and other health professions programs to practice primary care in underserved areas, because starting in the 1950s medical graduates began gravitating in large numbers to large cities to practice a medical specialty. The IHS is the principal federal healthcare provider and health advocate for American Indians and Alaska Natives, providing comprehensive health services to approximately 2.5 million individuals.

Furthermore, through their police powers, states directly regulate individual and corporate behavior in order to protect and promote the public's health. For example, states regulate the food supply and food establishments, enforce occupational safety rules, curb pollution, control the sale of firearms, restrict the marketing of tobacco products, and accredit healthcare professionals and facilities. Indeed, at the local, state, and federal levels, the law has played important roles in all of the 10 most noteworthy public health achievements of the 20th century, as selected by the CDC (1999): control of infectious diseases, motor vehicle safety, fluoridation of drinking water, tobacco use control, vaccinations, decline in deaths due to coronary heart disease and stroke, food safety, improvements in maternal and child health, family planning, and safer workplaces. (See **Box 7.5** for a group activity about the law and health-harming social needs.)

Taken together, the preceding list illustrates how using law to achieve better health is well suited to what is called a "health in all policies" (HIAP) strategy. This strategy is based on the recognition that several pressing health-related challenges—inequities, chronic disease, skyrocketing costs, the need for insurance reform, and so on—are often complex, multidimensional, and linked to one another. As a result, HIAP relies on a collaborative governmental (and sometimes nongovernmental) approach to health improvement by incorporating health considerations into an array of policy decisions, and by engaging governments and other stakeholders in a multisector approach to shaping the economic, physical, and social environments in which people live, work, and play.

In thinking about how law could be used to foster an HIAP approach, consider the number of rule-making departments and agencies at just the federal level that can (and do) serve healthcare and public health functions even though they are not commonly identified as health agencies. The Environmental Protection Agency plays an obviously important role in environmental health. Reducing injuries and hazards in the workplace is the key goal of the Occupational Safety and Health Administration, which is part of the Department of Labor. The Department of Homeland Security protects health when it prepares for and responds to disasters and terrorism. The Department of Agriculture (along with the Food and Drug Administration) plays an important role in the protection of the nation's food supply. The Department of Housing and Urban Development influences the built environment, which in turn influences health. The Department of Energy sets radiation safety standards for nuclear power plants and other sources of energy. Again, these are just federal agencies, and they are all part of the executive branch of government; in addition, legislative branch committees at the federal, state, and local levels that are also not typically considered "health" committees could also craft legislation with an HIAP approach in mind. The involvement of multiple branches and agencies in health-related matters plainly demonstrates that a variety of influences that impact individual and population health are outside the control of the health sector alone.

Right to Criminal Legal Representation vs. Civil Legal Assistance

Appreciating the law's power to ameliorate social conditions that negatively affect health requires an understanding of the difference between using law to design broad policies (e.g., Title VI of the Civil Rights Act, firearm regulations, federal housing policy, the ACA) and leveraging the legal system as an individual who is aiming to redress their own hardship. In the case of the latter, it helps to understand the difference between rights that attach in the area of criminal legal representation versus those that exist in the realm of civil legal assistance, because it is through civil legal assistance that many types of health-harming social drivers can been ameliorated.

Criminal Legal Representation

The government is required to provide legal counsel to all federal defendants who are unable to afford their own attorneys; this right is explicit in the Sixth Amendment to the U.S. Constitution. The right to counsel in state criminal prosecutions was established by the U.S. Supreme Court (although only for serious offences) in the famous 1963 case of *Gideon v. Wainwright*. The case arose out of an everyday burglary at a Florida pool hall, for which Clarence Earl Gideon was arrested notwithstanding the flimsy evidence against him. Because Gideon was indigent and could not afford private counsel, he appeared in court alone. He requested counsel but was denied, and as a result acted as his own lawyer at trial. A jury found him guilty and the Florida trial court sentenced Gideon to serve 5 years in state prison.

From prison, Gideon appealed his conviction to the U.S. Supreme Court, arguing that his constitutional rights had been violated when he was denied counsel. The Supreme Court agreed to hear Gideon's constitutional claim and assigned him a well-known lawyer, Abe Fortas, who himself would one day become a U.S. Supreme Court Justice. Building on previous right to counsel cases (for example, in the event of a state prosecution where the death penalty was sought), the court ruled that the assistance of counsel, if desired by an indigent defendant, was a fundamental right under the U.S. Constitution that was required in state prosecutions of serious crimes. Gideon received a new trial and—with the assistance of a lawyer supplied at government expense— was acquitted of all charges just 5 months after the Supreme Court's ruling.

The decision in *Gideon v. Wainwright* spawned many changes in the representation of indigent criminal defendants, including in misdemeanor and juvenile proceedings. The decision effectively created the need for public defenders (lawyers employed at public expense in criminal trials), and it lies at the heart of a series of cases dealing not only with legal representation at trial and on appeal, but also with police interrogation tactics and the right to remain silent.

Civil Legal Assistance

Although the right to legal representation exists in many criminal matters, no such right exists on the other side of the legal ledger: Generally speaking, there is no right to the assistance of a lawyer in civil matters, even when the most basic human needs are at stake. Common civil legal matters involve immigration status, domestic violence, disability law, family law (e.g., child custody cases), housing needs, public benefits (e.g., Medicaid, food stamps, Social Security), employment disputes, and special education needs. In all of these types of disputes—which can be incredibly complex from a legal perspective and which can have life-altering consequences—low-income individuals and families can have no expectation that an attorney will provide them with assistance. (We should note, however, that under some state laws individuals have a right to counsel in limited civil situations, such as with the termination of parental rights or involuntary commitments to mental health facilities.) In civil matters, indigent people (and, increasingly, more members of the middle class and a rising number of small businesses that cannot afford legal fees)[b] can apply for what is known as civil legal aid or civil legal services, which are provided by a network of publicly funded legal aid agencies, private lawyers, and law firms practicing on a pro bono basis, law school clinics, and professional organizations (the latter group includes organizations such as the American Bar Association, the National Legal Aid and Defender Association, and the American Bar Foundation).

This network is the heart and soul of what is termed the *access to justice* movement, which promotes strategies to address the severe gap in access to both criminal and civil justice for low-income and other vulnerable populations.[c] One of the goals of this movement is to establish a "civil *Gideon*"—in other words, to create a mandate for legal representation of the poor in civil lawsuits. For example, the American Bar Association's House of Delegates passed in 2006 a resolution backing the concept of "civil *Gideon*":

RESOLVED, That the American Bar Association urges state, territorial and federal jurisdictions to provide counsel as a matter of right at public expense to low-income persons in those categories of adversarial proceedings where basic human needs are at stake, such as those involving shelter, sustenance, safety, health or child custody, as determined by each jurisdiction.[d] (American Bar Association, 2006)

Because the combined resources of the civil legal services community are very limited, services are approved on the basis of financial need, meaning that only those individuals with very low incomes receive assistance. Indeed, reports on the legal aid community routinely describe situations in which 80% of civil legal needs for low-income families were not being met, and legal services programs typically turn away over half of the low-income individuals that seek assistance. Congress is most to blame for legal aid's financial predicament; it provides the vast majority of the budget for the Legal Services Corporation (LSC), a not-for-profit corporation established by federal law in 1974 as the single largest funder of civil legal aid for low-income Americans. Considering LSC's annual appropriations from Congress in constant 2015 dollars, its appropriation in 1976 was approximately $386 million; in 2015, its appropriation was $375 million (Legal Services Corporation, 2015).[e] So even as need has soared over time—the U.S. Census Bureau's statistics on poverty show that over 60 million Americans could qualify for civil legal assistance funded by LSC—the key element of legal aid funding has been treated as an afterthought (Legal Services Corporation, 2018).

The link between civil legal assistance and individual and population health is exemplified by a study of the civil justice experiences of the American public, called the Community Needs and Services Study (Sandefur, 2014). The study uncovers widespread incidence of events and situations that have civil legal aspects and for which people receive no formal or expert legal assistance: Fully two-thirds of a random sample of adults in a mid-sized American city reported experiencing at least one of 12 different categories of civil justice situations in the previous 18 months (the average number of situations reported was 3.3, and poor people, African Americans, and Hispanics were more likely to report civil justice situations than were middle- or high-income earners and White people). The most commonly reported situations concerned problems with employment, finances and government benefits, health insurance, and housing. Importantly, respondents indicated that almost half of the civil justice situations they experienced resulted in a significant negative consequence such as feelings of fear, a loss of confidence, damage to physical or mental health, or verbal or physical violence or threats of violence. In fact, adverse impacts on health were the most common negative consequence, reported for 27% of situations. Also important is the fact many of those who responded indicated that they did not even know that the problems they were experiencing were rightly considered "legal" in nature.

For all of the reasons just discussed—the lack of a right to needed civil legal services, the misunderstandings among those most in need, and the lack of resources in the civil legal aid community—it is paramount that the nation develop and implement innovative, upstream approaches to addressing social conditions that harm health. One such innovation that has taken root is medical–legal partnership, an approach described in the next section. Before turning to it, consider the discussion questions in **Box 7.6**.

Combating Health-Harming Social Conditions Through Medical–Legal Partnership[f]

"Do you have any concerns about your housing conditions? Are you concerned about having enough food to eat? Is your child receiving proper supports at school? Do you feel safe at home?" These types of questions are asked of low-income patients with regularity, and their medical care providers know well that the answers speak volumes about patients' health. When the answers come back, however, healthcare providers are too often powerless to do as much as they would like to help remedy these "life circumstances."

Training doctors, nurses, and allied health professionals to reframe these circumstances can help. By now, you probably recognize many of these types of health drivers for what they are—social conditions whose improvement would benefit from changes in the way in which law is designed or enforced, or from the provision of civil legal assistance. Yet despite the connection between poverty, health, and legal needs, and despite the fact that healthcare and civil legal aid professionals commonly provide services to overlapping vulnerable populations, the professions too infrequently attempt to address their populations' needs in a coordinated fashion.

Medical–legal partnership (MLP) aims to bridge this divide. At a practical level, MLPs function as a patient care team that includes both medical and legal professionals; a legal services attorney is literally embedded in a medical care setting (e.g., a hospital, community health center) to address underlying social conditions that negatively affect patient health but whose remediation is outside the expertise of traditional healthcare providers. At a more fundamental level, the goal of the MLP movement is to help create an interconnected care system that focuses on the whole patient (rather than just on biology and behavior), including the ways in which myriad social conditions factor into individual and population health. Thus, the work of MLP lawyers is quite different from that of a general counsel or compliance officer who normally inhabits hospitals and clinics; a general counsel typically provides legal advice to clinicians on matters of medical liability and informed consent and represents them in insurance and disciplinary matters, whereas corporate compliance officers ensure that the facility meets all governmental, environmental, and licensing regulations.

The Evolution of an "Upstream" Innovation

The modern MLP movement has its roots in the late 1960s, when visionary physicians H. Jack Geiger and Count Gibson were funded by the federal government to form the nation's first community health centers in Mississippi and Massachusetts. The government's community health center program grew out of the civil rights movement, when the federal Office of Economic Opportunity (the agency created to administer many of President Lyndon Johnson's War on Poverty programs, and whose programs continue in large part to this day under the auspices of the U.S. Department of Health and Human Services) established "neighborhood health centers" to provide health and social services to medically underserved populations. In designing the earliest centers, Drs. Geiger and Gibson recognized the importance of spending some of their federal funding on lawyers, who assisted African American health center patients who were battling housing discrimination.

The second prominent instance of the blending of medical and legal services for low-income populations occurred in the early 1980s when, faced with devastating death tolls from HIV/AIDS, some health clinics began providing on-site legal assistance to patients who needed to quickly grapple with end-of-life issues (e.g., medical decision-making, asset distribution, family and custody matters). A few pioneering clinics held on to this blended model even after the national AIDS crisis abated, offering comprehensive legal services to all patients in need.

Building on these examples, the first formal MLP was created in the early 1990s in a Boston hospital to intervene on behalf of pediatric patients with chronic conditions who were suffering the consequences of inadequate housing. From that point through 2006, MLPs sprouted up a few at a time, mainly in pediatric healthcare settings, where the model had proven effective in Boston. Since 2006, however, use of the MLP model has expanded considerably. Fueled by the creation of the National Center for Medical-Legal Partnership (NCMLP), the focus by social

scientists on the importance of social factors in determining health, and the ACA's focus on disease prevention and professional collaboration, MLP is now practiced in nearly all states by more than 450 hospitals and health centers, in settings as diverse as veteran care facilities, American Indian reservations, and correction facilities (National Center for Medical-Legal Partnership, 2018).

Under the MLP model, public interest lawyers work with healthcare workers to screen for health-related legal problems, often encompassing family matters (divorce, domestic violence), housing problems (eviction, habitability, utility advocacy), special education advocacy, immigration issues, disability issues, employment instability, receipt of public benefits (health insurance, Supplemental Security income), food security concerns, and additional problems that can lead to stress or injury or that can exacerbate existing health problems. **Figure 7.2** lays out the key

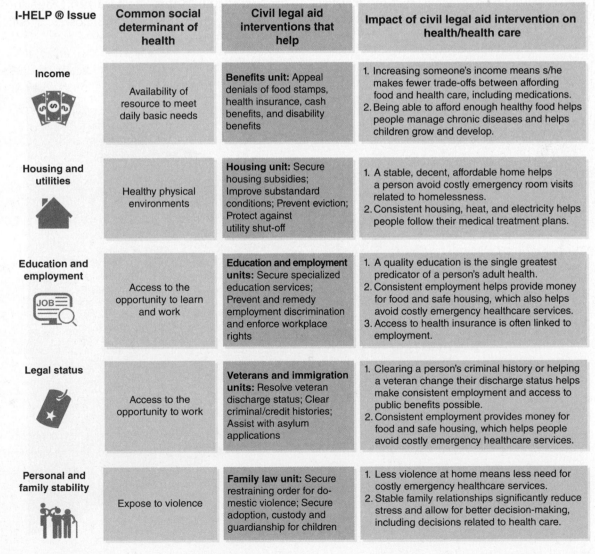

Figure 7.2 Framing Legal Care as Health Care

types of patient problems that make up the practice of a typical, comprehensive MLP, using the mnemonic "I-HELP": **I**ncome, **H**ousing and utilities, **E**ducation and employment, **L**egal status, and **P**ersonal and family stability (Marple, 2015).

The MLP approach is built on the understanding not only that many health-harming social drivers would benefit from legal interventions, but that moving "upstream" to assist vulnerable populations with legal needs is preferable to waiting until a legal crisis erupts (e.g., remediating a housing problem prior to the receipt of an eviction notice). It is similar to preventive health care: It is often more cost effective—and of course more beneficial to the patient, both physically and emotionally—to help a patient remain healthy, rather than treat the patient post-illness. At MLPs, healthcare and legal professionals are trained side by side about the intersection of health and legal needs and about ways to screen for health-harming legal needs. Because MLPs recognize that social factors contributing to poor health require both health system

and public policy change, MLP lawyers utilize on-site legal assistance provided to patients to identify patterns of systemic need, transform institutional practices, and advocate for improved population health policies. **Figure 7.3** portrays this upstream MLP approach. Similar to the movement to integrate behavioral healthcare services into primary care, the integration of civil legal aid with healthcare delivery can improve access to services, build team capacity, and promote patient-centered care.

MLPs have become more integrated over time, with healthcare and legal partners sharing patient and institutional data, jointly developing service and training priorities, and establishing cross-sector communication processes. The more collaboration and integration that occurs, the more likely it is that upstream detection of the social conditions that lead to poor health can occur. Deep collaboration and integration also present an opportunity for healthcare providers and lawyers—two learned professions that, historically, have not been the closest of colleagues

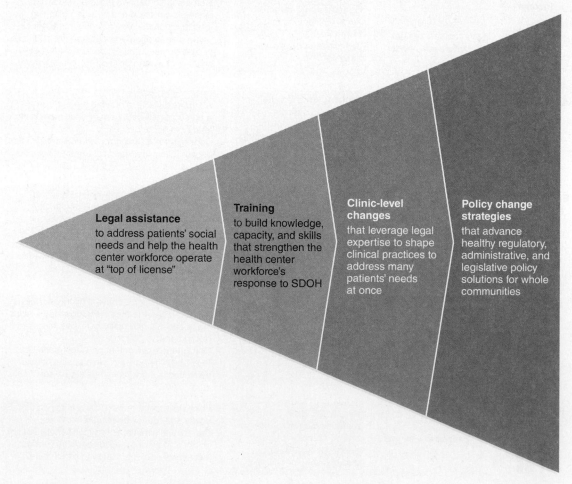

Figure 7.3 The Medical–Legal Partnership Approach to Social Drivers of Health

(Teitelbaum & Lawton, 2017)—to work together when policymakers design fixes for health-harming social and legal problems.

The Benefits of MLPs

Due to the relatively recent growth of MLPs, the effects of the MLP model have not been regularly tested in formal, large-scale studies. However, several small-scale studies have been conducted (Beeson et al., 2013; Martinez et al., 2017) and offer preliminary evidence of the benefits of the model in three areas: impact on patient health and well-being, financial impact on partners and patients, and impact on knowledge and training of health providers.

A handful of studies make the case for MLPs by demonstrating the positive impact they can have on patient health and well-being. One such study, focused on home visit/nurse-based interventions for prenatal and postpartum patients, demonstrated better prenatal health behaviors, better pregnancy outcomes, lower rates of child abuse and neglect, and higher rates of maternal employment among participants as a result of MLP services (Williams et al., 2008). A second study found a 91% reduction in emergency department visits and hospital admissions of inner-city asthmatic adults after a medical–legal intervention. In the same study, over 91% of patients also dropped two or more classes in asthma severity (O'Sullivan et al., 2012). Another study focused on cancer patients in an MLP showed a reduction in stress for 75% of the patients, an increase in treatment adherence for 30% of them, and greater ease in keeping appointments for 25% of patients (Fleishman et al., 2006). Yet another study showed that by redressing complex social issues through legal advocacy, patients experienced less stress, improved access to preventive health care, and gained a greater feeling of general well-being (Wang et al., 2009).

Several MLP studies have focused on the financial benefits of the model—in other words, on the "return on investment" that accrues to institutions that invest in an MLP. One such study found that an MLP targeting the needs of cancer patients generated nearly $1 million by resolving previously denied health insurance benefit claims (Rodabaugh et al., 2013). Similarly, a separate study highlighted four MLP programs, each of which demonstrated successful recovery of previously unreimbursed funds as a result of improperly denied Medicaid or Social Security Disability claims (Knight, 2008). More striking still is evidence of the financial impact that MLPs could have on patients: An MLP in Illinois helped to relieve $4 million in patients' healthcare debt, and claimed $2 million in additional awarded Social Security benefits for patients (Teufel et al., 2012).

Finally, multiple articles have addressed how MLPs can benefit practitioners and patients alike through interdisciplinary training and education. One article, focused on strategies for teaching cultural competence, interdisciplinary practice, and holistic problem solving in legal and medical curricula, describes a legal clinic that increased knowledge about avenues of legal assistance among doctors and of the clinical impact of social drivers of health among lawyers (Tobin-Tyler, 2008). A second paper describes how medical residents working in clinics with social/legal resources were more confident in their knowledge regarding public benefits and how these same residents were more likely than residents without these resources to ask patients about their social history, use of public benefits, and housing situation (O'Toole et al., 2012). Finally, medical residents who had social work or MLP resources on-site were more confident regarding their personal knowledge of social drivers of health, and as a result were found to screen for them more frequently than other residents (O'Toole et al., 2012).

Conclusion

Recall from the start of this chapter the concept of health equity—essentially, an environment in which all people have an equal opportunity to attain their full health potential. While the nation is far from achieving a state of health equity, it should be everyone's goal to orient society in this direction, even if incrementally. More evidence regarding whether this is in fact the case will come in a few years, when it will be more clear whether most Americans accept the ACA's main goals as ones worth striving for. (Note one final time the law's role as a structural driver of health: Should the ACA achieve near-complete implementation—and public acceptance along the lines of, say, the Medicare program—the nation, in our view, will be healthier than if the ACA continues to be subjected to political and legal attacks, and to implementation battles in at least a dozen states.)

Whether the nation strives for full health equity aggressively or half-heartedly, there is little doubt that increasing our collective focus on the link between structural drivers, social drivers, and health would benefit millions of individuals and, in turn, the public more generally. Considering that American children, in particular, experience a high prevalence of social conditions that compromise their care and development—including insufficient family income to meet basic living needs, food insecurity, unstable housing, environmental toxins, and a lack of high-quality child care—this type of reorientation is nothing less than a moral imperative (Miller et al., 2011).

One facet of this transformation is reframing civil legal services for vulnerable populations as a critical component of health care. Civil legal aid, after all, is first and foremost about promoting the

enforcement of existing laws that protect vulnerable populations (Houseman, 2015). If health is at the core of well-being for all people, then reducing barriers to good health should be an obvious societal goal, and for low-income and other vulnerable populations this means reducing the health-harming effects of social conditions that they struggle with disproportionately. To address this inequity, the civil legal community should closely align its activities and priorities with healthcare and public health partners.

References

American Bar Association. (2006). *Recommendation.* http://www.americanbar.org/content/dam/aba/administrative/legal_aid_indigent_defendants/ls_sclaid_06A112A.authcheckdam.pdf

Beeson, T., McAllister, B., & Regenstein, M. (2013). *Literature review: Making the case for medical-legal partnerships.* http://medical-legalpartnership.org/mlp-resources/literature-review/

Bradley, E. H., Elkins, B. R., Herrin, J., & Elbel, B. (2011). Health and social services expenditures: Associations with health outcomes. *BMJ Quality & Safety, 20*(10), 826–831.

Braveman, P., Egerter, S., & Barclay, C. (2011). *What shapes health-related behaviors? The role of social factors.* Robert Wood Johnson Foundation.

Braveman, P., & Gottlieb, L. (2014). The social determinants of health: It's time to consider the causes of the causes. *Public Health Reports, 129*(Suppl. 2), 19–31.

Burris, S. (2011). Law in a social determinants strategy: A public health law research perspective. *Public Health Reporter, 126*(Suppl. 3), 22–27.

Callahan, L. F., Martin, K. R., Shreffler, J., Kumar, D., Schoster, B., Kaufman, J., & Schwartz, T. (2011). Independent and combined influence of homeownership, occupation, education, income and community poverty on physical health in persons with arthritis. *Arthritis Care & Research, 63*(5), 643–653.

Centers for Disease Control and Prevention. (1999). Ten great public health achievements—United States, 1900–1999. *Morbidity and Mortality Weekly Report, 48*(12), 241–243.

Centers for Disease Control and Prevention. (2013). CDC health disparities and inequalities report. *Morbidity and Mortality Weekly Report, 62*(Suppl. 3), 1–187.

Corporation for Supportive Housing. (2014). *Housing is the best medicine: Supportive housing and the social determinants of health.* https://www.csh.org/wp-content/uploads/2014/07/Social DeterminantsofHealth_2014.pdf

Ferris State University. (2012). *What was Jim Crow.* http://www.ferris.edu/jimcrow/what.htm

Fleischhacker, S. E., Evenson, K. R., Rodriguez, D. A., & Ammerman, A. S. (2011). A systematic review of fast food access studies. *Obesity Review, 12*(5), e460–e471.

Fleishman, S. B., Retkin, R., Brandfield, J., & Braun, V. (2006). The attorney as the newest member of the cancer treatment team. *Journal of Clinical Oncology, 24*(13), 2123–2126.

Galea, S., Tracy, M., Hoggatt, K. J., DiMaggio, C., & Karpati, A. (2011).Estimated deaths attributable to social factors in the United States. *American Journal of Public Health, 101*(8), 1456–1465.

Gideon v. Wainwright, 372 U.S. 335 (1963).

Gostin, L. O., Jacobson, P. D., Record, K., & Hardcastle, L. (2011).Restoring health to health reform: Integrating medicine and public health to advance the population's well-being. *University of Pennsylvania Law Review, 159*, 1777–1823.

Hoffman, K. W., Trawalter, S., Axt, J. R., & Oliver, M. N. (2016).Racial bias in pain assessment and treatment recommendations, and false beliefs about biological differences between blacks and whites. *Proceedings of the National Academy of Sciences, 113*(6), 4296–4301.

Houseman, A. (2015). *Civil legal aid in the United States: An update for 2015.* https://repository.library.georgetown.edu/bitstream/handle/10822/761858/Houseman_Civil_Legal_Aid_US_2015.pdf

Jack, L., Jack, N. H., & Hayes, S. C. (2012). Social determinants of health in minority populations: A call for multidisciplinary approaches to eliminate diabetes-related health disparities. *Diabetes Spectrum, 25*(1), 9–13.

Jones, J. H. (1993). *Bad blood: The Tuskegee syphilis experiment.* The Free Press.

Kaiser Family Foundation. (2012). *Disparities in health and health care: Five key questions and answers.* https://kaiserfamilyfoundation.files.wordpress.com/2012/11/8396-disparities-in-health-and-health-care-five-key-questions-and-answers.pdf

Knight, R. (2008). *Health care recovery dollars: A sustainable strategy for medical-legal partnerships?* https://static1.squarespace.com/static/5373b088e4b02899e91e9392/t/53cd59cae4b02facb9407e39/1405966794425/Medical-Legal+Partnership+Health+Care+Recovery+Dollars.pdf

Layton, L. (2015, April 15). New brain science shows poor kids have smaller brains than affluent kids. *The Washington Post.* http://www.washingtonpost.com/local/education/new-brain-science-shows-poor-kids-have-smaller-brains-than-affluent-kids/2015/04/15/3b679858-e2bc-11e4-b510-962fcfabc310_story.html

Legal Services Corporation. (2015). *Congressional appropriations.* http://www.lsc.gov/about-lsc/who-we-are/congressional-oversight/congressional-appropriations

Legal Services Corporation. (2018). *Who we are.* http://www.lsc.gov/about/what-is-lsc

Marple, K. (2015). *Framing legal care as health care.* http://medical-legalpartnership.org/new-messaging-guide-helps-frame-legal-care-health-care/

Martinez, O., Boles, J., Muñoz-Laboy, M., Levine, E. C., Ayamele, C., Eisenberg, R., & Draine, J. (2017). Bridging health disparity gaps through the use of medical-legal partnerships in patient care: A systematic review. *Journal of Law, Medicine and Ethics, 45*(2), 260–273.

McGinnis, J. M., & Foege, W. H. (1993). Actual causes of death in the United States. *Journal of the American Medical Association, 270*(18), 2207–2212.

McGovern, L., Miller, G., & Hughes-Cromwick, P. (2014). *Health policy brief: The relative contribution of multiple determinants to health outcomes.* https://www.rwjf.org/content/dam/farm/reports/issue_briefs/2014/rwjf415185

Miller, W. D., Sadegh-Nobari, T., & Lillie-Blanton, M. (2011). Healthy starts for all: Policy prescriptions. *American Journal of Preventive Medicine, 40*(1 Suppl. 1), S19–S37.

Mokdad, A. H., Marks, J. S., Stroup, D. F., & Gerberding, J. L. (2004). Actual causes of death in the United States, 2000. *Journal of the American Medical Association, 291*(10), 1238–1245.

National Center for Medical-Legal Partnership. (2018). *Partnerships across the U.S.* http://medical-legalpartnership.org/partnerships/

National Federation of Independent Business v. Sebelius, 567 U.S. 519 (2012).

O'Sullivan, M. M., Brandfield, J., Hoskote, S. S., Segal, S. N., Chug, L., Modrykamien, A., & Eden, E. (2012). Environmental improvements brought by the legal interventions in the homes of poorly-controlled inner-city adult asthmatic patients: A proof-of-concept study. *Journal of Asthma, 49*(9), 911–917.

O'Toole, J. K., Burkhardt, M. C., Solan, L. G., Vaughn, L., & Klein, M. D. (2012). Resident confidence addressing social history: Is it influenced by availability of social and legal resources? *Clinical Pediatrics, 51*(7), 625–631.

Perlman, J., & Parvensky, J. (2006). *Denver housing first collaborative cost benefit analysis and program outcomes report.* http://shnny.org/uploads/Supportive_Housing_in_Denver.pdf

Powell, L. M., Slater, S., Mirtcheva, D., Bao, Y., & Chaloupka, F. J. (2007). Food store availability and neighborhood characteristics in the United States. *Preventive Medicine, 44*(3), 189–195.

Rodabaugh, K. J., Hammond, M., Myszka, D., & Sandel, M. (2013). A medical-legal partnership as a component of a palliative care model. *Journal of Palliative Medicine, 13*(1), 15–18.

Sandefur, R. L. (2014). *Accessing justice in the contemporary USA: Findings from the community needs and services study.* http://www.americanbarfoundation.org/uploads/cms/documents/sandefur_accessing_justice_in_the_contemporary_usa._aug._2014.pdf

Schneiderman, N., Ironson, G., & Siegel, S. D. (2005). Stress and health: Psychological, behavioral, and biological determinants. *Annual Review of Clinical Psychology, 1*, 607–628.

Schulman, K. A., Berlin, J. A., Harless, W., Kerner, J. F., Sistrunk, S., Gersh, B. J., Dubé, R., Taleghani, C. K., Burke, J. E., Williams, S., Eisenberg, J. M., Ayers, W., & Escarce, J. J. (1999). The effect of race and sex on physicians' recommendations for cardiac catheterization. *New England Journal of Medicine, 340*, 618–626.

Smedley, B. D., Stith, A. Y., & Nelson, A. R. (Eds.). (2003). *Unequal treatment: Confronting racial and ethnic disparities in health care.* The National Academies Press.

Stringhini, S., Sabia, S., Shipley, M., Brunner, E., Nabi, H., Kivimaki, M., & Sing-Manoux, A. (2010). Association of socioeconomic position with health behaviors and mortality. *Journal of the American Medical Association, 303*(12), 1159–1166.

Teitelbaum, J., & Lawton, E. (2017). The roots and branches of the medical-legal partnership approach to health: From collegiality to civil rights to health equity. *Yale Journal of Health Policy, Law, and Ethics, 17*(2), 343–347.

Teufel, J. A., Werner, D., Goffinet, D., Thorne, W., Brown, S. L., & Gettinger, L. (2012). Rural medical-legal partnership and advocacy: A three-year follow-up study. *Journal of Health Care for the Poor and Underserved, 23*(2), 705–714.

Tobin-Tyler, E. (2008). Allies not adversaries: Teaching collaboration to the next generation of doctors and lawyers to address social inequality. *Journal of Health Care Law and Policy, 11*, 249–294.

Tobin-Tyler, E. (2012). Aligning public health, health care, law and policy: Medical-legal partnership as a multilevel response to the social determinants of health. *Journal of Health and Biomedical Law, 8*(2), 211–247.

Tobin-Tyler, E., Lawton, E., Conroy, K., Sandel, M., & Zuckerman, B. (Eds.). (2011). *Poverty, health and law: Readings and cases for medical-legal partnership.* Carolina Academic Press.

Tobin-Tyler, E., & Teitelbaum, J. (2019). *Essentials of health justice: A primer.* Jones & Bartlett Learning.

U.S. Department of Agriculture. (2017). *Food access research atlas.* http://www.ers.usda.gov/data/fooddesert

U.S. Department of Health and Human Services, Office of Disease Prevention and Health Promotion. (2021). *Social determinants of health.* https://health.gov/healthypeople/objectives-and-data/social-determinants-health

U.S. Department of Justice. (n.d.). Office for Access to Justice. https://www.justice.gov/archives/atj

van Ryn, M., Burgess, D., Malat, J., & Griffin, J. (2006). Physicians' perceptions of patients' social and behavioral characteristics and race disparities in treatment recommendations for men with coronary artery disease. *American Journal of Public Health, 96*(2), 351–357.

Wang, C. J., Conroy, K. N., & Zuckerman, B. (2009). Payment reform for safety-net institutions—Improving quality and outcomes. *New England Journal of Medicine, 361*(19), 1821–1823.

Williams, D. R., Costa, M. V., Odunlami, A. O., & Mohammed, S. A. (2008). Moving upstream: How interventions that address the social determinants of health can improve health and reduce disparities. *Journal of Public Health Management and Practice, 14*, s8–s17.

World Health Organization. (2018). *Social determinants of health.* http://www.who.int/social_determinants/sdh_definition/en/

Yearby, R. (2013). Breaking the cycle of "unequal treatment" with health care reform: Acknowledging and addressing the continuation of racial bias. *Connecticut Law Review, 44*(4), 1281–1324.

Endnotes

a. For a full account of the Tuskegee Study, see Jones, 1993.

b. According to the World Justice Project, a not-for-profit group promoting the rule of law, the United States ranks 109th out of 128 countries in the access to and affordability of civil legal services.

c. For more information, see, for example, U.S. Department of Justice (n.d.).

d. See American Bar Association (2006) for the resolution and an accompanying report on achieving equal justice in the United States.

e. Note that LSC's heyday was back in the late 1970s and early 1980s, when their budget topped $800 million dollars in 2015 terms.

f. In the interest of disclosure, Professor Teitelbaum is co-principal investigator of the National Center for Medical-Legal Partnership at The George Washington University's Milken Institute School of Public Health. For more information about medical–legal partnership and the National Center, visit http://www.medical-legalpartnership.org/.

CHAPTER 8

Understanding Health Insurance

LEARNING OBJECTIVES

By the end of this chapter you will be able to:

1. Understand the role of risk and uncertainty in insurance
2. Define the basic elements of health insurance
3. Differentiate various insurance products
4. Discuss incentives created for providers and patients in various types of insurance arrangements
5. Discuss health policy issues relating to health insurance

Introduction

Unlike many other countries, the United States does not have a national healthcare delivery system; whether individuals have access to healthcare services—and whether they receive health care of appropriate quantity and quality—often depends on whether they are insured. Even if individuals are insured, the kind of coverage they have can affect their ability to obtain care. Understanding health insurance, however, requires more than understanding its importance to healthcare access.

Policymakers must also know how providers, suppliers, employers, states, and others respond to changes in the health insurance market. For example, if policymakers decide to reduce the number of uninsured by creating a new state health insurance exchange (essentially, an online marketplace) for the sale and purchase of private insurance coverage (as happened under the Patient Protection and Affordable Care Act [ACA]), they must know whether providers will participate in the program and what

features will make it more or less attractive to providers. Or, if policymakers want to reduce the number of uninsured by mandating that employers offer health insurance (as also happened under the ACA), they must know which requirements will make it more or less likely that more employees will be covered under such a mandate. In either case, policymakers might also want to know whether an initiative will affect the financial viability of public hospitals or health centers.

Several themes emerge when considering these types of health-insurance–related policy questions. First, insurance is rooted in the concepts of uncertainty and risk; reducing uncertainty and risk by, for example, offering a health insurance product, participating as a provider in a health insurance plan, or purchasing health insurance coverage as a consumer creates various incentives for insurers, the insured, providers, and governments to act or refrain from acting in certain ways. As noted in **Box 8.1**, one goal of the ACA is to reduce the risk of insuring small businesses and individuals by creating a large purchasing pool through state health insurance exchanges

Box 8.1 VIGNETTE

William owns a small farm that raises chickens and goats. He has nine employees and has always made it a priority to offer competitive benefits, including health insurance. Unfortunately, last year one of his employees was diagnosed with cancer, which he continues to fight. Due to the sharp increase in use of health services by his employee group, the insurance company doubled his group premiums for the upcoming year. When William contacted other carriers, several of them would not consider insuring his group, and most of the others gave him quotes that were just as expensive as his current carrier. One company gave him a lower quote, but it covered only catastrophic care; his employees would have to pay for the first $5000 of care out of their own pockets. After reviewing his company's finances, William is left with several unattractive options: stop offering health insurance; offer comprehensive health insurance but pass on the cost increase to his employees, which would make it unaffordable for most of them; offer the bare-bones catastrophic plan only; or significantly lower wages and other benefits to defray the rising health insurance costs. In addition to wanting to offer competitive benefits, William is concerned that adopting any of these options will cause his employees to leave and make it hard to attract others, threatening the sustainability of his company.

The 2010 health reform law (ACA) attempts to help small businesses like William's by creating state health insurance exchanges. Starting in 2014, these exchanges offered a variety of plans to individuals and small businesses that otherwise might not be able to afford health insurance coverage. By creating large groups of purchasers through the exchanges, it is possible to pool risk and keep prices lower than if individuals or small businesses were attempting to purchase insurance coverage on their own.

(Patient Protection and Affordable Care Act [ACA], 2010). Second, to a large extent, insurance carriers choose the design of their health insurance products, and employers and individuals choose whether to purchase health insurance—and, if so, what type. Indeed, insurance carriers have had wide latitude to determine the individuals or groups that may join a plan, employers have had broad discretion to determine whether to offer coverage and what type to offer, and individuals have had the choice whether to purchase health insurance coverage, although this choice

was often illusory due to the high cost of health care. The ACA attempts to change these choices and incentives. For example, many insurance plans will have to meet new requirements, such as offering a package of "essential health benefits"; most employers will have to provide health insurance coverage or pay a penalty; and most individuals will have to purchase health insurance or pay a penalty. For each choice, the question is: What policy goal (e.g., equity, universal coverage, fiscal restraint, market efficiency) should drive the design and regulation of health insurance?

This chapter begins with a short history of health insurance in the United States and then reviews the health insurance concepts key to understanding the structure and operation of health insurance. It concludes with an overview of managed care, a particular form of health insurance dominant in today's market.

A Brief History of the Rise of Health Insurance in the United States

Although about 92% of people in this country were insured in 2019, health insurance was not always an integral part of our society (U.S. Census Bureau, 2020, p. 3). The initial movement to bring health insurance to the United States was modeled after activities in Europe. In the late 1800s and early 1900s, the European social insurance movement resulted in the creation of "sickness" insurance throughout many countries: Germany in 1883, Austria in 1888, Hungary in 1891, Britain in 1911, and Russia in 1912, to name just a few examples. These programs varied in scope and structure, from a compulsory national system in Germany, to industry-based requirements in France and Italy, to extensive state aid in Sweden and Switzerland. Although the Socialist and Progressive parties advocated for the adoption of similar social insurance systems in the United States in the early 1900s, their efforts were unsuccessful (Starr, 1982).

In the absence of government-sponsored health insurance plans, the private sector insurance industry flourished with the growth of Blue Cross, Blue Shield, and commercial insurance carriers. Blue Cross established its first hospital insurance plan at Baylor University in 1929 by agreeing to provide 1500 teachers with 21 days of hospital care per year for the price of $6 per person (Starr, 1982, p. 295). The hospital industry supported the growth of private insurance as a way to secure payment for services during the Depression. Blue Shield, the physician-based insurance plan, began in 1939 as a way to forestall renewed efforts to enact compulsory national health insurance and to avoid growth in consumer-controlled prepaid health plans, both of which would have reduced the type of physician autonomy endemic at that time (Starr, 1982, p. 307).

World War II led to rapid growth in employer-sponsored health insurance. With employees scarce and a general wage freeze in effect, a 1942 War Labor Board ruling that employee fringe benefits of up to 5% of wages did not violate the wage freeze created a strong incentive for employers to provide health benefits to attract new workers and keep their current ones. After the war, labor unions gained the right to bargain collectively, leading to another expansion of employee health plans. In 1954, the Internal Revenue Service declared that employers could pay health insurance premiums for their employees with pretax dollars, further increasing the value of the fringe benefit to employers.[a] By 1949, 28 million people had commercial hospital insurance, 22 million had commercial physician insurance, and 4 million had independent hospital plans. At that time, over 31 million had Blue Cross hospital coverage and 12 million had Blue Shield coverage (Starr, 1982, p. 327). Employer-sponsored health insurance, not national health insurance, was well on its way to becoming entrenched as the primary form of health insurance.

The federal government first became a major player in health insurance with the passage of Medicaid and Medicare in 1965. These programs were created, in part, to fill in coverage gaps left by the private insurance market—namely, coverage for the elderly, disabled, and low-income populations who had too little income and too high health risks to be viable candidates for insurance coverage from the insurance carriers' point of view. Like many major policy changes, the passage of these programs was a multilayered compromise. Before the final design of these programs was established, several proposals were considered: the American Medical Association (AMA) supported a combination federal–state program to subsidize private insurance policies for older adults to cover hospital care, physician care, and prescription drugs; Representative John Byrnes (R-WI), ranking Republican on the House Ways and Means Committee, endorsed an AMA-like proposal but with federal, instead of federal–state, administration; the Johnson administration supported hospital insurance for older adults through Social Security; and Senator Jacob Javitz (R-NY) supported federal payments to state programs to provide health care to poor, elderly individuals (Stevens & Stevens, 2003, pp. 46–48). In the end, the Medicare and Medicaid programs were passed in one bill with features from all of these proposals. For example, Medicare was established as a federally funded program with two parts, one for hospital insurance and one for physician insurance, and Medicaid as a state–federal program for the poor.

By the 1970s a number of factors converged to place rising healthcare costs on the national agenda: advances had been made in medical technology, hospitals expanded and became more involved in high-tech care, physician specialties became more common, hospitals and physicians had a large new pool of paying patients due to Medicaid and Medicare, wages for medical staff increased, and an aging population required an increasing amount of services (Starr, 1982, pp. 383–384). In addition, the prevailing fee-for-service (FFS) insurance system rewarded healthcare professionals for providing a high quantity of services. As the name suggests, fee-for-service reimbursement means the providers are paid for each service they provide—the more services (and the more expensive the services) rendered, the more reimbursement the provider receives. From 1960 to 1970, hospital care expenditures tripled from $9.3 billion to $28 billion, and physician service expenditures almost matched that growth rate, increasing from $5.3 billion to $13.6 billion (Sultz & Young, 2001, pp. 257–258). Federal and state governments were also feeling the burden of high healthcare costs. From 1965 to 1970, federal and state governments collectively experienced a 21% annual rate of increase in their healthcare expenditures (Starr, 1982, p. 384).

As is discussed in more detail later in this chapter, managed care moves away from the FFS system by integrating the payment for services and the delivery of services into one place in an attempt to rein in healthcare costs and utilization. The federal Health Maintenance Organization Act of 1973 was intended to spur the growth of managed care by providing incentives to increase the use of health maintenance organizations (HMOs). The act relied on federal loans and grants and a mandate that employers with 25 or more employees offer an HMO option if one was available in their area (Sultz & Young, 2001, pp. 262–263). Even so, managed care did not flourish due to opposition by patients, who did not want their provider and service choices restricted, and by providers, who did not want to lose control over their practices.

As healthcare cost and quality concerns remained a national priority, the managed care industry eventually found a foothold in the health insurance market. Indeed, enrollment in managed care doubled during the 1990s, with almost 80 million enrollees by 1998. In 2020, only 3% of workers were in firms that offered conventional, nonmanaged-care arrangements (Kaiser

Most people in this country obtain health insurance through employer-sponsored plans. Although the historical background you just read explains *how* this system came about, it does not discuss whether it is a good or bad thing. Is our reliance on employer-sponsored health insurance ideal for individuals? Providers? Employers? Society? What are the benefits and drawbacks to having employers as the primary source of health insurance? How different are the benefits and drawbacks when considered from various stakeholder perspectives? Would it be better to have more federal government involvement in providing health insurance? What primary policy goal would you use to decide how to answer these questions?

Family Foundation [KFF], 2020). Although only about 34% of Medicare enrollees choose managed care arrangements (KFF, 2019), some 69% of Medicaid beneficiaries receive some or all of their services through managed care, although for many of them it is mandatory that they receive services through a managed care arrangement (KFF, 2018). Before moving on to the next section, consider the discussion questions in **Box 8.2**.

How Health Insurance Operates

This section provides an overview of the purpose and structure of health insurance. It begins with a review of basic health insurance terminology, considers the role of uncertainty and risk in insurance, and concludes with a discussion of how insurance companies set their premium rates.

Basic Terminology

As you read earlier, the health insurance industry first developed when the FFS system was standard. Under this system, not only do providers have incentive to conduct more and more expensive services, but patients are unbridled in their use of the healthcare system because FFS does not limit the use of services or accessibility to providers. As we will discuss later in this chapter, managed care developed as a response to the incentives created by the FFS system. However, even though there are numerous differences between FFS and managed care, many of the fundamental principles of how insurance operates are applicable to any type of health insurance contract. The following

discussion reviews how health insurance works generally, regardless of the type of insurance arrangement.

The health insurance consumer (also known as the *beneficiary* or *insured*) buys health insurance in advance for an annual fee, usually paid in monthly installments, called a *premium*. In return, the health insurance carrier (or company) pays for all or part of the beneficiary's healthcare costs if they become ill or injured and have a covered medical need. (A covered need is a medical good or service that the insurer is obligated to pay for because it is covered based on the terms of the insurance contract or policy. As discussed in detail elsewhere, the ACA requires many plans to cover all "essential health benefits.") Insurance contracts cannot identify every conceivable healthcare need of beneficiaries, so they are generally structured to include categories of care (e.g., outpatient, inpatient, vision, maternity) to be provided if deemed medically necessary (see **Box 8.3**). Definitions of the term *medically*

As a general matter, all types of insurance under traditional economic models cover expensive and unforeseen events, not events that have small financial risk or little uncertainty (Council of Economic Advisors, 2004, p. 195). For example, auto insurance does not cover regular maintenance, such as an oil change, and home insurance does not protect against normal wear and tear, such as the need to replace an old carpet. Accordingly, many economists argue that health insurance should not cover regular, foreseeable events such as physical exams or low-cost occurrences such as vaccinations. Other economists support a different school of thought. An alternative economic view is that health insurance should insure one's health, not just offer protection against the financial consequences of major adverse health events. Because people without health insurance are less likely to obtain preventive care such as physical exams or vaccinations, these economists believe that it is in everyone's best interest, ethically and financially, to promote preventive care. Therefore, it is appropriate for insurance to cover both unpredictable and expensive events as well as predictable and less expensive events. Which theory do you support? What do you think is the best use of insurance? If insurance does not cover low-cost and predictable events, should another resource be available to assist individuals, or should people pay out of their own pockets for these healthcare needs?

necessary vary by contract and are important when determining whether a procedure is covered.

Even if the beneficiary never needs healthcare services covered by the insurance policy, they still pay for the policy through premiums. The consumer benefits by having financial security in case of illness or injury, and the insurance company benefits by making money selling health insurance.

In addition to premiums, the beneficiary typically pays other costs under most health insurance policies. Many policies have *deductibles*, which is the amount of money the beneficiary must pay on their own for healthcare needs each year before the insurance carrier starts to help with the costs. For example, if a policyholder has a $500 deductible, the beneficiary must pay 100% of the first $500 of healthcare costs each year. The insurance carrier is not liable to cover any costs until the individual's healthcare bill reaches $501 in a given year. If the individual does not need more than $500 worth of health care in a specific year, the insurance carrier generally will not help that individual pay their healthcare costs.

Furthermore, a beneficiary generally continues to incur some costs in addition to the premiums even after the deductible has been met. Insurance carriers often impose cost sharing on the beneficiary through *copayment* or *coinsurance* requirements. A copayment is a set dollar amount the beneficiary pays when receiving a service from a provider. For example, many HMOs charge their beneficiaries $15 every time a beneficiary sees a primary care provider. Coinsurance refers to a percentage of the healthcare cost the individual must cover. For example, 20% is a common coinsurance amount. This arrangement means the beneficiary pays 20% of all healthcare costs after the deductible has been met, with the insurance carrier paying the other 80%.

Uncertainty

From a traditional economic perspective, insurance exists because of two basic concepts—risk and uncertainty. The world is full of risks—auto theft, house fires, physical disabilities—and uncertainty about whether any such events might affect a particular individual. As a result, people buy various forms of insurance (e.g., automobile insurance, home insurance, life or disability insurance) to protect themselves and their families against the financial consequences of these unfortunate and unforeseen events.

Although genetic predisposition or behavioral choices such as smoking or working a high-risk job may increase the chances that an individual will suffer from a health-related problem, in general there is a high level of uncertainty regarding whether a particular

person will become sick or injured and need medical assistance. Health insurance protects the consumer from medical costs associated with both expensive and unforeseen events. Even if the consumer does not experience a negative event, a benefit exists from the peace of mind and reduced uncertainty of financial exposure that insurance provides.

In terms of health status and wise use of resources, when insurance allows consumers to purchase necessary services they would not otherwise be able to afford, it functions in a positive manner. Conversely, when insurance leads consumers to purchase unnecessary healthcare goods or services of low value because the consumer is not paying full cost, it works in a negative manner. The difficult task is trying to figure out how to set the consumer's share of the burden at just the right point to encourage and make available the proper use of health care, while discouraging improper usage.

Risk

Risk is a central concern in insurance. Consumers buy insurance to protect themselves against the risk of unforeseen and costly events. But health insurers are also concerned about risk—the risk that their beneficiaries will experience a covered medical event.

Individuals purchase health insurance to protect themselves against the risk of financial consequences of healthcare needs. Because of differences in risk level, individuals who are generally healthy or otherwise do not anticipate having health expenses may place a lower value on insurance than individuals who are unhealthy or those who are healthy but expect to have medical expenses, such as pregnant women. Therefore, healthy individuals tend to seek out lower-cost insurance plans or refrain from obtaining insurance altogether if it is not, in their view, cost effective. Unhealthy individuals or healthy individuals who often use the healthcare system would obviously prefer a low-cost insurance plan (with comprehensive benefits) but are generally more willing to pay higher premiums because of the value they place on having insurance.

Health insurance carriers are businesses that need to cover their expenditures, including the cost of accessing capital needed to run their company, to stay in the market.[b] They earn money by collecting premiums from their beneficiaries, and they pay out money to cover their beneficiaries' healthcare costs above the deductible amount and to cover the costs of running a business (e.g., overhead, marketing, taxes). One way health insurance companies survive is to make sure the premiums charged to beneficiaries cover these costs. From the insurance carrier's perspective, it would be ideal to be able to charge lower premiums to attract healthy individuals who are less likely to use their benefits, and higher premiums to unhealthy individuals who are more likely to need medical care. See **Box 8.4**.

However, insurance companies have difficulty matching healthy people with low-cost plans and unhealthy people with high-cost plans because of the problem of *asymmetric information*. This is the term used by economists when one party to a transaction has more information than the other party. In the case of insurance, the imbalance often favors the consumer because insurance carriers generally do not know as much as the individual does about the individual's healthcare needs and personal habits. Although relatively healthy low-cost individuals want to make their status known because insurance carriers might be willing to sell them an insurance product for a lower price, relatively unhealthy individuals do not want their status known because insurance companies might charge them higher premiums. For this reason, when an insurance carrier lacks complete information, it is more beneficial to unhealthy beneficiaries than to healthy ones.

Together, uncertainty about risk and the presence of asymmetric information lead to the problem of *adverse selection*. In terms of health insurance, adverse selection is when unhealthy people overselect (that is, select beyond a random distribution) a particular plan. This occurs because people at risk for having high healthcare costs choose a particular plan because of that plan's attractive coverage rules (Penner, 2004, pp. 12–13). Consumers who know that they are a high risk for needing services will be more likely to choose a more comprehensive plan because it covers more services, even though it is probably a more expensive option. This overselection leaves the insurer that offers the comprehensive plan with a disproportionate number of high-risk beneficiaries. As a result of the relatively high-risk pool, beneficiaries will have high service utilization rates, requiring the insurance carrier to raise premiums to pay for the increased cost of covering services for beneficiaries. In turn, some of the healthier individuals might choose to leave the plan because of the higher premiums, resulting in an even riskier beneficiary pool and even higher premiums, and the cycle continues. The healthier consumers may find a lower-cost plan or may choose to go without health insurance (especially since the Tax Cut and Jobs Act of 2017 repealed, as of 2019, the penalty associated with violating the ACA's individual mandate; this is described in more detail in Chapter 11, "Health Reform and the Patient Protection and Affordable Care Act"), while the insurance plan is left with an increasingly higher percentage of relatively unhealthy people. This is the problem of adverse selection.

One instance where adverse selection is a key concern is with an increasingly popular type of health plan, the high-deductible health plan (HDHP). As the name suggests, these plans have very high deductibles (usually defined as at least $1000 for an individual or $2000 for a family). In 2020, annual premiums for the average HDHP were $6890 for individuals and $20,359 for families (KFF, 2020, Section 1). As with other insurance plans, consumers pay most of their healthcare expenses out-of-pocket until they reach the deductible. HDHPs are often used in conjunction with health reimbursement arrangements (HRAs) or health savings accounts (HSAs), which allow individuals to set aside money for future healthcare needs. Health reimbursement arrangements are funded solely by employers, who usually commit to making a specified amount of money available for healthcare expenses incurred by employees or their dependents, while HSAs are created by individuals, but employers may also contribute to HSAs if the employers offer a qualified HDHP. Individual contributions to HSAs are made with preincome tax dollars, and withdrawals

Box 8.4 DISCUSSION QUESTIONS

As discussed earlier, risk and uncertainty are important concepts in health insurance. Individuals purchase health insurance policies to protect themselves financially against healthcare costs, and insurance carriers try to set premiums that will cover the cost of the services used by their beneficiaries. Currently (when allowed by law), insurance carriers may consider factors such as medical history, demographics, type of occupation, size of the beneficiary pool, and similar criteria when setting the terms of an insurance policy. Should health insurance carriers also have access to and be able to use genetic testing results when deciding whether to insure an individual, what premiums to charge, or which services to cover? If you think the answer to that question should be "no," why is genetic information different from all of the other kinds of information insurance carriers may take into account when making those decisions? Conversely, what is the strongest argument you can make in favor of allowing insurance carriers to consider an applicant's genetic information? How would allowing genetic testing alter an individual's or a provider's diagnosis and treatment decisions? What is the primary policy goal that affects your view?

to pay for qualified healthcare expenses are also not taxed. As shown in **Figure 8.1** and **Figure 8.2**, HDHPs are increasingly popular with employers and employees.

Those who support HDHPs assert that plans with high deductibles promote personal responsibility because enrollees have a financial incentive to avoid overusing the healthcare system and to choose cost-effective treatment options. As a result, HDHPs are favored by employers and others as a cost-cutting strategy. Others are concerned that HDHPs will have a negative effect on enrollees' health because individuals

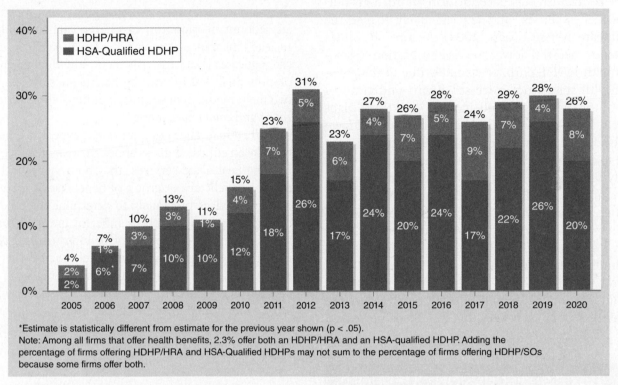

Figure 8.1 Percentage of Covered Workers Enrolled in a High-Deductible Health Plan (HDHP) or Health Reimbursement Arrangement, or in a Health Savings Account–Qualified HDHP, 2006–2020

Kaiser Family Foundation. (2020, October 8). *2020 Health benefits survey: Section 8: High-deductible health plans with savings option.* https://www.kff.org/report-section/ehbs-2020-section-8-high-deductible-health-plans-with-savings-option/

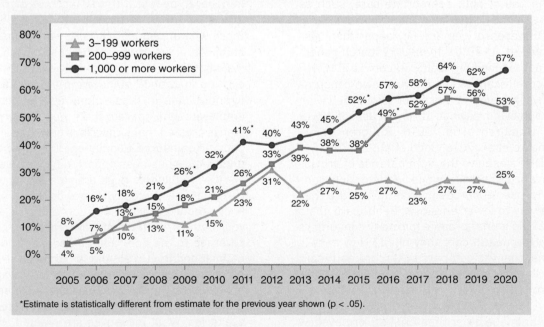

Figure 8.2 Among Firms Offering Health Benefits, Percentage That Offer an HDHP/SO, by Firm Size, 2005–2020

Kaiser Family Foundation. (2020, October 8). *2020 Health benefits survey: Section 8: High-deductible health plans with savings option.* https://www.kff.org/report-section/ehbs-2020-section-8-high-deductible-health-plans-with-savings-option/

cannot or will not price shop and are more likely to save money by simply avoiding needed care. As discussed in **Box 8.5**, researchers continue to evaluate these questions.

An enrollee's experience with an HDHP may depend, in part, on income level. Individuals who are wealthier and healthier are likely to have funds to place in a savings account, can afford high out-of-pocket expenses, and are less likely to use the healthcare system (Davis, 2004). As a result, critics contend that the lower service utilization associated with HDHP enrollees is likely due to their better health status, not price sensitivity, undermining one of the main arguments in support of these plans (Davis, 2004). Poorer individuals who may be drawn to the lower premium cost of HDHPs may not be able to afford care when they need it. In fact, a 2018 study found that HDHP enrollees without a savings account were less likely to obtain primary care, preventive services, or specialty care and more likely to be in poor or fair health as compared to enrollees with a savings account (Jetty et al., 2018). Finally, if healthier and wealthier individuals flock to HDHPs, poorer individuals in a comprehensive group plan (assuming one is available and affordable), face the possibility of adverse selection due to being part of a relatively high-risk insurance pool (Davis, 2004). Before moving on to the next section, consider the discussion questions in **Box 8.6**.

Setting Premiums

Assuming that insurance companies make their decisions in the context of asymmetric information, they cannot determine with certainty the appropriate amount of premium to charge each individual. Instead, insurance companies rely on making educated guesses about the risk each individual or group of individuals has of needing healthcare services. The two main methods of setting premiums are *experience rating* and *community rating*.

When insurance companies use experience rating to make an educated guess about the risk of someone's needing healthcare services, they are relying on how much a beneficiary or group of beneficiaries spent on medical services previously to determine the amount of the premium for each member or group. Thus, if an individual or group had very high medical costs in a given year, premiums are likely to rise the following year. Conversely, community rating does not take into account health status or claims history when setting premiums. In "pure" community rating, insurers use only geography and family composition to set rates; in "modified" community rating, insurers may

---

 Box 8.5 DISCUSSION QUESTIONS

A literature review of studies relating to consumer behavior with HDHPs found that these plans reduced the use of both appropriate care, such as preventive screenings, and inappropriate care, such as unnecessary emergency department visits (Agarwal et al., 2017). To date, research generally has not focused on health outcomes of HDHP users. Some recent studies have shown consumers rarely engaging in price-conscious behavior, instead achieving savings through use of fewer services (Kullgren et al., 2018; Kullgren et al., 2019; Sinaiko et al., 2016; Sood et al., 2013).

Do HDHPs achieve the right balance of providing insurance coverage while incentivizing consumers to use resources prudently? Or, are they simply a way to lower employer healthcare costs while making it unaffordable for many consumers to obtain the health care they need? How easy is it for consumers to compare costs for healthcare providers and services? What additional challenges might an HDHP present for individuals who are low income, live in rural areas, speak a primary language other than English, or have low health literacy?

Box 8.6 DISCUSSION QUESTIONS

In general, people with low incomes or no health insurance (or both) tend to be less healthy than those who are financially better off or insured (or both). As a result, policy proposals that suggest including poor, uninsured individuals in already-existing insurance plans are met with resistance by individuals in those plans and by carriers or employers who operate them. Yet, if an insurance plan is created that subscribes only a less-healthy, poor, or uninsured population, it is likely to be an unattractive business opportunity because beneficiaries are likely to need a high quantity of health care that will be costly to provide. Given what you know about adverse selection and risk, what, in your opinion, is the best way to provide insurance coverage to the poor and uninsured? Should they be included in current plans? Should the government provide financial incentives for private carriers to insure them? Should a separate plan or program be created to serve them? In these various scenarios, what incentives are created for plans, current plan members, government, and so on?

be allowed to consider other characteristics, such as age and sex.

Which rating system makes more sense from a policy perspective as a basis for setting premiums may depend on whether you evaluate the insurance market based on efficiency or equity (think back to discussions of competing conceptual frameworks). If the market is judged based on efficiency, then the key issue is whether the optimal amount of risk has shifted from consumers to insurers. If there are individuals willing to pay a higher amount for greater coverage and insurers willing to provide greater coverage for the higher amount, but something in the market prevents this transaction from occurring, then the optimal amount of risk shifting has not occurred. Or, if individuals value a certain level of insurance coverage at a price that is less than the price at which insurers are willing to provide that coverage, but individuals buy coverage anyway at the higher price, the market is not optimally efficient (due to excess coverage).

Conversely, the market may be judged based on equity or fairness. Even the most efficient market may result in some inequities. Some individuals may be uninsured, some may have to pay more than other individuals for the same level of insurance, some may not be able to purchase the level of coverage they desire, and some individuals may not be able to join a particular plan. These inequities are often a concern in the context of the uninsured, especially as uninsurance relates to low-income individuals or those with high health needs due to random events, such as an accident or genetic condition.

Regardless of the underwriting methodology used, premiums are cheaper for people purchasing insurance as part of a large group rather than buying health insurance individually or as part of a small group. Due to the law of averages, larger groups of people are more likely to have an average risk rate. When people join a group for reasons unrelated to health status, such as working for the same company, it is also more likely that the group will have an average risk rate. Groups with average risk rates are attractive to insurers because the cost of insuring a few unhealthy people will probably be offset by savings from insuring many healthy ones. Conversely, in smaller groups it is more likely that the group will have a relatively high risk rate and less likely that the cost of insuring an unhealthy person can be offset by the savings of insuring a few other healthy people. This is the problem faced by William, the small business owner described at the outset of the chapter who has one high-cost employee. Even though he would like to offer health insurance

coverage to his employees, William and other small business owners like him often are able to offer only expensive or limited coverage, if they can offer any health insurance benefit at all. To help individuals and small business owners like William, some states require insurers to use a community rating system to set premiums for these groups and in the state health insurance exchanges that were created by the ACA. (See **Box 8.7** for other considerations relating to rating systems.)

Carriers also prefer to insure large groups because most of the administrative costs associated with insurance are the same whether the carrier is covering a few people or a few thousand (Phelps, 2003, pp. 342–344). In fact, group coverage has traditionally required fewer marketing resources than individual coverage, which targets customers one at a time. However, the proliferation of information on the Internet may change this equation.

Medical Underwriting

The prior discussion about rate setting assumed asymmetric information (i.e., where the insurer has little information about the consumer's health status and the consumer has substantial information about their own healthcare needs). Of course, there are ways for insurers to gain information about the medical needs of a consumer looking to join a health plan: physical exams, questionnaires, medical records, occupation, and demographics all provide clues about the health status of the consumer. Although it is much more difficult to accomplish, insurers may also try to predict an individual's future costs through questionnaires that ask, for example, whether an individual engages in risky activities (e.g., riding a motorcycle) or through genetic testing (which is itself an emerging health policy and law issue).

💡 Box 8.7 DISCUSSION QUESTIONS

What populations or types of people pay more under experience rating? Does experience rating create any incentives for individuals to act in a certain way? What populations or types of people pay more under community rating? Does community rating create any incentives for individuals to act in a certain way? Which rating system seems preferable to you? What trade-offs are most important to you? Should the focus be on the good of the individual or the good of the community? Are these mutually exclusive concerns?

Whether companies are allowed to consider an applicant's medical history or other personal information to help assess risk of healthcare needs in the future—a practice referred to as medical underwriting—is a somewhat complicated legal question that involves both federal and state law. The Health Insurance Portability and Accountability Act of 1996 (HIPAA) includes an important protection for consumers by prohibiting group health plans from excluding or limiting otherwise qualified individuals due to preexisting conditions (a preexisting condition is a medical condition, such as cancer or diabetes, that is present at the time an individual applies to enroll in an insurance plan). The ACA expands this protection by requiring all health insurers to sell policies to all applicants, regardless of preexisting conditions. This requirement was in effect for children shortly after the ACA was signed into law, and took effect for adults in 2014; however, attempts are being made to chip away at this protection (as discussed in Chapter 11, "Health Reform and the Patient Protection and Affordable Care Act").

Prior to HIPAA, many individuals with preexisting conditions were denied insurance altogether, denied coverage for particular medical care, or charged very high premiums if they sought to purchase a policy. These practices led to a problem referred to as "job lock." Because most Americans receive insurance coverage through their employers, many employees with preexisting conditions could not switch jobs for fear that their new company's insurance policy would be denied to them on account of their preexisting condition. One study estimated that job lock resulted in a 4% reduction in voluntary turnover (Phelps, 2003, p. 341).

Although HIPAA and the ACA do not regulate the amount of premiums that may be charged, all members of a group generally pay the same premium due to the laws' nondiscrimination provisions. In HIPAA, these provisions prohibit plans or insurance carriers from requiring any individual to pay a higher premium or contribution than another "similarly situated" individual (Nondiscrimination in health coverage, 2001, p. 1382) in the plan based on eight health factors: health status, physical or mental medical conditions, claims experience (i.e., the individual has a history of high health claims), receipt of health care, medical history, genetic information, evidence of insurability, and disability (Nondiscrimination in health coverage, 2001, pp. 1378–1384, 1396–1403). However, because those who purchase individual health insurance plans are not covered by HIPAA's protections, the ACA protections were needed as well. The ACA also prohibits plans from charging individuals higher premiums due to their preexisting conditions.

Managed Care

The prior sections reviewed the history, basic structure, and purpose of health insurance generally. In this section, we discuss a specific kind of health insurance structure that has come to dominate the American market: managed care. We will describe why managed care emerged, some of the frequent cost-containment strategies used by managed care organizations, and the most common managed care structures in the market today.

Managed care became the predominant healthcare financing and delivery arrangement in the United States because healthcare costs had risen to alarming levels and there were few mechanisms for containing costs under the FFS system. As mentioned earlier, FFS does not create incentives for providers or patients to utilize healthcare services sparingly. Providers have an incentive under FFS to provide more services and more expensive services (but not necessarily higher-quality services) because their income rises with each procedure or office visit and fees are higher for more expensive services. As long as providers are accessible, insured patients can request services and assume their insurance company will pay most or all of the costs to the extent that the services are covered by the health plan and deemed medically necessary.

In addition, the FFS system does not create incentives for providers or patients to use the lowest-cost quality care available. Many people believe specialists provide higher-quality care and turn to them even for minor needs that do not truly require expensive specialty services, and the FFS system does not discourage this behavior. Furthermore, because traditional insurance coverage requires a specific diagnosis for reimbursement, patients are discouraged from seeking preventive services when they are symptom free under FFS. At the same time, traditional insurance companies do not have the ability to control costs or quality of care under FFS. Their job is limited to determining whether a service is covered and medically necessary and providing the agreed-upon reimbursement. They have little ability to measure or improve the quality of care provided by healthcare professionals and cannot control costs by limiting the amount or type of services received; instead, they can only raise premiums and other rates in the future to cover increasing costs.

To alter the inherent incentives under FFS and to grant insurers some ability to control the quality and utilization of services, managed care integrates the provision of and payment for healthcare services. Through various strategies discussed in the following sections, managed care organizations (MCOs) and managed care plans create incentives to provide fewer services and less expensive care, while still maintaining the appropriate level of healthcare quality. MCOs also attempt to alter patients' decision-making through cost-sharing requirements, cost-containment tools, utilization restrictions, and free or low-cost coverage for preventive care.

MCOs take various forms, but certain general features apply to all of them to varying degrees. All MCOs provide a comprehensive, defined package of benefits to the purchaser/member for a preset fee (including both monthly premium and cost-sharing requirements). Services are offered to members through a network of providers, all of whom have a contractual relationship with the MCO. The MCOs choose which providers to include in their networks and what services are rendered by network providers. Most notably, they also use financial incentives and other mechanisms to control the delivery, use, quality, and cost of services in ways that are not present in FFS insurance systems (Sultz & Young, 2001, p. 260).

Cost-Containment and Utilization Tools

Managed care introduced a variety of tools in its attempt to contain costs and control healthcare service utilization. The cost-containment strategies of *performance-based salary bonuses or withholdings*, *discounted fee schedules*, and *capitated payments* shift financial risk or limit payments to providers who, in turn, have an incentive to choose the least costly, but still effective, treatment option. The utilization control strategies of *gatekeeping* and *utilization review* focus on ensuring that only appropriate and necessary care is provided to patients. Another type of strategy, *case management*, is designed to ensure that necessary care is provided in the most coordinated and cost-effective way possible.

Provider Payment Tools

Depending on the structure of the MCO, provider salaries are based on a discounted fee schedule or capitation rate and include incentives to act or not act in certain ways. Providers in what are called staff-model MCOs are employees of the MCO and are paid an annual salary. The salary structure often includes bonuses or salary withholdings that are paid (or withheld) upon meeting (or not meeting) utilization or performance goals, thus shifting some financial risk from the MCO to the provider. A discounted fee schedule is a service-specific fee system, as is used in FFS. However, an MCO-style fee schedule pays lower reimbursement rates than is true in FFS systems; providers agree to accept less than their usual fee in return for the large volume of patients available to them by being a part of the MCO provider network. The MCO retains the financial risk in a discounted fee system, but the costs are lower for the company due to the discounted rate paid to providers. Finally, a capitated payment rate is a fixed monthly sum per member that the MCO uses to determine the provider salary. The capitation rate does not vary regardless of the number or type of services provided to patients. Physicians receiving a salary based on a capitated rate are responsible for providing all of the care needed by their MCO patients, within the provider's scope of practice. As a result, the financial risk in the case of capitated arrangements is shifted entirely from the MCO to the provider. Depending on the contract between the provider and the MCO, the insurance company may or may not guarantee the provider a minimum number of patients in exchange for accepting a capitated rate. These provider-focused cost-containment strategies are summarized in **Table 8.1**.

These payment methods lead to very different incentives for providers than is the case under the FFS system. Instead of being paid more for doing

Table 8.1 Provider Payment Cost-Containment Strategies

Strategy	Provider Payment Method	How Costs Are Controlled	Who Assumes Financial Risk
Salary and bonuses/withholdings	Provider receives a salary as an employee of an MCO	Incentive for provider to perform fewer and/or less-costly services	MCO and provider
Discounted fee schedule	Provider receives a lower fee than under FFS for each service to members	Pays provider less per service rendered than under FFS	MCO (but also has lower costs)
Capitation	Provider receives a set payment per month for each member regardless of services provided	Incentive for provider to perform fewer and/or less-costly services	Provider

Abbreviations: FFS = fee for service; MCO = managed care organization.

more, HMO providers are paid the same amount regardless of the number or type of services they provide. Given the use of bonuses and withholdings, salaried providers may be paid more if they make treatment decisions deemed favorable by an MCO. By using these incentives, MCOs encourage providers to render the fewest and most cost-effective services necessary.

Critics of managed care payment methodologies argue that MCO plan members will not receive all necessary care if providers are incentivized to provide fewer services and less-costly care. Instead of treating patients using both the most cost-efficient and medically necessary services, critics claim MCOs encourage providers to save money by providing fewer services and less specialized care than necessary; MCOs counter that their own incentive is to keep their members healthy so they do not need expensive services in the future. In addition, MCOs point to their ability to impose quality control measures on providers as a way to ensure that patients are properly treated. In response, critics argue that because members switch health plans relatively frequently, MCOs do not have an incentive to keep their members healthy because the MCOs will not realize the long-term savings as members come and go.

Which side has the better argument? There is no definitive answer. On the one hand, studies have found that treatment decisions under MCO arrangements are mostly influenced by clinical factors (not economic ones), that there is little or no measurable difference in the health outcomes of patients in FFS versus managed care plans, and that the quality of care provided under FFS and managed care plans is basically equal (Shi & Singh, 2017, p. 235; Shi & Singh, 2019, p. 382). In fact, patients in areas with a high market share of HMOs are more likely to engage in preventive care, receive diabetes care, and give high provider satisfaction ratings than are patients in areas with low HMO market share (Shi & Singh, 2017, p. 235). Researchers also have not found disparities based on race, ethnicity, and socioeconomic status in MCO versus FFS settings (Shi & Singh, 2017, p. 235; Shi & Singh, 2019, p. 382). While previous studies found that mental health patients did not fare as well in MCOs as in FFS plans, more recent research refutes that conclusion (Shi & Singh, 2019, p. 383).

On the other hand, nonprofit HMOs (a type of MCO) score better on quality measures than do for-profit ones, and HMO enrollees indicate lower patient satisfaction than do non-HMO patients (Shi & Singh, 2017, pp. 235–262; Shi & Singh, 2019,

p. 382). Also, due to low reimbursement rates, access is a particular concern for Medicaid MCO enrollees, who appear to have more limited access to certain services, higher emergency department use, and more unmet prescription drug needs (Shi & Singh, 2019, p. 381).

Utilization Control Tools

MCOs also employ other techniques, not related to provider payment methods, to control use of healthcare services. Once again, the goal in using these tools is to reduce the use of unnecessary and costly services. We review three common utilization control tools: gatekeeping, utilization review, and case management.

Gatekeepers monitor and control the services a patient receives. Members of managed care plans are often required to select a primary care provider from the MCO network upon enrollment. This provider acts as the member's "gatekeeper" and is responsible for providing primary care, referring patients for additional care, and generally coordinating the patient's care. Having a gatekeeper allows the MCO, not the patient or specialty provider, to determine when a patient needs additional or specialty services, diagnostic tests, hospital admissions, and the like. As with the cost-containment strategies discussed earlier, there are critics who contend that utilization-based bonuses or salary withholdings give gatekeepers financial incentive not to provide specialty referrals even when it is in the best interest of the patient.

Utilization review (UR) allows an MCO to evaluate the appropriateness of the services provided and to deny payment for unnecessary services. MCO personnel review and approve or deny the services performed or recommended by network providers. UR specialists are often healthcare professionals, and MCOs generally use existing clinical care guidelines to determine whether services are appropriate.

UR may occur prospectively, concurrently, or retrospectively. Prospective UR means that an MCO reviews the appropriateness of treatment before a service is rendered. A request for a recommended service is sent to a UR panel for approval or denial. A denial does not mean a patient cannot move forward with their preferred treatment plan; however, it does mean that the patient will have to pay for the treatment out-of-pocket. Prospective UR is distinguished from concurrent UR, which is when the MCO review of the appropriateness of treatment occurs while treatment is being rendered. For example, a patient may need a procedure that requires hospitalization. Even though the procedure is performed and covered, a UR specialist might still determine the number of days the patient may remain in the hospital or whether certain services, such as home care or physical therapy, will be covered upon discharge from the hospital. Finally, retrospective review means the MCO reviews the appropriateness of treatment (and therefore its coverage) after a service is rendered. In this case, a patient's medical records are reviewed to determine whether the care provided was appropriate and billed accurately; MCOs will not provide reimbursement for services deemed inappropriate or unnecessary. This latter type of review may also be used to uncover provider practice patterns and determine incentive compensation (Shi & Singh, 2019, pp. 373–374). Regardless of when the review occurs, the use of UR is controversial because it may interfere with the patient–provider relationship and allow for second-guessing of provider treatment decisions by a third party who is not part of the diagnosis and treatment discussions.

Case management is a service utilization approach that uses trained personnel to manage and coordinate patient care. Although gatekeeping serves as a basic form of case management for all members, many patients with complex or chronic conditions, such as HIV/AIDS or spinal cord injuries, may benefit from more intensive case management. These patients may have frequent need for care from various specialists and thus benefit from assistance by personnel who are familiar with the many resources available to care for the patient and who are able to provide information and assistance to patients and their families. A case manager works with providers to determine what care is necessary and to help arrange for patients to receive that care in the most appropriate and cost-effective settings (Shi & Singh, 2019, p. 370). Although the general idea of case management is not controversial, some people believe it can be implemented in a manner that acts more as a barrier than

an asset to care because additional approval is needed before a patient receives care and because another layer of bureaucracy is placed between the patient and the provider. **Table 8.2** summarizes the three service utilization control strategies just discussed.

As you might imagine, managed care's use of service utilization control mechanisms frequently leads to disputes between patients and their managed care company over whether the company is improperly affecting the provider–patient relationship (and negatively impacting the quality of care provided) by making decisions as to the type or quantity of care a patient should receive (see **Box 8.8**). This is both a highly charged health policy issue and a complicated legal issue, and one that is discussed in more detail in a review of individual rights in health care. For purposes of this chapter, it is enough to note that MCOs must have a grievance and appeal process to at least initially handle these sorts of disputes. Although companies' processes differ in their specifics, they generally allow members to appeal a coverage decision, provide evidence to support the appeal, and receive an expedited resolution when medically necessary. The ACA included a number of provisions relating to the appeals process required of insurance plans; these provisions establish a federal standard for state external appeals laws governing products in the individual and group markets and create a new federal appeals process for self-insured plans (the provisions do not affect Medicaid and Medicare, which have their own appeals processes) (National Conference of State Legislatures, 2018). The need for adequate grievance and appeal procedures can be particularly acute for patients with special healthcare needs, such as those with physical or mental disabilities, and patients who otherwise use the healthcare system more frequently than most people.

Table 8.2 Service Utilization Control Strategies

Strategy	Description	Potential Concerns
Gatekeeper	Uses a primary care provider to make sure only necessary and appropriate care is provided	Gatekeepers may have financial incentive to approve fewer services or less-costly care
Utilization review	Uses MCO personnel to review and approve or deny services requested by a provider to make sure only necessary and appropriate care is provided	Interferes with patient–provider relationship; someone other than the patient's provider decides whether treatment is appropriate
Case management	Uses MCO personnel to manage and coordinate patient care to make sure care is provided in the most cost-effective manner	May act as a barrier to receiving care if the case manager does not approve a desired service or service provider

Abbreviation: MCO = managed care organization.

Cost-containment strategies embraced by MCOs were a direct result of the FFS experience with ever-increasing utilization and healthcare costs. However, many consumers and providers chafe at the restrictions imposed by MCOs and are concerned that someone other than the provider is making treatment decisions. Are these restrictions appropriate and necessary? Do you favor some of the restrictions over others? Is it appropriate for one entity to be responsible for both paying for and providing care? Should someone other than an MCO—say the federal or state governments—have primary responsibility for making determinations about service utilization?

Common Managed Care Structures

There are three managed care structures common in the market today: health maintenance organizations (HMOs), preferred provider organizations (PPOs), and point-of-service (POS) plans. All three provide preventive and specialty care, but the rules relating to accessing care differ for each. In general, HMOs have the most restrictive rules pertaining to patients and providers, PPOs have the least restrictive rules, and POS plans fall in the middle.

As shown in **Figure 8.3**, PPOs are the most popular type of managed care plan, while very few people are still insured by a conventional FFS plan. In general, the more control an MCO has over its providers and

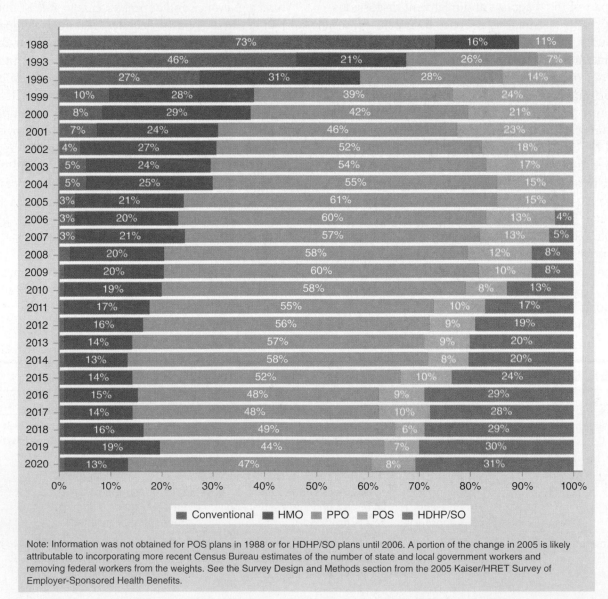

Note: Information was not obtained for POS plans in 1988 or for HDHP/SO plans until 2006. A portion of the change in 2005 is likely attributable to incorporating more recent Census Bureau estimates of the number of state and local government workers and removing federal workers from the weights. See the Survey Design and Methods section from the 2005 Kaiser/HRET Survey of Employer-Sponsored Health Benefits.

Figure 8.3 Distribution of Health Plan Enrollment for Covered Workers by Plan Type, 1988–2020

Kaiser Family Foundation. (2020, October 8). *2020 Employer health benefits survey: Section 5: Market shares of health plans.* https://www.kff.org/report-section/ehbs-2020-section-5-market-shares-of-health-plans/

members, the easier it is to control utilization of services and, therefore, healthcare costs and quality. Conversely, providers and patients prefer to have as much autonomy as possible, so the more restrictive MCO structures may be less desirable in that respect. However, the distinctions among managed care structures have become blurred recently because of the consumer and provider backlash against MCO restrictions.

Health Maintenance Organizations

When managed care first became prominent in the 1970s, HMOs were the most common type of MCO. There are several characteristics shared by all HMOs:

- They pay providers a salary to cover the cost of any and all services that beneficiaries need within a provider's scope of practice.

- They negotiate a capitated rate with plan purchasers (e.g., employers) that prices the plan based on a per-member, per-month amount for each type of provider.
- They coordinate and control receipt of services.
- They arrange for care using only their network providers.
- They are responsible for providing care according to established quality standards.

Despite these commonalities, HMOs may be structured through a variety of models, including the staff model/closed-panel model, group model, network model, individual practice association, and direct-contract model (Shi & Singh, 2019, pp. 374–377). Each model has advantages and disadvantages from the perspective of the HMO, its providers, and its members, as shown in **Table 8.3**.

Table 8.3 Key Characteristics of Common HMO Models

HMO Model	HMO–Provider Relationship and Payment Type	Provider Employment Arrangement	Must Members Seek Care from Network?	May Providers Care for Nonmembers?	General Comments
Staff model/closed-panel	HMO employs providers and pays a salary that often includes bonuses or withholdings	Employed by HMO	Yes	No	Provides services only in HMO's office and affiliated hospitals. Relatively speaking, HMO has the most control over providers and service utilization, but has fixed costs of building and staff. HMO may contract with outside providers if necessary. Providers and consumers often do not like restrictions imposed by HMO. Providers do not need to solicit patients. Consumers may find it to be the most cost-effective option.
Group	HMO contracts with one multispecialty group for a capitated rate	Employed by own provider group	Yes	Depends on terms of contract	HMO has less control over utilization. HMO contracts for hospital care on a prepaid or FFS basis. Providers may prefer this model because they remain independent as opposed to becoming an employee of the HMO and because they may serve nonmembers if their contract permits.

(continues)

Table 8.3 Key Characteristics of Common HMO Models   *(continued)*

HMO Model	HMO–Provider Relationship and Payment Type	Provider Employment Arrangement	Must Members Seek Care from Network?	May Providers Care for Nonmembers?	General Comments
Network	HMO contracts with several group practices (often primary care practices) for a capitated rate	Employed by own provider group	Yes	Depends on terms of contract	The group practices may make referrals but are financially responsible for reimbursing outside providers. HMO has less control over utilization due to greater number of contracts and ability of providers to subcontract. Providers may prefer additional autonomy, but also take on financial risk of providing primary and specialty care. Members may have a relatively greater choice of providers.
IPA	HMO contracts with IPA for a capitated rate	IPA is intermediary between HMO and solo practitioners and groups. IPA pays providers a capitated rate.	Yes	Depends on terms of contract	HMO has reduced control over providers but may have less malpractice liability because IPA is an intermediary. HMO may contract with specialty physicians as needed and for hospital care on a prepaid or FFS basis. Providers may prefer contracting with IPA instead of HMO to retain more autonomy. Members may have greater choice of providers.
Direct-contract	HMO contracts directly with individual providers for a capitated rate	Self-employed	Yes	Depends on terms of contract	HMO has more leverage over providers because it contracts with them as individuals, but its administrative costs are much higher than having one contract or a few contracts with groups. Providers have less leverage regarding practice restrictions when contracting on an individual basis.

Abbreviations: FFS = fee for service; HMO = health maintenance organization; IPA = individual practice association.

Preferred Provider Organizations

As is evident from Table 8.3, every form of HMO is fairly restrictive. In all models, the HMO provides coverage only if members seek care from network providers, and providers may or may not be limited to serving only HMO members. As both patients and providers began rebelling over these restrictions, new forms of MCOs emerged, often formed by providers and hospitals themselves.

Like HMOs, PPOs have a provider network, referred to as preferred providers. Unlike HMOs, however, PPOs provide coverage to patients seeking care from any provider, regardless of whether the provider is part of the member's PPO preferred provider network. However, the amount of the service price that the PPO will cover is greater for an in-network provider than an out-of-network provider. For example, a PPO may agree to cover 80% of the cost for an in-network physician visit, but only 70% of the cost for a similar, but out-of-network, physician visit. PPO patients thus have the option of paying more but choosing among a greater number of providers or paying less but choosing among a more limited number of (in-network) providers. In addition, a PPO member's cost-sharing responsibilities are often higher than is the case for HMO members.

In exchange for being in the network, providers agree to accept a discounted rate for their services, often 25%–35% below their usual rates (Shi & Singh, 2019, p. 378). Because PPO members have a financial incentive to seek providers who are in-network, these healthcare professionals find it worthwhile to accept a reduced rate from the PPO in exchange for the higher likelihood that PPO members will select them over non-network providers. Furthermore, unlike the capitation system found in HMOs, PPO providers do not assume financial risk for providing services. Depending on the terms of their contract with the PPO, preferred providers may or may not agree to limit their practice to PPO members. Although it is rare, PPOs may choose to guarantee preferred providers a minimum number of patients.

Even though an MCO has much less control over service utilization in the PPO model than in the HMO model, PPOs still provide more incentives to use care judiciously than is the case in an FFS system. For example, in-network PPO providers are paid less than their customary rate by the company when they provide care to PPO members and often agree to abide by quality control and UR strategies used by the PPO. In addition, PPO patients have an incentive to use certain providers who will cost them less and have cost-sharing requirements unlike anything found under FFS. The PPO model attempts to locate a middle ground between the very restrictive HMO models and the FFS structure that resulted in very high healthcare utilization and costs.

Point-of-Service Plans

In another effort to contain costs while still providing patients the freedom to choose their provider, POS plans combine features of HMOs and PPOs. Like an HMO, POS plans have a provider network, use a capitated or other payment system that shares financial risk with providers, and require members to use a gatekeeper to help control service utilization. However, designated services may be obtained from out-of-network providers who are paid on an FFS basis, but use of these providers costs the member more money, as with the PPO model. A POS gatekeeper must approve all in-network care and may also have some control over out-of-network care, depending on the terms of the plan. The call by many consumers for increased choice in providers has become forceful enough that some HMOs are now offering POS plans, which they may refer to as open-ended (as opposed to closed-panel) models.

The Future of Managed Care

Managed care is likely to remain an integral part of the health system despite its drawbacks. Patients chafe at utilization restrictions, as is evident by the increase in PPO popularity and the emergence of the hybrid HMO/POS plan. Accurate or not, there is a widespread perception that managed care plans deny necessary care and provide lower-quality care (Shi & Singh, 2017, pp. 218, 235). Providers also complain that managed care interferes with their ability to practice medicine in a manner of their choosing, placing them in ethical dilemmas due to the use of financial incentives and possibly lowering the quality of care they provide due to limits on tests and procedures they order. Yet, the key circumstance that led to the creation of managed care—high healthcare expenditures—has not abated. While the country struggles with ever-growing healthcare costs, even under managed care, the willingness to experiment with various cost and utilization containment strategies is likely to endure. See **Box 8.9** for more on this issue.

💡 Box 8.9 DISCUSSION QUESTIONS

In terms of containing healthcare costs and improving healthcare quality, do you think healthcare consumers and professionals need even more restrictions than are currently used in managed care? Are there any reasons to revert back to the FFS system, even knowing its inflationary qualities? If you think that managed care is not the answer to our still-rising healthcare costs and quality concerns, what other tools might help lower costs and improve the quality of care? Should any tools be imposed by government regulation or agreed to voluntarily by insurers and the insured?

Conclusion

This introduction to health insurance serves as a building block for additional study, which expands upon many of the key health policy and law themes mentioned here. It should be clear to readers that health policy analysts and decision makers must be particularly attuned to health insurance issues; without knowing both the basic structure of health insurance and how various incentives impact the actions of healthcare consumers, professionals, and insurance carriers, they cannot make informed recommendations and policies addressing the key health issues of the day.

References

Agarwal, R., Mazurenko, O., & Menachemi, N. (2017). Health deductible health plans reduce health care costs and utilization, including use of needed preventive services. *Health Affairs, 36*(10), 1762–1768. https://doi.org/10.1377/hlthaff.2017.0610

Council of Economic Advisors. (2004). *Economic report of the president.* U.S. Government Printing Office.

Davis, K. (2004). Consumer-directed health care: Will it improve system performance? *Health Services Research, 39,* 1219–1233.

Health Insurance Portability and Accountability Act of 1996, 42 U.S.C. §§ 18, 26, & 29.

Jetty, A., Petterson, S., Rabin, D. L., & Liaw, W. (2018). Privately insured adults in HDHP with higher deductibles reduce rates of primary care and preventive services. *Translational Behavioral Medicine, 8*(3), 375–385. https://doi.org/10.1093/tbm/ibx076

Kaiser Family Foundation. (2018). *Total Medicaid MCO enrollment.* https://www.kff.org/other/state-indicator/total-medicaid-mco-enrollment/?currentTimeframe=0&sortModel=%7B%22colId%22:%22Location%22,%22sort%22:%22asc%22%7D

Kaiser Family Foundation. (2019, February 13). *An overview of Medicare.* https://www.kff.org/medicare/issue-brief/an-overview-of-medicare/

Kaiser Family Foundation. (2020, October 8). *2020 Employer health benefits survey – section 4.* https://www.kff.org/report-section/ehbs-2020-section-4-types-of-plans-offered/

Kullgren, J. T., Cliff, E. Q., & Krenz, C. D. (2018). Consumer behaviors among individuals enrolled in high deductible health plans in the United States. *JAMA Internal Medicine, 178*(3), 424–426. https://doi.org/10.1001/jamainternmed.2017.6622

Kullgren, J. T., Cliff, E. Q., Krenz, C. D., Levy, H., West, B., Fendrick, A. M., So, J., & Fagerlin, A. (2019). A survey of Americans with high-deductible health plans identifies opportunities to enhance consumer behaviors. *Health Affairs, 38*(3), 416–424. https://doi.org/10.1377/hlthaff.2018.05018

National Conference of State Legislatures. (2018). *Right to health insurance appeals process.* http://www.ncsl.org/research/health/right-to-health-insurance-appeals-in-aca.aspx

Nondiscrimination in health coverage in the group market: Interim final rules and proposed rules, 66 Fed. Reg, 1378, 1382 (January 2001) (codified in 29 C.F.R. pt. 2590.702).

Patient Protection and Affordable Care Act of 2010, Pub. L. No. 111-148 (2010).

Penner, S. (2004). *Introduction to health care economics and financial management: Fundamental concepts with practical application.* Lippincott Williams & Wilkins.

Phelps, C. E. (2003). *Health economics* (3rd ed.). Addison-Wesley.

Shi, L., & Singh, D. A. (2017). *Essentials of the U.S. health care system* (4th ed.). Jones & Bartlett Learning.

Shi, L., & Singh, D. A. (2019). *Delivering health care in America: A systems approach* (7th ed.). Jones & Bartlett Learning.

Sinaiko, A. D., Mehrotra, A., & Sood, N. (2016). Cost-sharing obligations, high-deductible health plan growth, and shopping for health care: Enrollees with skin in the game. *JAMA Internal Medicine, 176*(3), 395–397. https://doi.org/10.1001/jamainternmed.2015.7554

Sood, N., Wagner, Z., Huckfeldt, P., & Haviland, A. (2013). Price-shopping in consumer-directed health plans. *Forum of Health Economics and Policy, 16*(1), 1–19. https://doi.org/10.1515/thep-2012-0028

Starr, P. (1982). *The social transformation of American medicine: The rise of a sovereign profession and the making of a vast industry.* Basic Books.

Stevens, R., & Stevens, R. (2003). *Welfare medicine in America: A case study of Medicaid.* Transaction Publishers.

Sultz, H. A., & Young, K. M. (2001). *Healthcare USA: Understanding its organization and delivery* (3rd ed.). Aspen Publishers.

Tax Cut and Jobs Act of 2017, Pub. L. No. 115-97 (2017).

U.S. Census Bureau. (2020). *Health insurance coverage in the United States: 2019.* (Current Population Reports, P60-271). U.S. Government Printing Office.

Endnotes

a. Section 106 of the IRS Code of 1954 states that employers who pay a share of premiums for employees' hospital and medical insurance may exclude that amount from the gross income of employees.

b. There are both for-profit and not-for-profit insurance companies. Both types of companies seek to earn enough revenues to cover expenses and the cost of accessing capital. However, for-profit companies return excess revenue to their investors, whereas not-for-profit companies put excess revenue back into the company.

CHAPTER 9

Health Economics in a Health Policy Context

LEARNING OBJECTIVES

By the end of this chapter you will be able to:

1. Understand why it is important for health policymakers to be familiar with basic economic concepts
2. Understand how economists view decision-making and options analysis
3. Describe the basic tenets of supply, demand, and markets
4. Understand how health insurance affects economic conditions
5. Apply economic concepts to health policy problems

Introduction

There are several disciplines that may be used to assist you in analyzing health policy problems; these include frameworks such as topical domains, historically dominant perspectives, and key stakeholder perspectives, along with political and legal analysis. Furthermore, throughout the text, issues are viewed through a social framework by asking you to consider what policies guide your decision-making—in other words, what do you think should happen? This chapter informs you about yet another discipline— economics—that is useful when conducting health policy analysis.

Students who are just beginning their health policy studies often question why it is necessary to study economics. Most would rather think about and discuss what policies they support and what values should govern decision-making, not about competitive markets, equilibriums, and externalities. What may not be clear initially to students is that economic theory provides one of the fundamental building blocks for making policy choices, both generally and in the context of health care and public health. For instance, economic tools help policymakers predict how consumers and producers will react if they implement certain policies. Knowing this may help policymakers choose the most effective and efficient policy to achieve their goals. The governor's request to Jaia in **Box 9.1** provides one example of how economic knowledge would prove helpful in health policy decision-making. Other examples include the following:

- When federal officials decide which communities should receive grants to support primary care clinics, they need to know if appropriate providers are available to staff clinics. Economic theory can help explain why some providers prefer to locate in urban or suburban Maryland instead of rural West Virginia, why there is a shortage of qualified nurses but an abundance of cardiologists, and how to change this situation and help a rural primary care clinic remain viable.

Box 9.1 VIGNETTE

Jaia is Governor Jara's chief health policy analyst. Governor Jara is interested in improving the health status of residents in the state but is concerned about the impact any new initiative will have on the state's economy. She asks Jaia to compare the economic consequences of three options: tax incentives for individuals to purchase exercise equipment or gym memberships, tax incentives for employers to offer wellness programs, and a mandate requiring that all stores selling food in the state provide fresh food and other healthy options. Fortunately, Jaia has a background in economics and knows that she needs to be concerned with basic principles of supply, demand, and market functions to help her governor make the best choice. This knowledge will lead her to ask questions such as: How big of a tax incentive is necessary to compel individuals or employers to act? Will tax incentives encourage behaviors, such as people joining a gym or employers offering wellness programs, that would not occur otherwise, or will the government simply be subsidizing transactions that would take place anyway? Is the problem that exercise options and healthy foods are not available and affordable, or are individuals simply making the choice not to engage in healthy behavior because they prefer to spend their time and money on other goods and activities? Will a mandate lead to the proliferation of healthy food stores or encourage stores to leave the state? The answers to these questions will help Jaia supply the governor with informed policy recommendations.

- In the face of a flu vaccine shortage, the president considers launching an initiative to ensure that every American can be vaccinated against the flu in the case of an epidemic. Economic theory sheds light on why there are so few vaccine producers supplying the United States currently and what could be done to entice manufacturers to participate in the flu vaccine market consistently over time.

Entire books and courses are devoted to the concept of health economics, and this chapter is not an attempt to distill all the theories and lessons of those texts and courses. Instead, our goal is to introduce you to the basic concepts of health economics because understanding how economists view health-related problems is one essential component of being a good health policy analyst and decision maker. This chapter begins with an overview of what health economics is, how economists view health care, and how individuals determine whether obtaining health insurance is a

priority in their lives. It then moves to a review of the basic economic principles of supply, demand, and market structure. As part of this discussion, you will learn what factors make supply and demand increase or decrease, how the presence of health insurance affects supply and demand, how different market structures function, and what interventions are available when the market fails to achieve desired policy goals.

Health Economics Defined

Economics is concerned with the allocation of scarce resources, as well as the production, distribution, and consumption of goods and services. Macroeconomics studies these areas on a broad level, such as how they relate to national production or national unemployment levels, while microeconomics studies the distribution and production of resources on a smaller level, including individual decisions to purchase a good or a firm's decision to hire an employee. Microeconomics also considers how smaller economic units, such as firms, combine to form larger units, such as industries or markets (Pindyck & Rubinfeld, 2003, p. 3). Health economics, then, is the study of economics as it relates to the health field.

How Economists View Decision-Making

Economists assume that people, given adequate information, are rational decision makers. Rational decision-making requires that people have the ability to rank their preferences (whichever preferences are relevant when any sort of decision is being made) and assumes that people will never purposely choose to make themselves worse off. Instead, individuals will make the decision that gives them the most satisfaction, by whatever criteria individuals use to rate their level of satisfaction. This satisfaction, referred to as *utility* by economists, may be achieved in many ways, including volunteering time or giving money to charities. Utility in a health context takes into account that individuals have different needs for and find different value in obtaining healthcare goods and services and that whether they purchase health resources—and, if so, which ones they purchase—will depend on the individual's preferences and resources.

Utility Analysis

What does utility mean in terms of health care? Most people do not enjoy going to the doctor or taking medicine. It seems strange to think of individuals as being "happy" as a result of, for example, receiving weekly allergy shots or getting chemotherapy treatments. Likewise, it seems odd to think of individuals as undergoing such regimens to "maximize the utility" of the interventions. However, health care can be discussed in terms of utility because most people enjoy being healthy.

Everyone has a different level of health, some due to their status at birth (e.g., infants born prematurely may have problems with their lungs or mental development) and others due to incidents that occur during their lives (e.g., an individual who was in a serious car crash may suffer from back pain). In addition, people have various tolerance levels for being unhealthy. In other words, the willingness to pay for a particular healthcare good or service will vary among individuals based on their circumstances and preferences.

Furthermore, at some point, obtaining additional "units" of a particular good will bring less satisfaction than the previous units did. For example, although icing a sore knee for 20 minutes may reduce swelling, icing the same knee for 40 minutes will not reduce swelling twice as much, or, although buying one pair of glasses may bring high satisfaction, buying two pairs of glasses will not double the consumer's satisfaction because the second pair of glasses cannot do more than the first. This concept is called *diminishing marginal utility*, and it also affects what goods and services a consumer purchases.

In addition, consumers must consider the *opportunity costs* of their decisions. Opportunity costs refer to the cost associated with the options that are not chosen. For example, if consumers decide not to purchase any medication to ease their back pain, there is zero accounting or monetary cost; that is, it did not cost consumers any money because they did not purchase the medication. However, there may be opportunity costs, monetary or otherwise, because the consumers are not pain-free. The consumers may endure a monetary loss if they have to take time off from work due to the injury. Or, consumers may endure a nonmonetary loss because they cannot enjoy walking or exercising due to the back pain. Opportunity costs are the hidden costs associated with every decision, and in order to fully assess the cost and benefits of any decision, these hidden costs must be included in the calculation.

In terms of healthcare goods only, utility can be thought of as a function of individuals' health and the healthcare goods and services they desire. Utility maximization in health care is the ideal set of health-related goods and services that an individual purchases. However, people need to purchase a variety of goods and services, not just those relating to health care. Overall, consumers maximize their utility by purchasing what they consider to be an ideal bundle of healthcare goods and services, as well as other goods and services, based on their desire for each good and service and subject to the income they have available to make these purchases.

Scarce Resources

In the healthcare arena, consumers have to make choices about the production, distribution, and consumption of healthcare resources. There are many types of healthcare resources. Healthcare goods include items such as eyeglasses, prescription drugs, and hospital beds; healthcare personnel include providers such as physicians, nurses, and midwives, as well as lab technicians, home healthcare workers, and countless others; and healthcare capital inputs (resources used in a production process) include items such as nursing homes, hospitals, and diagnostic equipment (such as an X-ray machine). All of these things (and others) are considered healthcare resources.

If there were unlimited healthcare resources and an unlimited ability to pay for goods and services, the questions confronted by health policy analysts about what healthcare items should be produced and who should have access to them would still exist, but the answers would be less dire because there would be enough health care available for everyone. In reality, however, there is a finite amount of healthcare goods, personnel, and capital inputs. The financial resources are not available to provide all of the health care demanded by the entire population and still provide other goods and services that are demanded. As a result of this scarcity of resources, choices and very apparent trade-offs must be made.

In general, consumer choices are based on individual preference, as discussed earlier, and the concept of efficiency. In economic terms, an efficient distribution of resources occurs when the resource distribution cannot be changed to make someone better off without making someone else worse off. This notion of efficiency in exchange is also referred to as Pareto-efficient, named after the Italian economist Vilfredo Pareto, who developed the concept. There are several types of efficiency, such as *allocative efficiency*, *production efficiency*, and *technical efficiency* (Penner, 2004, pp. 9–10; Santerre & Neun, 2004, p. 5). Allocative efficiency focuses on providing the most value or benefit with goods and services. Production efficiency focuses on reducing the cost of the inputs used to produce goods and services. Technical efficiency focuses on using the least amount of inputs to create goods or services.

The notion of efficiency raises many questions because there are always trade-offs to be made when producing goods and services. For example, should the production be more automated or more labor-intensive? Should the production sites be located in the United States or overseas? Can a service be provided in a less costly setting? Is there any additional or different service or product that will enhance the benefits of the goods or services consumers receive?

Although they may not use this technical economic jargon, public and private policymakers often consider concepts of efficiency when they answer these types of questions. The answers, in turn, help identify which goods and services should be produced overall in society and which of those goods and services should be related to health care. Because there is a finite amount of resources available, the choice to produce more healthcare goods and services would result in the production of fewer nonhealthcare goods and services, and vice versa. Similarly, the choice to produce more of one kind of healthcare good or service will lead to the production of fewer healthcare goods and services of other types.

Finally, policymakers must also decide whether equity or fairness concerns should be taken into account, and, in response, alter their production and distribution decisions in ways that may make some people better off at the expense of others. For example, during the COVID-19 pandemic, there was significant debate about which populations should have priority access to the initially limited supply of vaccine. Individuals who typically had access to healthcare goods and services but who were not in the high-priority groups were made worse off by the decision to limit access to the vaccine. On the other hand, some individuals in the high-priority groups who otherwise would not have been able to obtain the vaccine were made better off under the new policy. The point is not that efficiency is more important than equity or vice versa. It is important to understand, however, that these are distinct and not always complementary concerns, and whether and how one decides to influence the market will depend, in part, on how much the decision maker values efficiency and equity. In a world of limited resources, balancing consumer preferences, efficiency, and equity concerns can be a difficult task for policymakers.

How Economists View Health Care

Health economics helps explain how health-related choices are made, what choices should be made, and the ramifications of those choices. Evaluating the consequences of these choices is referred to as *positive* economics. Positive economics identifies, predicts, and evaluates who receives a benefit and who pays for a public policy choice. Positive economics answers the questions, "What is the current situation?" and "What already happened?" *Normative* economics discusses what public policy should be implemented based on the decision maker's values. It answers the question, "What should be?" (Feldstein, 2005, p. 5; Santerre & Neun, 2004, p. 14). For example:

> Positive statement: In 2019 approximately 26 million people in the United States did not have health insurance for the entire year.

> Normative statement: All people living in the United States should have health insurance.

As shown by the concepts of positive and normative economics, health economists, like other analysts, cannot avoid discussing how health care *should* be perceived. Is health care a good or service like any other good or service such as food, shelter, or clothing that consumers obtain or refrain from obtaining based on availability, price, resources, and preference? Or is health care a special and unique commodity for reasons such as its importance to individuals' quality of life or how the healthcare market is structured? Bear in mind that health policymakers take their own view of health care's place in the market into account when they argue for or against a policy.

The following sections identify two theories of how to view health care. Many economists' views fall somewhere in the middle of these two theories or combine aspects of the two theories to create a hybrid theory (see **Box 9.2**). These theories were not presented to be an either/or choice, but to illustrate that even within the field of economics there is a fundamental debate about how to view health care.

Economic Basics: Demand

Consumers, whether an individual, firm, or country, purchase goods and services. *Demand* is the quantity of goods and services that a consumer is willing and able to purchase over a specified time. In the case of health care, for example, demand equals the total demand for healthcare goods and services by all the consumers in a given market.

Demand Changers

In general, as the price of a good or service increases, demand for that good or service will fall. Conversely,

Box 9.2 DISCUSSION QUESTIONS | Consider each of the following issues and discuss whether you support Theory X, Theory Y, neither theory, or some combination of them.

Issue	Theory X	Theory Y
Your view about how an individual's health is determined	Whether a person is healthy or sick is determined randomly.	Whether a person is healthy or sick depends on lifestyle choices such as whether a person smokes, drinks, or wears a seat belt.
Your view of medical practice	Medicine is a science, and experts will ultimately discover the best means for treating every illness.	Medicine is an art and there will never be one best way to treat every illness because illnesses are often patient-specific and because there will always be a demand for lower-cost and less painful treatments.
Your view of medical care	Medical care is a unique commodity.	Medical care is similar to any other good or service.
Your view of the government's role in health care	Government regulations are necessary to protect this unique commodity, to control profiteering at the cost of patient care, to control resources spent on health care, and to improve information sharing.	Government regulations are not necessary; technological advances and more services are desirable; and competition, not regulation, should drive the market.

Musgrave, G. L. (1995). Health economics outlook: Two theories of health economics. *Business Economics, 30*(2), 7–13.

as the price of goods or services decreases, demand for those goods or services will rise.

Various factors in addition to price also increase or decrease the demand for a product. Insurance is an important factor relating to demand that is discussed separately later in this chapter. A few of the other factors that may change the demand for a product include the following:

- **Consumer's income:** As a consumer's income increases, demand for a product may increase. For example, a consumer may desire a new pair of eyeglasses but cannot afford it. Once the consumer's income increases, the consumer can purchase the eyeglasses.
- **Quality:** Consumers have preferences based on quality, both actual and perceived. In addition, a change in quality will likely result in a change in demand. A decrease in the quality of a product may result in a decrease in demand because consumers decide the product is no longer worth the price charged. For example, consumers may discover that the eyeglasses they want fall apart easily, thus they may decide not to buy the product.

- **Price of substitutes:** A substitute is a different product that satisfies the same demand. For example, contact lenses may be a substitute for eyeglasses. As the price of contact lenses drops, consumers may decide that they prefer contact lenses to eyeglasses.
- **Price of complements:** A complement is a product associated with another product. For example, cleaning solution is a complement to contact lenses. The price and quality of cleaning solution (the complement) may be an important factor when a consumer is debating whether to keep wearing glasses (the original product) or switch to contact lenses (the alternative product). If the price of cleaning solution increases, even though the price of contact lenses stays the same, the consumer may decide to purchase eyeglasses instead of contact lenses. In other words, demand for complements and alternative products shifts in opposite ways, so an increase in the price of a complement will decrease the demand for the alternative product, and vice versa.

The physical profile of a consumer has an impact on demand for healthcare services in some predictable ways. For example, women have higher per capita healthcare expenditures than men, mainly due to costs associated with maternity care and longer life expectancy (Cylus et al., 2011). Men and women also have demand for different types of healthcare services. For example, women use more heartburn and contraceptive medication, while men are more likely to purchase prescription drugs to treat attention deficit disorder and attention deficit hyperactivity disorder (Cylus et al., 2011). Regardless of sex, an individual who is born with a medical problem, or who develops one at a relatively young age, can be expected to have a higher than average demand for healthcare services. Aging consumers are more likely to have higher healthcare needs than younger consumers. Of course, any factor that usually leads to increases in demand for healthcare services may be offset by lack of financial resources or lack of access to providers.

In addition to the physical profile of a consumer, interesting research is being conducted in relation to consumers' level of education and their demand for services. Although there is no consensus on the direct impact of general education on demand for health services, some studies show a positive relationship between medical knowledge and demand for healthcare services; that is, the more the consumer knows about medicine, the higher the level of consumption of healthcare services. This association may indicate that consumers without as much medical knowledge underestimate the appropriate amount of health services they need, or it may mean that consumers with more medical education have a greater ability to purchase medical care. Other explanations are possible as well (Agency for Healthcare Research and Quality, n.d.; Cutler & Lleras-Muney, 2006; Fletcher & Frisvold, 2009; Santerre & Neun, 2004, p. 127).

Elasticity

Two of the demand changers discussed previously are shifts in price and shifts in income. *Elasticity* is the term used to describe how responsive the change in demand or supply is when there is either a change in price or a change in income. The concept of elasticity is important to understand as a policy analyst because it is essential to know whether changes in consumers' incomes (say, through a tax credit) or changes in the price of a product (perhaps through incentives given to producers) will result in the desired outcome. The desired outcome may be increased consumption, which might be the case if the service is well-child

checkups. Conversely, the desired outcome may be decreased consumption, which might be the case if cigarettes are the product being consumed.

Price Elasticity of Demand

Price elasticity of demand is based on the percentage change in the quantity demanded resulting from a 1% change in price. In other words, does consumer demand for a product, such as a vaccination, increase as the price of a product decreases by 1%, or vice versa? Elasticity is calculated as follows:

$$\text{Demand elasticity} = \frac{\% \text{ change in quantity demanded}}{\% \text{ change in price}}$$

(Economists often use the midpoint method, which averages the percentage change in quantity and price. This results in the same answer whether there is a price increase or decrease. Price elasticities are always negative because price and demand are inversely related. Even so, elasticities are reported in absolute values, not negative numbers.)

Demand for a product is considered elastic if the sum is greater than 1 and inelastic if the sum is less than 1. An elasticity of 0 is perfectly inelastic, meaning the demand does not change in response to a change in price.

For example, suppose a vaccine costs $20 per dose and at that price a family buys four doses, for a total of $80. The next year the price increases 20% to $24 per dose and the family buys only three doses for a total of $72. The midpoint of the two prices is $22 and the midpoint of the two quantities demanded is 3.5. Using the midpoint method, the calculation is as follows:

$$\frac{-\dfrac{1}{3.5}}{2/22} = -3.14 \ or \ |3.14|$$

Because elasticity equals 3.14, the product is considered elastic (because the result of the elasticity calculation is greater than 1). In this example, for every 1% increase in vaccine price, demand decreases by 3.14%. If the price decreases, the quantity demanded would be expected to increase.

Of course, goods may also be inelastic, which means the demand for the good is not as sensitive to a change in price. As a result, when price increases, the quantity demanded will not decrease at the same rate as the price increases. For example, some people will not reduce their consumption of cigarettes even if the price of cigarettes increases. However, at some point the price could become high enough that consumer behavior will change, resulting in a decrease in demand.

Supply elasticity works in much the same way as the price elasticity of demand and uses the same formula, except it refers to the relationship between the quantity of goods supplied and the price of the goods. Supply elasticity is often defined as the percentage change in quantity supplied resulting from a 1% increase in the price of buying the good. The change is usually positive because producers have an incentive to increase output as the price they will receive for the good rises. However, if supply elasticity refers to variables other than the price of the good, such as the cost of raw materials or wages, then the supply elasticity will be negative; that is, as prices of labor or other inputs rise, the quantity supplied will fall (all other things being equal).

Income Elasticity of Demand

Elasticity works in the opposite way in the case of *inferior goods*. An inferior good, as the name suggests, is less desirable than a *normal good*. As a result, as a consumer's income increases, demand for the inferior good will decrease. Instead of buying more of the inferior good, the consumer will prefer to buy the normal good. For example, suppose a generic over-the-counter pain medication is cheaper than a particular prescription pain medication, but the prescription pain medication is more effective. Consumers with low income may choose to purchase the over-the-counter medicine, the inferior good. If their income increases, they will not buy more of the inferior good, but instead will switch to the prescription pain medicine because it is a better good, for their purposes, than the inferior good.

Health Insurance and Demand

In addition to the general economic rules of demand for health services, the presence of health insurance affects demand for healthcare goods and services. Health insurance acts as a buffer between consumers and the cost of healthcare goods and services. In an insured consumer's view, healthcare goods or services cost less because instead of paying full price, the consumer may only have to pay, for example, a coinsurance rate of 20% (after satisfying the deductible). For example, if a surgical procedure normally costs $10,000, the insured consumer may have to pay only $2000 for the benefit of the surgery because the insurance company pays for the remainder. In this way, the presence of health insurance can have an effect on the

consumer—to increase demand—in the same way that an increase in the consumer's income can increase demand.

In general, insured consumers are less sensitive to the cost of healthcare goods and services than uninsured consumers (Penner, 2004, p. 38). Thus, the presence of health insurance creates the problem of *moral hazard*. Moral hazard can occur in a variety of economic situations when consumers buy more goods or services than necessary because they do not have to pay the full cost of acquiring the good or service. In relation to health insurance, moral hazard results when insured consumers use more services than they would otherwise because part of the cost is covered by insurance.

For example, if a consumer has a $500 health insurance deductible, the consumer pays 100% of the first $500 of health care received. If there is a 20% coinsurance charge after that, the consumer pays only $0.20 per dollar for every dollar spent after $500. If the consumer values a particular healthcare service, such as a preventive dental exam, at $50 but the service costs $100, the consumer will not purchase the service before meeting the deductible. However, after the deductible has been met, the dental exam (assuming it is a covered benefit) will cost the consumer $20 (20% of $100), so the consumer will purchase the service because it is under the consumer's $50 value threshold.

As the portion of the healthcare cost that a consumer pays based on copayments or coinsurance decreases, the consumer becomes less sensitive to changes in the price of the product. Say a consumer is unwilling to pay more than $2500 for surgery. If the consumer owes a 10% coinsurance charge, the consumer will be willing to pay for surgery as long as it is not priced at more than $25,000. At $25,000, the consumer would pay $2500 and the insurance company would pay $22,500. However, if the same consumer has a 20% coinsurance rate, he or she will not elect surgery once the price rises above $12,500 because the cost to the consumer would be more than the consumer's $2500 limit; for example, if the surgery costs $15,000, the consumer would owe $3000 and the insurance company would cover the other $12,000.

The problem of moral hazard is particularly relevant in health care because consumers have an incentive to seek out more medical care—they think it will make them feel better. And, as noted earlier, insured consumers are more likely to purchase a desirable healthcare good or service because the presence of insurance reduces their cost. The same cannot be said of owning a home or auto insurance; although consumers may be a little less careful because of the protection fire or car insurance affords them, it is unlikely that a person will allow an automotive center to replace a working fuel pump on his or her car just because he or she has car insurance.

Economic Basics: Supply

Supply is the amount of goods and services that producers are able and willing to sell at a given price over a given period of time. As with demand, the price of a product is a key factor in determining the level of supply. However, unlike demand, where there is often an inverse relationship between price and demand, an increase in the price a good is sold for usually leads to an increase in quantity supplied. Conversely, as the price consumers will pay for a product decreases, supply will often decrease as well. As with demand, there are many factors that affect the quantity of a good or service being supplied.

Costs

Costs are a key factor in determining the level of supply. Costs refer to what inputs are needed to produce a good or service. For example, the price of cotton may impact the cost of producing medical scrubs or bed linens made out of cotton, or the price of steel may affect the cost of producing an autoclave or X-ray machine made with steel. As the cost of these inputs increases, the cost of producing the final good increases as well. If the price for a good or service does not increase as the cost of inputs increases, the quantity supplied is likely to decrease. Thus, if it costs a manufacturer $100 more to build an X-ray machine because the cost of steel has risen, it is likely that the manufacturer will pass that production cost increase on to the consumer by raising the purchase price of the X-ray machine. Alternately, the manufacturer may choose to absorb the $100 cost increase and not raise the purchase price, which will lead the manufacturer to supply fewer X-ray machines, find a way to produce the good more cheaply using the same method, or find a different way to produce the good.

Costs are counted in many different ways. We focus here on *average costs* and *marginal costs*.

- **Average cost:** The cost of producing one product over a specific period of time. For example, if it costs a manufacturer $2 million to produce 2000

hospital beds in 1 year, the average cost is $1000 per bed during that year.

$$\text{Average cost} = \text{Total cost/Quantity}$$
$$= \$2,000,000/2000 \text{ hospital beds}$$
$$= \$1000 \text{ per hospital bed}$$

- **Marginal cost:** The price of producing one more unit of the output—in our example, one more hospital bed. Whatever additional labor, equipment, and supplies are needed to produce one more hospital bed is the marginal cost of production. As a general matter, the marginal cost increases as output increases.

Supply Changers

Other factors in addition to sale price and cost can increase or decrease the supply of a product. Two common factors are number of sellers and changes in technology:

- **Number of sellers:** As the number of sellers of a good increases, the supply of the good will increase as well because there are more companies producing the good. As long as the market is profitable, new sellers will be enticed to enter the market. This occurs until the market reaches equilibrium, where the quantity demanded equals the quantity supplied.
- **Change in technology:** New technology may mean a new way to produce a desired outcome, which may alter the supply of a good or service. For example, fiberglass has replaced plaster in most casts and the production of each material has shifted accordingly (fiberglass up, plaster down). New technology can also make a product more accessible than before. For example, many surgeries once handled on an inpatient basis may now be performed on an outpatient basis or in a physician's office due to new technology, such as arthroscopy. In addition, evolving technology has led to brand-new fields, such as robotic surgery. Technological improvements can increase demand for some services and reduce demand for others, leading to a change in the production of these goods and services.

Profit Maximization

Although consumers are driven by the desire to maximize their satisfaction, suppliers are driven by their desire to maximize revenues. For-profit companies seek to make profits to pass on to their shareholders, while not-for-profit companies face a variety of requirements regarding disposing of the revenue they generate in excess of expenses and the cost of acquiring capital to run the company. For ease of explanation, the term *profit* will be used here to discuss supplier incentives, even though the healthcare field includes a large share of not-for-profit companies.

Profit is the price per unit sold less the production cost per unit. In a competitive market, profit is maximized at the level of output where the marginal cost equals the price. If a hospital bed costs $1000 to produce and is sold for $1500, the profit per bed is $500. If the marginal cost of producing one more bed is $1400, the producer will make that additional bed because it can be sold for $1500, a $100 profit; however, if the marginal cost of producing an additional bed is $1600, the producer has no incentive to produce that additional bed because it can only be sold at a loss of $100. Due to the profit maximization goal, if the price of a product increases and a competitive market exists for the product, manufacturers will increase production of the product until the output level again reaches the point where the marginal cost equals the price.

When a profitable market exists, new producers will be drawn into the market so they can reap financial benefits. The new producer may price its hospital bed for less than $1500 to attract consumers, or the new producer may think there is a niche for a higher-priced bed that has additional features. Assume the new producer chooses to market a similar bed as the $1500 bed but sells it for $1250. If a consumer can purchase the bed from the competing company for $1250 with no additional opportunity costs, demand for the $1500 hospital bed is likely to fall. The manufacturer of the $1500 bed will have to lower its price or improve the product (or the perception of the product) to increase demand for a higher-priced bed. At the point where there is a balance between the quantity supplied and the quantity demanded and the price is set to the marginal cost of production, there is *equilibrium* in the market.

If such a balance does not occur, there is *disequilibrium* in the market. The disequilibrium could represent a surplus of a good or service due to excess supply or sudden drop in demand, or it could result from a product shortage due to inadequate supply or a sharp increase in demand. Surpluses occur when the market price in a competitive market is higher than the marginal cost of production; as a result, producers lower their prices to increase sales of their product. These price reductions will keep happening until market equilibrium is reached. For example, there

could be a sudden drop in demand for a food product due to a news report that eating the product more than three times per week may put people's health at risk. Due to the sudden drop in demand, excess product will be available. Producers will, in turn, lower the price of the product until equilibrium is reached. Shortages occur when the market price is lower than the marginal cost of production. As a result of the shortage, consumers might be willing to pay more for the product, so producers increase their prices until demand stops increasing and market equilibrium is reached. If an opposite news story appeared, hailing the food product as improving health if eaten at least four times per week, there may be a sudden surge in demand. As a result, consumers will likely be willing to pay more for the product and producers will raise the price until equilibrium is reached. Because producers often cannot make significant changes to their production schedule or products in a short amount of time, market equilibrium positions may take some time to achieve.

Health Insurance and Supply

Just as the presence of health insurance affects a consumer's demand for medical goods and services, it also may impact a healthcare provider's willingness to supply goods and services. This is a complicated issue because, on the one hand, a provider is expected to act as the patient's agent and thus should act in the patient's best interests. If providers encourage only appropriate care, insurance is working in a positive way.

On the other hand, providers may have a financial incentive to encourage or discourage the consumption of healthcare goods and services. Providers could recommend against treatment because of financial incentives resulting from the presence or absence of health insurance. For example, financial incentives found in managed care may discourage providers from recommending a particular treatment. Additionally, if a patient is both uninsured and unable to pay for services out-of-pocket, providers have a financial incentive not to provide potentially necessary services due to their inability to receive payment. Similarly, a provider may seek to increase his or her income by encouraging inappropriate or excessive care. This problem—the provider version of moral hazard—is referred to as *supplier-induced demand*. Supplier-induced demand is the level of demand that exists beyond what a well-informed consumer would have chosen. The theory behind supplier-induced demand is that instead of consumer demand leading to an increase in suppliers (healthcare providers), the suppliers create demand in the consumers (patients), often by relying on information only available to the supplier. However, economists debate whether supplier-induced demand actually exists because it is difficult to study empirically, and because behavior consistent with supplier-induced demand may also be consistent with appropriate medical treatment (Phelps, 2003, pp. 237–242).

Economic Basics: Markets

To this point, we have reviewed many basic aspects of economic theory—how consumers behave, how suppliers behave, what drives and shifts demand, and what drives and shifts supply. To understand how these theories work in the healthcare industry, it is necessary to explore how health insurance affects markets, what kind of market exists for health care, how market structure relates to the production and distribution of goods and services, and why markets fail and what can be done to alleviate the problems associated with market failure.

Health Insurance and Markets

Before delving into the basics of economic markets, it is necessary to highlight how the presence of health insurance alters the dynamics of a standard economic transaction. In a typical market transaction, such as buying food at the grocery store, there are only two parties involved—the consumer who buys the food and the supplier who sells the food. The cost to the consumer is the cost of the food; the consumer bears full responsibility for paying that cost and pays that cost directly to the supplier, the grocery store.

The typical medical transaction, however, does not follow these rules, both because of the types of events that lead to a medical transaction and because of the presence of health insurance. In health care, there are both routine and expected events (e.g., an annual physical) and unanticipated needs due to an unpredictable illness or injury. The exact diagnosis and treatment are often unknown initially and the patient's response to treatment is not guaranteed, resulting in an inability to predict exactly what resources will be needed. Without knowing what goods and services are required, it is impossible to estimate the cost to be incurred. This makes it very difficult for consumers to weigh their preferences for medical care as compared to other goods and services, and makes it difficult for suppliers to know which goods and services will be demanded and at what price they can sell their goods and services.

Another reason healthcare transactions often do not follow the typical market exchange is because the presence of health insurance means healthcare transactions involve three players, instead of two; these three players are (1) patients (the consumer), (2) healthcare providers (the supplier), and (3) insurers (who are often proxies for employers). Insurers are also known as "third-party payers" because they are the third party involved in addition to the two customary parties. In the public insurance system, the third-party payer is the government, and in the private sector, the third-party payers are private health insurance companies. Having the health insurance carrier as a third party means consumers do not pay the full cost of healthcare resources used and therefore may be less likely to choose the most cost-effective treatment option, to reduce the information gap between themselves and providers, or be as vigilant against supplier-induced demand as they might in other circumstances.

Market Structure

Understanding markets begins with the notion of a *perfectly competitive* market, because in economic theory a perfectly competitive market serves society by efficiently allocating the finite resources available. Due to specific market conditions that make up a perfectly competitive market, a competitive equilibrium is reached once quantities supplied equal the quantities demanded.

There are numerous types of market structures, ranging from perfectly competitive markets with many buyers and sellers to *monopolistic* markets with a single seller controlling the market. Other common market structures include oligopolies, which have a few dominant firms and substantial but not complete barriers to entry, and monopsonies, which have a limited number of consumers who control the price paid to suppliers. Based on the market structure, consumers and producers have varying degrees of power in terms of setting prices, choosing among products, and deciding whether to participate in the market. **Table 9.1** reviews the characteristics of three market structures that are most useful to understanding healthcare markets: perfectly competitive markets, monopolistic markets, and monopolistically competitive markets.

You know from the discussion of supply and demand that the healthcare market cannot be perfectly competitive based on the description in Table 9.1. (In fact, no markets are truly perfectly competitive.) Some consumers, such as the federal government, may have extensive market power as well as

Table 9.1 Characteristics of Key Market Structures

	Perfectly Competitive	Monopoly	Monopolistically Competitive
Number of firms	Many	One (in a pure monopoly)	Many
Market share	No dominant firms	One firm has all market share and price and output.	There may be many firms with market share and or a few dominant firms. Firms can set price because of product differentiation.
Barriers to entry for new firms into market	No	Yes—absolute barriers; no new firms may enter market.	Some barriers, due to differentiation of product, licensure, etc.
Product differentiation	No. Products are for each other.	No. Only one product; no substitutes are available.	Yes. Many products; they are not substitutes for each other (brand loyalty).
Access to information and resources	Consumers and producers have perfect information.	One firm controls all information (asymmetric information).	All firms have equal access to resources and technology unless there are a few dominant firms with more access to resources.
Cost of transaction	Consumers bear cost of consumption, and producers bear cost of production.	Higher price to consumer because firm has ability to reduce quantity, retain excess profits.	Blend of costs in perfectly competitive market and monopoly market.

the ability to set prices. Producers of patent-protected healthcare products are provided with supply power for a limited period of time, which gives them an ability to control prices. Consumers do not have perfect information regarding healthcare needs and healthcare costs, and providers and insurers do not have perfect information regarding patient illnesses. Given the presence of health insurance, consumers do not bear all the cost of using healthcare services. With these characteristics, the healthcare market is monopolistically competitive. In many areas of the healthcare market, there are a few dominant firms with a lot of market power and many smaller firms that participate in the market, but the smaller firms do not have the power to shape market conditions.

Market Failure

A *market failure* means resources are not produced or allocated efficiently. As you recall, we defined efficiency generally as the state of least cost production where the resource distribution cannot be changed to make someone better off without making someone else worse off, and we also described a few specific types of

efficiency. When something about the structure of the market prohibits it from being efficient, it is referred to as market failure; the question then becomes what interventions in the market, if any, should occur in an attempt to alleviate the market failure.

Before we turn to why markets fail, we must address one additional issue: Does an inequitable distribution of resources constitute a market failure? Under the traditional economic school of thought, the answer is no; a market failure refers to inefficiency, and concerns about equity are not part of the efficiency calculation. However, some economists consider equity a valid factor when evaluating the functioning of a market. Regardless, whether an inequitable distribution of resources fits under the economic designation of "market failure" is not as important as whether policymakers choose to intervene in a market based on equity concerns.

Some of the most salient reasons that market failures occur in health care include concentration of market power, imperfect information (producers or consumer not having complete and accurate information), the consumption of *public goods*, and the presence of *externalities*. We have already discussed concentration of market power and imperfect information; the next sections focus on public goods and externalities.

Public Goods

Public goods have two main features. First, public goods are *nonrival*, meaning that more than one person can enjoy the good simultaneously. An example of a rival private good would be a single pen, as two people may not use the same pen at the same time. Second, a public good is *nonexclusive*, because it is too costly to try to exclude nonpaying individuals from enjoying public goods (Santerre & Neun, 2004, p. 230).

Classic examples of public goods are national defense measures and lighthouses. Everyone simultaneously benefits from national defense, and it is not economically feasible to exclude nonpaying individuals (e.g., tax evaders) from enjoying the benefits. In the same way, multiple ships may benefit at the same time from a warning provided by a lighthouse, and it would be difficult to exclude a particular ship from enjoying the benefit. In the health field, examples of local public goods include clean water in a free public swimming area or a public health awareness campaign on city streets. Everyone enjoys the clean water (at least until it is overcrowded), and it would be costly to exclude nonpayers. Similarly, multiple people can benefit from a public health campaign simultaneously, and exclusion of nonpayers would be impossible or quite costly.

Public goods can be transformed into other types of goods. For example, a public good could be made exclusive by charging a fee; these are called *toll goods* (Weimer & Vining, 1999, p. 81). The public swimming water could be fenced off and a fee charged for admission, or the public health campaign could be placed in the subway, which would exclude those who could not afford the fare. Once public goods are transformed into toll goods, concerns arise about whether the price is set at the most efficient level. Toll goods may still lead to market failure if the cost of using the good excludes users who would gain more from enjoying the good than they would cost society by consuming the good (Weimer & Vining, 1999, pp. 81–82).

In addition, goods provided by local, state, and federal governments may be, but are not necessarily, public goods in the economic sense. For example, if a state funds a free healthcare clinic, it is not funding a public good. Even though nonpayers are, by definition, included, the benefits generally inure to the individual and, in most cases, more than one individual cannot enjoy the same healthcare good or service. It is possible, however, that other people will benefit from a healthcare service they do not receive; for example, if your neighbors receive a service that helps them quit smoking, you will receive the benefit of no longer being exposed to your neighbors' secondhand smoke.

Public goods also create the *free rider* problem, making it unprofitable for private firms to produce and sell goods due to the high cost of excluding nonpayers (Santerre & Neun, 2004, p. 230). The free rider is one who enjoys the benefit of the good without paying for the cost of producing the good. Because it is impossible to exclude users or force consumers to reveal their true demand for the public good, they do not have incentive to pay for the units of the good they use (Weimer & Vining, 1999, p. 86). For example, an individual cannot be prevented from gaining knowledge from a public health awareness campaign, so if a private company were responsible for providing the education campaign, it could not force a consumer to pay for it. Eventually, even though many people would like to take advantage of clean air or health education, the lack of people paying for it would result in an underproduction of these services unless some action were taken to alter the market dynamics.

Externalities

Externalities are much more common than public goods in the healthcare market. An *externality* is "any valued impact (positive or negative) resulting from any action (whether related to production or consumption) that affects someone who did not fully consent to it through participation in a voluntary exchange" (Weimer & Vining, 1999, p. 94). In a typical economic transaction, the costs and benefits associated with a transaction impact only those involved in the transaction. For example, remember our consumer buying food at the grocery store? The only two people affected by that transaction are the consumer, who pays money and receives food, and the grocer, who provides food and receives money. Situations with externalities, however, are different. Externalities exist when the action of one party impacts another party *who is not part of the transaction*; in other words, the parties to the transaction will find there is an "unpriced by-product" of producing or consuming a good or service (Santerre & Neun, 2004, p. 231).

Externalities may be positive or negative. An example of a positive externality is when one person gets vaccinated against the chicken pox and other people benefit because chicken pox is less likely to be transmitted in that community. If enough people get vaccinated, "herd immunity" will exist in the community.[a] In this case, the positive unpriced by-product is the additional protection received by others who were not vaccinated. An example of a negative externality is represented by illegal hazardous waste disposal. Say a hospital dumps biological waste such as blood, syringes, gauze with infected material on it, and the like into a public water source. The unpriced by-product is paid by the general public, who face an increased risk of illness from using the contaminated water source. The costs to the general public may not have been included in the hospital's cost–benefit analysis when it decided to dump the biological waste.

With both positive and negative externalities, the cost and benefits of production or consumption are borne by individuals who do not participate in the transaction. Due to the unpriced by-products, there are external costs and benefits that are not considered when deciding whether to make the transaction, leading to an under- or overproduction of the resource from society's perspective.

Government Intervention

When market failures occur, the government may intervene to promote efficiency or to promote equity (of course, it may also choose not to intervene at all; see **Box 9.3**). Some examples of government interventions include financing or directly providing public goods, creating incentives through tax breaks and subsidies, imposing mandates through regulation, prohibiting activities, and redistributing income. We discuss these options in the following sections.

Government Finances or Directly Provides Public Goods.
When market failure occurs, the government may choose to finance or provide a good or service directly instead of attempting to

---

Box 9.3 DISCUSSION QUESTIONS

Some people argue that the government should not intervene in the case of a market failure because the government itself is inefficient and will simply create new problems to replace the ones it is trying to fix. In addition, critics contend that the government is usually less efficient than the private sector. Do you think the government is less efficient than the private sector? Does it depend on the issue involved? If you think it is inefficient in a particular area, does that lead you to recommend against government intervention, or is there a reason that you would still support government intervention? If you think the government should intervene, which intervention options do you prefer and why?

---

influence the actions of private producers. For example, if the government wanted to increase access to health care, it could create new government-run health centers or provide financing to privately run health centers.

These are two different paths—direct provision or financing—with different sets of issues. The main difference when the government provides or finances care instead of a private sector is the lack of profit motive on the part of the government (Santerre & Neun, 2004, p. 252). Instead of focusing on the financial bottom line, public providers may focus on other goals, such as equity or assuring the presence of a particular good or service for everyone or for specific populations.

When the government creates or expands a public program, there is concern that *crowd-out* may occur. Whenever a program is established or expanded, the program has a particular goal and targets a particular audience. For example, the government may try to reduce the number of people without insurance by expanding an existing public program such as the Children's Health Insurance Program. Crowd-out occurs when instead of reaching only the target audience (in this case, the uninsured), the public program also creates an incentive for other individuals (in this case, privately insured people) to participate in the public program. Because the program has a finite amount of resources, some of the target audience (the uninsured) may be crowded out from participating in the program by the presence of the other, nontargeted individuals (the privately insured). This unintended development prevents programs from maximizing cost-effectiveness because instead of obtaining the largest change (in this case, the reduction in the number of uninsured) for the public dollar, some of the change is simply a result of a cost shift from a private payer (the privately insured) to a public payer (the expanded program). Crowd-out may also change incentives for other providers of services. In this example, the presence of the new or expanded government program may reduce the incentive for private employers to provide the same good or service (in this case, health insurance).

Government Increases Taxes, Tax Deductions, or Subsidies.
Taxes and subsidies can be used to alter the price, production, or consumption of goods in an effort to fix a market failure. For example, increasing a tax on a good raises the price of that good and discourages consumption; this strategy is often employed to discourage consumption of harmful products, such as cigarettes. Similarly, the government could choose to tax cigarette producers as a way to

encourage them to produce less of the harmful product or leave the market altogether.

Conversely, the government could subsidize a good, directly or through a tax deduction, when it wants to encourage the consumption and production of the good. For example, if the government wanted more low-income individuals to purchase healthy foods, it could choose to subsidize their purchase of fruits and vegetables by allowing individuals who use public benefits, such as food stamps, to purchase more fruits and vegetables than would normally be allowed by the face value of the food stamps (for example, $1 in food stamps would allow for the purchase of $2 of fruits or vegetables). Similarly, if the government wanted to encourage vaccine manufacturers to produce more vaccine doses, it could accomplish this goal through direct subsidies to or tax deductions for the manufacturers.

Note that the government has an economic incentive to tax goods that are price inelastic. This incentive exists because the amount purchased declines by a smaller percentage than the price increase. For example, if cigarettes are price inelastic, a 10% cigarette tax increase will result in less than a 10% decrease in cigarette consumption, meaning the cigarette tax will be a good revenue producer for the government because consumers will continue to purchase cigarettes despite the tax. However, taxing price-inelastic goods is less effective as a public health tool for the same reason. If the government desires a 10% reduction in cigarette consumption, the tax must be much higher than 10% if cigarettes are price inelastic. Of course, the government may choose to impose a higher cigarette tax, but it is likely that, for political reasons, a higher tax increase will be harder to obtain than a smaller one.

Government Issues Regulatory Mandates.
Regulations may be used to fix a market failure by controlling the price, quantity, or quality of goods and services, or the entry of new firms into the market (Santerre & Neun, 2004, p. 241). For example, healthcare consumers often have imperfect information when making their healthcare decisions. As a result, the government may choose to create a requirement that a type of provider, such as nursing homes, supply information to the public about the quality of care in their facilities to aid in consumers' decision-making. The government may also promulgate regulations that restrict entry of new firms into a market and regulate prices because it is cheaper for one or a few firms to produce a high level of output. Of course, government regulations could also be used to

achieve a policy goal like reducing carbon emissions by mandating that public transportation systems use alternative fuels that result in lower emissions.

The government could also set a cap on the price of a good and prohibit producers from selling that good above the set price. This will keep the good at a price the government deems socially acceptable. However, if the price is set below the market price, some unfavorable market consequences may occur because it is no longer profitable for the producer to supply the product. Possible consequences include the following:

- Suppliers exiting the market or reducing the quantity of the good supplied, resulting in a shortage
- Suppliers reducing the quality of the good by making cheaper products or providing less care
- Suppliers shifting cost from one product to another
- Suppliers engaging in unethical behavior because some consumers will be willing to pay more than the government price ceiling

Furthermore, regulations aimed at increasing the quality of a good or service will likely impose additional costs on producers of the good. As the cost of inputs rises, the price charged to consumers is likely to rise as well. As a result, some consumers will be priced out of the market for that good or service.

Government Prohibits Goods or Services.
Prohibiting the production of goods and services often is ineffective and leads to a "black market" for such products. Because the prohibited goods or services are not available legally, consumers may be tempted to purchase goods or services that are not protected by price or quality controls. This situation may occur with the use of drugs or supplements not approved by the Food and Drug Administration, including unapproved drugs from other countries entering the United States via the Internet or other sources. In addition, because other countries are producing the good or service, the United States may be at a competitive disadvantage. For example, if stem cell research is permitted abroad but not in this country, some scientists may leave the United States to work abroad and domestic companies may not remain competitive in certain fields.

Redistribution of Income.
In the case of market failure, the government may also act to redistribute income. Remember, efficient allocation of resources is not the same as equitable allocation of resources. A government may decide that every member

of society should obtain a certain minimum level of income or resources or health status. Redistributing income may occur by taxing the wealthier members of society and using the revenue to provide resources to poorer members of society. If the government sought to create more market equity through voluntary donations, it is likely that a free rider problem would exist because some citizens would volunteer to contribute resources while others would not, but the latter would still receive a benefit from the redistribution. For example, wealthier citizens who should be in the "donor group" but do not contribute may benefit from the donations given by other wealthy citizens that lead to increased productivity and welfare of those in the recipient group. Both the notion of income redistribution and the decisions regarding who should be providing versus receiving resources is open to debate. In addition, it is important to remember that income redistribution may reduce efficiency or have other undesirable market effects.

Conclusion

This introduction to economic concepts illustrates why health policy analysts and decision makers must understand how economists analyze healthcare problems. We have taken a broad look at the issues of supply, demand, and market structure with a focus on concerns that are relevant in the health policy field. In particular, it is essential to understand how health insurance affects both consumer and producer decisions. Although we only scratched the surface of healthcare economics in this chapter, you should now realize that without an understanding of the economic ramifications of a policy decision, a health policy analyst cannot know, for example, whether to recommend addressing a problem through a government-run program, subsidy, or the like, or if it would be better to let the free market set the production level and price of a resource.

References

Agency for Healthcare Research and Quality. (n.d.). *Population health: Behavioral and social science insights.* https://www.ahrq.gov/sites/default/files/publications/files/population-health.pdf

Cutler, D., & Lleras-Muney, A. (2006). *Education and health: Evaluating theories and evidence* (National Bureau of Economic Research Working Paper 12352). http://www.nber.org/papers/w12352.pdf

Cylus, J., Hartman, M., Washington, B., Andrews, K., & Catlin, A. (2011). Pronounced gender and age differences are evidence in personal health care spending per person. *Health Affairs, 30*(1), 153–160. https://doi.org/10.1377/hlthaff.2010.0216

Feldstein, P. (2005). *Health care economics* (6th ed.). Thomas Delmar Learning.

Fletcher, J. M., & Frisvold, D. E. (2009). Higher education and health investments: Does more schooling affect preventive health care use? *Journal of Human Capital, 3*(2), 144–176. https://doi.org/10.1086/645090

Gordis, L. (2000). *Epidemiology* (2nd ed.). WB Saunders; p. 19.

Penner, S. J. (2004). *Introduction to health care economics and financial management: Fundamental concepts with practical applications.* Lippincott Williams & Wilkins.

Phelps, C. E. (2003). *Health economics* (3rd ed.). Addison-Wesley.

Pindyck, R. S., & Rubinfeld, D. L. (2003). *Microeconomics* (5th ed.). Prentice Hall.

Santerre, R. E., & Neun, S. P. (2004). *Health economics: Theories, insights, and industry studies* (3rd ed.). Thomas South-Western.

Weimer, D., & Vining, A. (1999). *Policy analysis: Concepts and practice* (3rd ed.). Prentice Hall.

Endnotes

a. *Herd immunity* is "the resistance of a group to an attack by a disease to which a large proportion of the members of the group are immune" (Gordis, 2000). Once a certain portion of the group is immune, there is only a small chance that an infected person will find a susceptible person to whom the disease may be transmitted.

CHAPTER 10

Government Health Insurance Programs: Medicaid, CHIP, and Medicare

LEARNING OBJECTIVES

By the end of this chapter you will be able to:

1. Describe the basic structure, administration, financing, and eligibility rules for:
   - Medicaid
   - The Children's Health Insurance Program (CHIP)
   - Medicare
2. Understand how the Patient Protection and Affordable Care Act alters Medicaid, CHIP, and Medicare
3. Discuss key health policy questions and themes relating to each of these public programs

---

📝 Box 10.1 VIGNETTE Governor Sophia is in a quandary. She believes everyone should have access to health care and would like to support state policies that make care accessible and affordable. While she supported President Obama's goal of reducing the number of uninsured, she is concerned that some of the provisions in the Patient Protection and Affordable Care Act are too burdensome on the states, particularly in a fragile economy. The governor wonders how her state can afford the mandated Medicaid expansion when the recent trend has been to cut services across the board. How will state agencies cope with their new responsibilities when positions are being defunded and employees are being furloughed? Should she spend her state's time and resources to establish a health insurance exchange when the federal government will step in if she does not act? At the same time, does she want to leave decisions about how the exchange will be operated in her state to bureaucrats in Washington, D.C.?

Introduction

Employer-sponsored health insurance plays a significant role in financing health care; in addition, private insurers have flexibility in designing health insurance coverage and selecting who they will cover, and there are many reasons why private insurers do not have incentive to cover high-risk populations; prior chapters discussed these issues in detail. In this chapter, we focus on Medicaid, the Children's Health Insurance Program (CHIP), and Medicare, which were established in part because the private health insurance market was not developing affordable, comprehensive health insurance products for society's low-income, older, and disabled populations. Federal and state governments chose to fill some of those gaps through these public programs. The insurance coverage gaps were substantial, as shown by the over 130 million beneficiaries served by these three programs today (Department of Health and Human Services [HHS], 2017; Medicaid .gov, n.d.c). Due to the needs of vulnerable populations and the requirements necessary to make health insurance coverage for them viable, these programs are quite different from standard private health insurance plans.

There are numerous other important health insurance and direct service programs funded by federal, state, and local governments. Just a few examples include the Ryan White Care Act, which provides HIV/AIDS services to infected individuals and their families; the Women, Infants, and Children Supplemental Nutrition Program, which provides nutritional supplements and education to poor women and their children; and the Indian Health Service, which provides federal health services to American Indians and Alaska Natives. Although these and many other health programs are vital to the health of our population, this chapter focuses only on the three major government health insurance programs in this country, because in addition to providing health insurance to millions, these programs are also influential in terms of setting healthcare policy. For example, when Medicare, a program that serves almost 60 million people, makes a decision to cover a certain treatment, private insurance companies often follow suit, establishing a new standard for generally accepted practice in the insurance industry (HHS, 2017). Conversely, states may decide to try healthcare innovations with their Medicaid programs that, if successful, may become commonplace across the country. Thus, understanding these three major programs is essential in terms of both how this country finances and delivers health care and how it makes health policy decisions.

The Patient Protection and Affordable Care Act (ACA) made wide-ranging changes to Medicaid, CHIP, and Medicare (the ACA is discussed in more detail in Chapter 11, "Health Reform and the Patient Protection and Affordable Care Act"). In general, the ACA included a significant Medicaid eligibility expansion, altered which children are eligible for Medicaid and CHIP, added new benefits to Medicare, and included a host of changes intended to produce savings in the Medicare program. Overall, the ACA expansion has created a two-tier Medicaid program, with newly eligible individuals falling under one set of eligibility, financing, and benefit rules, and the rest of Medicaid beneficiaries adhering to different standards.

As you learn about specific rules for each program, keep in mind the numerous tensions that are present throughout the healthcare system as policymakers decide how to design and implement public insurance programs. This chapter touches on several recurring themes relating to these tensions, which were evident during the debate that led to passage of the ACA: choosing between state flexibility and national uniformity; determining the appropriate role for government, the private sector, and individuals in healthcare financing and delivery; defining a primary decision-making goal (e.g., fiscal restraint, equity/social justice, improved health outcomes, uniformity); and settling on the appropriate scope of coverage to offer beneficiaries.

Before delving into the details of each program, it is necessary to explain the difference between entitlement and block grant programs. Medicaid and Medicare are *entitlement* programs, whereas CHIP is a *block grant* program. Some of the themes listed earlier, such as the appropriate role of government and primary decision-making goals, are implicated in the decision of whether to establish a program as an entitlement or a block grant.

In an *entitlement* program, everyone who is eligible for and enrolled in the program is legally entitled to receive benefits from the program. In other words, the federal or state governments cannot refuse to provide program beneficiaries with all medically necessary and covered services due to lack of funds or for other reasons. Because everyone who is enrolled has a legal right to receive services, there cannot be a cap on spending. The absence of a spending cap has the advantage of allowing funds to be available to meet rising healthcare costs and unexpected needs, such as increased enrollment and use of services during recessions or natural or man-made disasters.

Opponents of entitlement programs focus on the open-ended budget obligation that entitlements create. With healthcare costs straining federal and state budgets, critics would prefer to establish a cap on the funds spent on entitlement programs such as Medicaid. It is impossible to determine how many people will enroll in the program or how many and what kind of healthcare services they will use in any given year, so governments cannot establish exact budgets for their Medicaid program. In addition to these fiscal objections, many opponents reject the notion that government should play a large role in providing health insurance, preferring to leave that function to the private market.

Entitlement programs are often contrasted with *block grant* programs, such as CHIP. A block grant is a defined sum of money that is allocated for a particular program (often, but not always, from the federal government to the states) over a certain amount of time. If program costs exceed available funds, additional money will not be made available and program changes have to be made. Such changes could include terminating the program, capping enrollment in the program, reducing program benefits, or finding additional resources. Unlike entitlement programs, individuals who qualify for block grant programs may be denied services or receive reduced services due to lack of funds.

The arguments for and against block grant programs are similar to those found with entitlement programs (see **Box 10.2**). Proponents of block grant programs laud the limited and certain fiscal obligation and reduced role of government in providing health insurance. Opponents of block grant programs object to the lack of legal entitlement to services and the finite amount of funds available to provide health insurance.

Medicaid

Medicaid is the country's federal–state public health insurance program for the indigent. In this section, we discuss fundamental aspects of the Medicaid program, including its structure, eligibility, benefits, and financing, as well as changes to Medicaid made by the ACA.

Box 10.2 DISCUSSION QUESTIONS

Do you think it makes more sense to structure government healthcare programs as entitlements or block grants? What are the economic and healthcare risks and benefits of each approach? Does your answer depend on who is paying for the program? Who the program serves? What kinds of benefits does the program provide? Do you think various stakeholders would answer these questions differently? How might the answers change if you ask a member of the federal government, a governor, a state legislator, an advocate, or a tax-paying citizen who is not eligible for benefits under the program?

Unlike private health insurance plans, which are based on actuarial risk, the Medicaid program is designed to ensure that funds are available to provide healthcare services to a poorer and generally less-healthy group of beneficiaries; to do so, Medicaid has several features that are not found in private health insurance plans.

Program Administration

Medicaid is jointly designed and operated by the federal and state governments. The Centers for Medicare and Medicaid Services (CMS) is the federal agency in charge of administering the Medicaid program. Each state, the District of Columbia, and certain U.S. territories,[a] as defined in the Social Security Act (SSA) of 1935, have the option to participate in the Medicaid program, and all have chosen to do so. The federal government sets certain requirements and policies for the Medicaid program through statutes (SSA, Title 19), regulations (Grants to States, 1988), a *State Medicaid Manual* (Medicaid.gov, n.d.h), and policy guidance such as letters to state Medicaid directors (Medicaid.gov, n.d.h). Each state has its own Medicaid agency that is responsible for implementing the program in the state. States file a Medicaid State Plan with the federal government outlining the state's own eligibility rules, benefits, and other program requirements; this plan is effectively a contract between states and the federal government and between states and program beneficiaries.

The federal and state governments jointly set rules concerning who is covered and which services are provided by Medicaid. The federal government outlines which populations must be covered (*mandatory populations*) and which ones may be covered (*optional populations*), as well as which benefits must be covered (*mandatory benefits*) and which ones may be covered (*optional benefits*). Between these floors and ceilings, states have significant flexibility to determine how Medicaid will operate in their particular state. In general, states must cover mandatory populations and benefits, and they may choose to cover any combination of optional populations or benefits, including the choice not to offer any optional coverage at all. In addition, states may seek a waiver from federal rules, allowing states to experiment with coverage and benefit design while still drawing federal funds to operate their program. Given all of these possible permutations, it is often said that "if you have seen one Medicaid program, you have seen one Medicaid program"; in other words, within the broad federal parameters, every state (and territory) has a unique Medicaid structure—no two programs are exactly alike. As a result, similarly situated individuals in different states may have very

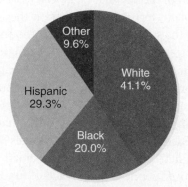

What are the benefits and drawbacks of having a health program that varies by state versus having one that is uniform across the country? Do you find that the positives of state flexibility outweigh the negatives, or vice versa? Does your analysis change depending on what populations are served? Does your analysis change depending on whose point of view you consider? Is it fair that similarly situated individuals may be treated differently in different states? Does this occur in other aspects of society?

different experiences in terms of the generosity of benefits they are entitled to or even whether they are eligible for the program at all (see **Box 10.3**).

Eligibility

Traditionally, Medicaid has covered low-income pregnant women, children, adults in families with dependent children, individuals with disabilities, and older adults. About 43% of all Medicaid beneficiaries are children, and another 40% are individuals with disabilities and older adults (Rudowitz & Garfield, 2018). Approximately 11 million people are called *dual enrollee* or *dual-eligible* older adults, meaning they qualify for both Medicaid and Medicare (Accius et al.,

2017). Although most dual enrollees are eligible for full Medicaid benefits, a small portion of them receives only premium and/or cost-sharing assistance to help them pay for Medicare, and not full Medicaid benefits.

Among all people with health insurance, members of ethnic or minority groups are more likely than Caucasians to have coverage through Medicaid. As shown in **Figure 10.1**, about 41% of Medicaid beneficiaries are White, non-Hispanic; almost 30% are Hispanic; and 20% are Black. **Figure 10.2** shows that Medicaid provides assistance to a variety of vulnerable populations.

Total nonelderly Medicaid enrollees: 55,903,220

Figure 10.1 Medicaid Beneficiaries by Race/Ethnicity, 2019

Kaiser Family Foundation. (2019). *Distribution of the nonelderly with Medicaid by race/ethnicity.* https://www.kff.org/medicaid/state-indicator/medicaid-distribution-nonelderly-by-raceethnicity/...

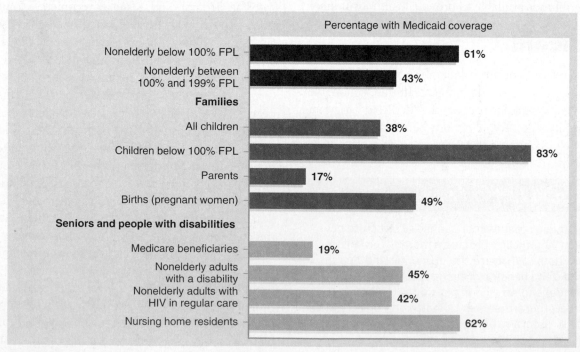

Note: FPL—Federal Poverty Level. The U.S. Census Bureau's poverty threshold for a family with two adults and one child was $20,420 in 2017.

Figure 10.2 Medicaid Plays a Key Role for Selected Populations, 2017

Rudowitz, R., Garfield, R., & Hinton, E. (2019). *10 Things to know about Medicaid: Setting the facts straight.* Kaiser Family Foundation. https://www.kff.org/medicaid/issue-brief/10-things-to-know-about-medicaid-setting-the-facts-straight/

While Medicaid covers both children and adults, coverage for children and pregnant women typically has been more generous than coverage for nonpregnant adults. Prior to ACA implementation, Medicaid covered 75% of children who lived below the poverty line, but only 35% of adults below that income level (Paradise et al., 2015, p. 3). Of adults who were covered by Medicaid, states were more generous when it came to pregnant women. While half the states provided coverage to pregnant women up to 200% of the federal poverty level (FPL; see **Box 10.4**), the median income eligibility limit for working parents was 61%, and many states did not cover childless adults at all (Paradise, 2015, p. 8; Paradise et al., 2015, p. 3). Traditionally left out of the program have been low-income adults without disabilities, women who are not pregnant, and the near-poor who earn too much money to qualify for Medicaid. However, the ACA included a significant eligibility expansion. As of July 2020, there were 18 million more Medicaid enrollees than prior to passage of the ACA (Medicaid and CHIP Payment and Access Commission [MACPAC], n.d.f). States that adopted the ACA Medicaid expansion option experienced an average enrollment increase of 42% as compared to nonexpansion states, with 27 states increasing enrollment by at least 25% (MACPAC, n.d.f). As discussed later in more detail, the expansion was designed to include the low-income groups that traditionally had been excluded from Medicaid.

Medicaid enrollment trends are responsive to national and state policy decisions, economic conditions, and significant national events (e.g., Hurricane Katrina, the terrorist attacks of September 11, 2001). Not surprisingly, the COVID-19 pandemic resulted in increased Medicaid enrollment as more individuals lost employment and became eligible for the program. In addition, the Families First Coronavirus Response Act (FFCRA) gave states additional federal Medicaid funds as long as they met certain "maintenance of eligibility" requirements, incentivizing states to keep coverage conditions stable (Hinton et al., 2021). Medicaid and CHIP enrollment increased from 71.3 million in February 2020 to 80.5 million in January 2021 (Galewitz, 2021). This increase stands in contrast to declining Medicaid and CHIP enrollment from 2016 to 2019 (Hinton et al., 2021). The prior enrollment loss was likely due to a variety of factors, including an improving economy, additional renewal barriers, tighter eligibility verification standards and new document requirements, reduced outreach assistance, and immigration policies that may have deterred individuals from enrolling or renewing coverage (Kaiser Family Foundation [KFF], 2019a).

Traditional Medicaid Eligibility Requirements

Eligibility requirements (as well as financing rules and benefits) differ for the groups that have been traditionally covered by Medicaid and those that are covered under the ACA expansion option. To help clarify these differences, when referring to the rules that existed prior to the ACA, we use the term *traditional Medicaid*, and when referring to rules that attach to the ACA, we use the term *expansion Medicaid*. It is important to remember that states may follow both traditional and expansion Medicaid rules; the ACA expansion did not replace traditional Medicaid, but rather added to it.

Under traditional Medicaid rules, everyone must meet *all five* of the following requirements to be eligible:

1. **Categorical:** An individual must fit within a category (e.g., pregnant women) covered by the program.
2. **Income:** An individual/family must earn no more than the relevant income limits, which are expressed as an FPL percentage (e.g., 133% of the FPL).
3. **Resources:** An individual/family must not have nonwage assets (e.g., car, household goods) that exceed eligibility limits.
4. **Residency:** An individual must be a U.S. resident and a resident of the state in which they are seeking benefits.
5. **Immigration status:** Immigrants must meet certain requirements, including having been in the country for at least 5 years (for most immigrants).

★ Box 10.4   Special Topic

Federal Poverty Level

Federal poverty guidelines are determined annually and calculated based on the number of individuals in a family. The guidelines are commonly referred to as the *federal poverty level*, but the U.S. Department of Health and Human Services (HHS) discourages the use of this term because the Census Bureau also calculates, using different methods, a figure referred to as the *federal poverty threshold*. However, because the term *federal poverty level* is still commonly used when discussing eligibility for federal and state programs, we use it here. The poverty guidelines are somewhat higher for Alaska and Hawaii due to administrative procedures adopted by the Office of Economic Opportunity.

Table 10.1 Select Medicaid Mandatory and Optional Eligibility Groups and Income Requirements Prior to ACA

Eligibility Category	Mandatory Coverage	Optional Coverage
Infants < 1 year	≤ 133% FPL	≤ 185% FPL
Children 1–5 years	≤ 133% FPL	> 133% FPL
Children 6–19 years	≤ 100% FPL	> 100% FPL
Pregnant women	≤ 133% FPL	≤ 185% FPL
Parents	Below state's 1996 AFDC limit	May use income level above state's 1996 AFDC limit
Parents in welfare-to-work families	≤ 185% FPL	
Older adults and disabled SSI beneficiaries	SSI limits	Above SSI limits, below 100% FPL
Certain working disabled	May not exceed specified amount	Variable, SSI level to 250% FPL
Older adults—Medicare assistance only[a]	Variable, up to 175% FPL	Variable up to 175% FPL
Nursing home residents		Above SSI limits, below 300% SSI
Medically needy		"Spend down" medical expenses to state-set income level

[a]Medicare assistance only = payment for Medicare cost-sharing requirements.

Abbreviations: AFDC = Aid to Families with Dependent Children; FPL = federal poverty level; SSI = Supplemental Security Income (a federal program that provides cash assistance to older adults and individuals who are blind or disabled who meet certain income and resource requirements).

As shown in **Table 10.1**, under traditional rules it is necessary to consider both categorical eligibility and income limits for all populations to understand who is covered by Medicaid and which populations are mandatory and which are optional. The groups in Table 10.1 represent some of the larger and more frequently mentioned categories of Medicaid beneficiaries, but it is not an exhaustive list. There are approximately 50 categories of mandatory and optional populations in the Medicaid program, with each state picking and choosing which optional populations to include and at what income level (see **Box 10.5**).

Medically Needy

Medicaid's *medically needy* category is an option that has been picked up by 34 states as of 2019 (KFF, 2018). As its name implies, this category is intended to cover individuals who have extremely high medical expenses. These individuals fit within a covered category but earn too much money to be otherwise eligible for Medicaid. Given who is in this population,

 Box 10.5 DISCUSSION QUESTIONS

Looking at Medicaid's traditional eligibility rules, you will notice numerous value/policy judgments—pregnant women and children are favored over childless adults, the medically needy are favored over other low-income individuals with high costs, nonimmigrants are favored over immigrants. Under the ACA expansion, these distinctions mostly disappear, and eligibility depends purely on income level in the case of the biggest expansion group. Which approach do you prefer? If the ACA approach were expanded beyond 133% of FPL, the costs of the Medicaid program would soar. Given limited resources, do you think it would be better to cover more people at a higher poverty level across the board or continue to favor some groups over others through the categorical requirement? Should we decide that, for some populations, the government should step in and provide coverage regardless of the cost? In other words, is there a point where equity trumps financial constraints?

it is not surprising that the medically needy experience high medical expenses: In 2009, this population accounted for only 5% of Medicaid beneficiaries but 11% of Medicaid expenditures (KFF, 2012a).

Medically needy programs have both income and asset requirements (see **Box 10.6**). In terms of income requirements, states subtract the costs of individuals' medical expenses from their income level. States have the choice of deducting the medical expenses as they are incurred each month, every 6 months, or any time in between. As soon as otherwise qualified individuals "spend down" enough money on medical expenses, they are eligible for Medicaid through the medically needy option based on their reduced income level for the remainder of the period.

The following is a simplified example of how the "spend down" process works. Let's say a state calculates incurred medical expenses every 3 months to determine eligibility for the medically needy option, and in this state an individual (whom we will call Peter) must earn no more than $8500 a year to qualify as medically needy. Peter earns $11,000 per year and has $6000 each year in medical expenses, incurred at a rate of $500 per month. After 3 months, Peter has spent $1500 on medical expenses. Instead of considering the income level to be the annual amount earned ($11,000), the state subtracts Peter's medical expenses as they occur. So, after 3 months the state considers Peter to earn $9500 annually ($11,000 – $1500). Because this amount is

still over the $8500 limit, Peter is not eligible under the medically needy option. In another 3 months, Peter will have spent $3000 in medical expenses over the past 6 months. At that time, the state considers Peter to earn $8000 annually ($11,000 – $3000), making him eligible because he earns less than the $8500 limit. For the rest of this period (i.e., 3 months), Peter is eligible for Medicaid. After another 3 months, the state recalculates his earnings and medical expenses. Each year, this entire calculation starts over. In the end, Peter will not be eligible for Medicaid for the first 6 months of the year but will be eligible for Medicaid for the second 6 months of the year.

Immigrants

There are also special Medicaid eligibility rules relating to immigrants. The Personal Responsibility and Work Opportunity Reconciliation Act of 1996 (PRWORA) severely restricted immigrant eligibility for Medicaid (and most of the same rules in PRWORA were later applied to CHIP eligibility in 1997). Prior to PRWORA, legal immigrants followed the same Medicaid eligibility rules as everyone else, but undocumented immigrants were not eligible at all. PRWORA instituted a 5-year bar, meaning that most immigrants who come to the United States after August 22, 1996, are not eligible for Medicaid (or CHIP) for the first 5 years after their arrival. After 5 years, legal immigrants are eligible on the same basis as U.S. citizens, while undocumented immigrants remain ineligible for full Medicaid (or CHIP) benefits. However, both legal and undocumented immigrants who are otherwise eligible for Medicaid may receive emergency Medicaid benefits without any temporal restrictions. Immigrant eligibility eased slightly when CHIP was reauthorized through the Children's Health Insurance Program Reauthorization Act of 2009. States now have the option to cover legal immigrant children and/or pregnant women through Medicaid and CHIP in the first 5 years that they are in the United States.

Proponents of the immigrant restrictions believe they discourage people who cannot support themselves from coming to the United States and prevent immigrants from taking advantage of publicly funded programs they did not support through taxes before their arrival. In addition, some proponents believe that healthcare resources should go first to U.S. citizens, not noncitizens.

Opponents of the restrictions assert that most immigrants pay taxes once they arrive in this country and therefore deserve to receive the full benefits of

---

💡 Box 10.6 DISCUSSION QUESTIONS

Does the medically needy category make sense to you? Do you think it is a good idea to discount medical expenses of high-need individuals so they can access the healthcare services they need through Medicaid? If so, is the process just described cumbersome and likely to result in people being on and off Medicaid (and therefore likely on and off treatment) because their eligibility is based on their spending patterns? Why should individuals with high medical needs have an avenue to Medicaid eligibility that is not available to other low-income people who have other high expenses, such as child care or transportation costs? Would it make more sense to simply raise the eligibility level for Medicaid so more low-income people are eligible for the program? Politically, which option would likely have more support? Does your view about the medically needy category vary depending on your primary decision-making goal (e.g., fiscal restraint, equity, improved health outcomes)?

those taxes (Fremstad & Cox, 2004, p. 15). They also find the restriction ill-suited as a deterrent because immigrants often come to the United States for economic opportunities, not social benefits (Passel, 2005). Furthermore, restricting immigrants' access to health care may be a public health hazard for all members of the community because contagious diseases do not discriminate by immigration status. Finally, opponents contend that having higher numbers of uninsured individuals in the United States will further strain the ability of providers to care for all vulnerable populations in a community and lead to rising healthcare costs because uninsured immigrants are much less likely to obtain preventive care or early treatment for illnesses or injuries (Fremstad & Cox, 2004, p. 15). As of 2019, 36 states and the District of Columbia cover legal immigrant children under Medicaid and/or CHIP (Centers for Medicare and Medicaid Services [CMS], 2019). Sixteen states use CHIP funding to cover pregnant women under the unborn child option, which allows for coverage regardless of immigration status. Also, 23 states cover legal immigrant pregnant women under Medicaid without the 5-year bar. Two states and the District of Columbia use state-only funds to cover pregnant women who qualify based on income, but not immigration status (Brooks et al., 2017). Even with these reforms and the ACA, of the 28 million individuals who remain uninsured as of 2018, 24% were noncitizens. Among all noncitizens, undocumented immigrants are most likely to be uninsured (KFF, 2020c).

Medicaid Eligibility Expansion Under the ACA

As mentioned earlier, the ACA significantly expanded Medicaid eligibility. As of 2014, all non–Medicare-eligible individuals younger than 65 years, with incomes up to 133% FPL,[b] are eligible for Medicaid in states that choose to expand their programs. This eligibility expansion option marks a drastic departure from how Medicaid has generally been structured. Unlike Medicaid's traditional eligibility structure, individuals eligible through the expansion only have to satisfy an income threshold and do not have to meet a resource test or fit within a preapproved category. In addition, in traditional Medicaid, states have significant flexibility to determine how individual income and other personal resources are calculated. Under the ACA expansion, however, all states are required to accept newly eligible individuals using the federal income level

calculation and without accounting for other assets (see **Box 10.7**).

The ACA Medicaid expansion was intended to be mandatory in all states, but the Supreme Court's decision in *National Federation of Independent Business v. Sebelius* (2012) held that the federal government could not force states to expand Medicaid in this way. This case is discussed in detail in Chapter 11, "Health Reform and the Patient Protection and Affordable Care Act." As of May 2021, 39 states and the District of Columbia have chosen to expand their Medicaid program under the ACA (KFF, 2021c). The American Rescue Plan Act of 2021 (ARPA) included financial incentives to entice the remaining states to expand Medicaid. Under ARPA, newly expanding states would receive a 2-year, 5% bump in the matching rate for their *traditional* Medicaid population. These funds are not only projected to offset the cost of expanding Medicaid, but also provide those states with a significant amount of additional revenue (Rudowitz, Corallo, et al., 2021). In addition to financial incentives, numerous studies have shown that Medicaid expansion has positive effects on mortality, cancer, chronic diseases, disabilities, sexual and reproductive health, behavioral health, state economies, health disparities, and social drivers of health (Guth & Ammula, 2021). While the new financial incentives are causing some states to reconsider their position, others remain opposed to expansion for political and ideological reasons. Medicaid expansion opponents argue that expansion is too costly, the federal government is an unreliable fiscal partner, and states should have greater flexibility in managing their program (Armour, 2021).

Lawmakers built the ACA coverage options assuming that all states would be required to expand Medicaid. After the Supreme Court ruled that Medicaid expansion was optional, coverage gaps emerged in those states that did not choose to expand their Medicaid program. In nonexpansion states there are approximately 2 million poor adults who remain

---

💡 Box 10.7 DISCUSSION QUESTIONS

What are the implications of a two-tiered Medicaid system? Is there justification for offering some beneficiaries a less generous benefit package than others? Is it fair to impose additional requirements (categorical, asset test) on only some beneficiaries? Why do you think policymakers created these distinctions? Do you think they will remain in place over time?

ineligible for Medicaid and who are also too poor to obtain subsidies to purchase health insurance through their state exchanges (Garfield et al., 2021). Eligibility for these subsidies begins at 100% FPL, resulting in the illogical situation in which a poorer individual (e.g., one who earns 75% FPL) cannot obtain a subsidy while an individual who earns more (e.g., 115% FPL) is able to purchase subsidized insurance in the state exchange.

In addition to the Medicaid expansion rule just described, the ACA also requires that children ages 6 to 19 years be covered up to 133% FPL, instead of up to only 100% FPL as under pre-ACA rules. Undocumented immigrants, as well as legal immigrants who have resided in the United States for fewer than 5 years, will not be eligible for Medicaid under the expansion, although states have the option to cover legal immigrant pregnant women and children who have been in the country fewer than 5 years (matching the new rules put in place under CHIP).

Benefits

Medicaid benefits are structured in the same way as Medicaid eligibility: Some are mandatory and some are optional, and the newly eligible individuals under the ACA expansion have their own set of rules. Again, this means that no two Medicaid programs are alike, as each state picks its own menu of optional benefits to provide (see **Box 10.8**).

Traditional Medicaid Benefits

Historically, Medicaid programs have offered a rich array of benefits, including preventive services,

Box 10.8 DISCUSSION QUESTIONS

States have enormous flexibility in designing their Medicaid programs. States spend significant resources on optional services or mandatory services for optional populations. Even so, states complain that Medicaid expenditures are unsustainable and that significant reform, such as the Deficit Reduction Act and expanded waiver options, are needed. If states have the ability to reduce Medicaid spending without any reforms, why do you think state politicians are focused on reforming the program? Why might states choose not to reduce their Medicaid program to cover only mandatory services and populations? Politically, what do you think is the most feasible way for states to reduce their Medicaid budgets?

behavioral health services, long-term care services, supportive services that allow people with disabilities to work, institutional services, family planning services, and more. In fact, the coverage provided by traditional Medicaid generally has been more generous than the typical private insurance plan, particularly in the case of children. While federal Medicaid regulations exclude very few services, there are some prohibitions. Since 1977, Congress has prohibited the use of federal funds to pay for the costs of an abortion or mifepristone (commonly known as RU-486), a drug that induces medical abortions. Also, drug addiction or alcohol dependency may not be used as reasons to qualify an individual as disabled under SSI (and therefore, under Medicaid); however, if an individual is eligible for Medicaid for another reason, Medicaid programs may pay for substance abuse treatment.

All states provide the mandatory services listed on the left side of **Table 10.2** as part of their traditional Medicaid program, and states may provide the optional services listed on the right side. In addition to requiring a wide array of services, traditional Medicaid also defines many service categories quite broadly. For example, under the category of medical or remedial services, a state may pay for diagnostic, screening, or preventive services provided in any settings that are recommended by a licensed practitioner "for the maximum reduction of physical or mental disability and restoration of an individual to the best possible functional level" (Grants to States, § 440.130, 1988). As shown in Table 10.2, in addition to expanding eligibility, the ACA and ARPA included a few changes to Medicaid benefits. The ACA also includes a variety of demonstration programs that target key health issues such as obesity, high cholesterol, high blood pressure, diabetes, and tobacco use.

One of the broadest service categories is the early and periodic screening, diagnosis, and treatment (EPSDT) package of services for beneficiaries younger than 21 years. As the *E* in EPSDT indicates, this package of benefits provides preventive care to children to catch problems before they advance and offers early treatment to promote healthy growth and development. EPSDT benefits include periodic and as-needed screening services, comprehensive health exams (to detect both physical and mental health conditions), immunizations, lab tests, health education, vision services, hearing services, dental services, *and* any other measure to *correct or ameliorate* physical or mental defects found during a screening, *whether or not those services are covered under a state plan.* In addition to these benefits, EPSDT also requires states to inform families about the importance of preventive

Table 10.2 Traditional Medicaid Benefits

Mandatory	Optional
Acute Care Benefits	
Physician services Laboratory and X-ray services Inpatient hospital services Outpatient hospital services Early and periodic screening, diagnostic, and treatment services for beneficiaries < 21 years Family planning services and supplies Federally qualified health center services Rural health clinic services Nurse–midwife services Certified pediatric and family nurse practitioner services Nonemergency transportation to medical care	Prescription drugs Medical care or remedial care furnished by nonphysician licensed practitioners Rehabilitation and other therapies Clinic services Dental services, including dentures Prosthetic devices, eyeglasses, and durable medical equipment Primary care case management Tuberculosis-related services Other specified medical or remedial care
Long-Term Care Benefits	
Nursing facility services for individuals ≥ 21 years Home healthcare services for individuals entitled to nursing facility care	Intermediate care facility services for the mentally retarded Inpatient/nursing facility services for individuals ≥ 65 years in an institution for mental disease Inpatient psychiatric hospital services for individuals < 21 years Home- and community-based waiver services Other home health care Targeted case management Respiratory care services for ventilator-dependent individuals Personal care services Hospice services Services furnished under a Program of All-Inclusive Care for the Elderly
New Benefits in ACA	
Tobacco cessation program for pregnant women Freestanding birth centers	New state option for community-based care New state option for home health care New state option for family planning services
New Benefits in American Rescue Plan Act	
	New state option to extend postpartum coverage to a full year New state option to provide community-based mobile crisis intervention services

Data from 42 U.S.C. 1396d; 42 CFR Parts 430-498; Musumeci, M., Rudowitz, R., & Neuman, T. (2021, June 10). *How might lowering the Medicare age affect Medicaid enrollees?* https://www.kff.org/medicaid/issue-brief/how-might-lowering-the-medicare-age-affect-medicaid-enrollees/

care, seek out children in need of comprehensive care, and offer families assistance in securing care.

The *correct or ameliorate* standard is very different from the medical necessity standard that is used for adults in Medicaid and is commonly found in private health insurance plans. Typically, medically necessary services are those that restore *normal* function after an illness or injury. Not only does this standard

generally preclude care before a diagnosis is made, but if recovery is not possible (e.g., as a result of blindness), services that improve the quality of life or prevent deterioration of a condition may be denied. By contrast, the EPSDT *correct or ameliorate* standard means a state must provide coverage for preventive and developmental treatment, as well as for services needed to treat a specific diagnosis. Combined with the requirement to provide services regardless of state plan limitations, the correct or ameliorate standard means that almost any accepted treatment should be covered under EPSDT.

Benefits for Expansion Population Under the ACA

Expansion Medicaid populations receive their benefits through an Alternative Benefit Plan (ABP). The ABP structure is based on a law called the Deficit Reduction Act (DRA) of 2005 (see **Box 10.9**). As shown in **Box 10.10**, states have a variety of options at their disposal to use for their "benchmark" or "benchmark-equivalent" package of services for certain populations, instead of following the mandatory and optional list of services identified in Table 10.2 (SSA, § 1937). These options include DRA benchmark options, DRA benchmark-equivalent options, and new benchmarks effective as of 2020.

 Box 10.9   **Special Topic**

Citizenship Verification

The DRA also included new rules on citizenship verification. Prior to the DRA, all but four states allowed beneficiaries to self-attest to their citizenship status. Under the DRA, Medicaid and CHIP applicants now have to prove their citizenship status by providing original or certified copies of citizenship documents, such as a U.S. passport, state-issued driver's license, or birth certificate. The exact requirements depend on what type of document is submitted. Subsequent laws eased this burden by giving states the option to conduct a data match with the Social Security Administration's database to verify citizenship. Under the ACA, the matching system must be used to verify citizenship for individuals purchasing insurance in an exchange. These rules were intended to ensure that only eligible beneficiaries received Medicaid benefits. Many individuals have had difficulty obtaining access to these documents and as a result were dropped from the program despite being eligible.

Do you think these rules are a good idea? Do you think this requirement is a reasonable burden? Does it matter that evidence was not available to support the claim that noncitizens or ineligible immigrants were accessing Medicaid benefits? Or, is the possibility that ineligible immigrants might enroll in Medicaid concerning enough to warrant the new documentation requirements?

Box 10.10 Benchmark Benefit Options

DRA Benchmark Plans
Federal Employees Health Benefits program
State employee health plan
Largest commercial non-Medicaid health maintenance organization in the state
HHS secretary–approved plan

DRA Benchmark-Equivalent Plan
Full actuarial value for the following services:

- Inpatient and outpatient hospital
- Physician (surgical and medical)
- Laboratory and X-ray
- Well-baby and well-child
- Other appropriate preventive services (defined by HHS secretary)

Additional DRA Optional Benchmark-Equivalent Services
75% actuarial value for the following services:

- Prescription drugs
- Mental health
- Vision
- Hearing

New Benchmark Options Effective 2020
The 2017 essential health benefit (EHB) benchmark plan from any state
An existing state benchmark with one or more EHB categories replaced by a benchmark from another state
A new benchmark that meets the "typical employer plan" requirement
Note: States must wrap around EPSDT coverage as necessary.

Benchmarks provide a state with a standard to follow when designing its Medicaid package of benefits; this system does not mean that Medicaid beneficiaries are enrolled in the plans identified as benchmarks. Furthermore, a state may instead choose to offer "benchmark-equivalent" coverage that includes certain basic services as shown in Box 10.10. These services must have the same actuarial value as the services provided by one of the three benchmarks listed earlier (i.e., the value of the services must be similar). States may choose to supplement their benchmark-equivalent plans with additional services, as listed in Box 10.10. These additional services are required to be worth only 75% of the actuarial value of the same service provided in a benchmark plan. Finally, while the DRA guaranteed the same set of EPSDT services for children younger than 19 years, these services may be more difficult to access if they are provided through wrap-around benefits that supplement the benchmark package instead of within the package itself. The DRA was later amended to require states to ensure that EPSDT services are available to children up to age 21 years, to cover non-emergency transportation to medical appointments, and to cover family planning services and supplies.

The benefit changes allowed by the DRA may be applied only to certain populations, and these groups had to be part of a state plan prior to the law's enactment to receive the new benefits package. DRA-eligible populations include most categorically needy children, as well as parents and caretakers who receive Medicaid but not Temporary Assistance to Needy Families (the new welfare program created by PRWORA). The list of populations excluded from the DRA is quite lengthy and includes medically frail beneficiary groups with high expenditures, such as the disabled, dual eligibles, and terminally ill hospice patients (SSA, § 1937). Very few states have used DRA options for populations other than Medicaid expansion (EveryCRSReport.com, 2018).

The ACA further amended the DRA benchmark options, which are now referred to as section 1937 State Flexibility in Benefits Packages (based on the section of the SSA that describes these plans). Under the ACA, ABPs are offered in accordance with section 1937 rules. The ACA requires section 1937 plans to provide EHB coverage and comply with the Mental Health Parity and Addiction Equity Act, which requires parity between physical and mental health/substance abuse benefits (Medicaid.gov, n.d.b). EHBs include coverage for 10 categories of services in a scope equal to that of a typical employer plan (discussed in more detail in Chapter 11, "Health Reform and the Patient Protection and Affordable Care Act"). Furthermore, ABPs must comply with additional Medicaid rules that include coverage for federally qualified health centers and rural healthcare services; compliance with traditional Medicaid cost-sharing rules, which significantly limit the level of cost-sharing required of beneficiaries; and a prohibition against coverage for beneficiaries in institutions for mental diseases (Medicaid.gov, n.d.b). Certain medically frail populations remain exempt from section 1937 plans and continue to have access to all traditional Medicaid benefits in their state. **Box 10.11** highlights the ABP requirements. Because ABPs are based on commercial plans, some benefits may be more generous than traditional Medicaid coverage, while others may be less generous. To simplify matters, most states have chosen to align their ABP coverage with the traditional Medicaid coverage for adults (EveryCRSReport.com, 2018).

Box 10.11 Technical Spotlight

Alternative Benefit Plan (Section 1937 Plan) Requirements

- Align with an approved benchmark or benchmark equivalent
- Provide essential health benefits
- Include early and periodic screening, diagnosis, and treatment for children up to age 21 years
- Cover federally qualified health center/rural healthcare services
- Cover nonemergency transportation to medical care
- Cover family planning services and supplies
- Comply with mental health parity law
- Comply with traditional Medicaid cost-sharing rules
- Do not cover care for beneficiaries in institutions for mental diseases
- Exempt certain medically frail populations from benefit limits

Amount, Duration, and Scope, and Reasonableness Requirements

Although states have a great deal of flexibility in designing their Medicaid benefit packages, states have always had to follow several federal requirements prior to the DRA. These rules, collectively referred to as "amount, duration, and scope" and "reasonableness" requirements, were intended to ensure that all Medicaid beneficiaries in a state received adequate, comparable, and nondiscriminatory coverage. Some of these rules changed through section 1937.

Private insurers typically are not drawn to Medicaid's population because of the likelihood that these individuals would have relatively high healthcare needs. In addition, private insurers use a variety of tools (such as limited open-enrollment periods, experience rating, medical condition–based limitations, and narrow medical necessity standards) to limit their financial exposure. Medicaid, on the other hand, was designed as a healthcare entitlement program, with the goal to provide services to a needy population that would otherwise be uninsurable through commercial plans (Rosenbaum, 2002). **Table 10.3** identifies some of the requirements that help the Medicaid program achieve this goal, as well as any changes to them found in section 1937.

Medicaid Spending

Health policymakers not only are concerned with how much money Medicaid costs, but also the distribution of program spending. In 2019, Medicaid spent over $613 billion, accounting for approximately 16% of total national health expenditures in the United States (CMS .gov, 2020c). Understanding which populations utilize the most services, which services are utilized most frequently, and which services and populations are most costly helps policymakers decide if they need to change the Medicaid program and, if so, what changes should be made.

As you can see from **Figure 10.3**, not all populations and services are equal when it comes to cost. Generally, children and adults are fairly inexpensive to cover, whereas older adults and individuals with disabilities use more, as well as more expensive, services. Over half of Medicaid spending goes to care for older adult and disabled beneficiaries even though they constituted only one-fifth of all enrollees (Rudowitz, Williams, et al., 2021). Dual eligibles—beneficiaries enrolled in both Medicaid and Medicare—are particularly expensive. While they constitute 20% of enrollees, they account for 34% of spending (MACPAC, n.d.d).

Table 10.3 "Reasonableness" and "Amount, Duration, and Scope" Requirements in Medicaid

Requirement	Requirement Purpose	Section 1937 Changes to the Requirement
Reasonableness	State must provide all services to categorically needy beneficiaries in sufficient amount, duration, and scope to achieve its purpose.	States have to meet only amount, duration, and scope requirements found in the named benchmark or benchmark-equivalent plan.
Comparability	All categorically needy beneficiaries in the state are entitled to receive the same benefit package in content, amount, duration, and scope.	States may apply benchmark or benchmark-equivalent packages to some, but not all, populations.
Statewideness	In most cases, states must provide same benefit package in all parts of the state.	States may apply benchmark or benchmark-equivalent packages to some, but not all, populations.
Nondiscrimination	States may not discriminate against a beneficiary based on diagnosis, illness, or type of condition by limiting or denying a mandatory service.	DRA does not include language changing Medicaid nondiscrimination rules, and ACA includes nondiscrimination protections regarding age, expected life span, diagnosis, disability, medical dependency, quality of life, or other health condition (42 CFR 440.347(e)).

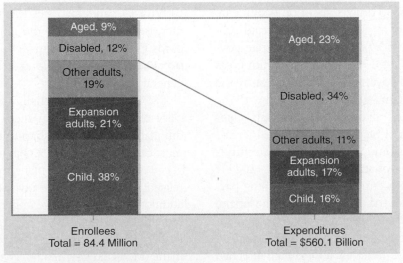

Note: Totals may not sum to 100% due to rounding.

Figure 10.3 Enrollment and Spending in Medicaid, 2018

Rudowitz, R., Williams, E., Hinton, E., & Garfield, R. (2021, May 7). *Medicaid financing: The basics.* Kaiser Family Foundation. https://www.kff.org/medicaid/issue-brief/medicaid-financing-the-basics/

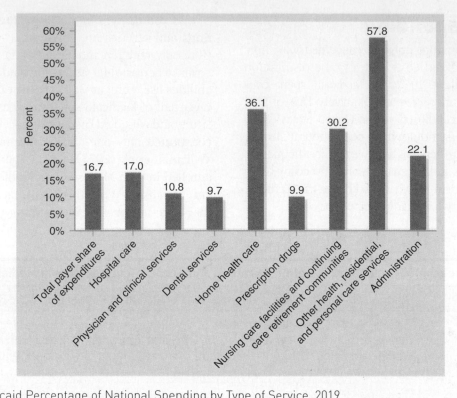

Figure 10.4 Medicaid Percentage of National Spending by Type of Service, 2019

Data from Medicaid and CHIP Payment and Access Commission. (2019, December). *MACSTATS: Medicaid and CHIP data book.* https://www.macpac.gov/wp-content/uploads/2015/12/MACStats-Medicaid-and-CHIP-Data-Book-December-2019.pdf

In addition, they are heavy users of prescription drugs and are relatively more likely to be hospitalized. **Figure 10.4** shows Medicaid's significant role in funding home health and nursing home care in this country, along with a variety of other services.

Medicaid Financing

Medicaid is responsible for a significant portion of health care spending in the United States, accounting for $1 out of every $6 dollars spent on health care (Rudowitz, Williams, et al., 2021). The Medicaid program is jointly financed by the federal and state governments, with about 64% of the total program costs paid for by the federal government and the rest by the states (Rudowitz, Williams, et al., 2021). Even with the federal government picking up over half the tab, states have found their share of Medicaid costs to be increasingly burdensome, encompassing 29% of state funds nationally in 2019 (Rudowitz, Williams, et al., 2021).

Program financing occurs through a matching payment system that divides the amount paid by the federal and state governments. The matching rate for most medical services, called the Federal Medical Assistance Percentage (FMAP), is determined by a formula that is tied to each state's per-capita income. Poorer states—those with lower per-capita incomes—receive more federal money for every state dollar spent on Medicaid, while the wealthier states receive less. The FMAP rate may not be lower than 50% for any state, meaning the costliest scenario for a state government is that it splits program costs evenly with the federal government. For FY 2022, FMAP rates range from 50% to 78% (Rudowitz, Williams, et al., 2021). In addition, the federal government periodically allows for temporary FMAP increases in times of national emergencies (e.g., Hurricane Katrina) or as incentives for specific providers (2-year increase for primary care providers). To assist states during the COVID-19 pandemic, FFCRA included a 6.2% FMAP increase as long as states did not reduce eligibility standards (Rudowitz, Williams, et al., 2021). As shown in **Box 10.12**, there are also long-standing exceptions to the general FMAP formula.

Medicaid is also partially financed through beneficiary copayments, coinsurance, and premiums. In traditional Medicaid, cost-sharing is extremely limited. In most cases, states may not charge cost-sharing for emergency services, family planning services, pregnancy-related services, or preventive services for children. In addition, states can charge only nominal cost-sharing for individuals under 100% FPL, such as $4 for a physician visit or $8 for nonemergency use of an emergency department (Medicaid.gov, n.d.f). The DRA included drastic changes to Medicaid's cost-sharing rules that now apply to ABPs through section 1937 (see **Box 10.13**). These changes allow for higher cost-sharing for individuals

Box 10.12   Technical Spotlight

FMAP Provision Details

In addition to the standard FMAP formula, there are several instances where states receive additional or different matching rates:

- Indian Health Service: 100%
- Family planning services: 90%
- Health homes: 90%
- Expansion Medicaid: 90%
- District of Columbia: 70%
- U.S. territories: capped at 55%
- Most administrative services: 50%
- Smoking cessation for pregnant women: FMAP +1%
- Specified preventive services and immunizations without cost-sharing: FMAP +1%

Box 10.13   DISCUSSION QUESTIONS

Is higher Medicaid cost-sharing a good idea? What are the strongest arguments you can make for and against higher cost-sharing? Should Medicaid beneficiaries have the same cost-sharing responsibilities as privately insured individuals, or should the government bear more of the cost because Medicaid beneficiaries are low-income individuals? What is the primary decision-making goal that led to the exclusion of so many populations and services from the new cost-sharing options?

who earn over 100% FPL, although out-of-pocket costs may not exceed 5% of a family's income. For example, beneficiaries between 101% and 150% FPL can pay up to a 10% copay for a physician visit, and beneficiaries over 151% FPL can pay up to a 20% copay for the same service (Medicaid.gov, n.d.f). Also, prior to the DRA, cost-sharing requirements were "unenforceable," meaning health professionals could not refuse to provide services if a beneficiary did not pay a required cost-share amount. Now states can deny services if enrollees do not pay the higher out-of-pocket costs. As with the DRA benefit changes, many groups and services are excluded from the new cost-sharing options.

As noted earlier, the federal government is picking up the bulk of the cost of the ACA Medicaid expansions. From 2014 to 2016, the federal government paid 100% of the cost of financing newly eligible enrollees. While the federal government's share will decrease over time, it will still cover 90% of the cost in 2020 and beyond. In 2019, the federal government paid almost $85 billion of the $94 billion tab for expansion enrollees. Expansion enrollees accounted for 20% of Medicaid beneficiaries and 16% of Medicaid spending that year (Rudowitz, Corallo, et al., 2021).

It was expected that the Medicaid expansion would reduce the uncompensated care burden of states—because fewer individuals will be uninsured—and this appears to be the case. Between 2013 and 2015, uncompensated care costs fell from 3.9% to 2.3% of hospital costs, for a savings of over $6 billion. Hospitals in expansion states that treat the highest proportion of low-income and uninsured patients experienced the largest savings (Dranove et al., 2017). However, as the uninsured rate increased in 2017 and 2018, the uncompensated care costs rose as well (Lukens, 2021). The ACA also included cuts to Disproportionate Share Hospital (DSH) payments (discussed in more detail in Chapter 11, "Health Reform and the Patient Protection and Affordable Care Act"). These payments provide additional funds to hospitals that care for a significant number of Medicaid and low-income uninsured patients. Because the ACA was supposed to reduce the number of low-income uninsured patients through universal Medicaid expansion, it was thought that fewer DSH payments would be needed. The combination of policies that have increased the number of uninsured individuals, and the Supreme Court's decision that made Medicaid expansion optional, mean that DSH payments continue to be a vital resource to help hospitals combat uncompensated care costs. To date, Congress has delayed DSH payment reductions until 2024.

Medicaid Provider Reimbursement

Medicaid's complex design also extends to its provider reimbursement methodology. States have broad discretion in setting provider rates (see **Box 10.14**). Not only

Box 10.14   DISCUSSION QUESTIONS

Who should determine Medicaid provider reimbursement rates, and how should they compare to other insurance programs or plans? Should the federal government play a stronger role in setting provider rates? Is this an area where it is better to have state variation or national uniformity? Should the federal or state governments be required to ensure that Medicaid reimbursement rates match private insurance reimbursement rates? What might occur if poorer states were required to provide higher reimbursement rates? What is the risk if reimbursement rates are very low?

do reimbursement rates vary by state, they also vary by whether services are provided in a fee-for-service (FFS) or managed care setting and by which type of provider (e.g., physicians, hospitals) renders a service.[c] In 2019, almost half (49%) of payments went to managed care organizations (MCOs), mostly to comprehensive managed care plans (Rudowitz, Williams, et al., 2021).

FFS Reimbursement

When reimbursing FFS care under Medicaid, states are required to set their payment rates to physicians at levels that are "sufficient" to ensure Medicaid patients have "equal access" to providers compared to the general population (SSA § 1396a(a)(30)(A)). Despite this language, Medicaid reimbursement rates are lower than Medicare or private insurance rates. In 2016, Medicaid paid physicians 38% less than Medicare (Holgash & Heberlein, 2019). A 2015 U.S. Supreme Court decision found that providers cannot sue a state to raise Medicaid reimbursement rates (*Armstrong v. Exceptional Child Center*, 2015).

Low reimbursement is the primary reason that many providers are wary of treating Medicaid patients, but other factors are important as well. Physicians also decline to participate in Medicaid due to extensive program requirements, delays in payment, and the burden of treating a complex patient population (Holgash & Heberlein, 2019; Rosenbaum, 2014). A 2014–2015 national review found that 71% of physicians would be willing to accept new Medicaid patients as compared to 85% and 90% of physicians who would accept new Medicare and privately insured patients, respectively (Holgash & Heberlein, 2019). Acceptance of new Medicaid patients varied greatly by physician specialty; 88% of general surgeons were willing to take on new Medicaid patients compared to just 36% of psychiatrists (Holgash & Heberlein, 2019).

Physicians who treat Medicaid patients are demographically different from those who serve privately insured patients. Medicaid patients are more likely to be seen by physicians who are younger, work in large practices, are graduates of foreign medical schools, are graduates from lower-ranked medical schools, and are not board-certified (Decker, 2018). Overall, relatively few physicians see the bulk of Medicaid patients across the country: From 2013 to 2015, approximately 20% of physicians saw 60% of Medicaid patients (Neprash et al., 2018).

Prior to the ACA, Medicaid reimbursement was 59% of Medicare rates (Decker, 2018). The ACA included a temporary bump in primary care payment rates for services provided in both FFS and managed care settings. For 2013 and 2014, primary care payment rates equaled 100% of Medicare payment rates,

with the federal government covering the cost of the increased reimbursement. On average, this change resulted in a 73% increase in Medicaid payments, but there was wide variation across the country (Decker, 2018). While this measure was intended to support primary care providers and boost access to primary care services, its temporary nature undermined the effectiveness of the policy. Research has found no significant increase in physician participation in Medicaid after the fee bump (Advisory Board, 2018; Decker, 2018).

Hospital FFS plans are reimbursed at a rate that is "consistent with efficiency, economy, and quality of care" (SSA, § 1902(a)(30)(a)). However, there is no specified minimum reimbursement level that states are required to meet, resulting in rates that are lower than what hospitals receive from Medicare and private insurance. While it is difficult to estimate Medicaid payments to hospitals due to data issues and differences in state payment methodologies, it appears Medicaid pays hospitals about 90% to 93% of costs on average, with significant variation across the country (Cunningham et al., 2016). Hospitals that serve a high number of Medicaid and uninsured individuals may receive additional Medicaid DSH payments.

States have flexibility in how they reimburse hospitals. For inpatient services, states may pay hospitals per diem (number of days a patient is in the hospital), by reported costs, or through the diagnosis-related group (DRG) system that is also used by Medicare. The DRG system, which includes a rate per discharge with additional costs for outlier cases, is the most common choice. States may also make supplemental payments, including quality or efficiency incentives, and adjust payments based on factors such as hospital type, geography, or outlier cases (MACPAC, 2018b). For outpatient hospital services, states reimburse hospitals through cost reimbursement, ambulatory patient classification (APC) groups, enhanced ambulatory patient groups (EAPGs), or state fee schedules (MACPAC, 2016). The APC system bundles similar services into one payment rate, although one visit can have multiple APCs and payments. EAPGs also bundle services and reimburse hospitals based on the complexity of the patient's needs (MACPAC, 2016). As with inpatient rates, states may add supplemental payments, including funds for safety-net hospitals and academic health centers, and adjust payments based on factors such as hospital type, geography, and services provided out of state (MACPAC, 2016).

Managed Care Reimbursement

As with the rest of the healthcare system, managed care has become an increasingly important part of the Medicaid program. In 2018, 83% of all Medicaid

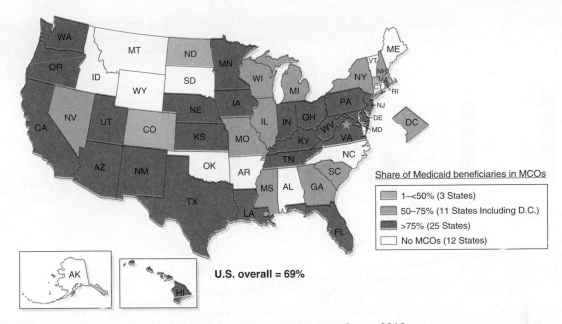

Figure 10.5 Share of Beneficiaries in Managed Care Organizations, by State, 2018

Hinton, E., Rudowitz, R., Stolyar, L., & Singer, N. (2020, October 29). *10 Things to know about Medicaid managed care.* Kaiser Family Foundation. https://www.kff.org/medicaid/issue-brief/10-things-to-know-about-medicaid-managed-care/

beneficiaries—mostly children and parents—obtained their care through MCOs, with 69% in comprehensive managed care plans (Hinton et al., 2020; **Figure 10.5**). In addition, seven states used a "medical home" or primary care case management (PCCM) model that year, while five other states offered both types of MCOs (Hinton et al., 2020). PCCM models pay a provider to coordinate care for beneficiaries, whether it is only primary care services or a range of services, such as physical, behavioral, long-term care, social supports, and so on. As with Medicaid enrollment overall, managed care enrollment increased in 2020, most likely due to loss of employment during the pandemic and maintenance of effort requirements to obtain the temporary FMAP increase (Stolyar et al., 2021). States may require managed care enrollment for all beneficiaries except children with special healthcare needs, Native Americans, and Medicare recipients (SSA, § 1936u-2).

MCOs that enroll Medicaid beneficiaries receive a monthly capitated rate per member and assume financial risk for providing services. In 2019, managed care payments to comprehensive MCOs accounted for 46% of Medicaid spending (Hinton et al., 2020). States and MCOs agree upon a set of services the MCOs will provide for the capitated rate. If there are any Medicaid-covered services that are not included in a state's managed care contract with MCOs, states reimburse them an amount in addition to the capitated rate or reimburse non-MCO providers on an FFS basis to provide those services. In other words, beneficiaries are still entitled to all

Medicaid services, even when they are enrolled in a managed care plan.

States are required to pay MCOs on an "actuarially sound basis," a term that is not defined in the Medicaid statute (SSA, § 1396b(m)(2)(iii)). As with other types of provider rates, capitation rates vary widely among states. However, it is difficult to compare capitation rates across states because of the variation in Medicaid programs generally and in the types of services and populations covered by the managed care contracts. Capitation rates for 2020 were set prior to the COVID-19 pandemic, leaving MCOs with high unanticipated testing and treatment costs and providers with revenue loss due to lower utilization. CMS has provided several methods for MCOs to address both payment concerns and provider rates (Hinton et al., 2020).

With the rapid growth of Medicaid managed care services, CMS issued rules in 2016 to improve the managed care component of the program. These rules covered a wide variety of issues, such as strengthening beneficiary protections, aligning Medicaid and CHIP requirements as necessary, improving payment provisions and program integrity, promoting quality of care, and creating network adequacy standards (Paradise & Musumeci, 2016). As shown in **Figure 10.6**, Medicaid MCOs are using a variety of quality initiatives to improve performance.

Medicaid Waivers

Much of the previous discussion about Medicaid highlighted both the numerous requirements placed on

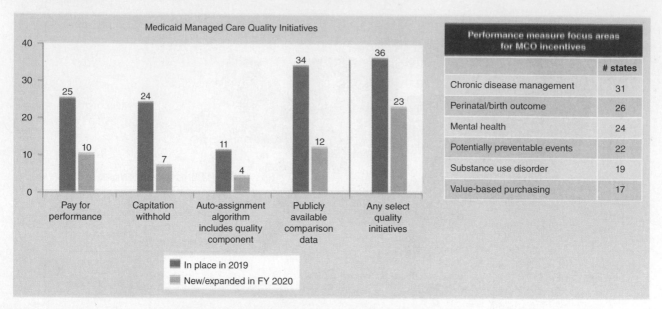

Notes: Medicaid Managed Care Quality initiatives: States with MCOs indicated if selected quality initiatives were in place in FY 2019, new or expanded in FY 2020. Performance Measure Focus Areas: States that employed a pay for performance bonus or penalty, a capitation withhold and/or an auto-assignment quality factor were asked to identify performance measure focus areas linked to these quality incentives.

Figure 10.6 State Managed Care Organization Quality Measures, 2019

Hinton, E., Rudowitz, R., Stolyar, L., & Singer, N. (2020, October 29). *10 Things to know about Medicaid managed care*. Kaiser Family Foundation. https://www.kff.org/medicaid/issue-brief/10-things-to-know-about-medicaid-managed-care/

states and the enormous amount of flexibility states have in operating their programs. Medicaid *waivers* provide still another level of flexibility for states. There are several different types of waivers under Medicaid; here, we focus only on the broadest one—the "section 1115" waiver. Under section 1115 of the SSA, states may apply to the secretary of HHS to waive certain requirements of health and welfare programs under the SSA, including both Medicaid and CHIP. The secretary may grant section 1115 waivers, also called demonstration projects, as long as the proposal "assists in promoting the objectives" of the federal program.[d] The Medicaid statute describes one main purpose of the program as furnishing medical assistance to those who cannot afford necessary care (SSA, § 1901). This broad standard has not been defined and leaves the secretary with enormous discretion to approve or reject waiver applications.

For decades, Medicaid waiver approvals have been a primary means for administrations from both parties to alter the Medicaid program to meet their priorities (**Figure 10.7**). President Carter focused on cost control, President Reagan expanded home and community-based care for individuals with disabilities, President Obama pursued delivery reforms, and President Trump supported work requirements and other enrollment and eligibility restrictions (Barker, 2020; KFF, 2021f). Because 1115 waivers are required to further the objectives of the Medicaid program, administrations have a stake in defining those objectives as much as possible within the confines of the statutory language. For

example, in 2015 the Obama administration released guidance that focused on increasing coverage, stabilizing provider networks, improving outcomes, and promoting delivery reforms (Solomon & Schubel, 2017). The Trump administration concentrated on supporting upward mobility, independence, responsible decision-making, and transitioning to private insurance (Medicaid.gov, n.d.a). While the Biden administration has not set out similar guidance at the time of this writing, it has withdrawn support of work requirement waivers due to concerns about coverage loss and skepticism about employment gains for beneficiaries (Rosenbaum, 2021).

As of December 2021, 46 states have approved 64 waivers (KFF, 2021f; see **Figure 10.8**). Waivers can be used to assist states during public health and national emergencies. For example, waivers were used to expand coverage after Hurricane Katrina and in response to the Flint, Michigan, water crisis. During the COVID-19 pandemic, CMS approved waivers to ease requirements relating to long-term services and supports (Guth et al., 2020). Waivers allowing work requirements have been contested in court. In *Stewart v. Azar*, the court held, in part, that the Secretary of HHS did not consider how Kentucky's waiver would promote affordable coverage, a key objective of the Medicaid program (Musumeci, 2018; see **Box 10.15**). The outcome of this and other court decisions will dictate how much leeway the administration has in changing the contours of the Medicaid program.

There is a long history of section 1115 waivers in Medicaid

1990s–2001 • **Broad coverage expansions:** Financed with savings from MCOs or DSH*

2001–2010 • **HIFA and other waivers:** Limited coverage expansions, with cost-sharing and reduced benefits to offset costs*

2010–2014 • **Pre-ACA expansion:** Early ACA implementation with regular match rate

2014–2017 • **Expansion waivers/delivery system reform:** Alternative ACA Medicaid expansion models and DSRIP

2017–2020 • **Condition eligibility and provide payment for IMD services:** Work requirements and other eligibility restrictions; paying for IMD services to treat SUD, SMI, SED

Over time: emergency waivers (e.g., 9/11, Katrina, Flint, COVID-19)

Notes: *These pre-2010 coverage expansions are no longer necessary due to the ACA.
MCO = Managed care organization
DSH = Disproportionate share hospital
HIFA = Health Insurance Flexibility and Accountability
ACA = Affordable Care Act
DSRIP = Delivery system reform incentive program
IMD = Institution for mental disease
SUD = Substance use disorder
SMI = Serious mental illness
SED = Serious emotional disturbance

Figure 10.7 History of Section 1115 Medicaid Waivers

Guth, M., Hinton, E., Musumeci, M., & Rudowitz, R. (2020, October 30). *The landscape of Medicaid demonstration waivers ahead of the 2020 election.* Kaiser Family Foundation. https://www.kff.org/medicaid/issue-brief/the-landscape-of-medicaid-demonstration-waivers-ahead-of-the-2020-election/

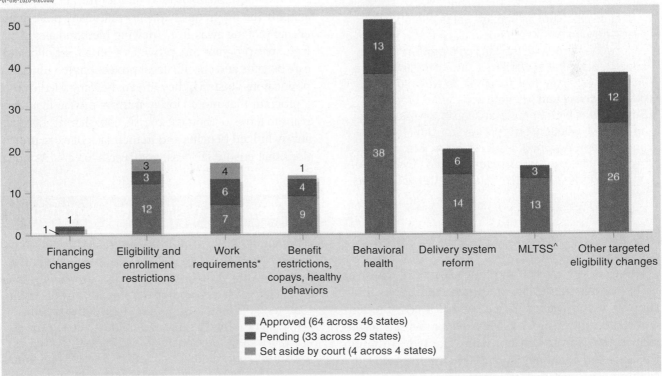

Notes: Some states have multiple approved and/or multiple pending waivers, and many waivers are comprehensive and may fall into a few different areas. Therefore, the total number of pending or approved waivers across states cannot be calculated by summing counts of waivers in each category. Pending waiver applications are not included here until they are officially accepted by CMS and posted on Medicaid.gov.

*On 2/12/21, CMS under the Biden administration sent letters to states with approved work requirements to begin the process of withdrawing these waiver authorities (see KFF Medical Waiver Tracker for more info).

^ "MLTSS" = Managed long-term services and supports.

Figure 10.8 Approved and Pending 1115 Medicaid Waivers, December 2021

Kaiser Family Foundation. (2021, December 20). *Medicaid waiver tracker: Approved and pending section 1115 waivers by state.* Kaiser Family Foundation. https://www.kff.org/medicaid/issue-brief/medicaid-waiver-tracker-approved-and-pending-section-1115-waivers-by-state/#Table3

⭐ Box 10.15   Special Topic

Work Requirement

Should states be allowed to impose work requirements as a condition for receiving Medicaid benefits? Do work requirements promote independence and upward mobility, and, if so, are those two goals legitimate objectives of the Medicaid program? Are work requirements unnecessary barriers to care?

Those who oppose work requirements argue that they do not further the objective of the Medicaid program, which is to provide coverage to those who cannot afford it. As a practical matter, most beneficiaries are already working, and most of those who are not working are in poor health or disabled, are acting as caregivers, or are students. Many of the nonworkers would be exempt even under the recently approved waivers. In addition, work requirements create extensive administrative obligations for beneficiaries and administrators alike. Of the 1 million to 4 million beneficiaries estimated to lose coverage if work requirements are imposed broadly, most would be disenrolled due to lack of reporting.

Those who support requirements contend that everyone who can work should be working, both to reduce the burden on the Medicaid program and to support personal upward mobility. According to this view, the ultimate goal should be to wean people off of Medicaid and promote work requirements. Some states with Republican legislatures, such as Virginia, would not support expanding Medicaid under the ACA without work requirements.

Do you support work requirements? Even if you oppose work requirements, is it better to expand coverage with work requirements than to not expand coverage at all?

One of the most important aspects of a waiver is the "budget neutrality" requirement. A state must show that the waiver project will not cost the federal government more money over a 5-year period than if the waiver had not been granted. Although the amount of money spent remains the same, by seeking a waiver, a state is agreeing to use itself as a "policy laboratory" in exchange for being able to operate its Medicaid program with fewer requirements. Ideally, other states and the federal government will learn from these demonstration projects and incorporate their positive aspects, while avoiding negative ones.

The Future of Medicaid

Due to the high cost of the Medicaid program, the large federal deficit, other pressures on federal and state budgets, and ideological differences among policymakers, Medicaid reform has been a hot topic in recent years (see **Box 10.16**). The stresses of the pandemic have shifted the focus of state Medicaid policies toward increasing provider support, addressing social drivers of health, improving long-term services and supports, and expanding telehealth (Gifford et al., 2020). Beyond pandemic-related issues, the Supreme Court's decision to make expansion optional has ensured that the battle over Medicaid and other entitlement programs will continue. Curtailing the Medicaid expansion and transforming Medicaid from an entitlement program to a block grant program were central features of the failed 2017 Republican ACA repeal and replacement efforts. Those plans may be revived if Republicans regain the White House and Congressional majorities.

Even if Medicaid remains effectively intact, with the Medicaid expansion population operating under different rules than traditional Medicaid enrollees, the administrative complexity of running a two-tiered system will undoubtedly lead to calls for further reforms to simplify the program. It appears that many policymakers are moving away from viewing Medicaid as a social insurance program that provides a certain set of healthcare benefits and specific legal protections to vulnerable populations. Instead, they are envisioning Medicaid as a program that more closely mirrors private insurance plans in terms of their use of risk, cost-sharing, comparatively limited benefits and in their lack of extra protections that ensure fairness, and access to care. As noted

💡 **Box 10.16** DISCUSSION QUESTIONS

What type of Medicaid reform, if any, do you support? Should Medicaid beneficiaries be treated like privately insured individuals, meaning increased cost-sharing requirements, fewer legal protections, and fewer guaranteed benefits than in the current Medicaid program? Is it fair to provide a more generous package of benefits to publicly insured individuals than most privately insured people receive? Can the country afford a more generous Medicaid program? Can it afford not to provide adequate health insurance and access to care for the poor and near-poor? Is it best to let states experiment with new ideas? If you could design a new Medicaid program, what would be your primary decision-making goal?

previously, some states are implementing these types of changes through waivers granted by HHS.

While the high number of Medicaid enrollees in expansion states speaks to the need for an affordable insurance option for many low-income individuals, the cost of the expansion is already making states question their ability to support a larger Medicaid program. Nonetheless, Medicaid remains quite popular with the public, with 75% of respondents having a favorable view of the program and 76% supporting expansion (KFF, 2020b; Lopes et al., 2021). Even so, Republicans are much less supportive than Democrats or Independents. These competing political views about what form Medicaid should take makes the future of the program uncertain at best.

Children's Health Insurance Program

Congress created the Children's Health Insurance Program (CHIP) in 1997 as a $40 billion, 10-year block grant program, codified as Title XXI of the SSA. When the program expired in 2007, Congress tried to extend it by passing two versions of the Children's Health Insurance Program Reauthorization Act (CHIPRA). Despite the bipartisan support for these bills, then-president George W. Bush vetoed both versions and instead signed a temporary extension of the program. In 2009, Congress again passed CHIPRA, and newly elected President Obama signed it into law as one of his first acts in office. CHIPRA included $33 billion in federal funds for children's coverage and extended the program and its funding through 2013 (KFF, 2012b). The ACA further extended the program until 2019, but only included funding through fiscal year 2015. In April 2015, Obama signed the Medicare Access and CHIP Reauthorization Act of 2015, which provided an additional 2 years of funding (through 2017) for CHIP. After a short lapse in funding, Congress extended funding until 2023 through the HEALTHY KIDS Act of 2018 and until 2027 through the Bipartisan Budget Act of 2018 (MACPAC, n.d.a).

CHIP is designed to provide health insurance to uninsured low-income children whose family income is above the eligibility level for Medicaid in their state. Overall, CHIP has been successful at insuring low-income children, enrolling more than 9.6 million children in 2019 (KFF, 2019c). Nonetheless, 5.2% of children younger than 19 years remained uninsured as of 2019, and many of them live in low-income families (U.S. Census, 2020, p. 6).

While the ACA and subsequent laws included maintenance of effort (MOE) provisions for CHIP, the pandemic relief acts did not. As opposed to Medicaid enrollment, which increased during the pandemic, CHIP enrollment fell overall in 2020 (Alker, 2020). Enrollment levels vary across states, with some states experiencing increased enrollment while enrollment declined in others. It is possible that some of the decrease in CHIP enrollment is due to children moving from CHIP to Medicaid as parents lost employment and wages. However, at least some of that loss should have been offset by newly eligible children who had been in families with higher incomes prior to the pandemic (Alker, 2020).

CHIP Structure and Financing

CHIP is an optional program for the states, but all 50 states and the District of Columbia have chosen to participate. States have three options regarding how their CHIP is structured:

1. States may incorporate CHIP into their existing Medicaid program by using CHIP children as an expansion population.
2. States may create an entirely separate CHIP program.
3. States may create a hybrid program in which lower-income children are part of Medicaid and higher-income children are in a separate CHIP program.

In 2020, two states had a separate program, eight states and the District of Columbia had a Medicaid expansion program, and 40 states had a hybrid program (MACPAC, 2020a). Combination programs became popular after the ACA's Medicaid and CHIP eligibility changes took effect.

As with Medicaid, federal CHIP funds are disbursed on a matching basis, although the federal match is higher for CHIP than for Medicaid. It is known as the E-FMAP, for enhanced-FMAP. The ACA included a significant but temporary increase in the CHIP match for states. As of 2021, the standard E-FMAP formula will be used, with a matching rate ranging from 65% to 88% (MACPAC, 2020b). Because the E-FMAP is based on the Medicaid FMAP amount, the temporary FMAP increase from the FFCRA resulted in higher CHIP matching rates as well (MACPAC, 2020b).

Originally, funding allotments were for 3 years and were based on state-specific estimates of the number of low-income uninsured children, the number of low-income children generally, and healthcare costs relative to other states. If states did not use their full

Table 10.4 Comparing Key Features of Medicaid and CHIP

Feature	Medicaid	CHIP
Structure	Entitlement	Block grant
Financing	Federal–state match	Enhanced federal–state match (higher rate than Medicaid)
Use of funds for premium assistance	No (without a waiver)	Yes
Benefits	Federally defined, with option to use benchmark or benchmark-equivalent benefits package; broad EPSDT services for children	Benefits undefined; uses benchmark package; limited "basic" services required for separate CHIP programs; full Medicaid benefits for Medicaid-expansion CHIP programs
Cost-sharing	Limited or prohibited for some populations and services, higher amounts allowed for some populations and services	Cost-sharing permitted within limits, but prohibited for well-baby and well-child exams
Antidiscrimination provision	Yes	No

Abbreviations: CHIP = Children's Health Insurance Program; EPSDT = early and periodic screening, diagnosis, and treatment.

allotment, the unused money reverted to the federal treasury and could be used by the federal government for any purpose. This system led to frequent fights to keep the money in the CHIP program, and over how the unused funds would be redistributed. Many states became dependent on receiving redistributed funds to keep their CHIP programs afloat.

Under the new system, 2-year state allotments are based on state CHIP spending, state child population growth, and medical inflation (MACPAC, 2018b). Unspent funds are redistributed to other states that have a funding shortfall in their own CHIP programs. If states exhaust their funding and they exceed target enrollment levels, they are eligible for contingency funding (MACPAC, n.d.c).

Table 10.4 highlights a number of differences between Medicaid and CHIP. One important difference is that whereas Medicaid is an entitlement program, CHIP is a block grant (see **Box 10.17**). As mentioned earlier, as a block grant, the federal matching funds are capped (through the allotments). Thus, a state is not entitled to limitless federal money under CHIP, and children, even if eligible, are not legally entitled to services once the allotted money has been spent. If a state runs out of funds and operates its CHIP separate from Medicaid, it will have to cut back its CHIP program by eliminating benefits, lowering provider reimbursement rates, unenrolling beneficiaries, or wait-listing children who want to enroll in the

 Box 10.17 DISCUSSION QUESTIONS

Why do you think that Medicaid was created as an entitlement program but CHIP was established as a block grant? Both programs are federal–state insurance programs for low-income individuals, so does the distinction make sense? Does it matter that one program is for children and the other is broader in scope? Should one program be changed so they are both either entitlements or block grants? Which structure do you prefer?

program. A state with a Medicaid expansion CHIP or a hybrid structure would not receive new CHIP money but would continue to receive federal funds for Medicaid-eligible children as allowed under the Medicaid rules and at the Medicaid matching rate.

CHIP Eligibility

Children are eligible for CHIP if they meet their state's income requirement, are younger than 19 years, do not have other health insurance coverage, and are not eligible for Medicaid (MACPAC, 2018a). CHIP originally allowed states to cover children up to 200% FPL, but CHIPRA expanded coverage to 300% FPL with the enhanced matching rate (KFF, 2012b).[e] If states go above 300% FPL, they receive the state's regular Medicaid match rate instead of the enhanced CHIP rate. Because

CHIP coverage is built on a state's Medicaid eligibility rules, when CHIP eligibility begins depends on when Medicaid eligibility ends. For example, if a state covers a child up to 150% FPL, CHIP eligibility in that state would start at over 150% FPL. If another state Medicaid program covers children at 200% FPL, CHIP eligibility would start at over 200% FPL. In 2021, CHIP eligibility ranges from 175% FPL in North Dakota to 405% FPL in New York. Only two states—North Dakota and Idaho at 190% FPL—have eligibility levels below 200% FPL. Twenty-one states cover children in families with incomes between 200% and 249% FPL, and 27 states and the District of Columbia cover children in families with incomes at or above 250% FPL (KFF, 2021a).

Under the ACA, states must cover all children ages 6 to 19 years up to 133% FPL in their Medicaid program, and children in families with incomes up to 133% who are currently in CHIP programs must be moved to the state's Medicaid program.[b] Variations may still exist above that level. As a result, children in families with the same income levels could be in CHIP in one state and in Medicaid in another state. States also have an MOE requirement under CHIP. They are required to maintain their 2010 eligibility levels through 2027 for children in families with income at or below 300% FPL (MACPAC, n.d.b).

Originally, pregnant women were not eligible for coverage under CHIP without a waiver. CHIPRA explicitly allows for coverage of pregnant women, and six states have used that option as of January 2021 (KFF, 2021c). In addition, 17 states have adopted an option to cover unborn children as a way to indirectly allow pregnant women to access the program (KFF, 2021b). As noted earlier in this chapter, CHIPRA also expanded eligibility by allowing states to cover lawfully residing immigrant pregnant women and children, even if they have not been in the United States for 5 years. Prior to CHIPRA, states could cover these populations only with state dollars. As of 2021, 35 states cover immigrant children and 25 states cover immigrant pregnant women without a 5-year waiting period (KFF, 2021b).

CHIPRA contained a number of provisions to streamline enrollment and improve outreach, including performance bonuses and other financial incentives for states that undertake these improvements (Ryan, 2009). While states must verify the citizenship status of CHIP enrollees, just as they must for Medicaid enrollees, states must do so through an electronic data match in most cases. They may request paper documentation only when electronic data are not available or are not "reasonably compatible" with information provided by the individual (Georgetown University, 2017). This option eases the administrative burden of the citizenship verification and other documentation requirements and makes it much less likely that eligible individuals will be dropped from the program. CHIPRA also allows states to use "express lane eligibility," which permits states to take information provided when individuals apply for other public programs and use that information to assess eligibility for CHIP.

Many states have adopted other measures to promote enrollment and coverage, such as presumptive eligibility (provides coverage while applications are processed), 12-month continuous eligibility (allows for small changes in income), and following up on returned mail (Brooks et al., 2020). During the pandemic, FFCRA required states to provide continuous eligibility through the end of a month to receive the new federal funding. As of 2020, all or almost all states use online applications, conduct rapid eligibility determinations, and have instituted automatic renewals (Brooks et al., 2020). On the other hand, just over half of the states conduct periodic data checks to confirm continued eligibility, and beneficiaries have only 10 days to provide necessary documentation (Brooks et al., 2020). Failure to do so may lead to disruption in coverage.

CHIP Benefits

As shown in **Table 10.5**, CHIP benefits vary by program type. All CHIP programs must cover well-baby and well-child care, dental care, behavioral health care, and vaccines (including COVID-19 vaccines during the pandemic). In addition, the Mental Health Parity and Addiction Equity Act of 2008 (MHPAEA, Pub. L. 110-343) mandates that behavioral health service requirements regarding cost-sharing, service limits, and treatment limits are not more restrictive than the same requirements for medical/surgical services (Medicaid .gov, n.d.d). States that use the Medicaid-CHIP structure must provide full Medicaid benefits to CHIP enrollees, including EPSDT up to age 21, and they must follow Medicaid cost-sharing rules (Medicaid.gov, n.d.d).

States with separate CHIP programs may choose a benefit package based on (1) one of three approved benchmarks; (2) a benchmark-equivalent plan that is actuarially equivalent to an approved benchmark; or (3) HHS Secretary–approved coverage, which is not specifically defined. Benchmark-equivalent plans must include inpatient and outpatient hospital services, physicians' surgical and medical services, lab services, and X-ray services (Medicaid.gov, n.d.f). Due to its flexibility, HHS Secretary–approved coverage is the most common choice for states, meaning that there is significant variation in CHIP benefits across the country (MACPAC, n.d.e; see **Box 10.18**). For dental coverage, states with

Table 10.5 Required CHIP Benefits

All Program Types	▪ Well-baby and well-child care ▪ Dental care ▪ Behavioral health care ▪ Vaccines
Medicaid-CHIP	Full Medicaid benefits (includes ESPDT up to age 21, cost-sharing limits)

Separate CHIP Program	▪ Approved benchmark:
	  • Health insurance plan that is offered by the HMO that has the largest commercial, non-Medicaid enrollment in the state
	  • Standard Blue Cross Blue Shield preferred provider plan for federal employees
	  • Health plan that is available to state employees
	▪ Actuarially equivalent benchmark
	▪ HHS Secretary–approved coverage
	Note: Benchmark-equivalent plans must include hospital, physician, lab, and X-ray services.
	▪ Dental
	  • Approved benchmark:
	    • Most popular federal employee dental plan for dependents
	    • Most popular state employee dental plan for dependents
	    • Most popular commercial dental insurer in the state
	  • HHS Secretary–approved coverage

Box 10.18 DISCUSSION QUESTIONS

When designing CHIP, policymakers chose to follow the private insurance model instead of the Medicaid model. Although states have the choice to create a generous Medicaid expansion program for their CHIP beneficiaries, they also have the choice to implement a more limited insurance program with fewer protections. Similar choices were made when the DRA options were created for Medicaid. These decisions raise essential questions about the role of government in public insurance programs. Does the government (federal or state) have a responsibility to provide additional benefits and protection to its low-income residents? Or, is the government satisfying any responsibility it has by providing insurance coverage that is equivalent to major private insurance plans? What if the standard for private insurance plans becomes lower—does that change your analysis? Is it fair for low-income individuals to receive more comprehensive health insurance coverage than other individuals? Is there a point where fiscal constraints trump equity or the likelihood of improved health outcomes when designing a public insurance program?

separate CHIP programs may select an approved dental benchmark plan or Secretary-approved dental services (Medicaid.gov, n.d.d). States may also provide additional benefits such as prescription drug coverage, vision services, hearing services, and other services needed by children. In fact, 11 states have chosen to include EPSDT in their separate CHIP benefit plan, and an additional two states provide services similar to EPSDT to certain populations (Brooks & Whitener, 2017). Even so, separate CHIP plans are generally more similar to an employer private plan than the more generous Medicaid programs (Rosenbaum et al., 2017). As with Medicaid, most CHIP enrollees are served through managed care plans. In 2018, 79% of CHIP beneficiaries in 32 states were enrolled in managed care (CMS.gov, 2020b).

CHIP Beneficiary Safeguards and Cost-Sharing

In addition to the benefit package options, there are other areas where CHIP provides states with more program flexibility and beneficiaries with less protection than is the case under Medicaid. CHIP does not have the same standards regarding reasonableness, benefit definitions, medical necessity, or nondiscrimination coverage on the basis of illness (although, as noted earlier, states may opt out of or alter some of these protections in Medicaid under section 1937 plans). States, however, may not exclude children based on preexisting conditions.

Cost-sharing includes enrollment fees, premiums, deductibles, coinsurance, and copayments. In general, CHIP enrollees face higher cost-sharing burdens than Medicaid enrollees. States with Medicaid-CHIP programs must follow Medicaid cost-sharing rules, which only allow for nominal cost-sharing in certain cases. States with separate CHIP programs may impose cost-sharing up to 5% of a family's annual income for families with incomes at or above 150% FPL (MACPAC, 2018a). For those below 150% FPL, Medicaid cost-sharing rules apply (Medicaid.gov, n.d.e). States may not include cost-sharing for well-baby or well-child services. In 2020, only four states charged premiums for Medicaid children as compared to 26 states with premiums for CHIP enrollees. Similarly, only one state imposed cost-sharing requirements on its Medicaid children, while 21 states have cost-sharing requirements for CHIP children (KFF, 2020a).

CHIP and Private Insurance Coverage

In devising CHIP, Congress was concerned that Medicaid-eligible children would enroll in CHIP instead of Medicaid without reducing the overall number of uninsured children in a state. To avoid this outcome, CHIP requires that all children be assessed for Medicaid eligibility and, if eligible, enrolled in Medicaid instead of CHIP (Medicaid.gov, n.d.g). With Medicaid expansion under the ACA, it is likely that some children in stand-alone CHIP programs will now be eligible for Medicaid. In addition, Congress wanted to make sure the government did not start funding health insurance coverage that was previously being paid for in the private sector. In other words, it did not want to give individuals or employers an incentive to move privately insured children to the new public program. To avoid private insurance crowd-out, Congress allowed states to institute enrollment waiting periods and impose cost-sharing requirements as a disincentive to switch to CHIP. As of 2021, 14 states have established waiting periods before enrollment. The most common time frame is 90 days. States that do not impose waiting periods may use heightened data evaluation to analyze movement from private insurance to CHIP (Medicaid.gov, 2021).

CHIP Waivers

States may apply to the secretary of HHS to waive CHIP requirements in exchange for experimenting with new ways to increase program eligibility or benefits. Initially, the most common use of CHIP waivers was to expand eligibility for uncovered populations, such as childless adults and parents and pregnant women who are not eligible under a state's Medicaid program. Using CHIP funds to provide coverage for adult populations was controversial because the program was designed to provide health insurance to children. While CHIPRA expands eligibility options for pregnant women, it also prohibits states from obtaining new waivers to cover adults with CHIP funds (Ryan, 2009). States have also used CHIP waivers to experiment with premium assistance programs, which are designed to keep families in private insurance plans by subsidizing their private insurance premiums. As with Medicaid, CHIP programs may use waivers to help beneficiaries during the pandemic by waiving or suspending premium payments, easing eligibility requirements, and expanding telehealth (Sokol, 2020).

The Future of CHIP

The future of CHIP is clouded by the politics ensnaring the ACA. CHIP has been a successful program, with consistent bipartisan support. CHIP could be strengthened by eliminating waiting periods for lower-income beneficiaries, reducing cost-sharing, continuing to fund outreach efforts, and developing policies to ensure seamless transitions as children move among various insurance products (MACPAC, 2017a). Many policy experts argued that CHIP remained necessary even with robust implementation of health reform that was supposed to include widespread expansion of Medicaid and strong marketplaces.

There are several reasons that CHIP remains vital in an ACA era: CHIP was designed for children, and CHIP providers specialize in treating children; CHIP is needed to assist low-income families in states that have not expanded Medicaid; CHIP is more affordable than many plans offered through state exchanges; and an estimated 2.8 million children would live in families who are not eligible for subsidies to purchase insurance through an exchange due to the "family glitch," which considers the cost of coverage for individual workers, not families, when assessing affordability (Cox et al., 2021; MACPAC, 2017a). The uncertainty surrounding the future of the ACA, the extent of Medicaid expansion, and the viability of the exchanges means the reasons CHIP was created in the first place—to provide insurance to uninsured low- to moderate-income children—continues today.

Medicare

Medicare is the federally funded health insurance program for older adults and some persons with disabilities. As a completely federally funded program with uniform national guidelines, Medicare's administration and financing is quite different from that found in Medicaid and CHIP (see **Box 10.19**). This section reviews who Medicare serves, what benefits the program provides, how Medicare is financed, and how Medicare providers are reimbursed. As with Medicaid and CHIP, the ACA included several provisions relating to Medicare. These changes include new coverage for preventive services, bonus payments for primary care services, and assistance in paying for prescription drugs. At the same time, a number of changes will result in reduced reimbursement for providers. When the ACA was passed, its Medicare-related provisions were projected to result in $533 billion in savings and $105 billion in new Medicare spending, for a net reduction of $428 billion in Medicare spending over 10 years (KFF, 2010).

💡 Box 10.19 DISCUSSION QUESTIONS

Although many Medicare beneficiaries are poor, there is no means test (income- or resource-specific eligibility level) to determine eligibility as there is with Medicaid and CHIP. Is there a good public policy reason for this difference? What would be the basis for making this distinction? Does the government have a different role to play in providing health care based on the population involved?

Medicare Eligibility

Medicare covers two main groups of people—older adults and the disabled. In 2019, there were 60.2 million Medicare enrollees, including 51.9 million older adults and 8.3 million persons with disabilities, end-stage renal disease (ESRD), or amyotrophic lateral sclerosis (ALS, also called Lou Gehrig disease; KFF, 2019b). These figures are expected to grow dramatically in the next few decades, as the baby boom population will result in the number of people age 65 years and older almost doubling from 52 million in 2018 to 95 million in 2060 (Mather et al., 2019). As shown in **Figure 10.9**, Medicare enrollment is projected to reach almost 80 million people by 2029.

To qualify for Medicare under the elderly category, individuals must be at least 65 years old and a U.S. citizen or permanent legal resident with at least 5 years of continuous residency. Individuals may enroll in Medicare under the disability category if they are totally and permanently disabled and receive Social Security Disability Insurance for at least 24 months, or have a diagnosis of either ESRD or ALS. There is no waiting period for individuals who qualify with an ALS or ESRD diagnosis. An individual may begin to receive disability at age 18 for those with ALS or age 20 for all other disabilities (CMS.gov, 2020a).

Unlike Medicaid and CHIP, Medicare eligibility is not based on an income or asset test; in other words, individuals of any income level are eligible for Medicare once they meet the eligibility requirements. As a result, Medicare enrollees vary greatly in terms of resources and health status. In 2016, half of Medicare

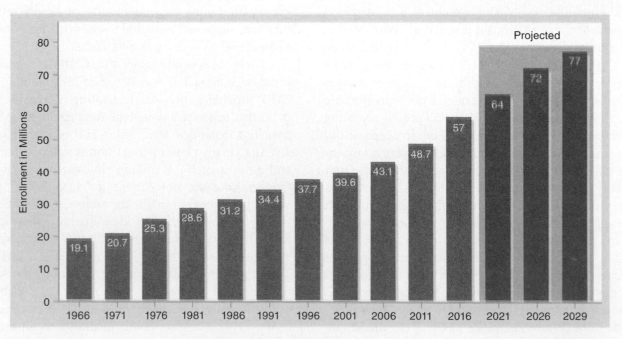

Figure 10.9 Projected Change in Medicare Enrollment, 2021–2029

enrollees had income under $26,200 and only 5% had income above $103,450 (Jacobson et al., 2017). Similarly, 25% of beneficiaries had savings below $14,550 and 8% had no savings or were in debt, while 5% had more than $1.3 million in savings (Jacobson et al., 2017). Higher income earners and savers are more likely to be White, married, highly educated, and between the ages of 65 and 74 (**Figure 10.10**) (Jacobson et al., 2017).

Health status also varies among Medicare enrollees. While just under half of Medicare enrollees (46%) reported having excellent or very good health in 2017, more than half are in poor, fair, or good health (**Figure 10.11**). As shown in **Figure 10.12**, six chronic conditions are reported by at least 25% of enrollees, with hypertension (59%) being the most common (Chronic Conditions Data Warehouse [CCDW], n.d.). Specific health needs vary by beneficiary demographic. For example, African-American and female enrollees are more likely to suffer from chronic kidney disease and diabetes than other diseases, while older enrollees tend to have Alzheimer disease, dementia, and heart failure (CCDW, n.d.).

In 2018, 2.2 million low-income older adults were considered dual eligibles (again, meaning they are eligible for both Medicaid and Medicare; CMS, 2020). All dual eligibles receive full Medicare benefits.

They may also receive either full Medicaid benefits or participate in a state Medicare Savings Program (MSP) that assists with Medicare's cost-sharing requirements and provides services not covered by Medicare, such as dental care and long-term care services and supports (CMS, n.d.). The level of coverage depends on the beneficiary's income level and state eligibility rules. Most dual eligibles receive full benefits, while just under one-third are eligible for partial benefits (CMS, 2020).

Not surprisingly, low-income beneficiaries tend to have significant healthcare needs. Medicare's dual eligibles are more likely than other beneficiaries to be in poor health, have several chronic conditions, require mental health services, and have long-term care needs (CMS, 2020). They are also more likely to be younger (39% v. 8.6%), female (59.6% v. 53%), and part of a racial or ethnic minority population (47.5% v. 21.1%) than Medicare beneficiaries overall (CMS, n.d.).

Given their frequent use of the healthcare system, dual eligibles consume a disproportionate share of resources. In 2012, this group constituted only 20% of Medicare beneficiaries but accounted for 34% of expenditures (CMS, 2020). Similarly, they made up 15% of the Medicaid population but were responsible for 33% of Medicaid spending (CMS, 2020). To assist

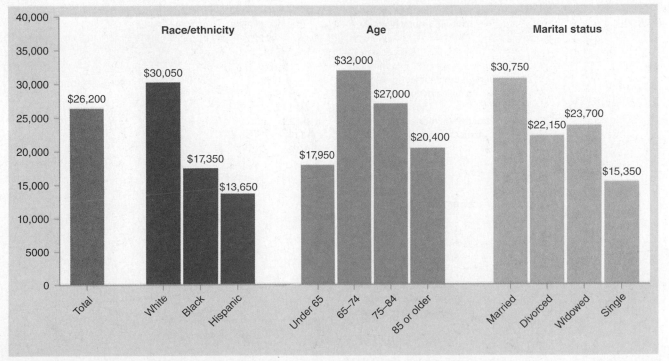

Note: Total household income for couples is split equally between husbands and wives to estimate income for married beneficiaries.

Figure 10.10 Income Levels by Beneficiary Characteristics, 2016

Jacobson, G., Griffin, S., Neuman, T., & Smith, K. (2017, April 21). *Income and assets of Medicare beneficiaries, 2016–2035.* Kaiser Family Foundation. https://www.kff.org/medicare/issue-brief/income-and-assets-of-medicare-beneficiaries-2016-2035/

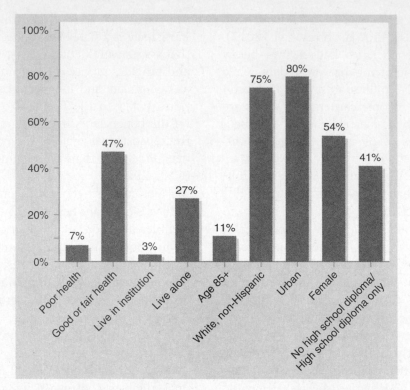

Figure 10.11 Characteristics of the Medicare Population

Kaiser Family Foundation. (2019). An overview of Medicare. https://www.kff.org/medicare/issue-brief/an-overview-of-medicare/

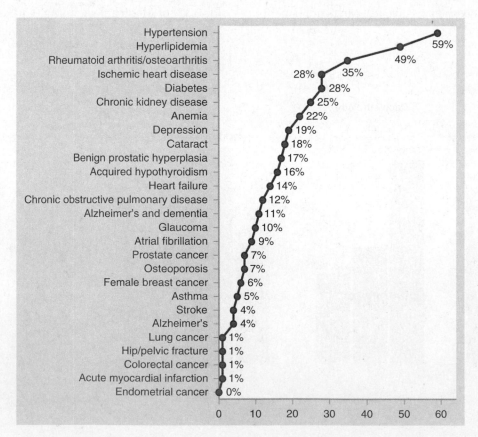

Figure 10.12 Percentage of Medicare Beneficiaries Reporting Select Chronic Diseases, 2018

Chronic Conditions Data Warehouse. (2018). *Medicare chronic conditions charts.* https://www2.ccwdata.org/web/guest/medicare-charts/medicare-chronic-condition-charts/#b1_age_current_year with this high-need, high-cost population, the ACA created the Federal Coordinated Health Care Office (referred to as the Medicaid–Medicare Coordination Office) within CMS to improve the integration of services for dual eligibles (CMS, 2020; **Figure 10.13**).

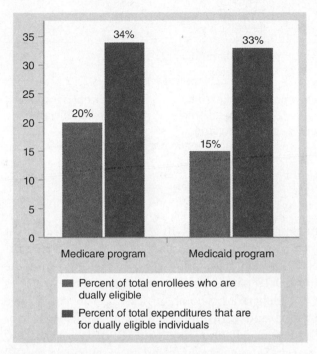

Figure 10.13 Share of Medicaid and Medicare Enrollment and Costs Associated with Dually Eligible Individuals, 2012

Centers for Medicare and Medicaid Services. (2020, March). *People dually eligible for Medicare and Medicaid.* https://www.cms.gov/Medicare-Medicaid-Coordination/Medicare-and-Medicaid-Coordination/Medicare-Medicaid-Coordination-Office/Downloads/MMCO_Factsheet.pdf

Medicare Benefits and Financing

As shown in **Tables 10.6** and **10.7**, Medicare is split into four parts, each covering a specified set of services. Parts A and B were originally included in Medicare when it was established in 1965. Part C was added in 1997, while Part D went into effect in 2006. Each part has a different enrollment process and financing mechanism (**Figure 10.14**). Part A, also known as Hospital Insurance (HI), covers inpatient care, while Part B, also known as Supplemental Medical Insurance (SMI), covers outpatient services. Parts A and B are provided on an FFS basis. Alternatively, enrollees may choose to receive their Part A and B benefits through Part C, the Medicare Advantage (MA) managed care program. Finally, Part D is the prescription drug benefit, which can be accessed through a stand-alone Prescription Drug Plan (PDP) or a managed care plan. (Because Part C is financed by Parts A and B and is an alternative to A and B, it is not included in Table 10.7. Whether beneficiaries have cost-sharing and other requirements under Part C depends on the specifics of each managed care plan.) Although Medicare benefits are quite extensive, coverage excludes services that one might expect to be part of a health insurance program targeting older adults, such as nursing home care, routine eye care, dental care, and hearing exams and hearing aids (Cubanski et al., 2015).

Table 10.6 Medicare Benefits

Part	Services Covered
A	Inpatient hospital, 100 days at skilled nursing facility, limited home health following stay at a hospital or skilled nursing facility, and hospice care
B	Physician, outpatient hospital, outpatient mental health, X-ray, laboratory, emergency department, and other ambulatory services; medical equipment; limited preventive services, including one preventive physical exam, mammography, pelvic exam, prostate exam, colorectal cancer screening, glaucoma screening for high-risk patients, prostate cancer screening, and cardiovascular screening blood test; diabetes screening and outpatient self-management; bone-mass measurement for high-risk patients; hepatitis B vaccine for high-risk patients; pap smear; and pneumococcal and flu vaccinations. ACA benefits: cost-sharing eliminated for select preventive services; coverage for personalized prevention plan, including comprehensive health assessment
C	Managed care plans, private fee-for-service plans, special needs plans, and medical savings accounts. The plans provide all services in Part A and Part B and generally must offer additional benefits or services
D	Prescription drug benefit

Table 10.7 Medicare Financing by Part

Medicare Part	Government Financing Scheme	Annual Deductible	Monthly Premium	Cost-Sharing
A	Trust fund through mandated employer and employee payroll taxes	Yes	No, if Social Security work requirements are met	Yes
B	General federal tax revenue	Yes	Yes—tiered by income	Yes
D	General federal tax revenue and state clawback payments for dual enrollees	Yes—except some low-income beneficiaries	Yes—tiered by income (some low-income beneficiaries do not pay premiums)	Yes—except some low-income beneficiaries

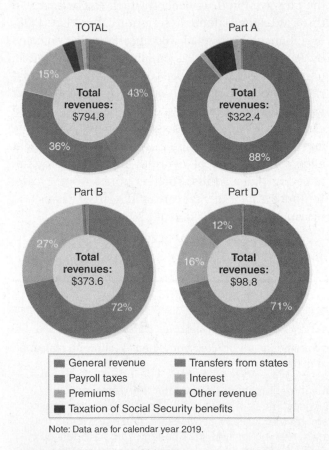

Note: Data are for calendar year 2019.

Figure 10.14 Sources of Medicare Revenue, 2019

Cubanski, J., & Neuman, T. (2021, March 16). *FAQs on Medicare financing and trust fund solvency*. Kaiser Family Foundation. https://www.kff.org/medicare/issue-brief/faqs-on-medicare-financing-and-trust-fund-solvency/

Part A

Part A covers a variety of inpatient needs for Medicare beneficiaries. While Medicare includes skilled nursing facility (SNF) coverage, it does not pay for long-term nursing home care. SNF coverage provides short-term benefits when daily care is needed that requires skilled nursing or therapy staff. In general, beneficiaries must have a qualifying hospital stay to receive SNF coverage, although that requirement was waived during the COVID-19 pandemic (Medicare.gov, n.d.e).

Beneficiaries who are at least age 65 years, have worked and contributed to Social Security (SS) or the Railroad Retirement Board (RRB) for at least 40 quarters (about 10 years), and are receiving SS or RRB benefits at least 4 months before becoming eligible, are automatically enrolled in Part A and receive Part A services without paying premiums. Those not yet receiving SS or RRB benefits must apply to enroll in Part A. Individuals who are age 65 years but do not meet the work requirements may become eligible for premium-free Part A benefits through earnings by a spouse, parent, or child (CMS.gov, 2020a). Elderly individuals who do not meet the work requirements may enroll in Part A during an open enrollment period. These individuals must pay Part A premiums and enroll in Part B. Beneficiaries who are eligible for Medicare based on the disability category may receive Part A benefits after receiving disability benefits for 24 months. If a beneficiary is determined to be disabled before collecting SS benefits, the waiting period is 29 months. Those with ALS do not have a waiting period and beneficiaries with ESRD may receive Part A coverage shortly after dialysis begins or a transplant occurs (CMS.gov, 2020a). Beneficiaries in the disabled category follow the same work requirement rules to determine whether they pay Part A premiums.

For those who have to pay Part A premiums, the amount varies by how many quarters the beneficiary worked and whether a late enrollment penalty is applicable. Beneficiaries who worked fewer than 30 quarters pay a higher premium than those who worked

30 quarters or more. For example, in 2021, beneficiaries who worked at least 30 quarters pay a $259 standard monthly premium, compared to $471 for those who worked fewer than 30 quarters (Medicare.gov, n.d.c). The late enrollment penalty applies when beneficiaries do not enroll during the initial enrollment period (IEP; which spans about 3 months before and after the individual turns 65, or 3 months before and after the 25th month of disability benefits). The late enrollment penalty is up to 10% of the monthly premium for two times the number of years the enrollee could have signed up but chose not to do so (CMS .gov, 2020a).

All Medicare beneficiaries are subject to Part A cost-sharing. Depending on the service, cost-sharing could include a deductible and/or a copayment. In addition, some copayments are tiered based on the length of stay. Each service has its own cost-sharing rules. For example, in 2021, there is no deductible for home health care, but beneficiaries pay a 20% copayment for approved durable medical equipment. Inpatient hospital stays are subject to a $1484 deductible plus a tiered copay after 60 days of $371 per day for days 61 through 90 and $742 per day from day 91 until all 60 lifetime reserve days are used (Medicare.gov, n.d.c).

Part A benefits are paid from the HI Trust Fund, funded through a mandatory payroll tax. Employers and employees each pay a tax of 1.45% of a worker's earnings (self-employed persons pay both shares, for a total tax of 2.9%), which is set aside for the HI Trust Fund. The ACA increases this rate for higher-income tax payers. Individuals who earn over $200,000 and couples who earn over $250,000 now pay a tax of 2.35% on their earnings (Cubanski & Neuman, 2018).

By relying on payroll taxes, Medicare Part A uses current workers and employers to pay for health benefits for the disabled and those older than 65 years, many of whom are already retired. This formula is problematic in the face of the looming retirement of those from the baby boom generation. As shown in **Figure 10.15**, from 2010 to 2050, the number of workers supporting each enrollee is expected to decline from 3.4 to 2.3. Because of this and for other reasons, the 2020 Medicare Board of Trustees estimated that the Part A HI Trust Fund will be exhausted by 2026 (Cubanski & Neuman, 2021a).

Part B

Part B covers a variety of outpatient services, including physician services, emergency department care, DME, and select services used as part of qualifying clinical research studies (Medicare.gov, n.d.a). Prior to the ACA, Medicare benefits included limited preventive services, such as select screenings and one preventive

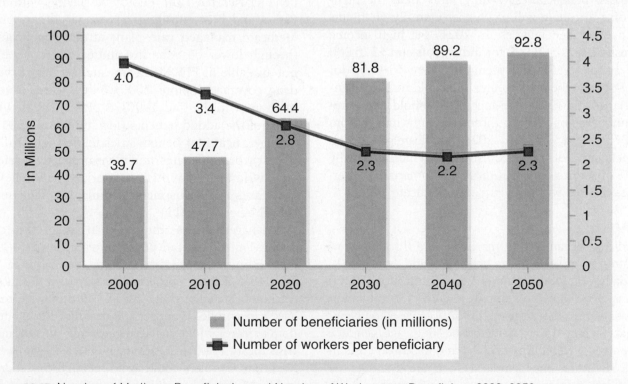

Figure 10.15 Number of Medicare Beneficiaries and Number of Workers per Beneficiary, 2000–2050

Kaiser Family Foundation, based on the 2014 Annual Report of the Boards of Trustees of the Federal Hospital Insurance and Federal Supplementary Medical Insurance Trust Funds.

exam annually. The ACA significantly expanded preventive services benefits by covering all U.S. Preventive Services Task Force A- and B-rated services without cost-sharing, including an annual comprehensive risk assessment, provided without cost-sharing when delivered in an outpatient setting. Under the various COVID-19 relief bills, Medicare will cover COVID-19 vaccines without cost-sharing and expanded telehealth services (Cubanski & Freed, 2020).

Part B is voluntary for enrollees, but most beneficiaries also opt to have Part B. Beneficiaries who receive Part A benefits without premiums are also eligible to enroll in Part B. If they have been receiving SS or RRB benefits for 4 months, they will be enrolled automatically, otherwise they must apply. To enroll in Part B, individuals who pay Part A premiums must be 65 or older, a U.S. resident, and a U.S citizen or permanent legal resident who has been in the United States for 5 years continuously (CMS.gov, 2020a). As with Part A, beneficiaries may pay a late enrollment penalty as long as they have Medicare if they do not enroll for Part B during the IEP. The penalty may increase premiums up to 10% for each 12-month period that the beneficiary chose not to enroll in Part B (CMS.gov, 2020a).

Part B is financed through general federal tax revenues and monthly premiums, deductibles, and cost-sharing paid by beneficiaries. The annual deductible was $203 in 2021. Overall, Medicare Part B premiums are set to cover 25% of the projected per-person Part B costs. Beneficiaries earning more than the high-income threshold will pay higher monthly premiums than other beneficiaries. In 2021, the high income threshold was $88,000 for individuals and $176,000 for couples. Monthly premiums were $148.50 for those below the high-income threshold in 2021. Beneficiaries above the high-income threshold pay a premium tiered by income; those premiums ranged from $207.90 to $505.90 in 2021 (Medicare.gov, n.d.c). Beneficiaries also pay coinsurance, which is usually 20% of service cost. **Figure 10.16** summarizes the services covered within each part of Medicare.

Part C

Medicare began testing managed care through demonstration projects in the late 1970s and early 1980s. Initially, only health maintenance organization (HMO) plans were allowed. Plans were paid on a capitation basis, using a risk adjustment formula based on beneficiary demographic characteristics (e.g., age, gender). The rates were county specific and based on costs in FFS Medicare. The formula sets the rate at 95% of the Medicare average, intending to provide savings to the Medicare program overall. As with managed care in

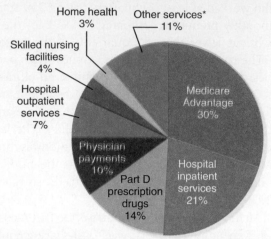

Total Medicare benefit payments, 2016: $675 billion

Note: *Consists of Medicare benefit spending on hospice, durable medical equipment, Part B drugs, outpatient dialysis, outpatient therapy, ambulance, lab, community mental health center, rural health clinic, federally qualified health center, and other Part B services.

Figure 10.16 Medicare Benefit Payments by Type of Service, 2016

Congressional Budget Office. (2017, June). *Medicare baseline.*

other parts of the health system, policymakers hoped Medicare's managed care program would increase consumer choice, provide more benefits, reduce costs, and increase efficiency (Barry & Kline, 2002; McGuire et al., 2011).

Unlike Medicaid beneficiaries, who are generally required to use managed care plans, Medicare beneficiaries have the choice of staying with FFS Part A and B or enrolling in a managed care plan. Medicare managed care plans attract beneficiaries through lower cost-sharing and/or added benefits not available in FFS Medicare, such as prescription drug coverage (before 2006) or eye care. Enrollment grew in the mid-1990s as plans increased the value of the added benefits (McGuire et al., 2011). Younger, healthier beneficiaries tended to enroll in the early plan offerings, and plans primarily serviced healthy, low-cost counties, indicating plans believed Medicare's risk adjustment formula was inadequate (McGuire et al., 2011).

Managed care was introduced, in part, to create cost savings for the Medicare program, yet during the 1990s Medicare was paying managed care plans 5% to 7% more than if those enrollees had stayed in traditional Medicare (McGuire et al., 2011). Not only were managed care enrollees younger and healthier, but the freedom to leave or join managed care plans on a monthly basis meant that Part C adversely selected against FFS Medicare. Enrollees could avoid the high cost-sharing in FFS Medicare by joining a managed care plan, but then return to FFS Medicare if a medical issue arose.

"In sum, on average, healthy, low-cost beneficiaries were joining MA and reducing TM [traditional Medicare] costs by less than the amount that Medicare was paying the plans" (McGuire et al., 2011). Policymakers have found it difficult to price managed care at a level that is high enough to allow plans to make a profit and be able to entice beneficiaries to enroll with additional benefits or lower cost-sharing, yet low enough so that Medicare saves money compared to using traditional FFS payments (McGuire et al., 2011).

In an attempt to improve the cost savings of Part C, the Balanced Budget Act of 1997 created the Medicare + Choice (M+C) managed care program. M+C added two additional managed care options: local preferred provider organizations (PPOs) and provider-sponsored organizations (PSOs), which were basically HMOs run by provider groups. In addition, Congress changed the risk adjustment model so managed care plans would receive higher reimbursement for sicker patients than healthier ones. There had been rapid growth of Medicare managed care plans in the mid-to-late 1990s, with plans heavily favoring urban areas. Rural areas were less profitable for insurers because the few providers in rural areas held most of the bargaining power, and marketing and administrative costs were high (McGuire et al., 2011). Congress also altered the payment formula because lower FFS reimbursement in rural areas also resulted in lower capitation rates. These changes resulted in higher reimbursement for

some counties and lower reimbursement in others. Accordingly, some plans reduced the added benefits and increased cost-sharing, while other plans left the program completely. Overall, plans retracted from M+C due to low federal reimbursement, burdensome administrative requirements, and various local factors, such as provider participation levels and costs of medical care (Barry & Kline, 2002). Not surprisingly, enrollment in Part C declined in the late 1990s and early 2000s; access in rural counties did not increase and rural county plans were often less generous than their urban counterparts (McGuire et al., 2011; **Figure 10.17**).

In another attempt to improve the managed care program and increase the private sector's role in Medicare, Congress passed the Medicare Prescription Drug, Improvement, and Modernization Act (MMA) in 2003. Once again, Congress altered the risk adjustment and reimbursement formula. These changes resulted in higher reimbursement in many counties and required health plans to receive at least the same reimbursement rate as FFS providers. Furthermore, the formula locked in plan payment growth in a way that widened the gap between lower FFS and higher managed care payments (McGuire et al., 2011). Once again, Part C, now referred to as Medicare Advantage (MA), did not save money for Medicare. In the early 2000s, managed care payments were 12% to 14% higher each year than FFS payments would have been for the same patients (McGuire et al., 2011).

Note: Includes cost plans as well as Medicare Advantage plans. About 62 million people are enrolled in Medicare in 2020.

Figure 10.17 Medicare Managed Care Enrollment, 1999–2020

Freed, M., Damico, A., & Neuman, T. (2021, January 13). *A dozen facts about Medicare Advantage in 2020.* Kaiser Family Foundation. https://www.kff.org/medicare/issue-brief/a-dozen-facts-about-medicare-advantage-in-2020/

The MMA also expanded Part C plan offerings in response to the managed care backlash being experienced in the private health insurance industry, with consumers rejecting the tight restrictions of HMOs in favor of the flexibility of PPOs (McGuire et al., 2011). Regional PPOs were established with the goal of increasing access for rural beneficiaries. These plans are similar to local PPOs but can cover an entire state or multiple states. Special needs plans (SNPs) serve dual-eligible beneficiaries and other high need populations with specialized care (McGuire et al., 2011). The combination of higher reimbursement and additional plan offerings resulted in rebounding enrollment in Part C.

In 2006, Congress added a bidding process to establish plan-capitated payment rates and the bids were compared to county-level benchmarks. Plans submit a bid to the federal government that estimates their cost per enrollee, and these bids are compared to benchmarks established by statute and that vary by county. The benchmark is the maximum amount Medicare will pay for services in that county. If the bid is below the benchmark, Medicare and the plan split the difference and the portion returned to the plan is referred to as a rebate and must be used to provide additional benefits to enrollees (Cubanski et al., 2015). Bids above the benchmark required enrollees to be charged higher premium rates (McGuire et al., 2011). Once a bid is accepted, a contract between plans and the federal government details the services the plan will provide and the premiums, deductibles, and cost-sharing it will charge beneficiaries.

The ACA adjusted the benchmark formula to reflect county-level spending in FFS Medicare. On average, MA plans had become 14% more expensive than FFS providers for comparable services (Cubanski et al., 2015). The ACA phased in reduced payments that bring MA plans closer to the benchmark payment for traditional Medicare services in their county. Additional reductions occurred due to changes in the risk-adjustment formula. Plans in higher spending areas receive a lower reimbursement rate under the new formula. Under the ACA, plans can also earn quality and performance bonuses (McGuire et al., 2011). MA plans are also required to follow the 85% medical loss ratio rule, limiting the amount of revenues that can be used for profits and administration (this rule is discussed in more detail in Chapter 11, "Health Reform and the Patient Protection and Affordable Care Act").

Enrollment has been increasing since 2007, and in 2020 24.1 million (39%) Medicare beneficiaries chose to enroll in Part C. The Congressional Budget Office (CBO) estimates that 51% of Medicare beneficiaries will enroll in Part C by 2030 (Freed et al., 2021). From 2009 to 2018, enrollment growth was highest for African-American and Hispanic enrollees, as well as dual eligibles (Meyers et al., 2021).

As shown in **Figure 10.18**, enrollment is not spread evenly throughout the country; 40% of MA enrollees are in plans in 19 states and Puerto Rico, while fewer than 20% are enrolled in plans in 9 states (Freed et al., 2021). In addition, many markets are highly concentrated. Insurance giants UnitedHealthcare and Humana signed 44% of all enrollees in 2020 (Freed et al., 2021). Plan offerings remain more numerous in urban areas, where beneficiaries have almost twice as many plan choices. Even so, the average beneficiary may choose from eight MA plans (Biniek et al., 2020).

MA plans continue to attract beneficiaries with additional benefits. Common benefits include eye care, telehealth, dental care, and fitness benefits (Freed et al., 2021; **Figure 10.19**). In 2019, CMS expanded the definition of the types of additional health benefits that plans may offer to include services such as meal delivery and nonmedical transportation (Kornfield et al., 2021). In addition, MA plans are allowed to offer special supplemental benefits to certain chronically ill enrollees. These are benefits indirectly that assist with health status, such as food and nonmedical transportation (Kornfield et al., 2021).

In 2021, most plans were HMOs (62%), while about one-third were local PPOs (Biniek et al., 2020). In addition, the availability of and enrollment in SNPs are on the rise (**Figure 10.20**). Most SNP enrollees are dual eligibles (86%), with fewer chronic condition (11%) or institutional care (3%) beneficiaries. Enrollees with chronic or disabling conditions are primarily enrolled in plans that focus on diabetes, heart disease, and lung conditions (Biniek et al., 2020).

Research regarding the quality of care provided in the MA program shows mixed results. Enrollees in MA plans use more preventive services, have fewer hospital admissions and emergency room visits, and stay in hospitals and SNFs for less time (Agarwal et al., 2021). Most beneficiaries are enrolled in high quality plans and overall MA plans performed as well or better than FFS Medicare on many quality of care measures (Meyers et al., 2021). Yet, African-American and Hispanic beneficiaries are often enrolled in lower quality plans and marginalized MA enrollees have worse health outcomes (Meyers et al., 2021). Even though MA plans receive higher payments than FFS Medicare, they did not perform better on readmission rates, mortality, or experience of care, and enrollees

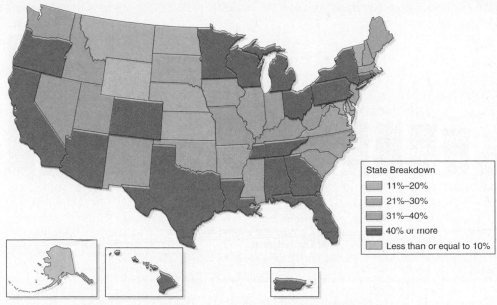

Note: Includes cost plans, as well as other Medicare Advantage plans. Excludes beneficiaries with unknown county addresses.

Figure 10.18 Medicare Advantage Penetration, by State, 2020

Freed, M., Damico, A., & Neuman, T. (2021, January 13). *A dozen facts about Medicare Advantage in 2020.* Kaiser Family Foundation. https://www.kff.org/medicare/issue-brief/a-dozen-facts-about-medicare-advantage-in-2020/

Note: Dental includes plans that only provide preventive benefits, such as cleanings.

Figure 10.19 Share of Medicare Advantage Enrollees in Plans with Extra Benefits, by Benefit Type, 2020

Freed, M., Damico, A., & Neuman, T. (2021, January 13). *A dozen facts about Medicare Advantage in 2020.* Kaiser Family Foundation. https://www.kff.org/medicare/issue-brief/a-dozen-facts-about-medicare-advantage-in-2020/

were more likely to use average quality hospitals and lower quality nursing facilities (Agarwal et al., 2021). These findings indicate that further quality improvements are needed and increased attention is required to address healthcare disparities in the MA program (Agarwal et al., 2021; Freed et al., 2021).

MA plans charge beneficiaries varying premiums and copayments. In addition, enrollees pay their regular Part B premiums unless the plan chooses to cover all or some of it (Medicare.gov, n.d.b). Most (89%) MA plans offer prescription drug coverage and about

half (54%) do not charge a Part C premium. Approximately 60% of enrollees do not pay any premium for their MA plan, but still pay a Part B premium (Biniek et al., 2020). Overall, the average monthly premium plan for 2021 was $21, down from $25 in 2020 (**Figure 10.21**).

Part D

The MMA also created Part D, Medicare's prescription drug benefit. The drug benefit was made

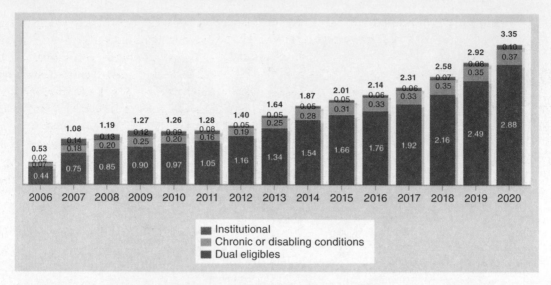

Note: Numbers may not sum to the total due to rounding. Includes enrollment in Puerto Rico.

Figure 10.20 Number of Beneficiaries in Special Needs Plans, 2006–2020

Freed, M., Damico, A., & Neuman, T. (2021, January 13). *A dozen facts about Medicare advantage in 2020.* Kaiser Family Foundation. https://www.kff.org/medicare/issue-brief/a-dozen-facts-about-medicare-advantage-in-2020/

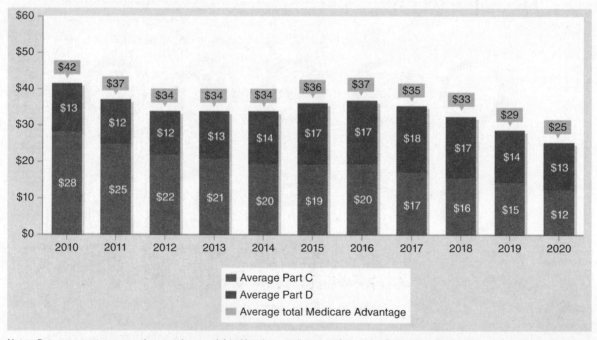

Notes: Data represent average plan premiums weighted by plan enrollment and are not adjusted by inflation. Data do not include Special Needs Plans, employer-sponsored plans, Part B–only plans, or plans not offering a Part D drug benefit. The Part C premium covers Medicare medical and hospital care; the Part D premium is a total (basic and supplemental) premium.

Figure 10.21 Average Medicare Advantage Premiums, 2010–2020

The Commonwealth Fund Medicare Data Hub. (n.d.). *Medicare Advantage.* https://www.commonwealthfund.org/medicare-data-hub/medicare-advantage

available to recipients beginning in 2006, and 48 million beneficiaries were enrolled in Part D in 2021 (Cubanski & Damico, 2021). To obtain prescription drugs through Medicare, beneficiaries have the choice of (1) remaining in traditional FFS Medicare under Parts A and B and enrolling in a separate private prescription drug plan (PDP), (2) enrolling in a Part C plan through MA that includes prescription drug coverage (MA-PD), or (3) enrolling in a plan for special populations, such as unions or MA SNPs. MA plans are required to offer basic prescription drug benefits and may offer supplemental prescription drug benefits for an additional premium. Some beneficiaries may also have access to employer-sponsored health insurance that includes prescription drug benefits. These beneficiaries may keep their employer coverage only, keep their employer coverage and enroll in Part D, or drop their employer coverage (see **Box 10.20**). Finally, beneficiaries may also choose not to obtain any prescription drug coverage. However, in certain circumstances, beneficiaries who decline to enroll in Part D during the allotted enrollment period and do not have other comparable prescription drug coverage will be charged a penalty of 1% of the national average premium for every month they do not enroll (Medicare .gov, n.d.d).

If at least two plans are not available in a region, the government contracts with a fallback plan (a private plan that is not an insurer) to serve that area. So far, fallback plans have not been needed. There were almost 1000 PDPs available across 34 PDP regions in 2021, and enrollees have a choice among multiple options in every state (KFF, 2021d). Three firms— Humana, UnitedHealthcare, and CVS Health—have signed up over half of all Part D enrollees, and the top five firms (also including Centene and Cigna) accounted for 74% of enrollment in 2021 (Cubanski & Damico, 2021). While 2021 enrollment was split almost evenly between PDPs and MA-PDs, enrollment is trending upward in MA plans and decreasing in PDPs (Cubanski & Damico, 2021).

Part D plans may choose to offer the defined standard benefit, an actuarially equivalent benefit package, or an enhanced benefit package. An enhanced benefit package may include a low or no deductible, lower cost-sharing, or increased initial coverage limit (Cubanski & Damico, 2021). All plans must cover at least two drugs in each therapeutic class or category of Part D drugs as well as all drugs in six "protected" classes: immunosuppressants, antidepressants antipsychotics, anticonvulsants, antiretrovirals, and antineoplastics (KFF, 2020a). Beyond that, Part D plans have flexibility to determine their formulary, formulary tiering, cost-sharing, and utilization management options.

Dual eligibles may no longer obtain prescription drug coverage under Medicaid; they must receive their prescription drug benefit through Medicare. Under the MMA, states are now required to help fund Medicare's prescription drug benefit for dual enrollees through an MOE or "clawback" provision (see **Box 10.21**). This provision requires states to pay the federal government a share of expenditures the states would have made to provide prescription drug coverage to dual enrollees. The state share began at 90% in 2006 and tapered down to 75% in 2015 and beyond. This represents the first time that states have assisted with Medicare financing. In 2021, the clawback provision cost states $10.7 billion, and would have been almost $2 billion higher without the FFCRA assistance (Federal Funds Information for States, 2020). If states choose to provide dual enrollees with prescription drug coverage through Medicaid, states must use 100% of their own dollars to finance the coverage, even if the beneficiary does not enroll in Part D.

A low-income subsidy (LIS) to assist with Part D premiums and cost-sharing is available to enrollees with incomes under 150% FPL who have limited assets (KFF, 2020c). In 2021, 12.8 million enrollees received these subsidies, with 26% of them receiving benefits through MA SNPs (Cubanski & Damico, 2021). A benchmark premium is the maximum amount CMS will pay for a Part D plan premium through the LIS

⭐ Box 10.20   Special Topic

Employer Subsidy

Lawmakers were concerned that adding a prescription drug benefit to Medicare would encourage employers to drop prescription drug coverage to the beneficiaries who receive prescription drugs through retiree health plans. In an effort to avoid a shift in older people who rely on public insurance instead of private insurance for their prescription drug coverage, Congress included in the MMA a tax-free subsidy to encourage employers to maintain prescription drug coverage. While the ACA eliminates the tax deduction, the subsidy remains in place. The amount of the subsidy is based on the prescription drug costs of individuals who remain with the employer's plan and do not enroll in Part D. In 2020, approximately 1.3 million beneficiaries purchased coverage through employer retiree plans and employers received a subsidy of 28% of their costs between $445 and $9200 per retiree. Employers receive an average of $575 per beneficiary from this subsidy (KFF, 2021e).

Is this subsidy a good idea? Is the proper role of government to pay private companies to maintain insurance coverage? If so, should it occur for other benefits? Do you have a preference regarding giving incentives for private entities to provide insurance coverage versus the government financing the coverage directly?

Clawback Provision

The clawback provision is controversial and highlights some of the tensions concerning state flexibility and national uniformity that policymakers face when designing public programs. The clawback seems to contradict the prior decision to provide states with flexibility and program design responsibilities under Medicaid. In addition, it changes the decision to use only federal funds to pay for Medicare. Given decisions made by states prior to the MMA, there are many variations among state prescription drug benefits that will be "frozen" in place with the clawback provision. At the same time, the MMA creates a uniform rule regarding how all states finance prescription drug funding in the future, and this could impact state-level decisions about dual enrollee coverage.

Is the clawback provision a good idea? Should states help pay for federal prescription drug coverage? Is there a better design? Should states or the federal government control Medicaid prescription drug coverage that is provided to dual enrollees? Should dual enrollees be treated differently than other Medicaid beneficiaries?

program. An LIS enrollee who chooses a benchmark plan will not pay a plan premium. If an LIS enrollee chooses a nonbenchmark basic plan, they have to pay the difference between the benchmark premium and their plan premium (as long as the difference is more than the *de minimis* threshold, which was $2 in 2021). If an LIS enrollee chooses an enhanced plan, they must pay a partial premium even if the plan premium is below the benchmark premium (Q1 Group, 2020).

Part D is financed through an annual deductible, monthly premiums, general revenues, and state payments for dual enrollees. Generally, premiums are set to cover 25% of Part D costs. Under Part D, deductibles, premiums, benefit limits, and catastrophic thresholds are not fixed; instead, they are indexed to increase with the growth in per-capita Medicare spending for Part D. As shown in **Figure 10.22**, beneficiaries pay an annual deductible ($445 in 2021), 25% of the cost of drugs up to a set amount ($4130 in 2021) during the initial coverage period and coverage gaps phase, and 5% of the cost above the catastrophic threshold. As with Part B, enrollees pay a tiered premium based on their income. Individuals with higher incomes (individuals over $87,000 and couples over $174,000 in 2021) pay a surcharge that ranges from 35% to 80% of Part D, depending on their income (Medicare.gov, n.d.d).

When Part D was first created, the coverage gap in Medicare between the initial coverage period and the catastrophic coverage period was referred to as the *doughnut hole*, because beneficiaries had to pay 100% of the costs of drugs. The ACA included provisions to close the doughnut hole, such that beneficiaries only pay 25% cost-sharing in that range of drug spending starting in 2020 (subsequent legislation moved the date to 2019). To close the coverage gap, beneficiaries

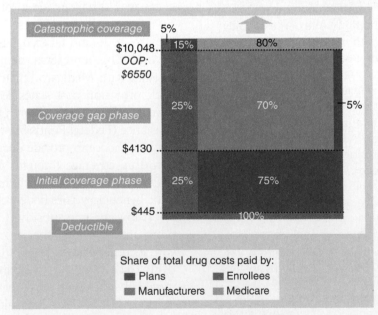

Note: Some amounts rounded to nearest dollar. OOP = out of pocket.

Figure 10.22 Standard Medicare Prescription Drug Benefit, 2022

Kaiser Family Foundation. (2021, October 13). *An overview of the Medicare Part D prescription drug benefit.* Kaiser Family Foundation. https://www.kff.org/medicare/fact-sheet/an-overview-of-the-medicare-part-d-prescription-drug-benefit/

received phased-in discounts for generic and brand-name drugs purchased in the doughnut hole.

As shown in **Figure 10.23** and **Figure 10.24**, premiums and cost-sharing tend to be higher in PDPs than MA-PDs because MA plans can use Medicare rebates (and possibly bonuses) for Part A and B coverage to lower Part D cost-sharing (Cubanski & Damico, 2021). In 2021, the average PDP premium was $38, compared to $12 for the Part D portion of MA benefits. Premiums for all types of plans have decreased

in recent years due to the increase in manufacturer rebates in the coverage gap phase (Cubanski & Damico, 2021). Most Part D enrollees chose enhanced plans in 2021. Not surprisingly, the premiums for enhanced plans are about 40% higher for PDPs (Cubanski & Damico, 2021). Enrollees in PDPs are also more likely to be in plans that charge a deductible than enrollees in MA-PDs. Even when MA-PD beneficiaries pay a deductible, it is much lower than PDP deductibles (Cubanski & Damico, 2021).

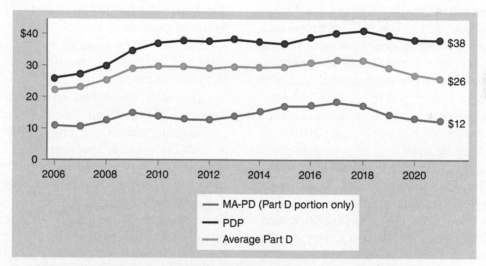

Note: PDP is stand-alone prescription drug plan. MA-PD is Medicare Advantage drug plan. Estimates are weighted by enrollment (March of the respective year) and exclude employer group plans and Special Needs Plans. The average premium for MA-PDs is for Part D drug coverage only; the average total MA-PD premium, including Part C and Part D benefits, is higher ($21.18 in 2021).

Figure 10.23 Monthly Part D Premiums by Plan Type, 2006–2021

Cubanski, J., & Damico, A. (2021, June 8). *Key facts about Medicare Part D enrollment, premiums, and cost sharing in 2021.* Kaiser Family Foundation. https://www.kff.org/medicare/issue-brief/medicare-part-d-in-2018-the-latest-on-enrollment-premiums-and-cost-sharing/

Note: PDP is stand-alone prescription drug plan. MA-PD is Medicare Advantage drug plan. Estimate weighted by enrollment (March of respective year). Average weighted Part D deductible amount excludes employer group plans and Special Needs Plans.

Figure 10.24 Average Part D Annual Deductibles by Plan Type, 2006–2021

Cubanski, J., & Damico, A. (2021, June 8). *Key facts about Medicare Part D enrollment, premiums, and cost sharing in 2021.* Kaiser Family Foundation. https://www.kff.org/medicare/issue-brief/medicare-part-d-in-2018-the-latest-on-enrollment-premiums-and-cost-sharing/

Medicare Spending

Medicare expenditures reached almost $814 billion in 2020 (The Commonwealth Fund Medicare Data Hub [MDH], 2020). Medicare spending is projected to double from 2019 to 2029, when it is expected to account for 18% of total federal spending (Cubanski et al., 2019; MDH, 2020; **Figure 10.25**). Even though Medicare spending will grow slowly compared to historical data, an aging population, longer life expectancy, and overall growth in healthcare costs will contribute to Medicare's rising expenditures (Peter G. Peterson Foundation, 2020). Spending levels would be even higher without savings created by the ACA and the Budget Control Act (BCA) of 2011. The ACA included both provider and plan payment reductions as well as health delivery reforms that were intended to slow growth and improve quality of care (these are discussed further in Chapter 11, "Health Reform and the Patient Protection and Affordable Care Act"). The BCA included additional payment reductions (Cubanski et al., 2019).

Medicare covers at least 20% of national spending on most major healthcare services (**Figure 10.26**). Within Medicare, the proportion of funds spent on hospital services has decreased over time, while spending on Part B and Part D services has increased. Prescription drug spending is concentrated in a relatively small group of drugs. In Part D, the 250 top-selling drugs that have a single manufacturer and no generic or biosimilar counterpart accounted for 60% of Part D spending in 2019. Similarly, in Part B, which covers prescription drugs provided in outpatient settings, the top 50 drugs were responsible for 80% of drug spending (Cubanski & Neuman, 2021b). Of course, as new drugs are approved, spending projections may change. For example, after the new Alzheimer drug, Aduhelm, was approved, experts estimated that Medicare and its beneficiaries could spend $6 billion to $29 billion *annually* on just that drug (Katz et al., 2021). Part C spending, which includes payments for Part B benefits, will rise as use of outpatient services and drugs increase. In addition, as MA enrollment climbs, payments to MA plans will increase (Cubanski et al., 2019; **Figures 10.27** and **10.28**).

The ACA established an Independent Payment Advisory Board, which had the task of submitting proposals to reduce the rate of Medicare spending if Medicare exceeds specified targets. The Secretary of HHS was required to implement proposals submitted by the board unless Congress enacts alternative proposals that achieve the same level of savings. Congress limited the board's options by prohibiting consideration of proposals that ration care, increase revenue, change benefits, change eligibility, or change

Figure 10.25 Medicare Spending, 1967–2029

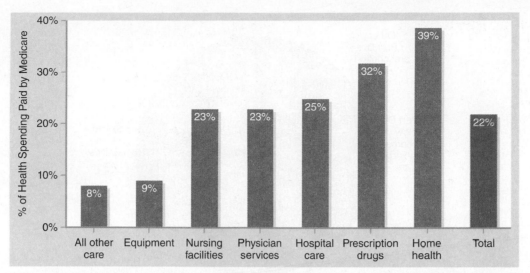

Notes: Data are for 2018. "Equipment" includes both durable medical equipment and other nondurable medical products. "All other care" includes dental services, other professional services, and other health, residential, and personal care expenditures.

Figure 10.26 Medicare Spending on Major Healthcare Services, 2019

Peter G. Peterson Foundation. (2020, July 29). *Budget basics: Medicare.* https://www.pgpf.org/budget-basics/medicare

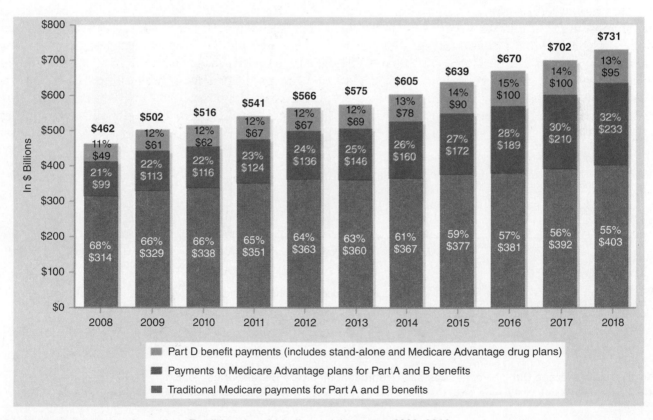

Figure 10.27 Medicare Spending, Traditional and Medicare Advantage, 2008–2018

Cubanski, J., Neuman, T., & Freed, M. (2019, August 20). *The facts on Medicare spending and financing.* Kaiser Family Foundation. https://www.kff.org/medicare/issue-brief/the-facts-on-medicare-spending-and-financing/

cost-sharing. This board, which was never constituted and was derided by policymakers and politicians from both sides of the aisle, was repealed as part of a budget bill in 2018.

Not all Medicare beneficiaries cost the same amount to care for because of the disparities in the amount and type of services they require (**Figures 10.29**, **10.30**, and **10.31**). As with Medicaid and private insurance, a relatively small group of beneficiaries uses a high proportion of these and other services. From 2007 to 2018, 10% of all beneficiaries accounted for 60% of Medicare expenditures (Wallis et al., 2021).

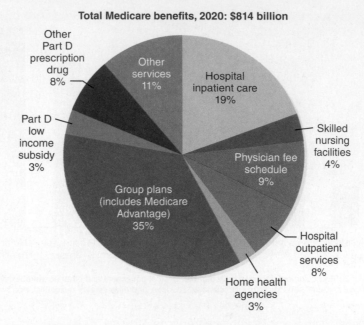

Total Medicare benefits, 2020: $814 billion

- Other Part D prescription drug 8%
- Other services 11%
- Hospital inpatient care 19%
- Part D low income subsidy 3%
- Physician fee schedule 9%
- Skilled nursing facilities 4%
- Group plans (includes Medicare Advantage) 35%
- Hospital outpatient services 8%
- Home health agencies 3%

Figure 10.28 Medicare Spending by Type of Service, 2020

The Commonwealth Fund Medicare Data Hub. (2020). *Solvency and spending* [slide 4]. https://www.commonwealthfund.org/medicare-data-hub-solvency-spending

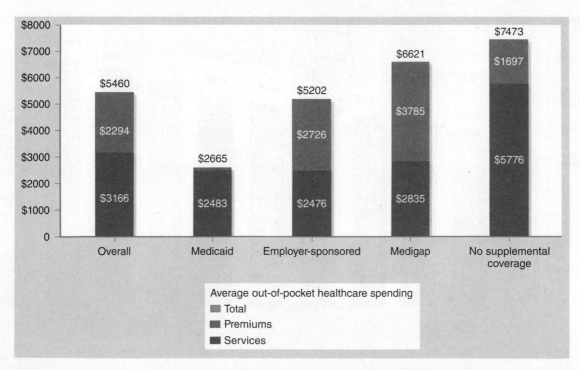

Figure 10.29 Average Out-of-Pocket Costs for Traditional Medicare Beneficiaries, 2016

Cubanski, J., Koma, W., Damico, A., & Neuman, T. (2019, November 4). *How much do Medicare beneficiaries spend out of pocket on health care?* Kaiser Family Foundation. https://www.kff.org/medicare/issue-brief/how-much-do-medicare-beneficiaries-spend-out-of-pocket-on-health-care/

Medicare Provider Reimbursement

Medicare's reimbursement rules vary by provider type and by whether care is provided through an FFS arrangement or an MA plan. Medicare payments are lower than private insurer rates for both hospital and physician services (Lopez et al., 2020; **Figure 10.32**). Medicaid reimbursement varies greatly by state. On average, Medicare reimbursement for physicians is about 44% higher than reimbursement rates provided by Medicaid (CBO, 2015). On the other hand, Medicaid pays hospitals as much or more than Medicare when supplemental payments are included (KFF, 2016;

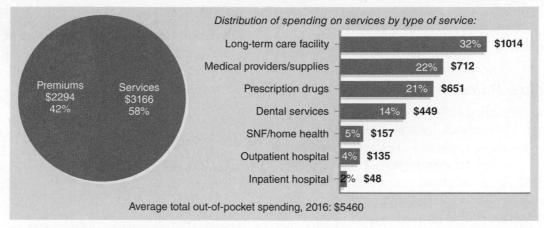

Notes: SNF is skilled nursing facility. Analysis includes beneficiaries living in the community and long-term care facility residents, and excludes beneficiaries with Part A only or Part B only for most of the year or Medicare as a secondary payer, and beneficiaries in Medicare Advantage.

Figure 10.30 Total Out-of-Pocket Spending on Services and Premiums, 2016

Cubanski. I , Koma, W., Damico, A., & Neuman, T. (2019, November 4). *How much do Medicare beneficiaries spend out of pocket on health care?* Kaiser Family Foundation. https://www.kff.org/medicare/issue-brief/how-much-do-medicare-beneficiaries-spend-out-of-pocket -on-health-care/

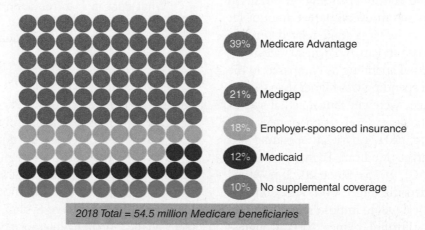

Note: Total excludes beneficiaries with Part A only or Part B only for most of the year (n = 4.7 million) or Medicare as a secondary payer (n = 1.7 million).

Figure 10.31 Medicare Enrollees with Supplemental Coverage, 2018

Koma, W., Cubanski, J., & Neuman, T. (2021, March 23). *A snapshot of sources of coverage among Medicare beneficiaries in 2018.* Kaiser Family Foundation. https://www.kff.org/medicare/issue-brief/a-snapshot-of-sources-of-coverage-among-medicare-beneficiaries-in-2018/

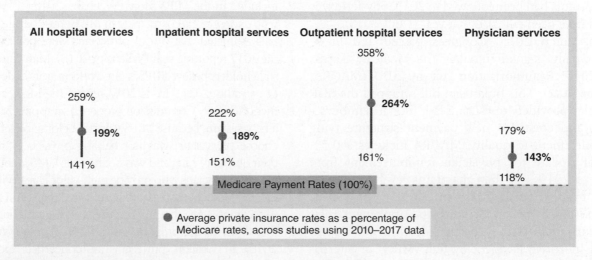

Figure 10.32 Comparison of Medicare and Private Insurer Payment Rates

Lopez, E., Neuman T., Jacobson, G., & Levitt, L. (2020, April 15). *How much more than Medicare do private insurers pay? A review of the literature.* Kaiser Family Foundation. https://www.kff.org/medicare/issue-brief/how-much-more-than-medicare-do-private-insurers-pay -a-review-of-the-literature/

MACPAC, 2017b). MA reimbursement was discussed in the prior section on Part C. This section reviews FFS physician and hospital reimbursement methodologies.

Physician Reimbursement

Physicians providing care on an FFS basis are paid according to the Medicare fee schedule. The fee schedule assigns a relative weight to every service to reflect the resources needed to provide the service. These weights are adjusted for geographical differences in costs and multiplied by a conversion factor (a way to convert the relative value that defines all medical services on the fee schedule into a dollar amount) to determine the final payment amount. Payment rates are changed through upward or downward shifts in the conversion factor.

In 1997 Congress established a formula for reimbursing physicians, referred to as the sustainable growth rate (SGR), as a way to control spending on physician services. The formula set an overall target amount for spending on physician services (and related services such as laboratory tests) in Part B. Payment rates were adjusted to reflect actual spending as compared to the target level—if actual spending was higher than the target level, payment rates were cut, but if actual spending was lower than the target level, payment rates were raised. From 1997 to 2001, physician spending was slightly below the target (Medicare Payment Advisory Commission [MedPAC], 2015). Since 2003, however, spending has exceeded the target level, and Congress has not had the political will to impose reimbursement cuts called for by the formula. Since 2003, Congress suspended the formula annually because it would have resulted in rate reductions, and instead legislated rate increases for physicians. Deferring reimbursement cuts year after year has led to an untenable situation. If the SGR formula had been followed in 2015, physician fees would have been cut 21% that year (CBO, 2015).

In March 2015, Congress passed and President Obama signed into law the Medicare Access and CHIP Reauthorization Act of 2015 (MACRA; see **Box 10.22**). This bipartisan bill scrapped the SGR formula, provided physicians additional reimbursement, and created a new payment structure tying reimbursement to quality. MACRA includes a 0.5% annual update for physician reimbursement from 2015 to 2019 and then maintains level reimbursement from 2019 to 2025. In addition, physicians will be given the opportunity to supplement their reimbursement if they participate in a new Merit-based Incentive Payment System (MIPS) or alternative payment model (APM; e.g., bundled payments or accountable care organizations; National Law

> ### Box 10.22 DISCUSSION QUESTIONS
>
> Controlling Medicare spending is a difficult task. Even if provider reimbursement rates are reduced, physicians and hospitals may increase volume and intensity of services to make up for lost revenue. The ACA included a number of pilot programs and demonstration projects to experiment with reforming the way health care is financed and delivered, and MACRA increased the incentives for physicians to participate in these experiments. Some of these projects include bundling payment for acute care services; using value-based purchasing, which ties payments to quality outcomes; and creating accountable care organizations that bring together providers across the healthcare spectrum and reward organizations with better outcomes. The ACA created the CMS Innovation Center to oversee these and other reform projects.
>
> What approach to reducing costs and improving quality do you prefer? What are the advantages and disadvantages of these ideas?

Review, 2015). After 2026, physicians participating in an APM will receive a 1% reimbursement update, instead of a 0.5% increase for nonparticipants.

The MIPS program is an attempt to streamline three existing programs that tie physician reimbursement to improved quality and use of electronic health records: the Physician Quality Reporting System, the Value-Based Modifier, and the Promoting Interoperability (originally named Meaningful Use) program for electronic records (National Law Review, 2015). Based on their scores, physicians can receive cuts or additions to their reimbursement updates, up to a capped amount. As of 2018, physician cost is included in the MIPS score (Wilensky, 2018). Physicians who choose not to participate in MIPS must pay a penalty. It is estimated that 3% of physicians were penalized for the 2017 reporting year (Wilensky, 2018). Many interested stakeholders believe MIPS is not working as intended (Liao & Navathe, 2021). In its 2017 report, the Medicare Payment Advisory Commission proposed scrapping MIPS for a new system, because MIPS was not helping beneficiaries choose physicians, was not helping physicians improve their quality of care, and was not helping CMS identify and reward physicians who provide high-value care (Wilensky, 2018). Medical associations and the American Hospital Association agree that MIPS is not working well but prefer that CMS fix the program instead of replace it (Wilensky, 2018). In addition, physicians are concerned about the costs and administrative burden of participating in MIPS (Khullar et al., 2021).

CMS released its final rule implementing MACRA in November 2016. These rules included a transition period in 2017 that gave providers more flexibility and fewer reporting requirements in the MIPS program, additional models to qualify as an APM, and eligibility thresholds that may exempt more physicians (Patel et al., 2016). CMS estimated that over half of physicians would be exempt from MIPS because they do not have patient contact, they have low Medicare revenue or patient volume, they are new Medicare providers, or they participate in an APM (Patel et al., 2016). Under MACRA, physicians who participate in and receive a significant amount of their revenue through APMs that include the risk of financial loss and a quality improvement component will receive a 5% bonus from 2019 to 2024. In addition, participation in an APM releases physicians from the requirement to participate in MIPS and most Promoting Interoperability programs (National Law Review, 2015). CMS continues to explore APM structures, including creating the Bundled Payments for Care Improvement Advanced Model that pays a retrospective amount for services over a 90-day period (Geilfuss & Romano, 2018) and allowing MA providers to qualify as APMs (Dickson, 2018). One suggestion for improving MIPS includes aligning MIPS with the APM practice of considering cost and quality concurrently, instead of separately (Liao & Navathe, 2021).

Hospital Reimbursement

Hospitals are paid for acute inpatient services on a prospective basis using diagnostic-related groups (DRGs). DRGs sort patients into more than 500 groups based on their diagnoses. Various diagnoses are grouped together if they have similar clinical profiles and costs. Each DRG is assigned a relative weight based on charges for cases in that group as compared to the national average for all groups. In addition, the part of the DRG covering hospitals' cost of labor is adjusted by a wage index to account for cost differences in different geographical areas (MedPAC, 2005, p. 43). Hospitals may also receive additional payments for providing high-cost outlier cases; incurring costs associated with use of new technology; incurring indirect medical education costs; serving a high proportion of low-income patients; or being a qualified sole community provider, a rural referral center, a small Medicare-dependent hospital, a rural hospital treating fewer than 200 admissions, or a critical access hospital (a qualified rural hospital that provides critical care services) (MedPAC, 2005, pp. 43–44).

For outpatient care, hospitals are reimbursed by Medicare using a different prospective system. Each outpatient service is assigned to one of about 800 ambulatory payment classification (APC) groups. APCs have a relative weight based on the median cost of the service compared to the national average. Again, a conversion factor is used to calculate the specific dollar amount per APC, and the labor cost portion is adjusted based on a hospital wage index to account for geographical cost differences. APC payments may be adjusted when hospitals use new technologies or biologicals and when they treat unusually high cost patients (MedPAC, 2005, p. 44).

The ACA included a number of provisions that reduced reimbursement for hospitals and other Medicare providers, including SNFs and hospices (discussed in Chapter 11, "Health Reform and the Patient Protection and Affordable Care Act"). These rate reductions include "market basket" updates, which set the prices for a mix of goods and services, and a lowering of DSH payments, which are given to hospitals that provide services to a relatively high proportion of Medicaid and uninsured patients. In addition, hospitals will receive reduced payments for services connected to preventable readmissions and hospital-acquired conditions.

The Future of Medicare

While there is broad agreement across the political spectrum that Medicare's financing is unsustainable going forward, there is less accord about how to address that problem. If Medicare is altered dramatically, one conservative proposal is to turn Medicare into a premium support program. In this type of program, the federal government provides beneficiaries with a set amount of funds to purchase health insurance, with the beneficiary making up the difference between the allotment and the cost of the premium (Glied, 2018). Of course, both the amount of savings for the federal government and the burden on beneficiaries would depend on the size of the premium support provided to beneficiaries. In any case, by shifting from an entitlement program to a specific allotment, much of the financial risk of rising healthcare costs would fall on beneficiaries, not the federal government (Glied, 2018). A less drastic program change would encourage more enrollment in managed care by automatically enrolling new beneficiaries into MA plans while offering an option to switch to FFS Medicare (Miller & Wilensky, 2020). On the other hand, progressives prefer to reform Medicare by reducing the eligibility age to 55 or 60, expanding benefits to include dental, vision, and hearing services, reducing cost-sharing, and allowing Medicare to negotiate drug prices (Broadwater, 2021; Cubanski et al., 2020). Given Medicare's financial trajectory, there are concerns regarding whether these changes are affordable. President Biden included a proposal to reduce Medicare eligibility age from 65 to 60 in his FY 2022 budget, but did not detail the cost or structural implications for the program (Musumeci et al., 2021). Given the closely divided Congress and the difficulty of reforming a popular social program, it is doubtful that a significant restructuring will happen any time soon. In the meantime, other policy changes—such as simplifying the program structure, increasing future beneficiaries' share of costs, increasing the eligibility age, and encouraging the use of private plans through competition—are more likely to become a central part of the debate over Medicare's future. Whatever structural and financial changes occur, policymakers must also account for the racial and ethnic health disparities that persist in the Medicare program.

Conclusion

This chapter provided an overview of the three main public programs that provide health insurance coverage to millions of people in the United States and raised a series of policy questions for your consideration.

Based on the size of the programs, their costs to the federal and state governments, and their importance to millions of (often low-income) individuals, the role and structure of Medicaid, CHIP, and Medicare are constantly being debated. Some people would like to see coverage expanded to ensure that everyone has adequate access to health insurance, others would like to dismantle the programs in the interest of eliminating government-funded entitlements, and still others suggest incremental changes to the programs. The debate continues even with the passage of the ACA. Some want to repeal the law, while others are discussing cuts to entitlement programs as a way to reduce the federal deficit. Each of these decisions, and many others, reflect the recurring themes that have been discussed throughout this chapter: choosing between state flexibility and national uniformity; determining the appropriate role for government, the private sector, and individuals in healthcare financing and delivery; defining a primary decision-making goal (e.g., fiscal restraint, equity/social justice, improved health outcomes, uniformity); and settling on the appropriate scope of coverage to offer beneficiaries. Given these programs' expected increase in beneficiaries and the complementary increase in their cost, it is likely that the debates over Medicaid, CHIP, and Medicare will continue vigorously in the foreseeable future.

References

Accius, J., Flowers, L., & Flinn, B. (2017, March). *Low-income Medicare beneficiaries rely on Medicaid for critical help.* https://www.aarp.org/ppi/info-2017/low-income-medicare-beneficiaries-rely-on-medicaid-for-critical-help.html

Advisory Board. (2018, July 24). *The ACA boosted Medicaid payments for two years. But doctors were no more likely to take Medicaid patients, studies find.* https://www.advisory.com/en/daily-briefing/2018/07/24/medicaid-payment

Agarwal, R., Connolly, J., Gupta, S., & Navathe, A. (2021, June). Comparing Medicare Advantage and traditional Medicare: A systematic review. *Health Affairs, 40*(6), 937–944. https://doi.org/10.1377/hlthaff.2020.02149

Alker, J. (2020, December 18). *What's happening to CHIP enrollment during the pandemic?* https://ccf.georgetown.edu/2020/12/18/whats-happening-to-chip-enrollment-during-the-pandemic/

Armour, S. (2021, April 3). *Medicaid expansion is under reconsideration in red states.* https://www.wsj.com/articles/medicaid-expansion-is-under-reconsideration-in-red-states-11617460071?page=1

Armstrong v. Exceptional Child Center, U.S., No. 14-15 (2015, March 31).

Barker, T. (2020, February 20). *Washington D.C. appellate court upholds prohibition on Medicaid work requirement waivers.* https://www.medicaidandthelaw.com/2020/02/20/washington-d-c-appellate-court-upholds-prohibition-on-medicaid-work-requirement-waivers/

Barry, C., & Kline, J. (2002, April 1). *Medicare managed care: Medicare+Choice at five years.* https://www.commonwealthfund.org/publications/issue-briefs/2002/apr/medicare-managed-care-medicarechoice-five-years

Biniek, J. F., Freed, M., Damico, A., & Neuman, T. (2020, October 29). *Medicare Advantage 2021 spotlight: First look.* https://www.kff.org/medicare/issue-brief/medicare-advantage-2021-spotlight-first-look/

Bipartisan Budget Act of 2018, Pub. L. No. 115-123, 132 Stat. 64 (2018).

Broadwater, L. (2021, May 27). *Broad coalition of Democrats presses Biden to expand Medicare.* https://www.nytimes.com/2021/05/27/us/politics/medicare-expansion-biden.html

Brooks, T., Roygardener, L., Artiga, S., Pham, O., & Dolan, R. (2020, March 26). *Medicaid and CHIP eligibility, enrollment, and cost sharing policies as of January 2020: Findings from a 50-state survey.* https://www.kff.org/coronavirus-covid-19/report/medicaid-and-chip-eligibility-enrollment-and-cost-sharing-policies-as-of-january-2020-findings-from-a-50-state-survey/

Brooks, T., Wagnerman, K., Artiga, S., Cornachione, E., & Ubri, P. (2017, January 12). *Medicaid and CHIP eligibility, enrollment, renewal, and cost sharing policies as of January 2017: Findings from a 50-state survey.* https://www.kff.org/report-section

/medicaid-and-chip-eligibility-enrollment-renewal-and-cost
-sharing-policies-as-of-january-2017-medicaid-and-chip
-eligibility/

Brooks, T., & Whitener, K. (2017, June). *At risk: Medicaid's child-focused benefit structure known as EPSDT.* https://ccf .georgetown.edu/wp-content/uploads/2017/06/EPSDT-At -Risk-Final.pdf

Centers for Medicare and Medicaid Services. (n.d.). *Dually eligible individuals - Categories.* https://www.cms.gov/Medicare -Medicaid-Coordination/Medicare-and-Medicaid-Coordina tion/Medicare-Medicaid-Coordination-Office/Downloads/ MedicareMedicaidEnrolleeCategories.pdf

Centers for Medicare and Medicaid Services. (2019, December 11). *Medicaid and CHIP coverage of lawfully residing children & pregnant women.* https://www.medicaid.gov/medicaid/enrollment-strategies /medicaid-and-chip-coverage-lawfully-residing-children -pregnant-women

Centers for Medicare and Medicaid Services. (2020, March). *People dually eligible for Medicare and Medicaid fact sheet.* https://www .cms.gov/Medicare-Medicaid-Coordination/Medicare-and -Medicaid-Coordination/Medicare-Medicaid-Coordination -Office/Downloads/MMCO_Factsheet.pdf

Children's Health Insurance Program Reauthorization Act of 2009, Pub. L. No. 111-3, 48 Stat. 998 (2009).

Chronic Conditions Data Warehouse. (n.d.). *Medicare chronic condition charts.* https://www2.ccwdata.org/web/guest/medicare -charts/medicare-chronic-condition-charts

CMS.gov. (2020a, July 8). *Original Medicare (Part A and B) eligibility and enrollment.* https://www.cms.gov/medicare/eligibility-and -enrollment/origmedicarepartabeligenrol

CMS.gov. (2020b, November 9). *Medicaid & Children's Health Insurance Program (CHIP) managed care final rule—CMS-2408-F.* https://www.cms.gov/newsroom/fact-sheets/medicaid -childrens-health-insurance-program-chip-managed-care -final-rule-cms-2408-f

CMS.gov. (2020c, December 16). *NHE fact sheet.* https://www.cms .gov/Research-Statistics-Data-and-Systems/Statistics-Trends -and-Reports/NationalHealthExpendData/NHE-Fact-Sheet

Congressional Budget Office. (2015). *Medicare's payment to physicians: The budgetary effects of alternative policies relative to CBO's January 2015 baseline.* https://www.cbo.gov/publication/49923

Cox, C., Amin, K., Claxton, G., & McDermott, D. (2021, April 7). *The ACA family glitch and affordability of employer coverage.* https://www.kff.org/health-reform/issue-brief/the-aca-family -glitch-and-affordability-of-employer-coverage/

Cubanski, J., & Damico, A. (2021, June 8). *Key facts about Medicare Part D enrollment, premiums, and cost sharing in 2021.* https:// www.kff.org/medicare/issue-brief/key-facts-about-medicare -part-d-enrollment-premiums-and-cost-sharing-in-2021/

Cubanski, J., & Freed, M. (2020, December 4). *Coverage and costs related to COVID-19 testing and treatment.* https://www.kff.org /medicare/issue-brief/faqs-on-medicare-coverage-and-costs -related-to-covid-19-testing-and-treatment/

Cubanski, J., Freed, M., Neuman, T., & Damico, A. (2020, December 8). *FAQs on Medicare coverage and costs related to Covid-19 testing and treatment.* https://www.kff.org/medicare /issue-brief/faqs-on-medicare-coverage-and-costs-related-to -covid-19-testing-and-treatment/

Cubanski, J., & Neuman, T. (2018, June 22). *The facts on Medicare spending and financing.* https://www.kff.org/medicare/issue -brief/the-facts-on-medicare-spending-and-financing/

Cubanski, J., & Neuman, T. (2021a, March 16). *FAQs on Medicare financing and trust fund solvency.* https://www.kff.org/medicare

/issue-brief/faqs-on-medicare-financing-and-trust-fund -solvency

Cubanski, J., & Neuman, T. (2021b, April 19). *Relatively few drugs account for a large share of Medicare prescription drug spending.* https://www.kff.org/medicare/issue-brief/relatively-few-drugs -account-for-a-large-share-of-medicare-prescription-drug -spending/

Cubanski, J., Neuman, T., & Freed, M. (2019, August 20). *The facts on Medicare spending and financing.* https://www.kff.org /medicare/issue-brief/the-facts-on-medicare-spending-and -financing/

Cubanski, J., Swoope, C., Bocutti, C., Jacobson, G., Casillas, G., Griffen, S., & Neuman, T. (2015, March 20). *A primer on Medicare: Key facts about the Medicare program and the people it covers.* https://www.kff.org/medicare/report/a-primer-on-medi care-key-facts-about-the-medicare-program-and-the-people -it-covers/

Cunningham, P., Rudowitz, R., Young, K., Garfield, R., & Foutz, J. (2016, January 9). *Understanding Medicaid hospital payments and the impact of recent policy changes.* https://www.kff.org /report-section/understanding-medicaid-hospital-payments -and-the-impact-of-recent-policy-changes-issue-brief/

Decker, S. L. (2018). No association found between the Medicaid primary care fee bump and physician-reported participation in Medicaid. *Health Affairs, 37*(7), 1092–1098. https://doi .org/10.1377/hlthaff.2018.0078

Deficit Reduction Act of 2005, Pub. L. No. 109-362, 107 Stat. 312 through 685 Stat. 1025 (2006).

Department of Health and Human Services. (2017, January 26). *HHS 2017 budget in brief—CMS—Medicare.* https://www .hhs.gov/about/budget/fy2017/budget-in-brief/cms/medicare /index.html

Dickson, V. (2018, June 29). *CMS to test Medicare Advantage as alternative payment model under MACRA.* https://www.modern healthcare.com/article/20180629/NEWS/180629900/cms-to -test-medicare-advantage-as-alternative-payment-model -under-macra

Dranove, D., Garthwaite, C., & Ody, C. (2017, May 3). *The impact of the ACA's Medicaid expansion on hospitals' uncompensated care burden and the potential effects of repeal.* https://www.commonwealthfund .org/publications/issue-briefs/2017/may/impact-acas-medicaid -expansion-hospitals-uncompensated-care

EveryCRSReport. (2018, November 26). *Medicaid alternative benefit coverage: Frequently asked questions.* https://www .everycrsreport.com/reports/R45412.html#_Toc531081957

Federal Funds Information for States. (2020, June 8). *Medicare clawback update: CY 2020 savings, CY 2021 estimates.* https://ffis .org/PUBS/issue-brief/20/15

Freed, M., Damico, A., & Neuman, T. (2021, January 13). *A dozen facts about Medicare Advantage in 2020.* https://www .kff.org/medicare/issue-brief/a-dozen-facts-about-medicare -advantage-in-2020/

Fremstad, S., & Cox, L. (2004, November). *Covering new Americans: A review of federal and state policies related to immigrants' eligibility and access to publicly funded health insurance.* https://www.kff.org/medicaid/report/covering-new -americans-a-review-of-federal/

Galewitz, P. (2021, June 17). *Pandemic swells Medicaid enrollment to 80 million people, a 'high-water mark'.* https://khn.org/news /article/medicaid-enrollment-record-80-million-pandemic/

Garfield, R., Damico, A., & Orgera, K. (2021, January 21). *The coverage gap: Uninsured poor adults in states that do not expand Medicaid.* https://www.kff.org/medicaid/issue-brief

/the-coverage-gap-uninsured-poor-adults-in-states-that-do-not-expand-medicaid/

Geilfuss, C. F. II, & Romano, D. H. (2018, January 12). *CMS announces advanced alternative payment model—BPCI advanced.* https://www.healthcarelawtoday.com/2018/01/12/cms-announces-an-advanced-alternative-payment-model-bpci-advanced/

Georgetown University Health Policy Institute. (2017, February 6). *The Children's Health Insurance Program.* https://ccf.georgetown.edu/2017/02/06/about-chip/

Gifford, K., Lashbrook, A., Barth, S., Hinton, E., Rudowitz, R., Guth, M., & Stolyar, L. (2020, October 14). *State Medicaid programs respond to meet COVID-19 challenges: Results from a 50-state Medicaid budget survey for state fiscal years 2020 and 2021.* https://www.kff.org/medicaid/report/state-medicaid-programs-respond-to-meet-covid-19-challenges/

Glied, S. (2018). Financing Medicare into the future: Premium support fails the risk-bearing test. *Health Affairs, 37*(7), 1073–1078. https://doi.org/10.1377/hlthaff.2018.0008

Grants to States for Medical Assistance Programs, 53 Fed. Reg. 36571 (September, 1988) (codified in 42 C.F.R. pts. 430-498).

Guth, M., & Ammula, M. (2021, May 6). *Building on the evidence base: Studies on the effects of Medicaid expansion, February 2020 to March 2021.* https://www.kff.org/medicaid/report/building-on-the-evidence-base-studies-on-the-effects-of-medicaid-expansion-february-2020-to-march-2021/

Guth, M., Hinton, E., Musumeci, M., & Rudowitz, R. (2020, October 30). *The landscape of Medicaid demonstration waivers ahead of the 2020 election.* https://www.kff.org/medicaid/issue-brief/the-landscape-of-medicaid-demonstration-waivers-ahead-of-the-2020-election/

Hinton, E., Rudowitz, R., Stolyar, L., & Singer, N. (2020, October 29). *10 Things to know about Medicaid managed care.* https://www.kff.org/medicaid/issue-brief/10-things-to-know-about-medicaid-managed-care/

Hinton, E., Stolyar, L., & Rudowitz, R. (2021, March 12). *Medicaid spending and enrollment trends amid the Covid-19 pandemic - Updated for the FY 2021 & looking ahead to FY 2022.* https://www.kff.org/coronavirus-covid-19/issue-brief/medicaid-spending-and-enrollment-trends-amid-the-covid-19-pandemic-updated-for-fy-2021-looking-ahead-to-fy-2022/

Holgash, K., & Heberlein, M. (2019, April 10). *Physician acceptance of new Medicaid patients: What matters and what doesn't.* https://www.healthaffairs.org/do/10.1377/hblog20190401.678690/full/

Jacobson, G., Griffin, S., Neuman, T., & Smith, K. (2017, April 21). *Income and assets of Medicare beneficiaries, 2016–2035.* https://www.kff.org/medicare/issue-brief/income-and-assets-of-medicare-beneficiaries-2016-2035/

Kaiser Family Foundation. (2010). *Summary of key changes to Medicare in the 2010 health reform law.* https://www.kff.org/health-reform/issue-brief/summary-of-key-changes-to-medicare-in/

Kaiser Family Foundation. (2012a). *The Medicaid medically needy program: Spending and enrollment update.* https://www.kff.org/medicaid/issue-brief/the-medicaid-medically-needy-program-spending-and/

Kaiser Family Foundation. (2012b). *State adoption of coverage and enrollment options in the Children's Health Insurance Reauthorization Act of 2009.* https://www.kff.org/medicaid/fact-sheet/state-adoption-of-coverage-and-enrollment-options/

Kaiser Family Foundation. (2016). *Medicaid-to-Medicare fee index.* https://www.kff.org/medicaid/state-indicator/medicaid-to-medicare-fee-index/?currentTimeframe=0&sortModel=%7B%22colId%22:%22Location%22,%22sort%22:%22asc%22%7D

Kaiser Family Foundation. (2018). *Medicaid eligibility through the medically needy pathway.* https://www.kff.org/other/state-indicator/medicaid-eligibility-through-the-medically-needy-pathway/?currentTimeframe=0&sortModel=%7B%22colId%22:%22Location%22,%22sort%22:%22asc%22%7D

Kaiser Family Foundation. (2019a, November 25). *Analysis of recent declines in Medicaid and CHIP enrollment.* https://www.kff.org/medicaid/fact-sheet/analysis-of-recent-declines-in-medicaid-and-chip-enrollment/

Kaiser Family Foundation. (2019b). *Distribution of Medicare beneficiaries by eligibility category.* https://www.kff.org/medicare/state-indicator/distribution-of-medicare-beneficiaries-by-eligibility-category-2/?dataView=1&currentTimeframe=0&sortModel=%7B%22colId%22:%22Location%22,%22sort%22:%22asc%22%7D

Kaiser Family Foundation. (2019c, June 11). *Total number of children ever enrolled in CHIP annually.* https://www.kff.org/other/state-indicator/annual-chip-enrollment/?currentTimeframe=0&sortModel=%7B%22colId%22:%22Location%22,%22sort%22:%22asc%22%7D

Kaiser Family Foundation. (2020a, January 1). *Premiums, enrollment fees, and cost-sharing requirements for children.* https://www.kff.org/medicaid/state-indicator/premiums-enrollment-fees-and-cost-sharing-requirements-for-children/?currentTimeframe=0&sortModel=%7B%22colId%22:%22Location%22,%22sort%22:%22asc%22%7D

Kaiser Family Foundation. (2020b, February 28). *Data note: 5 Charts about public opinion on Medicaid.* https://www.kff.org/medicaid/poll-finding/data-note-5-charts-about-public-opinion-on-medicaid/

Kaiser Family Foundation. (2020c, March 18). *Health coverage of immigrants.* https://www.kff.org/racial-equity-and-health-policy/fact-sheet/health-coverage-of-immigrants/

Kaiser Family Foundation. (2021a, January 1). *Medicaid and CHIP income eligibility limits for children as a percent of the federal poverty level.* https://www.kff.org/health-reform/state-indicator/medicaid-and-chip-income-eligibility-limits-for-children-as-a-percent-of-the-federal-poverty-level/?currentTimeframe=0&sortModel=%7B%22colId%22:%22Location%22,%22sort%22:%22asc%22%7D

Kaiser Family Foundation. (2021b, January 1). *Medicaid/CHIP coverage of lawfully-residing immigrant children and pregnant women.* https://www.kff.org/health-reform/state-indicator/medicaid-chip-coverage-of-lawfully-residing-immigrant-children-and-pregnant-women/?currentTimeframe=0&sortModel=%7B%22colId%22:%22Location%22,%22sort%22:%22asc%22%7D

Kaiser Family Foundation. (2021c, July 1). *Status of state Medicaid expansion decisions: Interactive map.* https://www.kff.org/medicaid/issue-brief/status-of-state-medicaid-expansion-decisions-interactive-map/

Kaiser Family Foundation. (2021d, October 13). *An overview of the Medicare Part D prescription drug benefit.* https://www.kff.org/medicare/fact-sheet/an-overview-of-the-medicare-part-d-prescription-drug-benefit/

Kaiser Family Foundation. (2021e, October 22). *Medicaid waiver tracker: Approved and pending section 1115 Medicaid waivers by state.* https://www.kff.org/medicaid/issue-brief/medicaid-waiver-tracker-approved-and-pending-section-1115-waivers-by-state

Kaiser Family Foundation. (2021f, December 20). *Medicaid waiver tracker: Approved and pending section 1115 waivers by state.* https://www.kff.org/medicaid/issue-brief/medicaid-waiver

-tracker-approved-and-pending-section-1115-waivers-by -state/#Table3

Katz, J., Kliff, S., & Sanger-Katz, M. (2021, June 22). *New drug could cost the government as much as it spends on NASA.* https:// www.nytimes.com/2021/06/22/upshot/alzheimers-aduhelm -medicare-cost.html

Khullar, D., Bond, A., & O'Donnell, E. (2021, May 14). Time and financial costs for physician practices to participate in the Medicare merit-based incentive payment system: A qualitative study. *JAMA Health Forum, 2*(5), e210527. https://doi.org /10.1001/jamahealthforum.2021.0527

Kornfield, T., Kazan, M., Frieder, M., Duddy-Tenbrunsel, R., Donthi, S., & Fix, A. (2021, February 10). *Medicare Advantage plans offering expanded supplemental benefits: A look at availability and enrollment.* https://www.commonwealthfund .org/publications/issue-briefs/2021/feb/medicare-advantage -plans-supplemental-benefits

Liao, J., & Navathe, A. (2021, March 2). Medicare should transform MIPS, not scrap it. *Health Affairs* [blog]. https://www .healthaffairs.org/do/10.1377/hblog20210226.949893/full/

Lopes, L., Kearney, A., Kirzinger, A., Hamel, L., & Brodie, M. (2021, March 3). *KFF health tracking poll: Economic hardship, health coverage, and the ACA.* https://www.kff.org /coronavirus-covid-19/poll-finding/kff-health-tracking-poll -late-february-2021/

Lopez, E., Neuman, T., Jacobson, G., & Levitt, L. (2020, April 15). *How much more than Medicare do private insurers pay? A review of the literature.* https://www.kff.org/medicare/issue-brief/how -much-more-than-medicare-do-private-insurers-pay-a -review-of-the-literature/

Lukens, G. (2021, April 20). *Medicaid expansion cuts hospitals' uncompensated care costs.* https://www.cbpp.org/blog/medicaid -expansion-cuts-hospitals-uncompensated-care-costs

Mather, M., Scommenga, P., & Kilduff, L. (2019, July 15). *Fact sheet: Aging in the United States.* https://www.prb.org/resources /fact-sheet-aging-in-the-united-states/

McGuire, T. G., Newhouse, J. P., & Sinaiko, A. D. (2011). An economic history of Medicare Part C. *Milbank Quarterly, 89*(2), 289–332. https://doi.org/10.1111/j.1468-0009.2011.00629.x

Medicaid and CHIP Payment and Access Commission. (n.d.a). *CHIP.* https://www.macpac.gov/topics/chip/

Medicaid and CHIP Payment and Access Commission. (n.d.b). *CHIP eligibility.* https://www.macpac.gov/subtopic/eligibility-2/

Medicaid and CHIP Payment and Access Commission. (n.d.c). *CHIP financing.* https://www.macpac.gov/subtopic/financing/

Medicaid and CHIP Payment and Access Commission. (n.d.d). *Dually eligible beneficiaries.* https://www.macpac.gov/topics /dually-eligible-beneficiaries/

Medicaid and CHIP Payment and Access Commission. (n.d.e). *Key CHIP design features.* https://www.macpac.gov/subtopic /key-design-features/

Medicaid and CHIP Payment and Access Commission. (n.d.f). *Medicaid enrollment changes following the ACA.* https:// www.macpac.gov/subtopic/medicaid-enrollment-changes -following-the-aca/

Medicaid and CHIP Payment and Access Commission. (2016, July). *Medicaid outpatient payment policy.* https://www.macpac .gov/wp-content/uploads/2016/07/Medicaid-Outpatient -Payment-Policies-Overview.pdf

Medicaid and CHIP Payment and Access Commission. (2017a, January). *Recommendations for the future of CHIP and children's coverage.* https://www.macpac.gov/publication/recommendations -for-the-future-of-chip-and-childrens-coverage/

Medicaid and CHIP Payment and Access Commission. (2017b, April). *Medicaid hospital payment: A comparison across states and to Medicare.* https://www.macpac.gov /wp-content/uploads/2017/04/Medicaid-Hospital-Payment-A -Comparison-across-States-and-to-Medicare.pdf

Medicaid and CHIP Payment and Access Commission. (2018a, February). *State Children's Health Insurance Program (CHIP).* https://www.macpac.gov/publication/state-childrens-health -insurance-program-chip-fact-sheet/

Medicaid and CHIP Payment and Access Commission. (2018b, December). *Medicaid inpatient hospital services fee-for-service payment policy.* https://www.macpac.gov/wp-content/uploads /2016/03/Medicaid-Inpatient-Hospital-Services-Fee-for -Service-Payment-Policy.pdf

Medicaid and CHIP Payment and Access Commission. (2020a, June 11). *CHIP program structure by state.* https://www .medicaid.gov/chip/downloads/chip-map.pdf

Medicaid and CHIP Payment and Access Commission. (2020b, December). *MACStats: Medicaid and CHIP Data Book, Exhibit 6.* https://www.macpac.gov/wp-content/uploads/2018/04/EXHIBIT -6.-Federal-Medical-Assistance-Percentages-and-Enhanced-Federal -Medical-Assistance-Percentages-by-State-FYs-2018-2021.pdf

Medicaid.gov. (n.d.a). *About section 1115 demonstrations.* https:// www.medicaid.gov/medicaid/section-1115-demo/about -1115/index.html

Medicaid.gov. (n.d.b). *Alternative benefit plan coverage.* https:// www.medicaid.gov/medicaid/benefits/abp/index.html

Medicaid.gov. (n.d.c). *April 2018 Medicaid and CHIP enrollment data highlights.* https://www.medicaid.gov/medicaid/program -information/medicaid-and-chip-enrollment-data/report -highlights/index.html

Medicaid.gov. (n.d.d). *Benefits.* https://www.medicaid.gov/chip /benefits/index.html

Medicaid.gov. (n.d.e). *CHIP cost sharing.* https://www.medicaid .gov/chip/benefits/index.html

Medicaid.gov. (n.d.f). *Cost sharing out of pocket costs.* https:// www.medicaid.gov/medicaid/cost-sharing/out-of-pocket -costs/index.html

Medicaid.gov. (n.d.g). *Eligibility.* https://www.medicaid.gov /chip/eligibility/index.html

Medicaid.gov. (n.d.h). *Federal policy guidance.* https://www .medicaid.gov/federal-policy-Guidance/index.html

Medicaid.gov. (2021, April). *Waiting periods in CHIP.* https://www .medicaid.gov/chip/eligibility-standards/waiting-periods -chip/index.html

Medicare Access and CHIP Reauthorization Act of 2015, Pub. L. No. 114-10, 129 Stat. 87 (2015).

Medicare.gov. (n.d.a). *Clinical research studies.* https://www .medicare.gov/coverage/clinical-research-studies

Medicare.gov. (n.d.b). *Costs for Medicare Advantage plans.* https:// www.medicare.gov/your-medicare-costs/costs-for-medicare -advantage-plans

Medicare.gov. (n.d.c). *Medicare costs at a glance.* https://www .medicare.gov/your-medicare-costs/medicare-costs-at-a-glance

Medicare.gov. (n.d.d). *Monthly premium for drug plans.* https://www .medicare.gov/drug-coverage-part-d/costs-for-medicare -drug-coverage/monthly-premium-for-drug-plans

Medicare.gov. (n.d.e). *Skilled nursing facility (SNF) care.* https:// www.medicare.gov/coverage/skilled-nursing-facility-snf-care

Medicare Payment Advisory Commission. (2005, March). *Report to the Congress: Medicare payment policy.* https://www.medpac .gov/wp-content/uploads/import_data/scrape_files/docs /default-source/reports/Mar05_EntireReport.pdf

Medicare Payment Advisory Commission. (2015, June). *Report to the Congress: Medicare and the health care delivery system.* https://www.medpac.gov/document/http-www-medpac-gov-docs-default-source-reports-june-2015-report-to-the-congress-medicare-and-the-health-care-delivery-system-pdf/

Mental Health Parity and Addiction Equity Act of 2008, Pub. L. 110-343.

Meyers, D. J., Mor, V., Rahman, M., & Trivedi, A. N. (2021, June 7). Growth in Medicare Advantage greatest among Black and Hispanic enrollees. *Health Affairs, 40*(6), 945–950. https://doi.org/10.1377/hlthaff.2021.00118

Miller, B., & Wilensky, G. (2020, September 16). *The next step in Medicare reform.* https://www.heritage.org/health-care-reform/report/the-next-step-medicare-reform

Musumeci, M. (2018, July 2). *Explaining* Stewart v. Azar: *Implications of the court's decision on Kentucky's Medicaid waiver.* https://www.kff.org/medicaid/issue-brief/explaining-stewart-v-azar-implications-of-the-courts-decision-on-kentuckys-medicaid-waiver/

Musumeci, M., Rudowitz, R., & Neuman, T. (2021, June 10). *How might lowering the Medicare age affect Medicaid enrollees?* https://www.kff.org/medicaid/issue-brief/how-might-lowering-the-medicare-age-affect-medicaid-enrollees/

National Federation of Independent Business v. Sebelius, 132 S. Ct. 2566 (2012).

National Law Review. (2015, April 20). *With SGR repealed, replacement policy creates new priorities—Sustainable growth rate.* https://www.natlawreview.com/article/sgr-repealed-replacement-policy-creates-new-priorities-sustainable-growth-rate

Neprash, H. T., Zink, A., Gray, J., & Hempstead, K. (2018). Physician participation in Medicaid increased only slightly following expansion. *Health Affairs, 37*(7), 1087–1091. https://doi.org/10.1377/hlthaff.2017.1085

Paradise, J. (2015, March 9). *Medicaid moving forward.* https://www.kff.org/health-reform/issue-brief/medicaid-moving-forward/

Paradise, J., Lyons, B., & Rowland, D. (2015, May 6). *Medicaid at 50.* https://www.kff.org/medicaid/report/medicaid-at-50/

Paradise, J., & Musumeci, M. (2016, June 9). *CMS's final rule on Medicaid managed care: A summary of major provisions.* https://www.kff.org/medicaid/issue-brief/cmss-final-rule-on-medicaid-managed-care-a-summary-of-major-provisions/

Passel, J. (2005, June 14). *Unauthorized migrants: Numbers and characteristics.* http://www.pewhispanic.org/2005/06/14/unauthorized-migrants/

Patel, K., Darling, M., & Ginsberg, P. (2016, December 15). *Key takeaways from the final MACRA rule, plus remaining challenges.* https://www.brookings.edu/blog/usc-brookings-schaeffer-on-health-policy/2016/12/15/key-takeaways-from-the-final-macra-rule-plus-remaining-challenges/

Personal Responsibility and Work Opportunity Reconciliation Act of 1996, Pub. L. No. 104-193, 100 Stat. 2105 (1996).

Peter G. Peterson Foundation. (2020, July 9). *Budget basics: Medicare.* https://www.pgpf.org/budget-basics/medicare

Q1 Group. (2020, July 3). *2021 State low-income subsidy benchmark premium amounts - with a comparison of benchmark changes since 2006.* https://q1medicare.com/q1group/MedicareAdvantagePartD/Blog.php?blog=Latest-Medicare-News&blog_id=832&category_id=8

Rosenbaum, S. (2002). Medicaid. *New England Journal of Medicine, 346*(8), 635–640. https://doi.org/10.1056/NEJM200202213460825

Rosenbaum, S. (2014). Medicaid payments and access to care. *New England Journal of Medicine, 371,* 2345–2347. https://doi.org/10.1056/NEJMp1412488

Rosenbaum, S. (2021, April 8). *Biden administration begins process of rolling back approval for Medicaid work experiments, but Supreme Court hangs on.* https://www.commonwealthfund.org/blog/2021/biden-administration-begins-process-rolling-back-approval-medicaid-work-experiments

Rosenbaum, S., Gunsalun, R., Rothenberg, S., & Schmucker, S. (2017, September 19). *Extending the Children's Health Insurance Program: High stakes for families and states.* https://www.commonwealthfund.org/publications/issue-briefs/2017/sep/extending-childrens-health-insurance-program-high-stakes

Rudowitz, R., Corallo, B., & Garfield, R. (2021, March 17). *New incentive for states to adopt the ACA Medicaid expansion: Implications for state spending.* https://www.kff.org/coronavirus-covid-19/issue-brief/new-incentive-for-states-to-adopt-the-aca-medicaid-expansion-implications-for-state-spending/

Rudowitz, R., & Garfield, R. (2018, April 12). *Ten things to know about Medicaid: Setting the facts straight.* https://www.kff.org/medicaid/issue-brief/10-things-to-know-about-medicaid-setting-the-facts-straight/

Rudowitz, R., Williams, E., Hinton, E., & Garfield, R. (2021, May 7). *Medicaid financing: The basics.* https://www.kff.org/medicaid/issue-brief/medicaid-financing-the-basics/

Ryan, J. (2009). *The Children's Health Insurance Program (CHIP): The fundamentals.* http://www.nhpf.org/library/background-papers/BP68_CHIPFundamentals_04-23-09.pdf

Social Security Act of 1935, Title XIX, 42 U.S.C. §1396 (1965).

Social Security Act of 1935, Title XIX, 42 U.S.C. §1901 (1965).

Social Security Act of 1935, Title XIX, 42 U.S.C. §1902 (1965).

Social Security Act of 1935, Title XIX, 42 U.S.C. §1936 (1965).

Social Security Act of 1935, Title XIX, 42 U.S.C. §1937 (1965).

Sokol, E. (2020, April 29). *Medicaid, CHIP amendments help states fight Covid-19 outbreak.* https://healthpayerintelligence.com/news/medicaid-chip-amendments-help-states-fight-covid-19-outbreak

Solomon, J., & Schubel, J. (2017, August 29). *Medicaid waivers should further program objectives, not impose barriers to coverage and care.* https://www.cbpp.org/research/health/medicaid-waivers-should-further-program-objectives-not-impose-barriers-to-coverage

Stewart v. Azar. 313 F.Supp.3d 237 (2018).

Stolyar, L., Hinton, E., Singer, N., & Rudowitz, R. (2021, June 24). *Growth in Medicaid MCO enrollment during the Covid 19 pandemic.* https://www.kff.org/coronavirus-covid-19/issue-brief/growth-in-medicaid-mco-enrollment-during-the-covid-19-pandemic/

The Commonwealth Fund Medicare Data Hub. (2020). *Solvency and spending* [slide 4]. https://www.commonwealthfund.org/medicare-data-hub-solvency-spending

U.S. Census Bureau. (2020, September). *Health insurance coverage in the United States: 2019* (Current Population Reports, P1–26). https://www.census.gov/content/dam/Census/library/publications/2020/demo/p60-271.pdf

Wallis, C. J., Poon, S. J., Lai, P., Podczerwinki, L., & Buntin, M. B. (2021). Trends in Medicare spending across strata of resource utilization among older individuals in the United States. *Lancet, 36,* 100873. https://doi.org/10.1016/j.eclinm.2021.100873

Wilensky, G. (2018, April 5). Will MACRA improve physician reimbursement? *New England Journal of Medicine, 378,* 1269–1271. https://doi.org/10.1056/NEJMp1801673

Endnotes

a. Puerto Rico, the U.S. Virgin Islands, Guam, Northern Mariana Islands, and American Samoa participate in Medicaid. However, financing rules are different in these territories than in the 50 states. Federal spending is capped and appropriated by Congress annually.

b. A special 5% adjustment allowed by law effectively brings the eligibility rate to 138% FPL.

c. Community health centers have their own per-visit prospective payment system for reimbursement under Medicaid.

d. Although federal law does not elaborate on the specifics of section 1115 waivers, other federal guidance does. In 1994, HHS prepared a nonbinding notice, "Demonstration Proposal Pursuant to Section 1115(a) of the Social Security Act," 59 Fed. Reg. 49249 (1994), and then the Health Care Financing Administration (now CMS) published "Review Guide for Section 1115 Research and Demonstration Waiver Proposals for State Health Care Reform." The *State Medicaid Manual* also contains information relating to Section 1115 waivers.

e. Because New Jersey and New York had already expanded coverage to children beyond 300% FPL prior to CHIPRA, those states are allowed to use their enhanced CHIP match up to their capped allotment.

CHAPTER 11

Health Reform and the Patient Protection and Affordable Care Act

LEARNING OBJECTIVES

By the end of this chapter you will be able to:

1. Describe previous national health reform attempts
2. Understand why national health reform has been difficult to achieve in the United States
3. Analyze why national health reform succeeded in 2010 when so many previous attempts had failed
4. Understand the key components of the Patient Protection and Affordable Care Act (ACA)
5. Understand the core rulings of multiple U.S. Supreme Court decisions related to the ACA
6. Evaluate the political climate regarding repealing and replacing the ACA, and understand the main features of legislation drafted toward that end
7. Discuss how the coronavirus pandemic has affected the U.S. healthcare system
8. Describe key issues going forward related to implementation of the ACA

Introduction

Over a decade after the Patient Protection and Affordable Care Act of 2010 (generally referred to as the Affordable Care Act or ACA) was passed, it finally appears safe to conclude that the ACA will remain the law of the land. Republicans were unable to repeal the law when they controlled Congress and the executive branch in 2017, Democrats found supporting the ACA to be a winning message in the 2020 elections, and in 2021 a conservative Supreme Court rejected a third attempt to strike down the law. While legal and political challenges to the ACA will surely continue, it seems the structure created by the ACA is now part of the fabric of the U.S. healthcare system.

The ACA is the most monumental piece of U.S. federal health policymaking in nearly 50 years. It reorders not only many aspects of the health insurance and healthcare delivery systems, but also long-standing relationships that underpin those systems. Over a decade in, there are clear successes, but there are also areas that need improvement. The ACA lowered the number of uninsured individuals in this country and increased access to care for millions of people. The ACA's expansion of the Medicaid program, in particular, increased coverage and access to care for vulnerable populations, reduced racial and ethnic disparities, and resulted in economic benefits for expansion states (Lantz & Rosenbaum, 2020; **Figure 11.1**). Another point is also clear: The ACA has flaws and even its

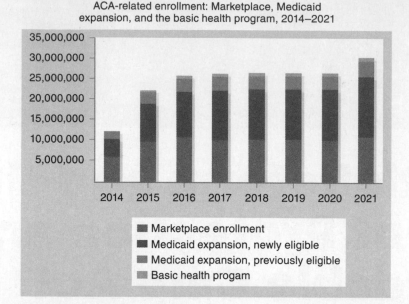

Figure 11.1 ACA Enrollment by Type of Coverage, 2014–2021

Assistant Secretary for Planning and Evaluation. (2021, June 5). *Health coverage under the Affordable Care Act: Enrollment trends and state estimates.* https://aspe.hhs.gov/system/files/pdf/265671/ASPE%20Issue%20Brief-ACA-Related%20Coverage%20by%20State.pdf

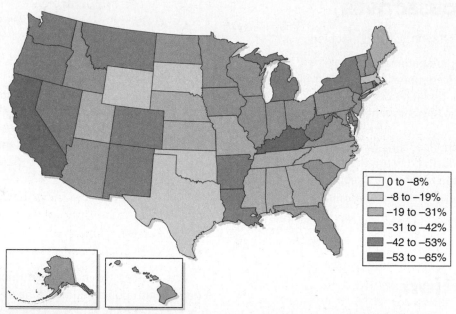

Notes: Percent change based on uninsured rate for the full population (all ages) in each state, comparing 2013 to 2019.

Figure 11.2 Relative Reduction in Uninsured Rate by State, 2013–2019

Assistant Secretary for Planning and Evaluation. (2021, June 5). *Health coverage under the Affordable Care Act: Enrollment trends and state estimates.* https://aspe.hhs.gov/system/files/pdf/265671/ASPE%20Issue%20Brief-ACA-Related%20Coverage%20by%20State.pdf

supporters recommend changes to improve afford-ability, increase access to care, strengthen insurance marketplaces, and contain healthcare costs (Blumberg et al., 2018a). Furthermore, the ACA's impact has not been uniform across the country due to state-level policy decisions. **Figure 11.2** shows the vast differences in changes to the uninsured rate since the ACA was implemented. Yet beyond the sheer scope and content

of the ACA and the policy trade-offs that led to its passage lies another story—its implementation and subsequent effects on the lives of tens of millions of Americans. Implementation of the ACA is an ongoing, dynamic process involving the federal government, states, employers, insurers, providers, patients, and others. In addition, there have been, and no doubt will continue to be, state and federal court decisions across the country that alter the trajectory of the law and its implementation.

The vignette in **Box 11.1** describes just a few of the competing viewpoints about the ACA and its role in creating a new and potentially more equitable health insurance system. As ACA implementation moves forward, bear in mind the many different ways that this round of health reform can be perceived and how it affects people differently.

The interplay between legal and political decisions makes it difficult to discern how implementation of the law will continue to be carried out. By way of example, the U.S. Supreme Court's landmark 2012 decision upholding the constitutionality of the ACA and its 2015 decision upholding subsidies to the federal insurance exchange provided through the ACA are described in the pages that follow, and

---

📝 Box 11.1 VIGNETTE

A group of friends were discussing the ACA, illustrating the wide-ranging viewpoints about the law. Katherine, whose friend Jadyn is struggling to make a living as a medical student is pleased that Jadyn has health insurance for the first time since graduating from college. Although Jadyn cannot stay on her parents' insurance because she just turned 27 years old, she can now afford a good health insurance plan that she found on her state's health exchange.

While Katherine has not noticed much of a change in her own health insurance coverage, which she obtains through her government employer, her cousin Mia is upset about health reform. She does not want the government forcing her to purchase health insurance (although she always chose to be insured in the past), and she recently found out that her old plan was cancelled because it did not meet the law's requirements. Mia found several new plan options to choose from, but none had her former plan's exact combination of benefits, providers, and price.

Katherine's uncle, Ethan, is 55 years old and self-employed. He purchases his health insurance on his state's exchange. Because he has preexisting conditions, he is grateful to be able to find a plan. Even so, Ethan's premiums will increase by 15% this year and his deductible is $5000, making health care difficult to afford even with insurance.

Katherine's husband, Calvin, thinks we should all be willing to pay a little more or change some aspects of our plans to help the millions of people who can now afford insurance for the first time as a result of the ACA. After witnessing her uncle's experience, however, Katherine is doubtful that the government will be able to keep its promises.

---

there remain many active ACA lawsuits, challenging everything from the ACA's contraceptive coverage mandate to its underpinning constitutionality. The practical consequences and legal rulings that actually manifest as a result of ACA implementation—not just the changes to American health care contemplated by Congress when they put pen to paper with the ACA—will, for years to come, need to be studied and understood by students across a range of disciplines, not just for academic purposes, but for healthcare and public health job market purposes as well.

Although there has been general agreement about the problems facing the U.S. healthcare system—high costs, high uninsured rates, health disparities, quality concerns—politicians and voters have disagreed about the best solutions. As a result, numerous attempts to pass national health reform legislation did not succeed. What was different in 2010? Why was Barack Obama's administration successful when several previous attempts had failed? This chapter begins with a discussion of why it has been so difficult to achieve broad health reform in the United States, and then examines the numerous failed attempts at national health reform made over the last century. Next, it analyzes how health reform was enacted in 2010, provides an overview of the law that eventually emerged, and covers the U.S. Supreme Court decision upholding its constitutionality. Finally, the discussion turns to the current political climate and what it means for health reform going forward, including a discussion of key political and implementation issues. Throughout this chapter we examine several key themes: choosing between state flexibility and national uniformity; determining the appropriate role for government, the private sector, and the healthcare financing and delivery entities; defining a primary decision-making goal (e.g., fiscal restraint, equity/social justice, improved health outcomes, uniformity); and settling on the appropriate scope of coverage to offer beneficiaries. In addition, we weave impacts of the COVID-19 pandemic through various discussions of health reform.

Difficulty Achieving Health Reform in the United States

The array of problems facing the U.S. healthcare system has led to numerous health reform proposals and implemented policies. The concept of *health reform* can be interpreted in several different ways. Given the patchwork health insurance system, health reform often refers to changes that seek to reduce the number of uninsured people. Due to the high and increasing cost of healthcare services, health reform might also include changes that seek to contain costs and control utilization. In addition, the notion of health reform could address other shortcomings, such as trying to reduce medical errors, strengthening patient rights, building the public health infrastructure, and confronting the rising cost of medical malpractice insurance. Unsurprisingly, the ACA touches on many of these issues.

We begin with a discussion of why health reform is difficult to achieve in the United States and then introduce some of the reforms that have been attempted, with varying degrees of success, on a national level. Numerous authors have addressed the main factors that deter significant social reform in this country, including health reform (Blake & Adolino, 2001; Gordon, 2003; Jost, 2004). Factors that are prominently discussed include the country's culture, the nature of U.S. political institutions, the power of interest groups, and path dependency (i.e., the notion that people are generally opposed to change).

Culture

This country's culture and lack of consensus about health reform have long impeded attempts to create universal coverage health plans. The twin concepts of entrepreneurialism and individualism have had a real impact on health policy decisions: Americans generally oppose government solutions to social welfare problems (Jost, 2004, p. 238). In addition, there is no agreement on the overall scope of the healthcare problems we face (Kaiser Family Foundation [KFF], 2008). Prior to the passage of the ACA, most Americans believed the extant health system needed major changes, yet 22% believed only minor changes were required and another

17% thought the system should basically stay the same (KFF, 2009a). Ten years later, a split exists even among Democrats and Democrat-leaning Independents, who are more likely to support health reform in general; during the 2020 presidential primary, 55% of these voters supported improving the ACA while 40% preferred the Medicare for All approach (Brodie et al., 2020).

Americans have a complicated and partisan view of the proper role of the federal government in the healthcare arena. In a 2019 survey, 53% of respondents indicated that the federal government has a responsibility to ensure healthcare coverage for all Americans (Dunn, 2019). While this is higher than the 47% who shared that view in 2010, at the height of the health reform debate (Newport, 2009), it is less than the 60% of respondents who felt that way in 2018 (Dunn, 2019). Of those who supported federal intervention in the 2019 survey, 27% reported they would like to see a single-payer system developed, while almost the same proportion (24%) preferred a mix of public and private payers (Dunn, 2019).

Interestingly, the COVID-19 pandemic has not (at least thus far) changed people's views. As of June 2020, there was no increase in those who preferred a single-payer plan or government leadership over private market actions in the areas of healthcare innovation, quality, and coverage (Swanson & Alonso-Zaldivar, 2020). This could be due to the public's generally negative view of federal government actions during the pandemic or "it simply could be a reflection of human nature to shelve ambitious schemes during a crisis" (Swanson & Alonso-Zaldivar, 2020, para. 9).

At the same time, there were stark differences of opinion regarding the government's role based on the respondents' political views (**Figure 11.3**). While 78% of Democrats and Democrat-leaning Independents

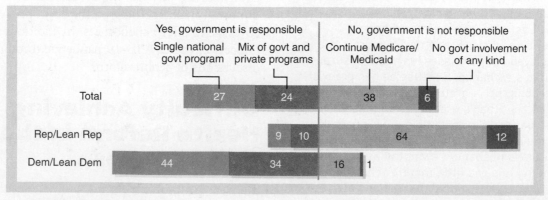

Note: Don't know responses not shown.

Figure 11.3 Democrats and Republicans Sharply Differ over Whether the Government Is Responsible for Ensuring That All Americans Have Healthcare Coverage

Dunn, A. (2019, July 26). *Democrats differ over best way to provide health coverage for all Americans.* Pew Research Center. https://www.pewresearch.org/fact-tank/2019/07/26/democrats-differ-over-best-way-to-provide-health-coverage-for-all-americans/

believed the federal government was responsible for ensuring healthcare coverage, only 19% of Republicans and Republican-leaning Independents agreed (Dunn, 2019). Even so, almost two-thirds (64%) of Republican/Republican-leaners supported the continuation of Medicaid and Medicare, the country's largest public health insurance programs. Furthermore, only 6% of all respondents thought the federal government should not have any role in ensuring healthcare coverage (Dunn, 2019).

It is accepted political dogma that it is difficult to take away benefits once they are established, and this has proven to be true with healthcare coverage (Steinhauer, 2017). The popularity of the ACA increased after the Republicans gained power in the 2016 elections and the threat of repealing the ACA became a realistic possibility. The ACA's favorability ratings passed 50% for the first time in 2017 and climbed slightly to 53% in 2021 (Brodie et al., 2020; KFF, 2021a). Furthermore, a majority of respondents opposed both the House (56% opposed; Magness, 2017) and Senate (55% opposed; Wynn, 2017) Republican replacement plans.

As shown in **Figure 11.4**, the partisan divide remains strong in relation to the ACA. A 2020 poll found that 85% of Democrats, 55% of Independents, and only 15% of Republicans held a favorable view of the ACA (KFF, 2021a). Similarly, a 2019 poll found that 76% of Democrats, 50% of Independents, and only 22% of Republicans did not want the Supreme Court to overturn the ACA (Kirzinger et al., 2019). While Republicans are more likely to oppose health reform, only 37% of Republicans say it is important to continue to try to repeal and replace the ACA (Cancryn, 2020). Despite this opposition, many of the ACA's major provisions (e.g., the health insurance exchanges, providing preventive services without cost-sharing, the Medicaid expansion) have had bipartisan support since its inception (Brodie et al., 2020; **Figure 11.5**). At the same time, regardless of political party, most people disliked the individual mandate from the beginning.

The public holds strong opinions about the ACA while also being misinformed about its contents. Despite being part of the healthcare landscape for a decade, fewer than half of respondents in one survey

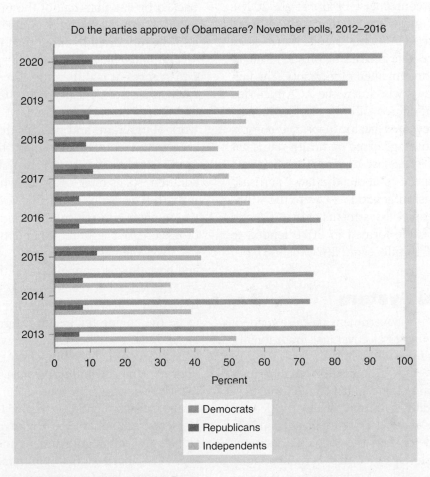

Figure 11.4 Approval of the Affordable Care Act, by Party

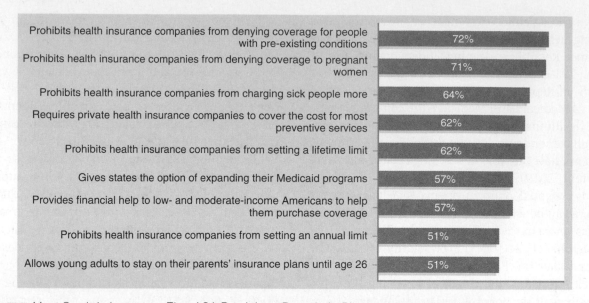

Figure 11.5 Most Say It Is Important That ACA Provisions Remain in Place

Kirzinger, A., Muñana, C., & Brodie, M. (2019, November 27). *6 Charts about public opinion on the Affordable Care Act.* Kaiser Family Foundation. https://www.kff.org/health-reform/poll-finding/6-charts-about-public-opinion-on-the-affordable-care-act

knew that the ACA would close the Medicare "doughnut hole," made it illegal for insurance companies to charge women more than men, or required insurance companies with high administrative costs to send premium rebates to consumers (Brodie et al., 2020). Furthermore, many individuals erroneously believed or were unsure if the ACA included end-of-life "death panels" for Medicare beneficiaries or provided financial assistance to undocumented immigrants. The percentage of respondents who knew the ACA included Medicaid expansion, offered subsidies to low-income individuals, and prevented health insurance companies from denying coverage based on health status has actually declined over the last 10 years (Brodie et al., 2020). Instead of specifics about the law, "partisanship and level of trust in government were the strongest predictors of people's assessments of the ACA and . . . the attitudes people formed in 2010 tended to become entrenched" (Brodie et al., 2020, p. 468).

U.S. Political System

The country's system of government has also made it difficult to achieve universal coverage. Traditionally, social welfare programs—including the provision of health care—have been the responsibility of the states. Initially, there was almost no federal involvement in the provision of health care, and when the federal government became more heavily involved in 1965, Medicaid continued to keep the locus of decision-making at the state level. Of course, certain populations, such as older adults (Medicare) and veterans (Veterans Health Administration), are covered by a

federalized health insurance system. However, support for federal involvement in health care depends on what language is used to describe the change. For example, "single-payer" or "socialized" health care was backed by less than half of the public in a 2019 poll, while "universal health coverage" and "Medicare-for-all" was supported by more than 60% (KFF, 2020).

Although states are generally home to social welfare changes, it is difficult to provide universal health care on a state-by-state basis. If state health reform efforts led the way, the country could have a patchwork of programs and policies that vary from state to state, with the potential to make health coverage even more complex and inefficient than it is currently. In addition, states must consider whether they are making policy decisions that will give employers an incentive to choose to relocate to another state with fewer or less onerous legal requirements. If employers leave the state, their departure could result in loss of jobs and have downstream effects on the state's economy.

The federal government also has resource advantages over states, making it easier for the federal level to be the engine for health reform. Individual states have a much smaller tax and revenue base than the federal government to draw from to implement health reform plans. In addition, once the federal government decides to tax a good or service, a state's ability to tax that same good or service is constrained by its residents' willingness and ability to pay a higher price. Unlike the federal government, most states have some type of balanced budget requirement (Garrett, 2011). While state legislatures may use accounting gimmicks and other maneuvers to avoid balanced budget requirements, states more often must make the difficult choices regarding resource allocation that federal policymakers often avoid (and thus generate enormous deficits). These restrictions, however, may help with reform efforts, by forcing states to a crisis point where a decision must be made to avoid an untenable situation. The federal government rarely reaches such a crisis point, which means tough decisions are often left for the next Congress, the next executive branch administration, or the next generation.

State reform efforts are also constrained by the Employee Retirement Income Security Act of 1974 (ERISA). ERISA is a federal law that regulates "welfare benefit programs," including health plans, operated by private employers. ERISA limits states' ability to undertake reform because (1) it broadly preempts state laws that "relate to" employer-sponsored plans, and (2) it applies to nearly all individuals who receive health benefits through a private employer. One effect of the law, for example, is that states have little regulatory control over the benefits covered in employer-sponsored health plans, because ERISA accords employers near-total discretion over the design of their benefit packages (Weissert & Weissert, 2002, p. 237).

Despite these hurdles, a health reform strategy that focuses on states has benefits as well. At its best, reform at the state level can be accomplished more rapidly and with more innovation than at the federal level. State legislatures may have an easier time convincing a narrower band of constituents important to the state than Congress has in accommodating the varied needs of stakeholders nationwide. Along the same lines, states are able to target reforms to meet the particular needs of their population, instead of covering more diverse needs across the entire country. Additionally, through the use of "direct democracy" (e.g., referenda, ballot initiatives), it is easier for citizens to have an impact on decisions made by state-level policymakers than those made by federal legislators. Finally, because the healthcare delivery system is run primarily on the state level, states have the expertise and ability to implement many parts of healthcare reform.

Some other aspects of the U.S. political system also make it difficult to institute sweeping reform. For example, although presidents have significant influence on setting the policy agenda and proposing budgets, they have limited power to make changes without the assistance of Congress. The federal government is often politically divided, with different parties holding power in the executive and legislative branches. This division frequently results in partisanship and policy inaction due to different policy priorities and views.

Furthermore, although members of Congress may ride the coattails of a popular president from their own party, they are not reliant on the president to keep their jobs. The issues and views that their constituents care about most may not align with the president's priorities. In those cases, members of Congress have a strong incentive to adhere to the wishes of the people who vote for them, instead of simply following the president's lead. Barring an overwhelming wave of discontent, as occurred in the 2010 midterm elections when Democrats suffered historic losses in Congress, it is usually difficult to unseat incumbents. Even when an unusual level of turnover occurs, reelection rates remain very high. Since 1990, there have been only two elections when fewer than 90% of House of Representatives incumbents successfully defended their seats (Murse, 2019). Even in the Senate, where turnover is relatively more common, on average 86% of incumbents have been reelected since 2000 (Center for Responsive Politics, n.d.). As a result, legislators in Congress may have confidence that they will retain their jobs when they put their district's or state's needs before those of the entire nation.

Federal legislative rules also support inaction or incremental reform over sweeping changes. In the Senate, 60 (of 100) votes are needed to break a filibuster in most cases. Thus, even the political party in the majority can have difficulty effecting change. In 2021, there were calls within the Democratic party to modify or eliminate the filibuster, as Republicans could block President Biden's agenda given the 50-50 split in the Senate. Those that supported changing the filibuster rule argued that the filibuster allows for minority rule and has been used historically to block civil rights legislation (Boston Globe, 2021). Others feared that without a tool for the minority to exert its influence, moderation and bipartisan compromise will be impossible to achieve (Segers, 2021)

One exception to the filibuster rule is the "reconciliation" process, which allows bills to pass with only 51 votes. Reconciliation is used as part of the budgetary process. Bills passed via reconciliation may not be filibustered (and so can pass with 51 votes), can pertain only to federal revenue and spending issues, must comply with spending and revenue targets set forth in the budget resolution, and must adhere to other budgetary rules (Tax Policy Center, n.d.). The reconciliation process is being increasingly used when one party maintains a slim majority and that party cannot find 60 votes to pass a bill. For example, the Democrats used a reconciliation bill to pass the ACA in 2010 after they lost their filibuster-proof majority. Likewise, the

Republicans attempted to use a reconciliation bill to pass their ACA repeal-and-replace bills. Also, because both the House and the Senate must pass bills containing the same policies and language to have any chance at becoming law, a large political majority in one chamber or the other does not guarantee the ability to enact a policy. As a result, members of Congress must often work together, at least to some degree, to devise a consensus policy that satisfies enough members to pass a bill. This need to build consensus makes radical change unlikely.

Interest Groups

Interest groups often influence the decisions of politicians. The role of interest groups is to represent their members' interests in policy decisions. These groups can be corporate for-profit entities or non-profit consumer-oriented organizations. They lobby politicians and the general public about the virtues or vices of specific proposals, work to improve proposals on the policy agenda, and attempt to defeat proposals they believe are not in the best interest of their group. By contributing to political campaigns or by helping to draw supportive voters out on Election Day, interest groups gain the ear, and often the influence, of politicians who vote on issues that are important to the group.

In terms of health reform, interest groups representing various providers, businesses, employer groups, insurance companies, and managed care organizations often have been opposed to comprehensive health reform (Jost, 2004, pp. 438–439). There are numerous points along the path—from developing a policy idea to voting for or against a bill—at which interest groups can attempt to affect politicians' views. The more radical the policy proposal, the more interest groups are likely to become engaged in the political decision-making process, making it difficult to pass a bill that includes comprehensive reform.

In general, it is easier to oppose a proposal than to develop one and pass a bill. Opponents of proposals are not required to provide a better alternative to whatever is on the table. Instead, they can simply point to aspects of the policy idea that are unpopular and call for the proposal to be rejected. This was the tactic used by the Health Insurance Association

of America in its well-known "Harry and Louise" television ads that opposed the Clinton administration's comprehensive health reform bill in 1993, the Health Security Act. In the ad, Harry and Louise, two "average" Americans, are seen discussing the healthcare system over breakfast. Although both agree the system needs to be improved, they highlight certain aspects of the Clinton plan that were particularly controversial, such as an overall cap on funds for healthcare needs and restrictions on provider choice. The tagline for the ad was, "There's got to be a better way" (West et al., 1996).

Similarly, before the 2016 elections, many Republicans promised to "repeal and replace" the health reform bill without specifying their favored replacement option. To be effective in opposing health reform, opponents did not have to propose an alternative that was scrutinized and compared with the existing proposal. Simply saying "the country can do better" was enough to help create significant opposition to the plan.

Path Dependency

The concept of path dependency has been another hindrance to major health reform. "The notion of path dependency emphasizes the power of inertia within political institutions" (Jost, 2004, p. 439). That is, once a certain way of doing things becomes the norm, it is hard to change course. Yet this theory does not mean that health reform is impossible. Inertia may be overcome at "critical moments or junctures" that open a window for change (Jost, 2004, p. 439). For example, the passage of Medicaid and Medicare in 1965 was a radical change from the past pattern of limited federal government involvement in health care. The catalysts for this change were the growing social pressure for improving the healthcare system and the landslide victory of Democrat Lyndon Johnson as president and of liberal and moderate Democrats in Congress.

The 1992 election of Democrat Bill Clinton, who ran on a platform emphasizing broad health reform, coupled with the Democratic majority in Congress (until 1994), also presented a window of opportunity. Although Clinton's plan was not ultimately successful, it appeared that the American public and politicians were open to changing the course of the healthcare "path" that had been taken to date. In 2010, another "critical moment" appeared, and President Obama took advantage of the circumstances to push through the health reform bill. Although path dependency suggests that inertia and fear of change have made broad reform difficult, it is not impossible to achieve.

Path dependency is also evident on the individual level; that is, once individuals are accustomed to having things a certain way, it is difficult for them to accept change. In 2010, prior to the passage of the ACA, approximately 84% of Americans had health insurance, most through employer-sponsored coverage (U.S. Census Bureau, 2010). It was assumed that comprehensive health reform would likely change the condition of the insured population to some degree by changing either their source of coverage, the benefits included in coverage, the cost of coverage, or some other factor. During the debate over the ACA, about one-third of people surveyed reported that the bill would probably make them worse off, and another third thought it would not make any difference to them (KFF, 2008). Professor Judith Feder (2004) refers to this problem as the "crowd-out" politics of health reform: "The fundamental barrier to universal coverage is that our success in insuring most of the nation's population has 'crowded out' our political capacity to insure the rest" (p. 461). In other words, many of the insured do not want a change in the healthcare system that will leave them worse off, even if it makes the uninsured better off.

According to Professor Feder, the way to solve the political crowd-out dilemma is by changing the very nature of American culture. The focus on individualism must be replaced with a concern for the community and recognition that all Americans are part of a single community. "The challenge to improving or achieving universal coverage is to decide whether we are a society in which it is every man, woman or child for him/herself or one in which we are all in it together" (Feder, 2004, p. 464). Clearly, the country remains divided about the extent to which "we are all in it together." Shortly before the ACA passed, more than half of people surveyed (54%) said they would not be willing to pay more so others could have access to health insurance (KFF, 2009b). The continued debate over the future of the ACA has highlighted fundamental disagreements about how our health system should be structured and the proper role of individuals and governments in ensuring the country's good health.

Unsuccessful Attempts to Pass National Health Insurance Reform

Since the early 1900s, when medical knowledge became advanced enough to make health care and health insurance desirable commodities, there have been periodic attempts to implement universal coverage through national health reform. The Socialist Party was the first U.S. political party to support health insurance in 1904, but the main engine behind early efforts for national reform was the American Association for Labor Legislation (AALL), a "social progressive" group that hoped to reform capitalism, not overthrow it (Starr, 1982, p. 243). In 1912, Progressive Party candidate Theodore Roosevelt supported a social insurance platform modeled on the European social insurance tradition that included health insurance, workers' compensation, old-age pensions, and unemployment insurance. After his loss to Woodrow Wilson, the national health insurance movement was without a strong national leader for three decades.

The AALL continued to support a form of health insurance after Roosevelt's defeat and drafted a model bill in 1915. This bill followed the European model, limiting participation to working-class employees and their dependents. Benefits included medical aid, sick pay, maternity benefits, and a death benefit. These costs were to be financed by employers, employees, and the state. The AALL believed that health insurance for the working population would reduce poverty and increase society's productivity and well-being through healthier workers and citizens.

Opposition to AALL's bill came from several sources (Starr, 1982, pp. 247–249). Although some members of the American Medical Association (AMA) approved of the bill conceptually, physician support rapidly evaporated when details emerged about aspects of the plan that would negatively impact their income and autonomy. The American Federation of

Labor (a labor union) opposed compulsory health insurance because it wanted workers to rely on their own economic strength, not the state, to obtain better wages and benefits. In addition, the federation was concerned that it would lose power if the government, not the union, secured benefits for workers. Employers were generally opposed to the bill, contending that supporting public health was a better way to ensure productivity. In addition, they feared that providing health insurance to employees might promote malingering instead of reducing lost workdays. After experiencing the high cost associated with workers' compensation, employers also were not eager to take on an additional expensive benefit. Of course, the part of the insurance industry that had already established a profitable niche in the death benefit business was strongly opposed to a bill that included a death benefit provision.

Employers, healthcare providers, and insurers have, in general, remained staunch opponents of national health reform over the years, while unions have supported national reform efforts. However, this dynamic has changed recently, with more provider groups, employers, and even some insurers calling for a national solution to the problems of rising healthcare costs and the number of uninsured.

The United States' entry into World War I in 1917 changed the tenor of the health reform debate. Many physicians who supported the AALL bill entered the military, shifting their focus away from the domestic health policy debate. Anti-German sentiment was high, so opponents of the bill gained traction by denouncing compulsory health insurance as anti-American. One pamphlet read as follows: "What is Compulsory Social Health Insurance? It is a dangerous device, invented in Germany, announced by the German Emperor from the throne the same year he started plotting and preparing to conquer the world" (Starr, 1982, p. 253).

The next time national health insurance might have taken hold was from the mid-1930s through the early 1940s, when the country was coping with the devastating effects of the Great Depression. During this time there was a significant increase in government programs, including the creation of Social Security in 1935, which provided old-age assistance, unemployment compensation, and public assistance. Yet the fourth prong of the social insurance package, health insurance, remained elusive. President Franklin Roosevelt heeded his staff's advice to leave health insurance out of Social Security because of the strong opposition it would create (Starr, 1982, p. 267). Opposition from the AMA was particularly strong.

The AMA believed that "socialized medicine" would increase bureaucracy, limit physician freedom, and interfere with the doctor–patient relationship.

Even so, members of Roosevelt's administration continued to push for national health insurance. The Interdepartmental Committee to Coordinate Health and Welfare Activities was created in 1935 and took on the task of studying the nation's healthcare needs. This job fell to its Technical Committee on Medical Care. Instead of supporting a federal program, the committee proposed subsidies to the states for operating health programs. Components of the proposal included expanding maternal and child health and public health programs under Social Security, expanding hospital construction, increasing aid for medical care for the indigent, studying a general medical care program, and creating a compensation program for those who lost wages due to disability.

Although President Roosevelt established a National Health Conference to discuss the recommendation, he never fully supported the medical care committee's proposal. With the success of conservatives in the 1938 election and the administration's concerns about fighting the powerful physician and state medical society lobbies, national health reform did not have a place on Roosevelt's priority list. Senator Robert Wagner (D-NY) introduced a bill that followed the committee's recommendations in 1939, and although it passed in the Senate, it did not garner support from the president or from the House.

World War II provided another opportunity for the opposition to label national health insurance as socialized medicine. But once the war neared an end, President Roosevelt finally called for an "economic bill of rights" that included medical care. President Truman picked up where Roosevelt left off, strongly advocating for national health insurance. President Truman's proposal included expanding hospitals, increasing public health and maternal and child health services, providing federal aid for medical research and education, and, for the first time, establishing a single health insurance program for all (Starr, 1982, p. 281). Heeding lessons from earlier reform failures, Truman emphasized that his plan was not socialized medicine and that the delivery system for medical and hospital care would not change.

Once again, the proposal for national health insurance drew strong opposition. The AMA vehemently rejected it, and most other healthcare groups opposed it as well. Although the public initially approved of it, there was no consensus about how national health insurance should be structured, and more people preferred modest voluntary plans over a national, compulsory, comprehensive health insurance program (Starr, 1982, p. 282). Additional opposition came from the American Bar Association, the Chamber of Commerce, and even some federal agencies concerned about losing control over their existing programs. In the end, only the hospital construction portion of the proposal was enacted.

When Truman won reelection on a national health insurance platform in 1948, it appeared the tide had turned. However, the AMA continued both its strong opposition and its attempts to link national health insurance to socialism. Congress considered various compromises but never reached a consensus. The public was uncertain about what kind of plan to favor. Employers maintained their opposition to compulsory insurance. In addition, one large group of potential supporters—veterans—was disinterested in the debate because they had already secured extensive medical coverage through the Veterans Administration. As the Korean War moved forward, Truman's focus shifted away from national health insurance and toward the war effort and other priorities.

National health insurance did not return to the national policy agenda until the 1970s. The landscape then was quite different from the Truman era. Medicaid and Medicare had been created, healthcare costs had begun to rise exponentially, and the economy was deteriorating. In 1969, President Richard Nixon declared that a "massive crisis" existed in health care and that unless it was fixed immediately, the country's medical system would collapse (Starr, 1982, p. 381). The general public seemed to agree, with 75% of respondents in one survey concurring that the healthcare system was in crisis (Starr, 1982, p. 381). Democrats still controlled Congress by a significant margin, and Senator Edward Kennedy (D-MA) and Representative Martha Griffiths (D-MI), the first woman to serve on the powerful House Committee on Ways and Means, proposed a comprehensive, federally operated health insurance system.

At the same time, support for broader health care and patient rights was gaining momentum. This movement advocated for rights to informed consent, to refuse treatment, to due process for involuntary commitment, and to equal access to health care (Starr, 1982, p. 389). The public was both anxious to obtain care and willing to challenge the authority of healthcare providers.

The Nixon administration's first attempt at health reform focused on changing the healthcare system's financing from one dominated by a fee-for-service system, which created incentives to provide more and more expensive services, to one that promoted restraint, efficiency, and the health of the patient. The result was a "health maintenance strategy" intended to stimulate the private sector to create health maintenance organizations (HMOs) through federal planning grants and loan guarantees, with the goal of enrolling 90% of the population in an HMO by the end of the 1970s (Starr, 1982, pp. 395–396). Ironically, group health plans, often labeled socialized medicine, had become the centerpiece of a Republican reform strategy.

Nixon's proposal included an employer mandate to provide a minimum package of benefits under a National Health Insurance Standards Act, a federally administered Family Health Insurance Program for low-income families that had a less generous benefits package than the one required by the National Health Insurance Standards Act, reductions in Medicare spending to help defray the costs, a call for an increase in the supply of physicians, and a change in how medical schools were subsidized. Opponents were plentiful, and ultimately this plan did not come to fruition. Some believed the plan was a gift to private insurance companies. Advocates for the poor were outraged at the second tier of benefits for low-income families. The AMA was concerned about HMOs interfering with physician practices and supported an alternative that provided tax credits for buying private insurance.

After the 1972 election, Nixon proposed a second plan that covered everyone and offered more comprehensive coverage. Private insurance companies would cover the employed and a government-run program would cover the rest of the population, with both groups receiving the same benefits package. Senator Kennedy and Representative Wilbur Mills (D-AR) supported a similar plan, and it appeared a compromise was close at hand. However, labor unions and liberal organizations preferred the original Kennedy plan and resisted compromising, in hopes of gaining greater power in the 1974 post-Watergate elections. Fearing the same political shift, insurance companies actually supported a catastrophic insurance plan proposed by Senator Russell Long (D-LA), believing it was better than any plan that would come out of a more liberal Congress after the elections. Once again, there was no majority support for any of the bills, and a national health insurance plan was not enacted.

Although President Jimmy Carter gave lip service to national health reform, he never fully supported a proposal. It was not until the election of Bill Clinton in 1992 that the next real attempt at national health insurance was made. The Clinton administration plan, dubbed the Health Security Act, was designed to create national health insurance without spending new federal funds or shifting coverage from private to public insurance. It relied on the concept of "managed competition," which combined elements of managed care and market competition.

Under the Health Security Act, a National Health Board would have established national and regional spending limits and regulated premium increases. "Health alliances" would have included a variety of plans that were competing for the business of employees and unemployed citizens in each geographical area. All plans were to have a guaranteed scope of benefits and uniform cost-sharing. Employers would have been required to provide coverage for their workers at a defined high level of benefits, and those with 5000 or fewer employees would have had to purchase plans through the health alliance. Subsidies were provided for low-income individuals and small businesses. Funding was to be provided from cost-containment measures that were reinvested. Forced by the Congressional Budget Office to provide an alternative funding strategy should the cost containment not create enough funds, the plan also included the option of capping insurance premium growth and reducing provider payments.

Like the national health insurance plans before it, the Health Security Act drew opponents from many directions. The health alliances were attacked as big government; employers resisted mandates and interference with their fringe benefits; some advocates feared that cost containment would lead to care rationing; the insured were concerned about losing some of their existing benefits or cost-sharing arrangements; older adults feared losing Medicare; and academic health centers were concerned about losing funds based on new graduate medical education provisions (Starr, 1982, p. 463). In addition, the usually strong support from unions was lacking because of an earlier disagreement with the president on trade matters. It is also generally accepted that the Clinton administration made several political mistakes that made a difficult political chore nearly impossible. In the end, the Health Security Act never made it to a vote in Congress.

⏱ The Stars Align (Barely): How the ACA Became Law

In many ways, 2010 was a very unlikely year to pass a national health reform plan. The ideological divisions in the country's populace had been growing ever

sharper, with the popular and electoral votes almost evenly split in both the 2000 and 2004 presidential elections. George W. Bush beat Al Gore despite losing the popular vote in 2000, and Bush beat John Kerry in 2004 with only 51% of the popular vote. Even though Barack Obama won the electoral vote in a landslide over John McCain (365 to 173), only 53% of the population voted for Obama in 2008 (Encyclopaedia Britannica, n.d.).

In addition to the ideological divide, a financial crisis erupted toward the end of the 2008 presidential election. In October 2008, President Bush signed into law the Emergency Economic Stabilization Act, which included the $700 billion Troubled Asset Relief Program (TARP) that allowed the federal government to take over distressed assets—primarily bad mortgage loans—from private financial institutions. It was argued that TARP was necessary to save the financial industry from collapsing, which could have led to another Great Depression. Even with TARP, the United States (and many other countries) entered into a recessionary period. Many individuals lived in homes they could no longer afford, banks limited lending opportunities, and employers laid off millions of workers due to the drop in consumer spending.

In an effort to improve the economy, Obama signed into law the American Recovery and Reinvestment Act of 2009, also known as the stimulus bill. This almost $800 billion effort was intended to save existing jobs, create new jobs, and spur long-term growth of the U.S. economy. Although TARP was not popular with politicians or the general public, it was seen as necessary by members of both political parties and signed into law by a Republican president. Unlike TARP, however, the stimulus bill was not a bipartisan effort. Republicans in the House unanimously opposed the stimulus bill, and only three Republicans voted for the bill in the Senate.

Not surprisingly, health care was not the sole issue on voters' minds during the election campaign. Shortly before the election, 43% of registered voters ranked the economy as their number one priority, with healthcare reform trailing by an almost two-to-one margin (Jones, 2010). Although voters from both political parties considered the economy to be their top priority, differences emerged along party lines regarding the next most important issue. Democratic voters ranked health care second, while both Republican and Independent voters were more concerned about the size and power of the federal government. These results were not surprising; Democrats had ranked health care as a higher priority than Republican and Independent voters in every presidential election from 1988 to 2016 (Blendon et al., 2008, p. 2053; Jones, 2010; Pew Research Center, 2016, section 4).

It was against this backdrop of a faltering economy, partisan differences, and the recent passage of two massive government spending bills that President Obama pursued a national health reform plan. Given the history of failed reform efforts, it would have been a major accomplishment to pass health reform in the best of times—and clearly this was not the best of times. How did Obama and the 111th Congress succeed? It was a combination of having commitment, exhibiting leadership, applying lessons from past failures, and being pragmatic that led to the passage of health reform.

Commitment and Leadership

It is highly unlikely that the 2010 health reform effort would have succeeded without a passionate and committed president willing to make health reform a priority. Health care has long been a priority for Democrats, and President Obama was no exception. Perhaps Obama's dedication to passing health reform stemmed in part from his personal experience: Obama's mother died of ovarian cancer, and he had seen her worry about paying her medical bills as much as beating the disease (Kornreich, 2007). Thus, for Obama, signing comprehensive health reform legislation into law would represent the opportunity to make sure others would not endure the same experience.

Some of Obama's political advisors suggested waiting to tackle health reform until after taking action to address the poor economy and rising unemployment. The economy was a top priority not just for Obama voters, but for *all* voters (Pew Research Center, 2008, section 3). Obama, however, felt the economy and health reform were intertwined:

> Some may ask how, at this moment of economic challenge, we can afford to invest in reforming our health care system. . . . I ask how we can afford not to. . . . If we want to overcome our economic challenges, we also must finally address our healthcare challenge. (Coll, 2008, para. 1)

Health reform efforts did not begin smoothly. President Obama initially wanted former U.S. Senator Tom Daschle to run both the Department of Health and Human Services (HHS) and the White House Office on Health Reform. It was thought that Daschle's experience in the Senate and relationships with legislators were the right combination to take the lead on health reform. When his nomination was derailed due to personal tax problems, it was not a good omen. As deliberations in Congress lagged, Democrats were not able to present a bill to President Obama before recessing for the summer. During the summer of 2009, members of Congress went home to their constituents and held town hall meetings to discuss health reform. Some of the meetings erupted in vocal opposition to health reform, and the media focused on these town hall meetings throughout the summer. Obama and the Democrats were criticized for losing the momentum for reform by letting the debate linger.

At the same time, there were several instances when the health reform effort appeared politically doomed, and President Obama's leadership made a clear difference in maintaining the momentum. Obama attempted to reclaim the upper hand on health reform with a speech to a joint session of Congress in September 2009. He memorably proclaimed, "I am not the first president to take up health reform, but I intend to be the last" (White House, 2009b). Although public support for health reform had been on the decline for several months, September 2009 polls showed that 62% still thought it was important to address health reform at that time, and 53% thought the country as a whole would be better off if health reform passed (KFF, 2009a). Less support existed for any specific congressional action, and two-thirds of Americans thought Congress did not have a "good understanding" of health reform issues (Newport, 2009, section 5).

In January 2010, an event occurred that some assumed was the death knell of health reform. In the 2008 elections, Democrats had made significant gains in Congress, earning a 59–41 majority in the Senate and a 257–178 majority in the House of Representatives. Furthermore, Senator Arlen Specter of Pennsylvania switched parties, giving Democrats the crucial 60th vote needed for a filibuster-proof majority. Although the numbers were now in their favor, President Obama, Senate Majority Leader Harry Reid (D-NV), and House Speaker Nancy Pelosi (D-CA) would have to balance the competing interests of conservative Democrats, who were concerned with having too much government intervention; progressive Democrats, who sought a public insurance option to compete with private companies; Blue Dog Democrats, who were most concerned with fiscal discipline; and pro-life and pro-choice factions, who would battle over whether and how abortion services would be included in any health reform bill.

Then, in August 2009, Senator Ted Kennedy (D-MA) died. In office for 47 years, Kennedy was not only a lifelong supporter of health reform but also an expert negotiator who could work with Republicans and possibly achieve a bipartisan consensus. The January 2010 special election to fill his seat was won by Republican Scott Brown, who campaigned against the Democrats' health reform plan. In a postelection poll, 42% of voters said they voted for Brown to stop health reform from moving ahead (Condon, 2010).

Despite this setback and concerns by some that health reform efforts should be abandoned, Obama, along with Reid and Pelosi, remained strong in his conviction to pursue reform. President Obama's senior advisors said it would be a "terrible mistake" to walk away from the process based on Brown's victory, and Pelosi reminded her caucus how detrimental it was when Democrats abandoned the health reform effort during the Clinton administration (Brown & O'Connor, 2010). In his 2010 State of the Union address, made just a week after Senator Brown claimed the special election, President Obama tied his health reform efforts to fixing the economy and reiterated his commitment to the issue:

> And it is precisely to relieve the burden on middle-class families that we still need health reform. Now let's be clear, I did not choose to tackle this issue to get some legislative victory under my belt. And by now it should be fairly obvious that I didn't take on health reform because it was good politics. . . . Here is what I ask of Congress though: Do not walk away from reform. Not now. Not when we are so close. Let us find a way to come together and finish the job for the American people. (White House, 2010)

Obama was not alone in providing leadership on health reform. Reid's and Pelosi's determination to see health reform succeed, and their skill in mobilizing and controlling their caucuses, were essential to the passage of the ACA. It is likely that health reform would not have passed without the adroit efforts of all three leaders working together. Even so, it is clear that the health reform effort would not even have begun without a president who put health reform at the top of the agenda and stuck with it despite the pitfalls and political opposition.

Lessons from Failed Health Reform Efforts

The Obama administration tried to avoid the types of events that had doomed earlier health reform efforts. Although the failed effort by the Clinton administration probably provided the most relevant lessons, Obama confronted some of the same obstacles that reformers had faced decades earlier. At times, President Obama was accused of learning some of the lessons too well, swinging the pendulum too far to the other side. Although that debate may continue, clearly the way in which the Obama administration applied those lessons brought him success where others had failed before him.

President Clinton was criticized for not moving quickly enough to try to enact health reform after he was elected in 1992. He did not present a plan to Congress until a year into his presidency, having been sidetracked by other issues such as the economy, including a budget showdown with Republicans, and whether gay people should be allowed to serve in the military. Even after he finally sent his healthcare proposal to Congress, Clinton was preoccupied with other issues that sapped his political capital, such as passing the North American Free Trade Agreement and the fallout from the deaths of 18 American soldiers in Somalia.

President Obama, over the objection of some aides, chose to address health reform as quickly as possible, despite also having to tackle the poor economy and possible collapse of the financial sector. Obama was elected to office with a 70% approval rating, and he moved to capitalize on his popularity (Saad, 2008). It was almost inevitable that his approval rating would decline as he shifted from the promise of a campaign to the reality of running the country. As Lyndon Johnson said after winning the 1964 election in a landslide, "Every day while I'm in office, I'm gonna lose votes" (Blumenthal & Morone, 2009, p. 172). In addition, it is almost universally expected that the president's party will lose seats in the midterm elections due to both lower voter turnout, which gives more clout to partisan voters, and a loss of popularity as the president moves from candidate to elected official (Wihbey, 2014). Obama was correct to assume his Democratic majorities in Congress would not last long. After the 2010 midterm elections, the Democrats lost control of the House and several seats in the Senate.

President Obama also dealt with interest groups in a different way from his predecessors. Previous failed efforts at health reform have shown that those vested interests can be important players in the debate. In general, although not in all instances, provider groups, insurers, and employers have opposed health reform, while unions have supported health reform efforts. All of these stakeholders have been known to devote significant resources and apply pressure on their representatives to support their point of view. During its reform effort, the Clinton administration warred with many stakeholder groups, with insurance companies and small businesses taking a leading role in the opposition to the Clinton proposal (West et al., 1996).

Obama took a different approach than Clinton, by making deals with various stakeholders at the outset of the health reform debate. The lure of millions of newly insured customers helped convince the Pharmaceutical Research and Manufacturers of America and the American Hospital Association to contribute to health reform financing through reduced Medicare and Medicaid payments. In addition, the health insurance industry supported universal insurance coverage under health reform. After being credited with helping derail the Clinton health plan, the Health Insurance Association of America favored the general idea of health reform, though it disagreed with Obama and the Democrats on some of the specifics. To be fair, Clinton may not have been able to broker deals with these stakeholders in the 1990s no matter how hard he tried. A combination of a changing healthcare environment, the likelihood that some type of health reform was likely to pass, and the uncertain future of employer-sponsored insurance made it more palatable for interest groups to try to influence—instead of oppose—the 2010 legislation (Oberlander, 2010).

Clinton was also criticized for failing to master the legislative process. The Clinton administration chose to design the health reform plan itself and developed a complicated and secretive process, headlined by the Health Care Task Force run by Hillary Clinton, to do so. Although naming Hillary Clinton as the leader of the task force signaled the administration's commitment to the issue, she became a lightning rod for criticism, and questions about the appropriateness of the First Lady taking on such a significant policy role detracted from the substance of the health reform debate. Instead of negotiating with Congress, the administration debated the specifics of health reform among its own advisors and then asked Congress to pass the bill they had developed. Shutting out members of Congress, instead of negotiating with them,

and taking over Congress's role in developing legislation was not, it turned out, a formula for success.

President Obama learned from Clinton's mistakes as well as from other presidents' legislative achievements. Instead of presenting a detailed plan or written legislation to Congress, success has often been found in outlining ideas and principles and letting Congress work through the details. When President Johnson was trying to get a Medicare bill passed, he told key members of Congress that he would not delve into the details of the bill but generally pushed for a larger package. When President George W. Bush was pursuing a new Medicare prescription drug benefit, he outlined his desire for an approach that worked with the private sector and encouraged competition, but let Congress find the exact formula that would pass (Morone, 2010, p. 1097).

Similarly, Obama set out his principles but left the work of drafting a bill and fleshing out the details to Congress. On June 2, 2009, he sent a letter to Senators Ted Kennedy and Max Baucus (D-MT), two leaders in the health reform effort, outlining his "core belief" that Americans deserved better and more affordable health insurance choices and that a health reform bill must not add to the federal deficit (White House, 2009a). Although he let the negotiators know what his priorities were, Obama stayed above the fray during the legislative process. While he preferred a public option to compete with private insurers, he did not insist on it. Although Obama campaigned against an individual mandate as a presidential candidate, he was open to including it in the bill. The president refused to be drawn into the debate over taxing generous health plans or creating a Medicare cost-containment commission. Instead, he focused his efforts on persuading Congress not to give up on the effort, bringing together various factions of the Democratic caucus, and reaching out to the public to garner support for health reform.

The legislative process for completing the bill was long, rocky, and ultimately partisan. The House of Representatives moved more quickly and with less fractious debate than did the Senate. Instead of having multiple House committees work on competing bills, as occurred during the Clinton administration, House Democratic leaders created a "Tri-Committee" bill jointly sponsored by Charles Rangel (D-NY), Henry Waxman (D-CA), and George Miller (D-CA), the chairmen of the House Ways and Means, Energy and Commerce, and Education and Labor (later renamed the Education and Workforce Committee) Committees, respectively. On November 7, 2009, the House passed its health reform bill with only two votes to spare, 220–215 (Affordable Health Care for America Act, 2009). Only one Republican voted for it, and 39 conservative Democrats voted against it. The bill from the then-more-liberal House contained several provisions that were likely to be rejected by the Senate: a public health insurance option to compete with private plans, a national health insurance exchange instead of state-based exchanges, more generous subsidies for low-income individuals, a broader expansion of Medicaid, and higher taxes on wealthier Americans.

Senator Baucus, the Finance Committee chairman, led the effort in the Senate. The legislative process he established was lengthy, and some observers believed he compromised on too many issues in an attempt to forge a bipartisan bill. For a time, Senator Charles Grassley (R-IA) actively participated in the health reform deliberations, and a few other Republican senators appeared willing to consider a bipartisan measure. Ultimately, however, a bipartisan agreement could not be reached. In a 2009 Christmas Eve vote, the Baucus bill passed 60–39, with all Democrats and two Independents voting for the measure and all Republicans voting against it (Patient Protection and Affordable Care Act, 2010).

Shortly after the New Year, members of the House and Senate began meeting to resolve the differences between the bills passed in the House and the Senate. Before those differences were resolved, however, Scott Brown was elected to fill Kennedy's seat in the Senate and the Democrats no longer had a filibuster-proof majority. Before the special election that led to Brown's victory, it was assumed that after the Senate passed a health reform measure, House and Senate negotiators would work out their differences in a conference committee, with each chamber then voting to pass the compromise bill. With Brown's election and his opposition to health reform, however, this plan became unworkable. Democratic congressional leaders were left with few options, all of them unpalatable: (1) The House could pass the Senate version of the bill; (2) Democrats could try to use the reconciliation process—which does not allow for the use of filibusters and requires only a simple majority vote—to pass a new comprehensive bill; (3) the House and Senate could compromise on a much smaller, more incremental health reform bill that focused on areas where a bipartisan agreement could be reached; or (4) Democrats could abandon their efforts to pass a health reform bill. The day after Brown's election, House Speaker Pelosi appeared to eliminate the easiest (legislatively speaking) of these paths by declaring that the House would not pass the Senate version of the bill: "I don't think it's possible to pass the Senate bill in the House. I don't see the votes for it at this time" (Barrett et al., 2010).

In the end, a compromise was reached. House and Senate leaders agreed to use the budget reconciliation process to amend the Senate bill. The House then passed the Senate version of the bill along with a companion reconciliation bill that amended certain aspects of the Senate bill. The reconciliation bill included more generous subsidies for individuals to purchase insurance than existed in the stand-alone Senate bill, the closure of the Medicare Part D doughnut hole, a tax on more generous insurance plans, changes to the penalties levied on individuals who did not buy insurance and on employers that did not offer insurance, and an increase in Medicare and investment taxes for higher earners. The Senate then passed the reconciliation bill. Once again, the final vote to approve the bills was along party lines. The House approved the Senate bill by a vote of 219–212, with all Republicans and 34 Democrats voting against it (Kahn, 2010). President Obama signed the bill into law on March 23, 2010 (Patient Protection and Affordable Care Act, 2010).

Some observers argue that Obama may have overlearned the lesson about working with Congress and that in doing so, he did not provide enough guidance to legislators and allowed the debate over health reform to linger for too long (Morone, 2010, p. 1097). On the one hand, it is difficult to criticize Obama's approach because he was ultimately successful. On the other hand, could the problems stemming from the 2009 town halls and Scott Brown's election have been avoided, and would public opinion of the health reform effort have been higher, if the process had been better managed? Only time will tell whether Obama was successful over the long term (e.g., Is the law effective? Will the public support it over time? Will it be repealed?) and whether the political cost of the lengthy battle hurt the Democrats more than passing the bill helped them.

Political Pragmatism

President Obama is both credited and criticized for being as pragmatic as necessary to help ensure that a health reform law came to fruition. He was comfortable making deals with industry stakeholders, even though those agreements limited the savings and other changes that could have been achieved in the health reform bill. Obama ultimately signed a bill that did not include a public option, even though he preferred that one be included, and his liberal base thought health reform without such an option was not true reform.

An argument over abortion nearly derailed the bill in its final days, and Obama supported a compromise on abortion language to keep enough Democrats in the fold. Even his goal of creating universal insurance coverage was not recognized. Yet Obama's willingness to be pragmatic instead of staunchly principled, taking some victories instead of an all-or-nothing approach, allowed him to succeed in passing a health reform bill where others had failed (Oberlander, 2010, p. 1116). Some people argued that it was worse to pass a flawed bill than not pass a bill at all, but Obama believed that the promise of reducing the uninsured rate and gaining numerous health insurance market reforms were worth the compromises he made.

Overview of the ACA

As noted earlier, while President Obama left the details of health reform legislation to Congress, he set forth what he believed to be the most important principles that should guide the legislation's development. Soon after becoming president in 2009, Obama delineated those principles, saying that any health reform measure should do the following:

1. Protect families' financial health (by slowing the growth of out-of-pocket expenses and protecting people from bankruptcy due to catastrophic illness).
2. Make health insurance coverage more affordable (by reducing administrative costs, wiping out unnecessary tests and services, and limiting insurers' ability to charge higher premiums for certain populations).
3. Aim for insurance coverage universality.
4. Provide portability of insurance coverage.
5. Guarantee choice of health plans and providers (including keeping current ones).
6. Invest in disease prevention and wellness initiatives.
7. Improve patient safety and healthcare quality.
8. Maintain long-term fiscal sustainability (by reducing cost growth, improving productivity, and adding new revenue sources).

The extent to which these principles were brought to life in what eventually became the ACA falls along a spectrum. For example, health insurance was absolutely made more affordable for millions of people; disease prevention and wellness initiatives seem to be gaining momentum, although slowly; and universal insurance coverage was absolutely not achieved. Whatever the case with any particular principle, it is instructive to look to four key reforms that became law under the ACA as having paved the way for President Obama's overall vision to come to fruition. These four reforms essentially reordered long-standing relationships among health system stakeholders, including individuals, providers, insurers, employers, and governments. As a result of this reordering, all of these stakeholders were legally obligated to alter normative behaviors.

The first major change, known as the individual mandate, is a requirement that individuals either maintain "minimum essential health coverage" (i.e., health insurance) or face the financial penalties that are spelled out in the ACA. This requirement was thought to be a critically important beam in the ACA architecture because it created a new, large pool of individuals who pay premiums to insurance companies, and it created leverage for policymakers who were eager for the private insurers to accept many of the ACA's other insurance reforms that might have otherwise been unpalatable. For certain individuals whose socioeconomic status makes it impossible for them to purchase (or gain through an employer) the type of minimum coverage mandated by the ACA, and who do not qualify for Medicaid (even under the ACA expansion), federal subsidies are made available under the law. As discussed in more detail later in this chapter, in 2017 Congress repealed the penalties associated with the individual mandate as part of the Tax Cut and Jobs Act.

The second fundamental change results from reforms that prohibit or curtail existing health insurer and health plan practices. These are the types of reforms that all insurers—not just those that sell products through the new exchanges, described in the following paragraph—were forced to accept to reciprocate for the new group of premium payers whom they would insure as a result of the individual mandate. For example, the ACA prohibits insurers from considering an applicant's preexisting conditions when determining whether to insure the applicant, guarantees the renewability of an individual's existing insurance plan, requires insurers to cover certain preventive and immunization services, and guarantees coverage for dependent children who are 26 years or younger. The Trump administration has weakened this important aspect of the ACA by providing options for health insurers to provide plans that do not meet all of these requirements.

The third key change is the creation of health insurance "exchanges" or "marketplaces" in each state. These are essentially online shopping sites, intended to make it easier for individuals and small employers to compare and purchase health insurance. Because the

ACA requires everyone to carry health insurance, and because the insurance marketplace has not historically been easy to navigate, policymakers forced the creation of regulated state-based exchanges to help with the purchase of individual and small-group insurance plans.

The final major reform is expansion of the existing Medicaid program (this is discussed in detail in Chapter 10, "Government Health Insurance Programs: Medicaid, CHIP, and Medicare"). This reform has the potential to dramatically increase the number of individuals who can gain access to insurance coverage—and thus access to better and more appropriate health care. Because states cannot be forced to implement this expansion (more on this later in the discussion of the U.S. Supreme Court's decision regarding the constitutionality of the ACA), and because many states have thus far declined to implement the expansion, this potential has yet to become a reality.

Although the ACA does not completely alter the way health insurance is provided by, say, establishing a single-payer system or even a large government-run insurance plan to compete with private insurers, the law makes significant philosophical and practical changes in how health insurance is regulated, structured, and administered in the United States. Indeed, as a result of the reforms and reordering just described, the ACA resulted in 20 million people gaining insurance between 2010 and 2020 (Goodnough et al., 2020). Given the expected increase in uninsured rates without the ACA, it is estimated that 30 million more people were insured in 2020 than had been forecasted in 2009 (Glied et al., 2020). The uninsured rate dropped from 16% in 2010 to 11.1% in early 2017 (Blumberg et al., 2018b). In 2018, however, the uninsured rate rose for the first time in a decade. Nearly 2 million more people reported being uninsured in 2018, and 400,000 children lost coverage between 2016 and 2018 (Galewitz, 2019; Goodnough et al., 2020). These losses are due largely to a sharp decline in Medicaid coverage and a high rate of coverage loss among noncitizens. The downturn is likely due to policies and processes that created barriers to enrolling in and maintaining Medicaid coverage, a reduction in outreach and enrollment funding, and immigration-related policy changes made during the Trump administration (Finegold et al., 2021). As of the time of this writing, the COVID-19 pandemic did not appear to significantly alter the uninsured rate because more individuals enrolled in Medicaid, the ACA provided options for those who lost job-related coverage, many of the newly unemployed were already uninsured, and some employers furloughed employees instead of firing them so the employees could retain benefits (Finegold et al., 2021). In addition, as a result of the essential health benefits requirement, a large segment of the population is no longer underinsured because their insurance plans do not offer comprehensive benefits.

Even so, many people contend that the ACA falls short in its reform of the healthcare delivery system. In many cases they are correct. The ACA is most notable for the transformations it makes to health insurance—both access to it and its content—rather than for structural reforms made to the delivery system. Many provisions that focus on improving the healthcare delivery system, increasing the quality of care received by patients, reducing healthcare costs, and incentivizing providers to reconsider traditional methods of delivering care often exist in the form of temporary pilot programs that may never be enacted permanently, even if they prove to be valuable. Other analysts contend that these provisions were written as strongly as they could be at the time, given the political environment and the data available to policymakers. According to this view, the ACA provides the secretary of HHS with unprecedented authority to make the pilot programs permanent, and it would have been irresponsible to implement more permanent, wholesale changes without more evidence supporting their effectiveness. Not surprisingly, analyses of various demonstration projects and reforms show mixed results. Some programs may have reduced cost and increased quality, while often resulting in modest changes (Lewis et al., 2020). Ideally, policymakers will continue to learn from and improve upon the results of these attempts to reform the healthcare payment and delivery system. In any case, as sweeping as the ACA is, it most certainly is not the last step that needs to be taken to improve how health care is provided in the United States.

Even though the ACA appears safe from legislative repeal or judicial demise, opportunities remain to expand or restrict the law's effect on the health system. The American Rescue Plan Act (ARPA) of 2021 made changes to the law that are discussed later in this chapter (Pub. L. 117-2). However, the bill that eventually became law only passed Congress by use of the reconciliation process. Given the closely divided Congress and lack of consensus about how to improve the ACA, future changes are likely to come via administrative action. The Trump administration demonstrated the significant impact the executive branch can have on the law. Examples include shortening the enrollment period, reducing navigator and advertising funding, expanding the contraception accommodation rules, increasing the opportunity to offer plans that are exempt from ACA requirements, and removing antidiscrimination provisions (Center on Budget and Policy Priorities, 2021). Early in its term, the Biden administration focused on expanding access, protecting individuals with preexisting conditions, limiting plans that do not have to meet ACA requirements, creating a special enrollment period, and increasing outreach and education funding (Keith, 2021b; Sheen, 2021)

Individual Mandate

An individual mandate is a requirement that individuals purchase health insurance. This is not a new idea. President Clinton proposed an individual mandate in 1993 as part of his Health Security Act, and other competing proposals at the time, including those supported by Republicans, also included an individual mandate. Massachusetts, the only state in the country to require, prior to passage of the ACA, that everyone older than 18 years have health insurance, included an individual mandate as one way to achieve that goal. A number of other countries, including the Netherlands, Switzerland, Germany, Japan, and Australia, have some form of an insurance mandate in their healthcare systems (Eibner & Nowak, 2018). During the 2008 election, Obama originally supported a mandate for children to be covered but suggested waiting to see if a mandate was necessary for adults after implementing other major health reform changes.

Even though the individual mandate *penalty* was repealed as of 2019, the mandate itself is still part of the ACA. It is important to understand the mechanics and policy issues relating to the individual mandate because it explains some of the animosity toward the ACA, provides insights into why policymakers made certain decisions, and could be reinstated in the future. President Biden has already asserted that he supports restoring the individual mandate penalty (Bursztynsky, 2019; see **Box 11.2** for a related discussion question).

While the individual mandate is not a new idea and has been championed by both Republicans and Democrats at different times in history, it has proved to be a politically perilous route to reducing the number of

Box 11.2 DISCUSSION QUESTIONS

Are there alternatives to the individual mandate that accomplish the same goals without engendering so much political turmoil? Could policymakers have designed an incentive system that would be as effective as a mandate? What are the pros and cons of using a mandate versus an incentive? Can you think of incentives to encourage enrollment that have occurred in other parts of the healthcare system? If you were President Biden, would you support reinstating the individual mandate penalty? Do you think the benefits would be worth the political risks?

uninsured. Opposition to the individual mandate has remained steady at 63% to 64% over the last several years (Kirzinger et al., 2019). In general, Republicans are more likely to oppose the individual mandate than are Democrats (Agiesta, 2017). In 2019, only about half (54%) of adults knew the individual mandate penalty had been eliminated. Of the uninsured adults who were aware of the change, 24% chose not to purchase insurance because there was no penalty, which translated to 11% of all uninsured adults (Collins & Gunja, 2019). It appears that some individuals prefer not to be told they have to purchase health insurance by the government, even if it is a choice they made on their own prior to the passage of the ACA.

Affordability has been, and continues to be, the main reason that people do not purchase insurance. In a poll conducted shortly after the first ACA enrollment period closed, most people who remained uninsured cited affordability (39%) or job-related reasons (22%) for that decision, while only 9% said that they did not want or need health insurance (Hamel et al., 2014). A decade later, the situation is unchanged. Of adults who visited a marketplace to look for insurance plans in 2019 but did not purchase one, more than half (51%) cited affordability as the reason for remaining uninsured, while only 4% decided they did not need coverage (Collins & Gunja, 2019). Understandably, affordability remains a top issue for the public, with prescription drugs, out-of-pocket costs, and surprise medical billing ranking as primary concerns (Brodie et al., 2020). In a recent study, almost 60% of those surveyed were worried about not being able to afford healthcare services in the future (Brodie et al., 2020).

Individual mandates can be set up in a variety of ways, but usually individuals who do not comply are required to pay some sort of penalty. The penalty is intended to provide both an incentive to comply with the law and a means to raise funds to cover the cost of health care for those individuals who choose not to carry health insurance. Individual mandates are considered to be a cornerstone of health reform efforts because they ensure that everyone subject to the mandate will be in an insurance pool to help cover costs and share risk.

Starting in 2014, the ACA's individual mandate required that almost everyone purchase health insurance or pay a penalty. This penalty was phased in over time, beginning at the greater of $95 or 1% of taxable income per person in 2014, and growing to the greater of $695 or 2.5% of taxable income per person in 2016 and 2017. In subsequent years, the penalty amount would have increased through cost-of-living adjustments. The maximum penalty is the cost of the national average bronze plan sold through the marketplace.

The mandate was considered essential because without it, people who are in poor health or otherwise expect to use more healthcare services would be more likely to purchase health insurance, while healthier people would be more likely to opt out of insurance coverage. This situation would lead to an insurance pool that is relatively sick and thus more expensive, a problem referred to as *adverse selection*. Adverse selection leads to a "death spiral" as the insurance pool gets continually sicker and more expensive, encouraging more healthy people to opt out of coverage.

While the exact impact of the recent decision to remove the penalties associated with the individual mandate remains uncertain, it is generally agreed that both the uninsured rate and premiums will increase due to adverse selection. Estimates of the extent of those effects vary significantly (Fiedler, 2020), and early returns have shown little impact on the individual insurance market (Fehr et al., 2020). At least in the first year after elimination of the mandate, the individual insurance market remained stable, without a significant increase in premiums or a marked decrease in health-care insurance enrollees (Fehr et al., 2020). Given the concerns about the possible negative effect of eliminating the individual mandate, 11 states have passed state-wide individual mandates in 2021 (ACAwise, n.d.).

Some policy experts consider the ACA's mandate to be too weak to be effective in any event, thus reducing, in their view, the impact of eliminating the penalties. In 2016, 6.5 million people paid an average fine of $70 for lack of coverage (Scott, 2018). Under the ACA, the penalties may not have been significant enough, or the premium subsidies generous enough, to compel people to buy insurance. In addition, the United States does not enforce the mandate as vigorously as other countries do (Scott, 2018).

Due to fears of adverse selection, analysts have been closely watching how many young adults (ages 18–34 years), who are more likely to be healthy, sign up for health insurance. Ideally, 40% of enrollees would be in this age range to prevent adverse selection. Only about 25% of the 11 million enrollees who signed up at the end of the 2019 enrollment period in were young adults, which is similar to the young adult enrollment rate from the ACA's first enrollment period (Galewitz, n.d.; Gunja et al., 2019). Even as overall insurance enrollment grew in 2020—mostly due to growth in Medicaid—the proportion of young adults enrolled in coverage remained stable (Keith, 2020b) Despite not reaching the ideal level of enrollment to prevent adverse selection, young adults experienced a dramatic reduction in their uninsured rate from 2010 to 2019, with this rate falling from 33.8% to 15.6% for 19- to 25-year-olds and from 27.8% to 16.1% for 26- to 34-year-olds (Elflein 2021; Gunja et al., 2019). As with other populations, the uninsured rate for young adults increased after 2016 (Gunja et al., 2019; **Figure 11.6**).

The individual mandate is also an essential feature of health reform because healthy individuals who choose not to purchase health insurance but then later need health care will likely receive some care even though they are uninsured. This is especially true if the individuals have the resources to pay for health-care services. These individuals are referred to as *free riders* because they avoid paying premiums for health insurance during their healthy years, but then enjoy the benefits of healthcare services when they become sick. In 2018, more than 8 million people who earned more than $75,000 per year were uninsured (U.S. Census Bureau, 2019). Because it is likely that many of these

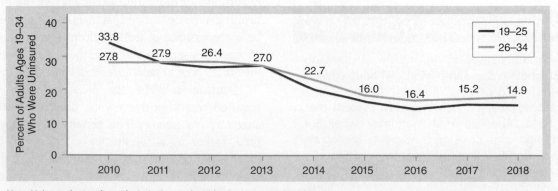

Note: Uninsured rates do not include those whose insurance status is unknown.
Data: Commonwealth Fund analysis of National Health Interview Survey (2010–2018).

Figure 11.6 Percentage of Adults Ages 19–34 Years Who Were Uninsured

Reproduced from Gunja, M. Z., Aboulafia, G. N., & Collins, S. R. (2019, October 31). *What young adults should know about open enrollment*. To the Point [blog]. Commonwealth Fund. https://doi.org/10.26099/va8n-cw45

individuals could have afforded to purchase health insurance, some analysts consider this evidence of the free-rider problem.

Politically, the individual mandate was essential to passing the ACA because it was the carrot that enticed health insurers to support health reform. The ACA includes a prohibition against excluding individuals who have preexisting conditions as a way to make health insurance available for those with health needs. Health insurers would have balked at being forced to enroll sicker individuals without a mandate intended to draw healthier consumers into the insurance plans as well. In addition, the mandate guaranteed new premium dollars from the new enrollees. Given that—thus far, at least—the repeal of the individual mandate penalty has had minimal effects, it is possible that the individual mandate will be best remembered for getting the health insurers on board at the outset.

A number of exceptions to the individual mandate requirement were specified in the ACA (**Box 11.3**). Some have criticized the exemptions for being so broad as to swallow the individual mandate, while others believe the exemptions will have minimal impact (Andrews, 2018). Of course, individuals have less incentive to apply for an exemption as long as the penalty remains repealed.

To some, the individual mandate remains controversial. In addition to believing that it represents unwarranted government intrusion into private decision-making, opponents of the individual mandate argued after the ACA was passed that Congress did not have the legal authority to impose such a requirement. This argument is grounded in jurisprudence relating to the U.S. Constitution's Commerce Clause, which gives Congress the power to "regulate commerce with foreign nations, and among the several states, and with the Indian tribes" (U.S. Constitution, article I, § 8). Since the 1940s, the Supreme Court has interpreted the Commerce Clause to permit Congress to regulate economic activity that carries across state lines or local concerns that substantially affect interstate commerce, and several Commerce Clause cases have allowed the regulation of individual conduct. For example, the U.S. Supreme Court has upheld laws that prohibit an individual from refusing to interact with a minority and laws that regulate an individual's ability to grow wheat or marijuana for home consumption (*Heart of Atlanta Motel v. United States*, 1964). Moreover, the regulation of health insurance has been deemed within the scope of the Commerce Clause (*Gonzales v. Raich*, 2005; *Wickard v. Filburn*, 1942).

Box 11.3 Technical Spotlight

Individual Mandate Exemptions

Individuals are exempt from purchasing insurance if their income is below the tax-filing threshold (in 2020, this amount was $12,200 for single people younger than 65 years and $24,400 for couples younger than 65 years), the lowest-cost plan option exceeds 8.24% of their income in 2020, they qualify for a religious exemption, they are incarcerated, they are undocumented immigrants, they were without coverage for less than 3 months, they are Native Americans, or they qualify as having a hardship. Based on a June 2013 HHS rule, hardship exemptions must be granted for individuals who experience an event that resulted in an unexpected increase in expenses such that purchasing health insurance would make it impossible to pay for necessities, such as food and shelter. The rule cites circumstances that would be considered under this exemption: homelessness, eviction, domestic violence, death of a close family member, bankruptcy, substantial recent medical debt, and disasters that substantially changed the individual's property (Exchange Establishment Standards, 2012). Hardship exemptions are also allowed for individuals who would have qualified for Medicaid had their state chosen to expand the program under the ACA, and other exemptions exist based on projected low income (Jost, 2013). In 2018, the Trump administration created four new exemption categories (Center for Consumer Information and Insurance Oversight, 2018; HHS Notice of Benefit and Payment Parameters [HHS Benefit and Payment Rule], 2018). Individuals may apply for a hardship exemption if they (1) live in counties without marketplace plans, (2) live in counties with a single insurer, (3) object to abortion coverage, or (4) meet additional hardship circumstances, such as needing specialty care from out-of-network providers (Andrews, 2018).

Data from Andrews, M. (2018, April 24). *4 New exemptions to the tax penalty for lacking health insurance*. NPR. https://www.npr.org/sections/health-shots/2018/04/24/605007498/4-new-exemptions-to-the-tax-penalty-for-lacking-health-insurance; Center for Consumer Information and Insurance Oversight, Centers for Medicare and Medicaid Services. (2018, April 9). *Guidance on hardship exemptions from the individual shared responsibility provision for persons experiencing limited issuer options or other circumstances.* https://www.cms.gov/CCIIO/Resources/Regulations-and-Guidance/Downloads/2018-Hardship-Exemption-Guidance.pdf; HHS Notice of Benefit and Payment Parameters for 2019. 83 Fed. Reg. 74, 16930–17071 (2018, April 17); and Exchange Establishment Standards and Other Related Standards Under the Affordable Care Act, 177 Fed. Reg. 11718, 2012.

Notwithstanding these cases, those who argued against the individual mandate contended that the Commerce Clause does not permit Congress to require an individual to purchase a service or good such as health insurance. In other words, the argument goes, an individual's decision not to purchase health insurance cannot be considered "economic activity" that Congress may regulate. Instead, it is argued, Congress is trying to regulate economic *inactivity*—the decision *not* to purchase health insurance—and that this is not permitted under the Commerce Clause (Shapiro, 2010).

In contrast, those who contend that the Commerce Clause permits Congress to establish an individual mandate to purchase health insurance argue that everyone uses healthcare services at some point in their lives. Decisions regarding health insurance are an economic activity because no one can opt out of the healthcare market; that is, the decision individuals make is not *whether* to participate but rather *how* to participate in it. People can participate by purchasing health insurance now to cover the cost of future services or by paying out-of-pocket later at the time services are needed.

In the end, the Supreme Court upheld the individual mandate as a valid exercise of congressional *taxing* power; the court did, however, agree with those who maintained that the mandate was not permitted under the Commerce Clause. This outcome is described more fully later, when we provide an overview of the Supreme Court's June 2012 ruling on the constitutionality of the ACA.

State Health Insurance Exchanges/Marketplaces

The ACA established a new series of entities called health insurance exchanges (also referred to as "marketplaces" in federal documents) that are intended to create a more organized and competitive market for purchasing health insurance. These state-based exchanges are geared toward those consumers who purchase health insurance as individuals (through American Health Benefit Exchanges) or through small businesses (through the Small Business Health Options Program [SHOP]). (See **Box 11.4** for details about a public option, an idea Congress rejected before settling on state exchanges.)

The SHOP exchange struggled from the start, with implementation delays and much lower than anticipated enrollment rates (Aron-Dine, 2017). Subsequently, the Trump administration announced a rule that effectively ended the federally facilitated SHOP

⊛ Box 11.4   Special Topic

Public Option

There was a lengthy debate about whether to include a public option in health reform. A public option is some type of government-run health plan that would be available to compete with private plans. A public option could exist either within the health exchange model or outside of it. Instead of a public option, Congress voted to require the Office of Personnel Management, which runs the Federal Employees Health Benefits program, to contract with at least two multistate plans in every state health insurance exchange. While President Biden has voiced support for a public option, it has not been a top priority to date and is unlikely to be politically feasible at the federal level (Lieberman, 2021).

States are stepping into the gap left by federal policy. As of June 2021, three states (Colorado, Nevada, and Washington) have created a public option with the hope of reducing healthcare costs. While each state public option varies in the details, the general idea is the same. In the state version of a public option, states contract with private companies to create new insurance options that are regulated by the state government. Public option plans sell products in the ACA marketplace and follow ACA private insurance rules.

In state public option plans, costs are lowered by requiring premiums that are lower than the state exchange benchmark plan and linking provider reimbursement to Medicare or Medicare-plus-a-percentage, instead of using higher private insurance rates. Of course, providers may balk at joining a plan with lower reimbursement, so states must find ways to incentivize participation. In Nevada, for example, insurers that offer Medicaid managed care plans also need to participate in the public option. Similarly, Nevada providers who accept Medicaid, workers' compensation, or the state employee health plan must also accept the public option plan. States would prefer to keep the savings to reinvest in their healthcare systems and are requesting federal waivers to do so.

What are the pros and cons of having a public option? Does the Office of Personnel Management compromise achieve all or some of the goals of having a public option? Why do you believe the Office of Personnel Management compromise was acceptable to legislators but the public option was not? Is it preferable to have public options developed at the state level? What are the pros and cons of a state versus federal public option?

Data from Scott, D. (2021, June 17). *The public option is now a reality in three states.* Vox. https://www.msn.com/en-us/news/politics/the-public-option-is-now-a-reality-in-3-states/ar-AAL9ac; Lieberman, T. (2021, June 16). *Is Biden opting out of a 'public option' for the Affordable Care Act?* Center for Health Journalism. https://centerforhealthjournalism.org/2021/06/15/biden-opting-out-public-option -affordable-care-act; and Luhby, T. (2021, June 7). *Biden has paused a public option. Nevada is about to try its own.* CNN. https://www.cnn.com/2021/06/07/politics/public-option-nevada-biden/index.html

exchange as of January 2018 (HHS Notice of Benefit and Payment, 2018; Jost, 2017; Luhby, 2017). The small employer tax credit will remain in place, but businesses will purchase SHOP-qualified plans directly from insurers instead of on the exchange. As of 2017, only 39,000 people had enrolled in SHOP coverage in the states with federally run SHOP exchanges (Norris, 2021c). While overall SHOP participation is limited, there is healthy enrollment in a handful of state-run exchanges. For example, California projected that 62,000 state residents would be enrolled by the end of the 2020 fiscal year, and the District of Columbia had over 80,000 enrollees in 2019 (Norris, 2021c).

Starting in 2014, the exchanges for individuals began offering a variety of health insurance plans that meet ACA criteria regarding plan benefits, payments, and consumer information. The Congressional Budget Office (CBO, 2020) projects that by 2030 just under 10 million individuals will purchase their own health insurance through an exchange or Basic Health Program (a state option to provide subsidized health insurance for residents with incomes between 138% and 200% of the federal poverty level [FPL]). A slight increase in enrollment is expected in 2020 due to pandemic-related unemployment and the subsequent loss of employer-sponsored coverage. These gains are projected to be short-lived as individuals will enroll in Medicaid or become uninsured over time (CBO, 2020). In addition, CBO expects 4 million fewer individuals to purchase nongroup coverage, including marketplace coverage, as a result of the repeal of the individual mandate penalty (CBO, 2019a).

The exchanges are a critical component of health reform because it would be untenable to require individuals to purchase health insurance without also making comprehensive and affordable health insurance options available. Individuals often face expensive and less comprehensive health insurance choices because their insurance pools are not extensive enough that the premiums paid by healthy individuals offset the costs associated with sicker individuals. The exchanges are intended to create a new market by bringing together large numbers of individuals to create wider insurance pools. Individuals are eligible to purchase health insurance through an exchange if they live in the state where the exchange operates, are U.S. citizens or legal immigrants, and are not incarcerated. Additional requirements must be met, however, to obtain subsidies that reduce the cost of health insurance. Subsidies are available to individuals who meet the previously mentioned requirements and who also do not have access to affordable (as defined by the ACA) employer-sponsored insurance, meet specified income requirements, file taxes jointly (if married), and

are not eligible for Medicaid, Medicare, or the Children's Health Insurance Program (CHIP; KFF, n.d.).

Under the ACA, states have three main options when it comes to exchanges: They can build their own, enter into a partnership with the federal government, or ignore the process altogether and thus default into a federally facilitated marketplace (FFM). The last of these, the FFM, is a federally facilitated exchange that was mandated by the ACA for states that were not willing or able to establish a state exchange or a partnership exchange. In a state-run exchange, the state either handles all functions or may use the federal information technology (IT) platform. In a federal–state partnership exchange, states may administer plan management functions, in-person consumer assistance functions, or both, with HHS performing the remaining responsibilities. In the FFM, HHS performs all of these functions. Whatever the structure, the exchanges for individuals were required to be up and running by January 1, 2014. In 2021, the breakdown was as follows: 14 states and the District of Columbia built their own exchange; 6 states have a state-based exchange, but use the federal IT platform; 6 states set up partnership exchanges; and 24 states use the FFM, although 5 of those states retain plan oversight responsibilities (Norris, 2021b). States also may form a regional exchange with other states or allow multiple exchanges within one state as long as each exchange covers a distinct geographical area. In addition, the federal Office of Personnel Management is required to offer at least two multistate plans within each exchange to provide individuals and businesses with additional choices.

The ACA requires the exchanges to ensure that the plans offered there meet other requirements of participating in the exchange. These requirements relate to marketing practices, provider networks (**Box 11.5**), outreach and enrollment, insurance market regulations, and the provision of information in plain language. In addition, the entity running the exchange must provide a call center for customers, maintain a website, develop uniform applications, provide information regarding eligibility for public programs, assist individuals in calculating their tax credits, and certify individuals who are exempt from the individual mandate requirement.

As noted earlier, the Trump administration's actions to undermine the ACA have focused on strategies that weaken the ACA marketplaces. One way to accomplish this goal is to allow cheaper alternatives that enable individuals to purchase health insurance in the nongroup market outside of the exchanges. In general, a cheaper alternative is likely to have less comprehensive benefits and/or

---

(★) Box 11.5   **Special Topic**

Provider Networks

An emerging policy and care delivery issue has been the question of whether provider networks available in plans offered in the exchanges are adequate. Prior to the ACA, insurers could control costs through a variety of mechanisms, including limiting benefits, excluding consumers with preexisting conditions, and using medical underwriting to charge higher premiums to higher-risk individuals and groups. Plans would compete with each other based on price, benefits, cost-sharing, and other features. The ACA includes a variety of rules that eliminate these options, such as prohibition of exclusions based on preexisting conditions, guaranteed issue requirements, community rating requirements, essential health benefits requirements, and actuarial tiering of plans.

As a result of ACA restrictions, many plans are trying to control costs by limiting provider networks and/or provider reimbursement. More expensive providers—such as teaching hospitals and large, urban hospitals—may be more likely to be excluded from narrow networks. Of course, some providers may choose not to participate in exchange plans if the reimbursement is not sufficient.

On the one hand, many consumers who purchase plans in an exchange choose plans based on the premium price and indicate they would prefer cheaper plans with narrow networks as opposed to more expensive plans with broader networks. One study found that ACA silver plans with narrow networks cost consumers 16% less than their broader network counterparts. On the other hand, consumers who purchase plans through employer-sponsored insurance often prefer broader networks, even if the coverage is more expensive. Complaints about narrow networks range from consumers being disappointed that their usual doctor or local hospital is not in network, to questions about access to care, network transparency, and quality of care. In addition, patients who have rare conditions, who need specialized treatment, or who live in rural areas could find that narrow networks create barriers to accessing care.

Several lawsuits have been filed against plans regarding network transparency and provider terminations. In 2014, the Office of the Insurance Commissioner issued federal rules regarding network adequacy in individual and small-group plans, and the Centers for Medicare and Medicaid Services (CMS) continues to issue guidance regarding network adequacy for qualified health plans. State responses to network adequacy concerns have spanned the gamut from Massachusetts' requirement that plans develop tiered and narrow networks to promote cost savings, to state laws requiring updated provider directories, to several failed attempts by state legislatures to pass "any willing provider" laws that require insurers to include any provider willing to accept the insurers' terms.

McDermott Will & Emery. (2015, April 20). *Challenges facing "narrow" provider networks on the ACA health insurance exchanges.* http://www.mwe.com/files/Uploads/Documents/News/Challengs-Facing-Narrow-Provider-Networks.pdf; and Masterson, L. (2018, January 9). *Could narrow networks be the next big cost cutter?* Healthcare Dive. https://www.healthcaredive.com/news/could-narrow-networks-be-the-next-big-cost-cutter/512298/

---

higher cost-sharing for the individual. The administration's rule expanding both association health plans (AHPs) and short-term limited-duration plans (STLDs) are part of this strategy. AHPs allow business associations and other organizations to join together to provide fringe benefits, including health insurance (CBO, 2018). STLDs are designed to fill in a temporary insurance coverage gap, are limited to 3 months of coverage, and are not renewable (Politz et al., 2018). While the Biden administration has reversed this rule, regulations regarding these types of health plans may be the subject of future modifications as the party in charge of the executive branch changes (**Box 11.6**).

Essential Health Benefits Requirement

All qualified health plans that participate in an exchange (as well as individual and small-group plans outside of the exchanges) must offer a standard benefits package, called essential health benefits (EHBs) (Giovannelli et al., 2014). Diagnosis and treatment for COVID-19 are covered under EHBs, although the coverage details and cost-sharing may vary by plan (Centers for Medicare and Medicaid Services [CMS], 2020a). This requirement represents the first time that private health insurance plans have been subject to a federal standard regarding what benefits must be offered. The ACA requires the secretary of HHS to ensure the scope of benefits is equal to the benefits level found in a "typical employer plan." Plans may not design their benefits or reimbursement packages in ways that discriminate based on age, disability, or expected length of life (Rosenbaum et al., 2011).

While the ACA outlines 10 categories of services that must be provided in the EHB package (**Box 11.7**), the federal regulatory process left states with significant discretion about how they implemented this requirement. States have a choice of 10 federally approved health plans to serve as a benchmark to

Box 11.6 | **Technical Spotlight**

AHPs and STLDs

Both AHPs and STLDs are likely to "limit benefits, be priced on the basis of an individual's health status, and impose lifetime and annual spending limits, and insurers could reject applicants on the basis of their health and any preexisting condition" (CBO, 2018, p. 10). One review of short-term plans found that 71% did not cover outpatient prescription drugs, 62% did not cover substance abuse services, 43% did not cover mental health services, and no plans covered maternity care (Pollitz et al., 2018). Concerns about STLD plans have led 12 states to prohibit insurers from using health status as a factor in medical underwriting, effectively eliminating those plans. Another 13 states and the District of Columbia limit plan duration to the original 3-month time frame (National Association of Insurance Commissioners [NAIC], 2020). CBO and the Joint Committee on Taxation (JCT) estimate that approximately 5 million people will enroll in AHPs or short-term plans each year from 2019 to 2028 (CBO, 2019b). Of those 5 million individuals, approximately 75% will enroll in an AHP and 80% will have been previously insured (CBO, 2019b).

When insurers are allowed to offer nongroup plans that do not have to comply with the ACA provisions, it becomes possible to create cheaper and skimpier insurance products. As a result, adverse selection is likely to occur in the exchange plans as healthier individuals who do not believe they need a comprehensive plan—or do not want to pay a higher premium to participate in one—leave the exchange plan and move to a cheaper nongroup option. Furthermore, the repeal of the individual mandate penalty makes it likely that some healthier individuals will choose a cheaper, less comprehensive option, leaving the ACA-compliant plans with a sicker and more expensive pool of enrollees. An analysis of insurers that detailed the policy and legislative reasons for requesting rate changes found that in 2019, premiums would "be an average of 6% higher, as a direct result of individual mandate repeal and expansion of more loosely regulated plans, than would otherwise be the case" (Kamal et al., 2018). In addition, states without STLD plan limits are expected to experience a 4% increase in ACA premiums and a 6% decrease in enrollment in ACA-compliant plans (NAIC, 2020).

Congressional Budget Office. (2018). *Federal subsidies for health insurance coverage for people under age 65: Tables from CBOs spring 2018 projections.* https://www.cbo.gov/system/files?file=2018-06/51298-2018-05-healthinsurance.pdf; CBO. (2019). *How CBO and JCT analyzed coverage effects of new rules for association health plans and short-term plans.* https://www.cbo.gov/system/files/2019-01/54915-New_Rules_for_AHPs_STPs.pdf; Kamal, R., Cox, C., Fehr, R., Ramirez, M., Hortsman, K., & Levitt, L. (2018, October 26). *How repeal of the individual mandate and expansion of loosely regulated plans are affecting 2019 premiums.* Kaiser Family Foundation. https://www.kff.org/health-costs/issue-brief/how-repeal-of-the-individual-mandate-and-expansion-of-loosely-regulated-plans-are-affecting-2019-premiums/; NAIC. (2020, April 17). *Short-term limited-duration health plans.* https://content.naic.org/cipr_topics/topic_short_term_limited_duration_health_plans.htm; and Pollitz, K., Long, M., Semanskee, A., & Kamal, R. (2018, April 23). *Understanding short-term limited-duration health insurance.* Kaiser Family Foundation. https://www.kff.org/health-reform/issue-brief/understanding-short-term-limited-duration-health-insurance/

 Box 11.7 | **Technical Spotlight**

Essential Health Benefits

All plans in the state exchanges must offer the following benefits:

- Ambulatory patient services
- Emergency services
- Hospitalization
- Maternity and newborn care
- Mental health services and substance use disorder services, including behavioral health treatment
- Prescription drugs
- Rehabilitative and habilitative services and devices (rehabilitative therapies improve, maintain, or prevent deterioration of functions that have been acquired [e.g., after an adult has surgery], while habilitative therapies are provided to achieve functions and skills never acquired [e.g., as with a developmentally disabled child])
- Laboratory services
- Prevention and wellness services and chronic disease management services
- Pediatric services, including vision and dental services

determine the breadth of the services covered under the EHB categories. These approved benchmark plans include the largest three small-group plans available in the state, the largest three state-employee health plans in the state, the largest three Federal Employees Health Benefits program plan options for federal employees, or the state's largest commercial HMO (Giovannelli et al., 2014). Most states select the small-group market as their benchmark plan (CMS, n.d.). The Trump administration added another benchmarking option through its definition of a "typical employer plan," effective in 2020. In addition to the 10 benchmark plans just discussed, states may use any of the five largest (by enrollment) group health insurance products in the state that meet certain requirements (Keith, 2018b). The Trump administration further expanded state choices in 2020 by allowing states to select annually whether to (1) use another state's entire 2017 benchmark plan, (2) replace one or more of its EHB categories with another state's EHB categories, or (3) choose a new EHB benchmark plan (Keith, 2018b; **Box 11.8**).

Benchmark plans are subject to both minimum and maximum standards. At a minimum, the benchmark plans must meet the "typical employer plan" standard. At a maximum, also known as the generosity test, the benchmark plan cannot offer more generous benefits than the most generous comparison plan (Keith, 2018a). The comparison plans are the state's

---

Box 11.8   Technical Spotlight

EHB Benefit Substitution

The Trump administration changed the rules regarding substituting benefits. Under the Obama administration, insurers were allowed to substitute benefits *within* an EHB category, but not *across* EHB categories, as long as the substitution was actuarially equivalent to the benefit it was replacing. Under the Trump administration, states may substitute actuarially equivalent benefits both *within* and *across* EHB categories (Keith, 2018a). An example of a *within*-EHB substitution could be replacing a blood screen (lab test) for ovarian cancer with coverage of a blood screen for high cholesterol—a different, but actuarially equivalent, laboratory test (Giovannelli et al., 2014). An *across*-EHB substitution would be replacing one type of service (e.g., an inpatient hospital service) with a completely different type of service (e.g., an outpatient physician service). Substitution is not permitted for prescription drugs. No state has chosen to substitute across EHB categories for its 2020 or 2021 plans (CMS, n.d.).

Centers for Medicare and Medicaid Services. (n.d.). *Information on essential health benefits (EHB) benchmark plans.* https://www.cms.gov/CCIIO/Resources/Data-Resources/ehb; Giovannelli, J., Lucia, K. W., & Corlette, S. (2014, October 31). *Implementing the Affordable Care Act: Revisiting the ACA's essential health benefits requirements.* Commonwealth Fund. https://www.commonwealthfund.org/publications/issue-briefs/2014/oct/implementing-affordable-care-act-revisiting-acas-essential; and Keith, K. (2018, April 10). *Unpacking the 2019 final payment notice (part 1).* Health Affairs. https://www.healthaffairs.org/do/10.1377/hblog20180410.631773/full/

2017 benchmark and the state's three or four largest (by enrollment) small-group health plans (Keith, 2018a). The federal government will defer to the state's interpretation of plan benefits and limits (Keith, 2018a).

Critics of the *across* substitution rule are concerned that plans will substitute for specific benefits so that they do not appeal to certain high-risk individuals. In addition, once a service is not considered an EHB, it is no longer subject to ACA protections, such as lifetime or annual dollar limits, nor is it used to calculate premium subsidies and cost-sharing reductions (Keith, 2018a). Nine states and the District of Columbia prohibited *within*-category substitution in 2014 (Giovannelli et al., 2014). As with many of the Trump administration changes, states will have the final say over whether and how they choose to take advantage of this flexibility.

Variation across the states may occur with habilitative services coverage and state benefits mandates. Habilitative services assist individuals with gaining or maintaining functional skills (e.g., speaking, walking). Prior to the ACA's passage, the coverage for and definition of habilitative services varied significantly. As part of ACA implementation, federal regulators permitted states to use the habilitative services definition in their benchmark plan (if there was such coverage), create their own coverage definition, or let the insurers define the coverage benefit (Giovannelli et al., 2014). As a result, the definition of habilitative services may differ across states and within states.

In addition, some states passed laws that required insurers in their states to cover a particular benefit, such as obesity management services. Any benefit mandates that were in place before 2012 were incorporated into that state's EHB package, meaning the variation that was in place prior to health reform is likely to continue. It is less likely that states will add new benefit mandates at this time because if a state plans to include any services beyond the EHB package that were not mandated prior to 2012, the state must defray the cost of the additional service through a payment to the enrollee or the plan. In addition, the new generosity test means that it may be more difficult for states to choose a benchmark that includes an expensive mandate (Keith, 2018a). Some states have avoided the extra costs associated with new mandates by exempting ACA-compliant plans or plans where the mandate would increase premiums by a specific percentage (Andrews, 2014).

In the lead-up to the passage of the ACA, significant debate arose over whether to allow or require plans to offer abortion and contraceptive services. In fact, the abortion debate was so divisive that it almost doomed the entire health reform bill at the 11th hour. A compromise was reached with the intent of keeping the status quo regarding federal funding for abortion services (i.e., limit federal funding for abortion services to cases where the life of the pregnant woman is in danger or the pregnancy is a result of rape or incest). Under the compromise, states may enact a law that prohibits plans that participate in their state exchanges from providing abortion services.

The ACA also provides coverage, without any cost-sharing, for all contraception methods approved by the Food and Drug Administration (FDA). Even though contraception is considered a preventive service under the EHB standard, it is not specifically listed in the statute. (Nor are other preventive services; instead, the statute references guidelines such as the U.S. Preventive Services Task Force's A and B recommendations.) Contraceptive coverage is part of a separate provision that includes women's preventive services identified by the Health Resources and Services Administration. Because this guideline is created by an administrative agency, each successive presidential administration has the power to change the list of approved women's preventive services without needing congressional approval. The Obama administration exempted religious employers and other nonprofit entities from being required to provide contraception coverage due to religious objections (Coverage of Certain Preventive Services, 2013). These entities could submit a form to self-certify that they objected to providing contraceptive coverage, and their insurer or third-party administrator would

then provide coverage for contraception at no cost to enrollees (Keith, 2020c). The Trump administration significantly broadened the list of employers, insurers, and individuals who would qualify for the exemption based on religious or moral grounds (Keith & Jost, 2017; **Figure 11.7**). Its revisions to the rule spurred numerous lawsuits, and several lower courts issued injunctions to prevent the rules from becoming effective.

In July 2020, the U.S. Supreme Court upheld the Trump administration's rules in the consolidated cases of *Little Sisters of the Poor v. Pennsylvania* and *Trump v. Pennsylvania*. The court concluded that the federal government had the legal authority to issue a broad religious and moral exemption to the contraceptive mandate (Keith, 2020e). For the moment, the court also ruled that the regulation did not violate the Administrative Procedures Act (APA), but it did not decide whether the rules were arbitrary and capricious under the APA. In addition, the court did not reach the question of whether the exemption was required or authorized by the Religious Freedom Restoration Act (RFRA; Keith, 2020e). As a result, litigation will continue over the exemption. Based on the court's ruling, the Trump administration's rules are now in effect and employers are no longer required to provide an accommodation if they choose not to provide contraceptive coverage. In those situations, women will have to find coverage elsewhere, if they can, and will likely have to pay out-of-pocket costs for

Notes: This requirement applies to employers with 50+ employees unless they offer a grandfathered plan.

Figure 11.7 Employers Objecting to Contraceptive Coverage: Exemptions and Accommodations Under the Trump Administration Final Regulations

Sobel, L., Salganicoff, A., & Rosenzweig, C. (2018, November 9). *New regulations broadening employer exemptions to contraceptive coverage: Impact on women.* Kaiser Family Foundation. https://www.kff.org/health-reform/issue-brief/new-regulations-broadening-employer-exemptions-to-contraceptive-coverage-impact-on-women/

that coverage. The federal government itself has estimated that between 70,500 and 126,400 women will lose access to cost-free contraceptive coverage under this rule (Keith, 2020f). During the presidential campaign, Biden promised to revert to Obama-era policies on contraception (Biden, 2020).

The Trump administration enacted policies that restricted contraceptive devices (e.g., by broadening the religious objection exemption) and access to abortion services (e.g., supporting the defunding of Planned Parenthood). The Biden administration has different priorities and has taken steps to remove the "gag rule," which prohibits federal funding for international organizations that provide abortion information; reinstate the original ACA contraceptive rules; and support Planned Parenthood (Hui, 2021). The newly constituted Supreme Court is even more conservative than recent iterations, leading to speculation about the future of *Roe v. Wade* and other women's health issues.

Given the changing dynamics at the federal level, many states have passed laws in these areas. As of June 2021, 29 states and the District of Columbia required insurance plans to cover the full range of contraceptive drugs, 16 states and D.C. banned cost-sharing for contraceptives, and 9 states and D.C. prohibited other restrictions and delays by insurers. At the same time, 20 states and D.C. exempted select employers and insurers from providing contraceptive coverage based on religious objections (Guttmacher Institute, 2021a). Regarding abortion services, 45 states allow healthcare providers to refuse to perform an abortion, and 42 states allow institutions to do so. Patients must pause until a waiting period passes between counseling and the procedure in 25 states (Guttmacher Institute, 2021a). Twelve states had enacted laws that restrict abortion coverage in private plans as of June 2021; plans usually provide coverage only if the patient's life is endangered, although consumers may often purchase additional abortion coverage (Guttmacher Institute, 2021b). If a state does not enact such a law and a plan chooses to offer abortion services in other circumstances, the plan must create separate financial accounts to ensure that federal premium and cost-sharing subsidies are not used toward those abortion services. At least one of the multistate plans is required not to provide abortion services beyond those that are currently allowed with federal funding. As with most compromises, neither side was entirely pleased with the ACA's abortion rules. Those who want more restrictive abortion policies found the separate accounting process to be a meaningless exercise, while those who want more permissive abortion policies were disturbed by states' ability to prohibit plans from offering abortion services.

The ACA also created a "catastrophic coverage" option that must include the EHBs (KFF, n.d.). A catastrophic plan may be offered only to individuals younger than 30 years who would be exempt from the individual mandate requirement due to hardship or affordability exemptions. These plans require coverage of EHBs, certain preventive services without cost-sharing, and at least three primary care visits each year before meeting the deductible (KFF, n.d.). Individuals may not use premium tax credits to subsidize catastrophic plans, which typically have low premiums but very high deductibles. CMS announced that catastrophic coverage plans must cover COVID-19 diagnosis and treatment services as an EHB and may provide coverage before enrollees meet their deductible (CMS, 2020b).

Premium and Cost-Sharing Subsidies

One key difference among the various exchange plans is the cost to the enrollee. Four levels of plans may be offered, which are distinguished by their actuarial value. Actuarial value is the average share of covered benefits generally paid by the insurer based on the cost-sharing provisions in the plan. The higher the actuarial value, the more the plan pays for a given set of services. For example, in a plan with a 70% actuarial value, the plan pays 70% of the cost of services on average across all enrollees, while enrollees pay 30%. Actuarial value is based on average cost, but any single enrollee in that plan may pay more or less than 30% of the cost of services. In general, plans with a higher actuarial value will also have higher premiums to cover the cost of providing services to enrollees. A plan with a lower premium could have higher cost-sharing (copayments or deductibles) to offset the lower premium. The four ACA-approved plan levels by actuarial value are bronze (60% actuarial value), silver (70% actuarial value), gold (80% actuarial value), and platinum (90% actuarial value). Plans must offer at least one silver-level and one gold-level option in each exchange in which they participate.

The ACA includes premium tax credits and cost-sharing subsidies, also known as cost-sharing reductions (CSRs), to help make it affordable for people to purchase health insurance in a state exchange (see **Box 11.9**, **Box 11.10**, and **Box 11.11**). Given the mandate to purchase insurance, it was necessary to include some assistance to make it possible for low-income individuals to comply with the new requirement.

Box 11.9 **Technical Spotlight**

Premium Tax Credit Calculation

The amount of the premium tax credit is tiered based on income and is set so that individuals will not have to pay more than a certain percentage of their income for premiums (see **Table 11.1**). The tax credit amount is based on the cost of the second-lowest-cost silver plan in the exchange and the location where the individual is eligible to purchase insurance. Individuals who want to purchase a more expensive plan have to pay the difference in cost between the second-lowest-cost silver plan and the plan they prefer to purchase. Under the ACA, HHS will adjust the premium people are expected to pay to reflect that premium costs typically grow faster than income levels. As an example, suppose Bob's income is 250% of the FPL (about $32,200 for an individual), and the cost of the second-lowest-cost silver plan in Bob's area is $5700. Under the premium tax credit schedule, Bob will pay no more than 8.05% of his income, or $2737. Bob's tax credit is $2963, which is $5700 minus $2737.

Kaiser Family Foundation. (n.d.). *Health reform FAQs.* https://www.kff.org/health-reform/faq/health-reform-frequently-asked-questions/#question-who-is-eligible-for-marketplace-premium-tax-credits

Box 11.10 **Technical Spotlight**

CSR Calculation

CSRs raise the actuarial value of a plan and limit the maximum out-of-pocket costs (Norris, 2019). As shown in **Table 11.2**, CSRs increase the actuarial value by having plans pay a higher percentage of service costs based on income level. The standard maximum out-of-pocket costs are based on health savings accounts limits and are indexed annually. CSRs set lower out-of-pocket maximums based on the scale in **Table 11.3**, which results in lower cost-sharing obligations (i.e., deductibles, copayments, coinsurance). For example, in 2020, enrollees with incomes between 100% and 200% of the FPL have a maximum out-of-pocket limit of $2700, compared to $8150 for an unsubsidized individual (Norris, 2019).

Unlike premium subsidies, CSRs are available only if enrollees sign up for a silver plan. The subsidy is automatically included in the cost when an eligible individual shops for a plan. Low-income individuals may be better off choosing a higher-premium silver plan than a low- or zero-premium bronze plan, based on the value of the CSR (Norris, 2019).

Norris, L. (2019, September 23). *ACA's cost-sharing subsidies: Key takeaways.* Healthinsurance.org. https://www.healthinsurance.org/obamacare/the-acas-cost-sharing-subsidies/

Box 11.11 DISCUSSION QUESTIONS

CBO estimates that premium subsidies and CSRs will cost the federal government $851 billion from 2018 to 2027 (CBO, 2017c). Is this a good use of resources? Are these subsidies well designed? Are they sufficient to make health insurance affordable? Do they cover people with incomes that are too high? Should they cover more people?

Congressional Budget Office. (2017). *Federal subsidies under the Affordable Care Act for health insurance coverage related to the expansion of Medicaid and nongroup health insurance: Tables from CBOs January 2017 baseline.* http://acasignups.net/sites/default/files/CBO-2017-01-healthinsurance.pdf

The tax credits and subsidies became available starting in 2014, the same year the individual mandate and the state health insurance exchanges went into effect. In 2020, 9.2 million people (87% of marketplace enrollees) received a premium tax credit, and 5.3 million people (50% of marketplace enrollees) received a CSR (Norris, 2021a).

Under the ACA, premium tax credits are available to individuals who are (1) eligible to purchase health insurance in state exchanges; (2) have incomes between 100% and 400% of the FPL (in 2021, 400% of the FPL was $51,520 for an individual and $106,000 for a family of four [Office of Assistant Secretary for Planning and Evaluation, 2021]); (3) not eligible for Medicaid, the CHIP, or Medicare; and (4) do not have access to affordable employer-sponsored health insurance. An employer plan is not considered affordable if it does not cover at least 60% of covered benefits or if the employee's share of premium contributions exceeds 9.83% of the employee's income in 2021. The premium contribution amount that determines whether contributions exceed the affordability threshold are based on individual coverage. Of course, many people purchase family coverage and the premiums for family coverage are higher than the premiums for individual coverage. This problem, only using individual premium costs, is referred to

Table 11.1 Premium Tax Credit Schedule

Income Level by Federal Poverty Level (FPL)	Premium as a Percentage of Income
100%–133%	2%
133%–150%	3%–4%
150%–200%	4%–6.3%
200%–250%	6.3%–8.05%
250%–300%	8.05%–9.5%
300%–400%	9.5%

Table 11.2 Cost-Sharing Subsidy Schedule

Income Level by Federal Poverty Level (FPL)	Actuarial Value
100%–150%	94%
150%–200%	87%
200%–250%	73%

Table 11.3 Out-of-Pocket Spending Limits

Income Level by Federal Poverty Level (FPL)	Out-of-Pocket Spending Limit
100%–200%	2/3 of maximum
200%–300%	1/2 of maximum
300%–400%	1/3 of maximum

(★) **Box 11.12** **Special Topic**

American Rescue Plan Act

ARPA was passed on March 11, 2021, almost 11 years after Obama signed the ACA into law. The Democrats used the reconciliation process to pass the almost $2 trillion COVID-19 relief bill. ARPA included a variety of provisions, such as stimulus payments to individuals, unemployment benefit extension, small business aid, and vaccine and testing funding. Related to the ACA, ARPA expanded the premium tax credit rules to include more individuals and provide higher payments. These provisions are temporary, only covering FY 2021 and 2022. The next Congress will determine whether the provisions are extended or whether the original ACA rules will return. Specifically, ARPA changes the premium tax credits by doing the following:

- Extended eligibility beyond 400% FPL. Individuals will receive financial assistance if they would otherwise spend more than 8.5% of their family income on individual market premiums. This provision is expected to reach 3.6 million uninsured individuals.

- Increase the premium tax credit for individuals between 100% and 400% FPL. For example, individuals earning 100%–125% FPL must contribute 2%–4% of their income under the ACA. Under ARPA, they can enroll in a $0 premium plan. This provision is expected to provide savings for 9 million current enrollees as well as additional new enrollees.

- The premium expansion is estimated to cost $34.2 billion over 10 years.

Data from Keith, K. (2021). The American Rescue Plan expands the ACA. *Health Affairs, 40*(5), 696–697. https://doi.org/10.1377/hlthaff.2021.00597

---

as the "family glitch" and is expected to affect over 5 million people (Cox et al., 2021).

The exact amount of the premium subsidy depends on the individual's income level (Table 11.1). The tax credits are advanceable and refundable, meaning they are available when health insurance is purchased and regardless of whether the individual owes any taxes. Temporary changes have been made to the premium tax credit rules under the American Rescue Plan Act (ARPA; **Box 11.12**).

CSRs are available to help low-income people reduce the amount of out-of-pocket spending on health insurance (Table 11.2). CSRs are available to people who earn between 100% and 250% of the FPL and are tiered by income (Box 11.10). Under the ACA, individuals with incomes less than 133% of the FPL were eligible for Medicaid beginning in 2014 in those states that elected to expand their Medicaid programs under the ACA.

Under the ACA, insurers receive CSR payments from the federal government to cover the expense of providing these subsidies to their low-income enrollees. These payments to insurers have been the subject of litigation brought by House Republicans, originally during the Obama administration (the case was first known as *House v. Burwell*, then it was retitled *House v. Price* to account for a new HHS Secretary, and finally the case was designated *House v. Azar* for the same reason). Initially, the federal trial court agreed with the plaintiffs' claim that the subsidies should not be funded because Congress did not appropriate money for that purpose. The Obama administration appealed, after which the case was put on hold during multiple delays. In October 2017, the Trump administration announced that it would no longer make CSR payments to insurers. As a result, the various parties to the lawsuit—House Republicans, the Trump administration, and several states (which had been granted a request along the way to intervene in the case)—started to negotiate a settlement. Having reached a conditional settlement in December 2017, the parties asked the original trial judge to issue an "indicative ruling" that she would vacate her original order on CSR payments if the case were sent back to her from the appellate court (to which the Obama administration had appealed some years earlier) without a ruling on the merits. At the request of the parties, the appellate court did just that; it dismissed the appeal and sent the case back to the trial court. In turn, the trial judge vacated her initial decision.

That said, the CSR saga is not over: Several state attorneys general filed a lawsuit against HHS over its decision to end the CSR payments, and some insurers have done the same. CSR litigation was stayed while the Supreme Court considered a similar case regarding risk corridor payments that Congress refused to fund. In April 2020, the court ruled that the federal government was obligated to pay the full risk payment amount—more than $12 billion—owed to insurers (Keith, 2020d). With that case decided, the lower federal courts turned their attention back to the CSR litigation. For example, in twin August 2020 cases (*Sanford Health Plan v. United States* and *Community Health Choice, Inc. v. United States*), the Court of Appeals for the Federal Circuit stated that while insurers were entitled to unpaid CSRs, they were not entitled to a windfall; as a result, the court ruled that any CSR payments received had to be reduced by the excess amount of premium tax credits that insurers received due to premium loading.

Without CSR payments to cover the costs of charging lower cost-sharing amounts to low-income consumers, insurers will increase premiums to make up for lost revenue and/or leave the insurance market altogether (Liptak et al., 2017). While the amount varies by state, CBO estimates that benchmark premiums will be 20% higher in 2021 if CSR payments are not resumed, as compared to a scenario where CSR payments are reinstated (Rao & Nowak, 2019). Many insurers are targeting their premium increase just to the silver plan, a strategy known as "silver loading" (Keith, 2018c). By doing so, they will maximize the premium tax credits they receive, which are tied to silver plan costs. In addition, because consumers may use their tax credits for any plan, many could enroll

in a bronze or gold plan at a lower cost than in prior years. Ironically, it is estimated that the cost to the federal government for not making the CSR payments will be $2 billion *more* than it would be if it simply made the payments, because of the higher premium tax credits owed (Fise, 2017). Undoing the freeze on CSR payments would have implications for cost and enrollment; that is, moving from CSRs to silver loading increased premium tax credits, and therefore, reduced plan costs for some individuals, leading to increased enrollment.

These subsidies—and, in turn, the viability of the ACA overall—were put at risk by a lawsuit that challenged the legality of subsidies provided to the millions of people in the states that use a federally operated insurance exchange instead of setting up a state-based exchange (Taylor et al., 2015). Congress wrote in the ACA that federal subsidies were available to individuals who purchased health insurance through exchanges that were "established by the State." As part of the law's implementation process, the Internal Revenue Service (IRS) issued a regulation indicating that federal subsidies were available to individuals who purchased health insurance in either state-run or federally operated exchanges (Health Insurance Premium Tax Credit, 2012). The individuals who brought the lawsuit argued that the IRS regulation was unlawful because it contradicted the language of the ACA. In essence, the court case boiled down to the meaning of the four words "established by the State": When read contextually against the rest of the ACA, were federally operated exchanges included in exchanges "established by the State," or were federal subsidies reserved only for individuals in states that established their own state-run exchange?

In a 6–3 decision in *King v. Burwell*, the U.S. Supreme Court upheld the ACA's statutory and regulatory scheme, allowing federal subsidies to flow to individuals who purchase insurance in both state-run and federally operated exchanges. Instead of reading the four words in question in a vacuum, Chief Justice Roberts, writing for the majority, viewed the phrase "established by the State" in the context of the overall purpose of the law. Doing otherwise, according to the court, would bring about "the type of calamitous result [insurance market failure] that Congress plainly meant to avoid" in crafting the ACA in the first place. Noting that the court's duty is to construe statutes as a whole, not "isolated provisions," Chief Justice Roberts wrote the following:

Congress passed the Affordable Care Act to improve health insurance markets, not to destroy them. If at all possible, we must interpret the [ACA] in a way that is consistent with the former, and avoids the latter. [The IRS regulation] can fairly be read consistent with what we see as Congress's plan, and that is the reading we adopt. (*King v. Burwell*, 2015)

In upholding the subsidies, the court differed in its reasoning from some lower federal courts that nonetheless also upheld the subsidies across all exchanges. These lower courts found the ACA's subsidy language ambiguous and therefore deferred to the agency (the IRS) that was tasked with interpreting the statute. In a critical move, the Supreme Court instead ruled that because the availability of tax credits was an issue with "deep economic and political significance" to the country, the meaning of the subsidy language should be interpreted by the court itself, rather than left to agency discretion. This decision means that the only way the subsidy language can be altered in the future is through congressional action, rather than by a future president whose administration might reinterpret the language more narrowly. Thus, it is far more likely that the subsidies will remain available in all exchanges—regardless of whether a state or the federal government operates them—going forward.

In addition to saving insurance subsidies for millions of Americans, the decision in *King v. Burwell* could have other ramifications. Taken in conjunction with *National Federation of Independent Business v. Sebelius* (the 2012 Supreme Court decision that upheld the constitutionality of the ACA), lower courts may read *King*'s direction to interpret the ACA as a congressional effort to improve insurance markets as a signal to forestall future litigation against the law. Furthermore, in states that have had difficulty setting up or operating their own exchanges, the decision may encourage them to rely on the federal exchange apparatus because there is no longer the threat that insurance subsidies could be easily untethered from federally facilitated exchanges (as of summer 2020, six states relied on the federal platform to operationalize their insurance exchanges).

Employer Mandate

Under the ACA, employers with 50 or more employees and at least 1 employee who qualifies for a tax credit were required to offer affordable health insurance or pay a penalty beginning in 2014. The Obama administration twice delayed implementation of this mandate to smooth the transition, but the mandate itself did not change. Under the employer mandate, covered employers have three options: (1) provide

affordable health insurance and not pay a penalty, (2) provide health insurance not considered affordable and pay a penalty, or (3) do not provide health insurance and pay a penalty. The penalties are based on whether an employer offers health insurance and whether any full-time employees take a premium tax credit. The amount of the penalty increases over time based on the national increase in premium costs (**Box 11.13**). The employer mandate was intended to encourage employers to continue offering or start offering health insurance. Without such a mandate, employers may have found it profitable not to offer health insurance and instead let their employees purchase health insurance through state exchanges, thereby shifting more of the costs of health reform to the public sector and taxpayers.

Employers that offer health insurance do not pay a penalty if the insurance is considered affordable. Insurance is deemed affordable if the plan has an actuarial value of at least 60% or if the premiums do not cost more than 9.83% of an employee's income in 2021. Employees who would have to pay more than 9.83% of their income on premiums have the option to purchase insurance through an exchange and receive a premium tax credit.

Employers that provide unaffordable insurance have to pay a penalty for each employee who takes a tax credit, not counting the first 30 employees (the 30-employee exception was included in the law due to Congress's concern about the impact of the employer mandate on small businesses). The penalty is $3000 per employee who takes a tax credit but may not exceed $2000 times the number of employees over 30. For example, if the employer has 50 employees and offers unaffordable coverage, the employer would pay a maximum penalty of $40,000 (50 − 30 = 20 employees; $2000 × 20). If only 10 employees take a tax credit, the penalty would be $30,000 ($3000 × 10). If all 50 employees take a tax credit, the penalty

---

👆 Box 11.13 **Technical Spotlight**

Calculating Employer Mandate Penalty

For employers that do not offer health insurance and have at least one full-time employee who takes the premium tax credit, the penalty is $2000 per employee after the first 30 employees. For example, if such an employer has 50 employees, the employer would pay a $40,000 penalty: 50 − 30 = 20 employees; $2000 × 20 employees.

would be $40,000, which is the maximum penalty allowed, rather than $150,000 ($3000 × 50).

Given their smaller pool of employees, small businesses have often found it quite expensive to offer health insurance to their employees. In addition to exempting businesses with fewer than 50 employees from the employer mandate (and creating a health insurance exchange for small businesses), Congress included a small business tax credit to encourage these employers to provide coverage. Employers are eligible for the tax credit if they have fewer than 25 full-time-equivalent employees, average annual wages less than $50,000, and pay for at least half of the cost of health insurance coverage for their employees. The tax credit covers a portion of the cost of the employer's contribution toward employees' premiums. It is capped based on the average premium costs in the employer's geographical area and phases out as firm size and annual wages increase.

Because the employer mandate (and other provisions) will lead to increased costs for certain employers, there was concern that some of these employers might potentially try to offset the new costs by employing more part-time workers (at the expense of full-time employment) and/or capping the number of workers they hire at 49 to avoid the mandate (Blumberg et al., 2014). While several analyses indicate that the ACA's effects on the labor market may be quite modest (Abraham & Royalty, 2017; Blumberg et al., 2014; Gorlick, 2017), the authors of one study (Blumberg et al., 2014) nonetheless advocate for eliminating the employer mandate altogether. They argue that doing so would actually not reduce overall insurance coverage significantly, would eliminate any market distortions that could result from changes in employer hiring practices, and would have the added benefit of lessening employer opposition to the ACA (Blumberg et al., 2014).

Changes to the Private Insurance Market

In addition to creating a new marketplace for private insurance through state exchanges, the ACA makes several changes to private health insurance rules and requirements. These requirements cover everything from rate setting, to benefits, to who must be covered. Although the overall health reform law is controversial, many of these private market reforms have overwhelming support. Together, these changes filled in gaps left by the private market that many people believed were unfair to consumers.

The following coverage changes took effect in 2010:

- **Preexisting conditions:** Individual and group plans may not exclude children due to their health status or based on preexisting conditions.
- **Dependent coverage:** Individual and group plans must provide dependent coverage up to age 26 years.
- **Preventive services:** New health plans may not impose cost-sharing for certain preventive services, including the following:
  - Preventive services with an A or B rating from the U.S. Preventive Services Task Force
  - Immunizations recommended by the Centers for Disease Control and Prevention's Advisory Committee on Immunization Practice
  - Preventive care and screening for women based on guidelines to be issued by the Health Resources and Services Administration
- **Coverage limits:** Individual and group plans may not impose lifetime dollar limits on coverage (and the ability to impose annual limits on the dollar value of coverage was prohibited as of 2014).
- **Rescission:** Individual and group plans may not rescind coverage except in the case of fraud.
- **Appeals:** New health insurance plans must have an effective appeals process that includes an external review option.

Congress also focused on the issue of how insurers determine premium rates and what they spend those resources on within their plans. The ACA charged HHS with establishing an annual process to review "unreasonable" increases in premiums (ACA, 2010, § 1003). The 2019 benefit and payment rules changed the definition of "unreasonable" from a 10% increase to a 15% increase and exempted student health services from the review requirements (Keith, 2018b). As of March 2017, 47 states and the District of Columbia had an effective rate review law in place for their individual or small-group insurance markets, and the federal government will conduct effective rate reviews in three states that need to improve their state processes. In general, the federal process is intended to work with—not preempt—those state laws (CMS, 2017). These states must post all proposed increases at the same time and all final rate increases at the same time and must provide CMS with 5 days' notice of rate increases (Keith, 2018b).

In addition, the ACA requires that plans spend at least 85% (large-group plans) or 80% (small-group or individual plans) of their premium dollars on medical care and quality improvement services, rather than administrative or other expenses (e.g., profits). Regulations clarifying this medical loss ratio

(MLR), as it is called, took effect on January 1, 2011 (Health Insurance Issuers, 2010). Insurers must provide enrollees with a rebate if they do not spend the requisite percentage on clinical and quality improvement services. These rebates are based on an average of the prior 3 years of financial data. Initially, insurers paid significant rebates to consumers ($1 billion in 2011), but by 2016 only 1.5% of enrollees received rebates as insurers improved their MLR to 92% in the individual market and 86% in the small-group market (Keith, 2018b). The MLR dropped significantly in the individual market between 2015 and 2018 as insurers adjusted to the new regulations and were better able to match premium revenue with the cost of claims.

Based on preliminary data, insurers were expected to pay $2.1 billion in rebates for 2021 with $1.5 billion stemming from individual market plans (McDermott & Cox, 2021). While somewhat lower than the 2020 level, the 2021 rebates are 50% higher than the 2019 rebates. The high rebate levels in 2020 and 2021 are likely due to the decreased use of and spending on healthcare services during the COVID-19 pandemic. While hospitals were overwhelmed with coronavirus patients, lucrative elective procedures were cancelled. In addition, many patients did not visit providers for nonemergent care and preventive screenings (**Box 11.14**). As a result, insurers had more premium profits than anticipated, resulting in the high level of rebates (McDermott & Cox, 2021).

Under the 2019 benefit and payment rules, insurers may automatically claim 0.8% of earned premiums for quality improvement without supplying verifying documentation. This will raise the MLR rate for most insurers (Keith, 2018b). The rule also eases standards for seeking an MLR adjustment in the individual market. CMS projects that 22 states will seek such an adjustment, resulting in consumer rebate reductions of $52 million to $64 million annually (Keith, 2018b).

A number of significant insurance changes took place in 2014 alongside implementation of the individual mandate and health insurance exchanges:

- **Guaranteed issue and renewability:** Individual and group plans may not exclude or charge more to individuals based on preexisting conditions or health status in the individual market, small-group market, and exchanges.
- **Rate variation limits:** Premium rates may vary based only on age, geographical area, family composition, and tobacco use in the individual market, small-group market, and exchanges.
- **Coverage limits:** Individual and group plans may not place annual dollar limits on coverage.

> ⊛ **Box 11.14** **Special Topic**
>
> ### Health Insurance Loss and the Pandemic
>
> The coronavirus pandemic created significant health insurance challenges for both individuals and insurers. In May 2020, the U.S. unemployment rate jumped to 13.3%, meaning 21 million people who wanted to work did not have a job (Bureau of Labor Statistics, 2020). To put this staggering number into perspective, the unemployment rate was 10% at the height of the Great Recession in 2009 (Gangopadhyaya & Garrett, 2020). One obvious consequence of these extensive job losses is that many individuals will lose their employment-based health insurance. An estimated 5.4 million workers lost their health insurance between February and May 2020. Overall, 27 million people (including dependents) have lost employer coverage due to the pandemic (Stolberg, 2020). Affected individuals may turn to Consolidated Omnibus Budget Reconciliation Act (COBRA) coverage, marketplace plans, or Medicaid (for those who are eligible) for coverage. Of course, COBRA and marketplace plans can be expensive, and individuals are less likely to be eligible for Medicaid in the nonexpansion states. Even in Medicaid expansion states, 20% of unemployed workers were uninsured in 2018 (Gangopadhyaya & Garrett, 2020).

Bureau of Labor Statistics. (June 19, 2020). *State employment and unemployment (monthly) new release.* https://www.bls.gov/news.release/archives/laus_06192020.htm; Gangopadhyaya, A., & Garrett, B. (2020, April). *Unemployment, health insurance, and the Covid 19 recession.* Robert Wood Johnson Foundation & Urban Institute. https://www.urban.org/sites/default/files/publication/101946/unemployment-health-insurance-and-the-covid-19-recession_1.pdf; and Stolberg, S. (2020, July 13). Millions have lost health insurance in pandemic driven recession. *The New York Times.* https://www.nytimes.com/2020/07/13/us/politics/coronavirus-health-insurance-trump.html?utm_campaign=KHN%3A%20Daily%20Health%20Policy%20Report&utm_medium=email&_hsmi=91340265&_hsenc=p2ANqtz-8C5D9eg4MGWuVxd1v_RkPDtWq9kswibn7iVH4nulEdtXkbdt7hd65pb6x_ClkrJc6hdMvYDVWGRT85Kq7Ykxyf4ZOzBw&utm_content=91340265&utm_source=hs_email

- **Essential health benefits:** Insurers providing coverage to small businesses or individuals and in the exchanges have to provide essential health benefits through one of four plan categories (bronze, silver, gold, or platinum) and adhere to annual cost-sharing limits.
- **Wellness programs:** Employers may offer rewards that reduce the cost of coverage to employees for participating in a wellness program (**Box 11.15**).

These private market changes do not affect all plans equally. In particular, plans in small-group or nongroup

⊛ Box 11.15   Special Topic

Wellness Programs

Workplace wellness programs are intended to entice employees to engage in healthy behaviors (e.g., more exercise, less smoking). Not only can such behaviors improve the individual's health, but employers also hope to save money through lower healthcare costs and less absenteeism. Participation requirements can range from taking a health assessment or joining a workout class to providing detailed health information and submitting to blood tests.

Under the ACA, employers may offer incentives to participate in wellness programs that are worth up to 30% of the cost of health insurance. Given the costs of health insurance, this could result in significant savings for employees. Perhaps not surprisingly, the popularity of these programs has skyrocketed. In 2020, 51% of small firms and 81% of large firms offered some type of wellness program. A small percentage of employers provide benefits or enforce penalties based on health outcomes.

The research on the effectiveness of wellness programs has been inconclusive. One of the first large-scale studies found that while employees self-reported improved health behaviors and benefited from reduced costs, there were no discernible effects on health outcomes, healthcare costs for employers, or absenteeism. That study reviewed initial outcomes after 18 months, which may not be enough time to achieve results. Another study also found no change in healthcare costs or outcomes. Researchers in that study noted that program participants were employees who were already healthier and motivated, and employers may benefit from keeping those employees in the organization over the long run.

Appleby, J. (2019, April 6). *How well do workplace wellness programs work?* NPR. https://www.npr.org/sections/health-shots/2019/04/16/713902890/how-well-do-workplace-wellness-programs-work; Kaiser Family Foundation. (2020). *2020 employer health benefits survey, section 12.* https://www.kff.org/report-section/ehbs-2020-section-12-health-screening-and-health-promotion-and-wellness-programs/; and Lueck, S. (2019, October 23). *Trump wellness programs would gut protections for people with pre-existing conditions.* Center on Budget and Policy Priorities. https://www.cbpp.org/blog/trump-wellness-programs-would-gut-protections-for-people-with-pre-existing-conditions

markets must follow these rules whether or not they are offered in an exchange. However, the ACA included two significant exceptions to these reforms. First, insurance plans that were in existence when the ACA was signed into law are referred to as "grandfathered plans" and are subject to some, but not all, of the new rules. The grandfathered plans must follow new requirements relating to preexisting conditions, lifetime and annual limits, waiting period limits, and dependent coverage rules. These plans are exempt, however, from having to provide essential health benefits, preventive services without copayments, and limited cost-sharing—although many of the large employer plans already have some of these features (Healthcare.gov, n.d.). A plan may retain its grandfathered status as long as it does not make significant changes to plan benefits or cost-sharing rules. If it loses its grandfathered status, the plan will have to meet all applicable requirements. In 2019, 22% of all employers offered at least one grandfathered plan, and 13% of covered workers were enrolled in one (KFF, 2019, section 13).

The second major exception is for self-funded plans. In these plans, an employer does not buy insurance from a company, but instead takes on the insurance risk itself. Self-funded plans are exempt from state law and subject to federal rules under the Employee Retirement Income Security Act of 1974 (ERISA). Self-funded plans must adhere to the ACA rules regarding dependent coverage, cost-sharing for preventive services, annual and lifetime limits, and waiting period limits, but do not need to comply with essential health benefit requirements (Commercial Insurance, 2012).

Financing Health Reform

Congress financed health reform primarily through Medicare and Medicaid savings, excise taxes and fees on the healthcare industry, changes to the income tax code, a tax on some health insurance plans, and expected individual and employer payments for violating insurance mandates. Several of these financing changes were made as part of the deals the Obama administration struck with various stakeholders.

The ACA's main financing features are as follows:

- **Medicare provider reimbursement:** Reduces "market basket" or cost updates for inpatient and outpatient hospital reimbursement and reduces payments for preventable hospital readmissions and hospital-acquired infections. This feature includes productivity adjustments (an adjustment in the Medicare physician fee schedule pertaining to physician productivity) for certain providers that will result in lower reimbursement rates.
- **Medicare Advantage payments:** Reduces reimbursement rates and imposes cost-sharing limits for Medicare's managed care plans.
- **Medicare Part A (hospital insurance):** Increases the Medicare Part A tax rate for high-income earners.

- **Medicare premiums:** Reduces the Medicare Part D (prescription drug) premium subsidy for high-income beneficiaries.
- **Medicare employer subsidy:** Eliminates the tax deduction for employers that receive a Medicare Part D (prescription drug coverage) subsidy.
- **Disproportionate share hospital (DSH) payments:** Reduces Medicare payments to DSH hospitals. Payments may increase over time based on the percentage of uninsured served and uncompensated care provided. This feature reduces Medicaid DSH payments and requires HHS to develop a new funding formula. The effective date of the reduction was repeatedly delayed; it is now slated to occur from 2024–2027 at $8 million per year. While hospitals likely welcome the delay, the aggregated amount of reduction increased from $18 billion to $32 billion (Congressional Research Service [CRS], 2021).
- **Medicaid prescription drugs:** Increases the rebates that drug manufacturers give to state Medicaid programs.
- **Income tax code provisions:** Increases the threshold from 7.5% to 10% of adjusted gross income to claim the deduction for unreimbursed medical expenses, prohibits purchasing over-the-counter drugs with tax-free savings accounts, increases the tax burden on distributions not used for qualified medical expenses, and limits the amount that individuals may put in accounts toward medical expenses.
- **Health industry fees:** Imposes a 10% tax on indoor tanning services, a 2.3% tax on all taxable medical devices, annual fees on the pharmaceutical manufacturing sector, and fees on the health insurance sector (repealed).
- **Health insurance plans:** Imposes a tax (referred to as the "Cadillac tax") on employer-sponsored health insurance plans with aggregate expenses that exceed $10,800 for individual coverage or $29,050 for family coverage (repealed).

Although the CBO is responsible for estimating the cost of legislation as it is written, time-bound cost estimates (e.g., a 10-year estimate) have their limitations. First, the CBO must assume that all the provisions in the bill will be implemented as written. This is not the case with the ACA. For example, Congress passed a 2019 spending bill that eliminated the ACA's main tax provisions (Cadillac tax, health insurance tax, and medical device tax), resulting in a projected revenue loss of $373 billion over 10 years (Keith, 2019). Second, because the 10-year estimate, by design, does not consider costs beyond the first decade, some expected costs are not included in

the estimate. Third, different methodologies may be used to calculate costs. Fourth, cost estimates cannot account for provisions that are left out of a bill. For these reasons, cost estimates should not be taken as the final word on the cost of any bill, because changes in political will can undermine the best projections.

Public Health, the Healthcare Workforce, Prevention, and Quality

Overall, the United States spends less than 3% of its total national health spending—less than $300 per person—on public health concerns (Trust for America's Health [TFAH], 2021). The ACA includes a variety of programs and pilot projects that focus on improving the quality of care, increasing access to preventive care, and addressing public health issues. These provisions show both a commitment to these issues and the limitations of that commitment. For example, the ACA's Prevention and Public Health Fund (PPHF) was "the first dedicated and mandatory funding source for prevention and public health within the federal budget" (TFAH, 2019, p. 8). Most of the CDC's portion of the fund is directed to state and local prevention efforts. The PPHF is scheduled to provide $16.2 billion to support these activities from 2022 to 2031 (TFAH, n.d.). Congress, however, has the ability to redirect resources, and the PPHF has been cut by more than $11 billion from 2013 to 2027 (TFAH, n.d.). In FY 2021, PPHF is due to receive about half the amount it was intended to receive originally (TFAH, 2021; **Figure 11.8**). In addition, while task forces and pilot programs can be useful tools to try out new ideas and gather data to inform future changes, their temporary nature can also mean that progress ends once the experiment is over, especially in tight budgetary times. Whether these steps lead to lasting reform and needed change in the delivery of health care and in public health practice remains to be seen.

As of July 2021, Congress had passed four pieces of legislation in response to the pandemic: an $8.3 billion emergency funding bill, the $192 billion Families First Coronavirus Response Act (Families First), the $2.2 trillion Coronavirus Aid, Relief, Economic Security Act (CARES) (Keith, 2020a), and the $1.9 trillion ARPA (**Box 11.16**). Together, these relief laws include over $75 billion in public health funding (Nicholson & Wile, 2021; TFAH, 2021). A large portion of the resources are one-time allocations directed toward pandemic relief. While necessary, this infusion of resources will not compensate for the years for

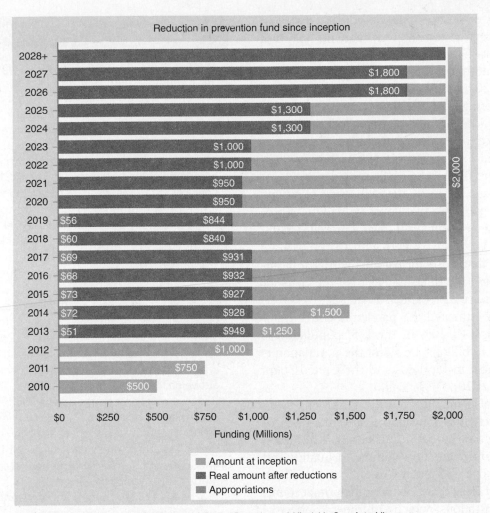

Notes: Original distributions (blue bars) from the Patient Protection and Affordable Care Act while cuts (orange bars) are from the Bipartisan Budget Act of 2018.

Figure 11.8 Prevention Funding Has Experienced a String of Cuts Since Creation of the Prevention and Public Health Fund

Data from Trust for America's Health. (2021, May). *The impact of chronic underfunding on America's public health system: Trends, risks, and recommendations, 2021.* https://www.tfah.org/wp-content/uploads/2021/05/2021_PHFunding_FnI.pdf

---

💡 Box 11.16 DISCUSSION QUESTIONS

Congress passed the various pandemic laws without paying for them. The federal deficit is projected to be $2.3 trillion in 2021, equaling 10.3% of GDP. This is the second largest deficit since 1945, only bested by the 2020 deficit (CBO, 2021). Even though in mid-2021 the U.S. economy is showing signs of recovery, unemployment remains high, millions of people are facing eviction, businesses are struggling to survive, and inflation fears are increasing. Were these laws the best use of resources? Does the country need additional federal aid given the ongoing pandemic? Who should be receiving aid? How will the U.S. economy recover?

Congressional Budget Office. (2021). *The budget and economic outlook: 2021 to 2031.* https://www.cbo.gov/system/files/2021-02/56970-Outlook.pdf; and Bipartisan Policy Center. (2020, May). *Deficit tracker.* https://bipartisanpolicy.org/report/deficit-tracker/

which the public health system has been underfunded (TFAH, 2021). While these acts have a wide range of provisions, we will highlight the ones related to public health and healthcare services.

Overall, these laws attempt to reduce the costs associated with diagnosing and treating COVID-19 and to provide relief to individuals and families affected by the coronavirus. Congress not only aimed to reduce the financial consequences of the pandemic for individuals, but also to limit the spread of the virus by removing a barrier to accessing care. Many insurance companies voluntarily assumed obligations for testing coverage, and states clarified their testing coverage rules for state-regulated plans. Even so, federal policy was necessary both to achieve uniformity and to cover group health plans that are subject to federal regulation (Keith, 2020a). All comprehensive health plans must cover FDA-approved testing, along with any items or services provided during a visit in which a coronavirus test is given. Patients may not be charged cost-sharing fees or be subject to barriers such as prior authorization requirements (Cochrane & Tankersley, 2020; Keith, 2020a).

While coverage for testing is important, treatment of COVID-19 can be expensive. Federal officials issued guidance reiterating that the major medical treatments used for coronavirus (e.g., lab tests, hospitalizations) are part of the EHBs provided by ACA-compliant plans (Keith, 2020a). Of course, having coverage does not mean that coverage will be affordable. Due to higher hospitalization and mortality rates, direct medical costs for patients with COVID-19 are 4 times higher than costs for patients with symptomatic influenza and 5.5 times higher than the costs for patients with pertussis (Bartsch et al., 2020). Overall, researchers estimated the pandemic could result in $163.4 billion (if 20% of the U.S. population is infected) to $654 billion (if 80% of the population is infected) in direct medical costs in the United States (Bartsch et al., 2020).

The ACA also includes a wide range of quality improvement activities that fall into three main categories: evaluating new models of delivering health care, shifting reimbursement from volume to quality, and improving the overall system (Abrams et al., 2015). New models of healthcare delivery include accountable care organizations, which combine a variety of providers who collectively assume responsibility for the cost and quality of patient care, and patient-centered medical homes, which provide comprehensive and coordinated primary care. Reimbursement reforms include strategies such as penalizing hospitals with high rates of hospital-acquired infections and providing bonuses or penalties based on performance on quality measurements.

Finally, overall system improvement efforts are highlighted by the National Strategy for Quality Improvement and the Patient-Centered Outcomes Research Institute (PCORI). The priorities of the National Strategy for Quality Improvement include improving delivery of healthcare services, patient outcomes, and population health. PCORI, a comparative effectiveness institute, was created to evaluate the clinical effectiveness of medical treatments. The idea behind comparative effectiveness is to determine which procedures, devices, and pharmaceuticals provide the best value for a given outcome (**Box 11.17**). PCORI is charged with supplying information to help providers, patients, and others make sound healthcare decisions; Congress has stipulated, however, that findings from the institute may not be construed as

---

☀ **Box 11.17** DISCUSSION QUESTIONS

There is a debate about the proper age at which to start regular mammogram screenings to detect breast cancer in women who do not have specific risk factors for the disease. As of 2009, the U.S. Preventive Services Task Force recommended waiting until age 50 years to begin mammogram screening for breast cancer and further recommended that screening should occur every 2 years. It also stated, however, that the final decision about the initial timing and frequency of breast cancer screening should be made by the patient and her physician. In making its recommendations, the Task Force found that physicians would need to screen 1000 women to save one woman's life and concluded that earlier and/or more frequent screening was not worth the harm associated with false positives (anxiety, unnecessary biopsies, overtreatment). Other organizations disagree with the U.S. Preventive Services Task Force and conclude that the life-saving effects of more routine mammogram screening outweigh the potential harm. Thus, the American Cancer Society recommends having routine annual mammograms from age 45 to 54 years (or at age 40 if the patient so chooses) and then every 2 years thereafter. The American College of Obstetricians and Gynecologists recommends starting annual mammograms at age 40 years.

The idea of comparative effectiveness research is to provide information about the value of different tools. Once that information is available, however, who should make the decisions about whether to provide coverage and reimbursement for a particular good or service? Can one objectively assess the potential harms and benefits associated with mammograms or other services or medications? Should decisions be made solely by the patient and the treating provider? Does it matter if decisions affect taxpayers (e.g., if a patient is covered by a government program such as Medicare or the Veterans Administration)?

U.S. Preventive Services Taskforce. (2016, January). *Breast cancer: Screening*. https://www.uspreventiveservicestaskforce.org/uspstf/document/RecommendationStatementFinal/breast-cancer-screening; American College of Obstetricians and Gynecologists. (2016, January 11). *ACOG statement on breast cancer screening guidelines*. https://www.acog.org/news/news-releases/2016/01/acog-statement-on-breast-cancer-screening-guidelines; and American Cancer Society. (n.d.). *Recommendations for the early detection of cancer*. https://www.cancer.org/cancer/breast-cancer/screening-tests-and-early-detection/american-cancer-society-recommendations-for-the-early-detection-of-breast-cancer.html

---

mandates or recommendations for payment, coverage, or treatment decisions.

The ACA also provides funds to promote public health, wellness, and a stable and high-quality healthcare workforce. In addition to the PPHF, the law calls for the creation of a new regular corps and a ready reserve corps to assist when public health emergencies occur. Unfortunately, the ready reserve corps was not funded until the CARES Act was passed in March 2020 (Lawrence, 2020). The ability of the Public Health Service's 6300-member commissioned officer corps to respond to the pandemic was limited by their current assignments. About half of the regular corps was already working in agencies—such as the Indian Health Service, the Bureau of Prisons, and Immigration and Customs Enforcement—treating underserved populations who have been hit hard by the pandemic (Lawrence, 2020).

Also, a variety of programs and incentives are in place to promote employer wellness programs. The workforce shortage is being addressed through graduate medical education reforms that promote primary care training; increases in scholarships and loans to support primary care providers and workforce diversity; and education, training, and loan repayment programs to address the primary care nursing shortage.

The U.S. Supreme Court's Decision in *National Federation of Independent Business v. Sebelius*

In November 2011, in the first of what would be several ACA-related decisions, the U.S. Supreme Court agreed to decide four issues related to the legality of the ACA, two of which remain relevant for purposes of this text: (1) whether Congress had the power under the federal Constitution to enact the individual insurance coverage requirement and (2) whether it was unconstitutionally coercive for Congress, through the ACA, to threaten to take away existing federal Medicaid funding from states that did not want to implement the Medicaid expansion.

In June of the following year, the Court handed down a remarkable 5–4 decision in the case of *National Federation of Independent Business, et al., [NFIB] v. Sebelius, Secretary of Health and Human Services, et al.* The opinion was surprising for two reasons. First, it defied expectations—few people thought that the entirety of the ACA would be found constitutional by a majority of the Court. Second, Chief Justice Roberts, a conservative, ended up in the majority with the court's relatively liberal members (Justices Ginsburg, Breyer, Sotomayor, and Kagan).

The Court first tackled the question of whether Congress exceeded its authority in effectively forcing almost everyone to carry health insurance. It concluded—not totally unexpectedly, given the outcome of the Court's more recent Commerce Clause decisions (e.g., *United States v. Lopez*, 1995)—that the "individual mandate" amounted to an unconstitutional reach on the part of federal legislators:

> The individual mandate . . . does not regulate existing commercial activity. It instead compels individuals to become active in commerce by purchasing a product, on the ground that their failure to do so affects interstate commerce. Construing the Commerce Clause to permit Congress to regulate individuals precisely because they are doing nothing would open a new and potentially vast domain to congressional authority. (*NFIB v. Sebelius*, 2012, p. 2587)

Surprisingly, however, the Court's analysis of the constitutionality of the individual mandate did not end there. The Court majority pivoted to Congress's power to tax, and ruled that under this separate power, the individual mandate passed constitutional muster. The court wrote

> The exaction the Affordable Care Act imposes on those without health insurance [i.e., the financial penalty assessed on those who do not obtain minimum health insurance coverage] looks like a tax in many respects. . . . In distinguishing penalties from taxes, this Court has explained that "if the concept of penalty means anything, it means punishment for an unlawful actor omission." While the individual mandate clearly aims to induce the purchase of health insurance, it need not be read to declare that failing to do so is unlawful. Neither the Act nor any other law attaches negative legal consequences to not buying health insurance, beyond requiring a payment to the IRS. (*NFIB v. Sebelius*, 2012, p. 2595)

Read together, the Supreme Court's analysis of the individual mandate under the Commerce Clause and the Taxing and Spending Clause leads to the following conclusion: Although Congress cannot outright *command* Americans to buy health insurance, it can *tax* those who choose not to.

Next, the Court turned its attention to whether the ACA's Medicaid expansion was structured in a way that effectively, and unlawfully, coerced states into adopting it. Fully half of the 50 states—the 26 that sued to halt implementation of the ACA—believed the answer to be "yes." As originally passed into law, the ACA allowed the secretary of HHS to terminate *all* of a state's Medicaid funding in the event that the state failed to implement the Medicaid expansion— even those Medicaid funds that a state would receive that were unconnected to the expansion. This, the states argued, amounted to a coercively unacceptable choice: either adopt the ACA Medicaid expansion or potentially receive no federal Medicaid financing at all. As a result, they asked the court to rule that the Medicaid expansion itself was unconstitutional.

The Court responded to this argument in two ways. On the one hand, it determined that the Medicaid expansion itself was perfectly constitutional. On the other hand, it ruled that it was indeed unconstitutional for HHS to penalize states that did not adopt the expansion by terminating all Medicaid funding:

> The Constitution simply does not give Congress the authority to require the States to regulate. That is true whether Congress directly commands a State to regulate or indirectly coerces a State to adopt a federal regulatory system as its own. . . . When, for example, such conditions take the form of threats to terminate other significant independent grants, the conditions are properly viewed as a means of pressuring the States to accept policy changes. . . . Nothing in our opinion precludes Congress from offering funds under the Affordable Care Act to expand the availability of healthcare, and requiring that States accepting such funds comply with the conditions on their use. What Congress is not free to do is to penalize States that choose not to participate in that new program by taking away their existing Medicaid funding. (*NFIB v. Sebelius*, 2012, pp. 2602–2607)

This twin ruling had the effect of making the ACA Medicaid expansion optional rather than mandatory, and states have been deciding individually whether to implement it. As of the time of this writing, 39 states and the District of Columbia had adopted the ACA's Medicaid expansion, while 11 states had not adopted the expansion (KFF, 2021b). Note that the latter number is dramatically smaller than the number of states (26) that originally argued in *NFIB v. Sebelius* that the Medicaid expansion was unconstitutionally coercive.

States and Health Reform

Before the ACA and in the wake of numerous failed attempts at national health reform, states had been active players in health reform. Filling the gap left by the lack of federal action, states took steps to experiment with individual mandates, employer mandates, small business pools, and programs to reduce the number of uninsured. As noted previously, some states are now implementing their own public option. Although the ACA is a federal law, it is full of state obligations and opportunities for state innovation. Even though governors in many states have expressed opposition to health reform, numerous states will expend significant efforts toward continued implementation of the ACA over the next several years. States will have their hands full developing and running health insurance exchanges, regulating the private health insurance market, and implementing Medicaid changes.

The Supreme Court's decision to transform the ACA's Medicaid expansion from a mandatory program change to a state option has significant ramifications. As noted earlier, 39 states and the District of Columbia have chosen to expand their Medicaid programs (KFF, 2021b). As a result, by July 2020 there were 15.9 million more enrollees than prior to the ACA, with most new enrollment occurring in expansion states (Medicaid, CHIP Payment and Access Commission, n.d.). Not surprisingly, expansion states have witnessed significant increases in Medicaid enrollment, both among newly eligible enrollees and among individuals who were previously eligible but nonetheless unenrolled. This latter group is a result of the "welcome mat" or "woodwork" effect, as broader eligibility rules, incentives, and outreach resulted in more previously eligible individuals joining the program (Antonisse et al., 2018). The number of new Medicaid beneficiaries will ultimately depend on how many states eventually choose to expand their Medicaid programs.

The Supreme Court's *NFIB v. Sebelius* decision drastically changed the blueprint of health reform. The ACA was designed assuming Medicaid expansion occurred in every state, meaning there would be uniform coverage across the country for individuals earning less than 138% of the FPL. Under this plan, Medicaid would provide insurance for the lowest-income individuals, while state exchanges (with the assistance of federal subsidies) and employer-sponsored insurance would provide coverage for those who had higher earnings. A "coverage gap" now exists in nonexpansion states for individuals with incomes below the poverty line. Their incomes are too high to qualify for the state's traditional Medicaid program, yet too low to be able to afford private insurance in the exchanges because they do not qualify for subsidies. (Because it was assumed Medicaid would be expanded nationally, premium subsidies are available only for individuals earning at least 100% of the FPL.) It is estimated that if nonexpansion states expanded their Medicaid programs, over 2 million people in the coverage gap would gain insurance, along with 2.1 million uninsured adults with incomes between 100% and 138% of the FPL (most of whom are already eligible for marketplace coverage; Garfield et al., 2021). Approximately 97% of those in the coverage gap live in the South, and over one-third of these individuals live in Texas. The distribution of individuals in the coverage gap reflects that region's population demographics (e.g., more poor uninsured adults, higher uninsured rates) and resistance to Medicaid expansion (Garfield et al., 2021).

Key Issues Going Forward

As noted at the outset of this chapter, it appears that the ACA is here to stay. With a Democrat in the White House until at least 2024, the law is safe in the near term. Furthermore, several things could help entrench the ACA in the long term: the increasing popularity of the law, the difficulty Republicans had campaigning against the ACA, Supreme Court decisions upholding the law, and over a decade of health system change in response to the law's requirements. Here, we discuss a few of the major political and implementation issues that will likely dominate the health reform discussion in the near term (see **Box 11.18**).

Health Reform Politics and the Pandemic

While the ACA has gained popularity overall, it is still not well regarded among Republicans. In May 2021, 85% of Democrats and 54% of Independents viewed the law favorably, compared to just 15% of Republicans (KFF, 2021d). Even prior to the COVID-19 outbreak, Democrats and Independents ranked health care as their most important issue going into the 2020 election, while Republicans listed it third after the economy and immigration (Bipartisan Policy Center, 2020; ProCon .org, 2020). Voters from across the political spectrum name prescription drug costs, preexisting condition protections, and surprise medical bills as their primary healthcare concerns (Bipartisan Policy Center, 2020). Although the ACA is not at risk at this time, it is worth considering the main features of Republican efforts to repeal the ACA to understand their policy priorities. Republicans are likely to continue pursuing these changes through administrative actions (if they regain

ⓐ Box 11.18   Special Topic

Medicare for All

While Democrats passed the ACA and remain its strongest supporters, not all Democrats and progressive constituents believe the ACA's approach was the best way to reform the healthcare system. During the 2020 election, Medicare-for-All (M4A) plans received unprecedented attention. A number of 2020 election polls found support for a national health plan called Medicare for All ranged from 56% to 70%. Nevertheless, the level of support dropped significantly when specific consequences were highlighted. For example, support dropped to 37% if private insurance companies were eliminated or taxes were increased, 32% if it endangered the current Medicare program, and 26% if testing and treatment delays occurred.

Ten different M4A plans were proposed in 2019, making it even more difficult to gauge public opinion accurately. The approaches included a true single-payer system for everyone, a national health plan with an opt-out option, a new public option to compete in the ACA marketplace, a Medicare buy-in option for elderly who did not qualify for the current program, and a Medicaid buy-in option for individuals purchasing insurance through an ACA marketplace. Of course, with all of these options, the details about the cost, financing, eligibility, benefits, changes to current programs, role of the federal government, and role of private insurance varied depending on the proposal.

If the experience of the ACA has made anything clear, it is that finding support for plans that promise comprehensive, affordable coverage is not too difficult, but maintaining that support is much more challenging once details are released and changes to the current system occur. M4A is a part of the national conversation in a way that even its supporters could not have imagined a decade ago. That being said, passing the ACA was a herculean task when the Democrats were mostly aligned. Having the Democrats divided over M4A versus ACA, let alone which M4A plan to support, makes it highly unlikely that an M4A plan will become reality in the near future.

Data from Kirzinger, A., Muñana, C., & Brodie, M. (2019). *KFF Health Tracking Poll – January 2019: The public on next steps for the ACA and proposals to expand coverage.* https://www .kff.org/health-reform/poll-finding/kff-health-tracking-poll-january-2019/?utm_source=link _newsv9&utm_campaign=item_257711&utm_medium=copy; Newport, F. (2019, May 21). *Americans' mixed views of healthcare and healthcare reform.* Gallup. https://news.gallup .com/opinion/polling-matters/257711/americans-mixed-views-healthcare-healthcare -reform.aspx; Kaiser Family Foundation. (2019). *Compare Medicare-for-all and public plan proposals.* https://www.kff.org/interactive/compare-medicare-for-all-public-plan-proposals/

control of the executive branch), legislative compromises, and, where possible, state laws.

Overall, the 2017 Republican repeal-and-replace bills reduced taxes, eliminated government mandates, lowered federal government spending, lowered premiums for some people while increasing them for others, phased out the Medicaid expansion under the ACA, and ended Medicaid as an entitlement program (**Table 11.4**). According to the CBO, the effect of the replacement bills would be to significantly increase the number of uninsured, significantly reduce the deficit, lower costs for young and healthy consumers, and increase costs for older and poorer consumers (CBO, 2017a, 2017b). As noted earlier, some aspects of these bills have been achieved through other legislation (individual mandate penalty repeal, tax repeals) or attempted through administrative actions (waivers for Medicaid work requirements, Medicaid block grants, weakening of EHBs).

One thing Congress has not tried yet is a bipartisan approach. A 2019 poll found that more respondents supported improving the current healthcare system (39%) than repealing the ACA (23%). In addition, bipartisan support was strongest for improving the current system, with 46% of Democrats, 38% of Independents, and 32% of Republicans favoring that approach (Bipartisan Policy Center, 2020). It is worth noting, however, that there is not majority support for any one approach, underlining the difficulty of achieving consensus. A bipartisan group of health leaders support a proposal that focuses on the following principles: Everyone should have meaningful and affordable health insurance (private or public); further reform should avoid major disruption of the current healthcare system; insurance markets must be stable; further reform should reduce excessive and unnecessary cost growth; and policies should be politically and financially sustainable over the long run (Bipartisan Policy Center, 2020).

The political difficulty of repealing and replacing the ACA is not surprising. It is always difficult to take away benefits once people have started to use them. Supporting a bill that would result in more than 20 million people losing insurance is clearly more politically perilous than not supporting legislation (i.e., the ACA) that would deliver health insurance to 20 million people for the first time. This is particularly true for federal legislators who hail from states that (1) implemented the ACA's Medicaid expansion and (2) have Republican governors. Why? Much of the savings from the House and Senate bills came from reduced Medicaid spending, both through the elimination of the expansion and by changing the entire program from an entitlement program to a block grant or per-capita allotment. In turn, states would either have had to absorb the federal spending reductions in their own budgets or absorb the healthcare costs of having more uninsured residents. Indeed, the proposed changes to Medicaid, which went well beyond repealing and replacing the ACA, resulted in many of the biggest criticisms from moderate Republicans.

Medicaid became even more important to the nation as the country grappled early on with the COVID-19 pandemic. State resources have been strained by increased healthcare needs due to the pandemic, and Medicaid provides a source of federal funding that can be crucial to state efforts. In addition, Medicaid rolls increased as residents became (or stayed) unemployed owing to the pandemic (Corallo & Rudowitz, 2021). In expansion states, Medicaid covers 35.8% of all unemployed adults (ages 19–64 years), compared to 16.4% in nonexpansion states (Mann, 2020). Overall, the unemployed uninsured rate in nonexpansion states is almost twice that of expansion states.

The coronavirus pandemic has also laid bare the extant racial and ethnic disparities in our healthcare system (**Figure 11.9** and **Figure 11.10**). Black, Indigenous, and People of Color (BIPOC) populations have suffered disproportionately during the pandemic. These populations have a high burden of COVID-19 cases overall, severe cases, hospitalizations, and deaths (Artiga et al., 2020). At the same time, BIPOC individuals were less likely to get tested for the virus, experienced longer wait times for testing, and had farther to travel to reach a testing site (Artiga et al., 2020). Yet, BIPOC populations are also less likely to be vaccinated than White individuals.

Although unpacking the myriad causes of racial and ethnic health disparities is beyond the scope of this chapter (see Tobin-Tyler & Teitelbaum, 2019), it is worth identifying a few of the structural factors that have led to disproportionate infection and mortality rates from COVID-19 among populations of color. Some of these reasons include living in densely populated areas and crowded living conditions; working in low-wage jobs that are considered essential; working in service-sector jobs that cannot be performed remotely; traveling by public transportation; having less access to healthcare services and health insurance; having higher rates of comorbidities that make the virus more lethal; facing language and health literacy barriers; having reduced access to the Internet; and living in areas of the country that are hardest hit by the pandemic (Bryan et al., 2020; Ford et al., 2020; Johns Hopkins University & Medicine, 2020). Families with noncitizen members face additional structural barriers, such as exclusions from public health programs, policies that discourage families from applying for public assistance even if they are eligible, and restrictions in coronavirus assistance legislation (Gonzalez,

Table 11.4 Comparison of U.S. House of Representatives and Senate Bills Designed to Replace the Affordable Care Act

	American Health Care Act (House)	Better Care Reconciliation Act (Senate)
Premium tax credits	Replace with tax credits based on age only, not income or geographical area	Keep tax credits, lower eligibility to 350% of the FPL, include those with incomes less than 100% of the FPL, tied to less expensive benchmark, change individual contribution levels so older consumers pay more
Individual mandate	Eliminate penalties, replace with 1-year 30% premium surcharge in case of a lapse in coverage	Eliminate penalties, replace with 6-month waiting period in case of a lapse in coverage
Employer mandate	Eliminate penalties	Eliminate penalties
Medicaid expansion	Phase out at end of 2019	Phase out by end of 2024
ACA taxes	Eliminate most key taxes	Eliminate many key taxes, keep the Medicare surtax and investment tax on high-income earners
Essential health benefits (EHBs)	Allow state waivers to redefine EHBs	Allow state waivers to redefine EHBs
Medicaid program	Changes to block grant or per-capita allotment in 2020, allow work requirements	Changes to block grant or per-capita allotment in 2020, allow work requirements
Cost-sharing reduction (CSR) funds	Fund through 2019, repeal in 2020	Fund through 2019, repeal in 2020
Women's health services	Defund Planned Parenthood for 1 year; redefine qualified plan to exclude plans that provide abortion services except for rape, incest, or life of mother in danger	Defund Planned Parenthood for 1 year; redefine qualified plan to exclude plans that provide abortion services except for rape, incest, or life of mother in danger
Private market rules	Keep guaranteed issue, dependent coverage until 26; keep preexisting condition protection	Keep guaranteed issue, dependent coverage until 26; keep preexisting condition protection; permit sale of noncompliant plans as long as selling one ACA-compliant plan
State stabilization pool	Provide $123 billion over 9 years	Provide $182 billion over 9 years
Prevention and Public Health Fund	Eliminate	Eliminate
Age rating band	Change to 5-to-1 but allow for state variation	Change to 5-to-1 but allow for state variation
CBO estimate: uninsured	23 million more uninsured by 2026	22 million more uninsured by 2026
CBO estimate: federal savings	$119 billion	$321 billion

Abbreviations: ACA = Affordable Care Act; CBO = Congressional Budget Office; FPL = federal poverty level.

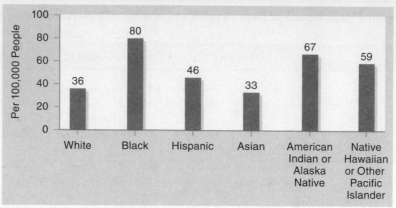

Note: Persons of Hispanic origin may be of any race, but are categorized as Hispanic; other groups are non-Hispanic.

Figure 11.9 COVID-19 Mortality Rates by Race/Ethnicity, as of August 2020

Artiga, S., Corallo, B., & Pham, O. (2020, August 17). *Racial disparities in Covid-19: Key findings from available data and analysis.* Kaiser Family Foundation. https://www.kff.org/report-section/racial-disparities-in-covid-19-key-findings-from-available-data-and-analysis-issue-brief/

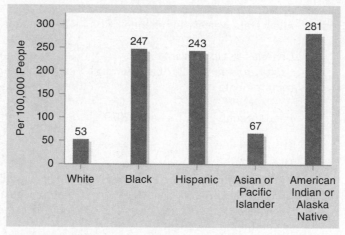

Note: Persons of Hispanic origin may be of any race, but are categorized as Hispanic; other groups are non-Hispanic.

Figure 11.10 Age-Adjusted COVID-19–Associated Hospitalization Rates by Race and Ethnicity, March 1–July 18, 2020

Artiga, S., Corallo, B., & Pham, O. (2020, August 17). *Racial disparities in Covid-19: Key findings from available data and analysis.* Kaiser Family Foundation. https://www.kff.org/report-section/racial-disparities-in-covid-19-key-findings-from-available-data-and-analysis-issue-brief/

2020). While some of the vaccination disparity is due to distrust of the government and the healthcare system due to past transgressions, other obstacles remain. BIPOC populations are less likely to be vaccinated because of access barriers such as lack of transportation, inability to leave work, fear of losing workdays due to side effects, low health literacy, fear of deportation among undocumented immigrants, and concerns about the safety of the vaccines (Lopez, 2021; Volpe, 2021). Under the ACA, low-income individuals and racial and ethnic minorities made significant strides in gaining health insurance, reducing healthcare costs, increasing access to care, having a consistent source of

care, and improving health outcomes (Lantz & Rosenbaum, 2020). Thus, overturning or weakening the ACA would exacerbate the inequities that are already present in our healthcare system and that are preyed upon by the novel coronavirus.

Affordability

One of the key issues to monitor going forward is the affordability of health insurance plans under the ACA. Most people were pleasantly surprised by their premium rates for 2014 and 2015, although there was great variation across the country. Insurers had an incentive to keep premiums low because they wanted to encourage people to enroll in their health plans. In addition, limited information was available about who would be in the insurance pools; this information could have assisted insurers with premium rate setting. Also, many plans contracted with a narrower set of providers as a way to keep premiums low. After moving past the initial enrollment period, will insurance companies hike premiums in future years?

In general, premiums decreased for the third year in a row in 2021, but variations by income level and choice of plan exist across the country. The average benchmark silver premium shrank by 2.2%, while bronze plan premiums decreased 1% and gold plan premiums were 4% lower (McDermott & Cox, 2021). Premium subsidies are based on the benchmark silver premium plans, so a lower premium for these plans may result in lower subsidies for some enrollees. Bronze plans with $0 premiums are available to low-income subsidized enrollees in 84% of counties. Even so, low-income individuals may be better off paying a silver plan premium and taking the cost-sharing subsidy, since CSRs are only available to silver plan enrollees (McDermott & Cox, 2021). These averages, however, hide variations across the country. For example, in 2021 premiums fell by 31% in Iowa, but increased by almost 6% in Arkansas (Ollove, 2021).

Many consumers focus on premiums when purchasing a plan; however, cost-sharing rates significantly affect affordability. In fact, surveys have concluded that the cost of deductibles are enrollees' biggest concern (Goodnough et al., 2020). In 2021, marketplace deductibles' limits were $8550 in unsubsidized individual plans and $17,100 in family plans (Obamacare Facts, 2020). In 2020, the most popular and more affordable bronze and silver plans had deductibles averaging more than $4000 (**Figure 11.11** and **Figure 11.12**). Again, there is great variation across the country. Among 36 reporting states, the average marketplace deductibles in 2021 ranged from $4786 in Ohio to $1902 in Alabama (KFF, 2021c). This problem is not isolated to the ACA; deductibles for employer-based health plans have quadrupled over the last decade (Levey, 2019). Even so, high out-of-pocket costs make it unaffordable for many to use their health insurance, dragging down the popularity of the ACA. These affordability concerns were foreseeable, but lawmakers and policy advisors were constrained by the need to keep the overall cost as low as possible to pass the ACA. Some hoped that cost-sharing subsidies would be increased in future years, but the damaged economy and the current focus on the pandemic make such a significant long-term

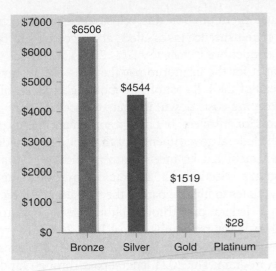

Figure 11.11 Average Medical Deductible in Plans with Combined Medical and Prescription Drug Deductibles, 2020

Kaiser Family Foundation analysis of marketplace plans in states with federally facilitated or partnership exchanges in 2020 (including Arkansas, New Mexico, Oregon, and Kentucky). Data are from Healthcare.gov. Health plan information for individuals and families available here: https://www.healthcare.gov/health-plan-information-2020/

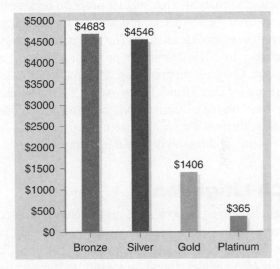

Figure 11.12 Average Medical Deductible in Plans with Separate Medical and Prescription Drug Deductibles, 2020

Kaiser Family Foundation analysis of marketplace plans in states with federally facilitated or partnership exchanges in 2020 (including Arkansas, New Mexico, Oregon, and Kentucky). Data are from Healthcare.gov. Health plan information for individuals and families available here: https://www.healthcare.gov/health-plan-information-2020/

investment unlikely. The alternative path to reducing deductibles—lowering healthcare prices—will be even harder to achieve (Goodnough et al., 2020).

Reinsurance is another tool that could help insurers reduce premiums. Insurers or companies may purchase reinsurance to protect themselves against losses from high-cost enrollees—losses that would lead to premium increases for everyone in the pool (Swartz, 2017). Essentially, insurers take out a policy to protect against costs in a certain segment of an individual's coverage (e.g., costs between $100,000 and $200,000). As with most insurance, the health insurer pays an annual premium for this reinsurance, a deductible before reinsurance takes effect, and a copayment once the deductible is met (Swartz, 2017). Even so, it is cheaper for the insurer to pay the costs of reinsurance instead of the full cost of care for a high-risk enrollee. By keeping costs down, insurers reduce not only premiums for enrollees, but also premium tax credits paid by the federal government. For that reason, the federal government has an incentive to promote reinsurance programs. Section 1332 State Innovation Waivers allow states to finance part of the reinsurance program with a "federal pass-through" from the savings attributed to lower premiums. As of June 2021, 14 states had an approved § 1332 waiver to create a reinsurance program. The 2021 federal pass-through funding is expected to be $1.29 billion, although it is unclear if the additional subsidies available through ARPA will increase that amount (Keith, 2021a).

While early results are promising, many states cannot afford to establish a reinsurance program because they have to front the entire cost and wait for the federal government to reimburse its share. The programs are, indeed, expensive: In 2019, Maryland's program cost $462 million and Oregon's program cost $95 million (National Academy for State Health Policy, 2019). Even if states are able to establish a reinsurance program and obtain federal funding, there is always a concern about whether state and federal funding will be available in future years.

ACA Litigation

Legal challenges in both state and federal courts concerning the ACA have been a fixture since the law's passage in 2010. Some challenges focus on specific aspects of the ACA, while others are existential provocations aimed at striking down the law in its entirety. Several ACA cases have already reached the U.S. Supreme Court—a rarity for a law that is still relatively young. First came the Supreme Court's 2012 decision in *NFIB v. Sebelius*, which was described earlier in this chapter. Then the court decided a case that answered whether, under a federal statute called the Religious Freedom Restoration Act (RFRA), closely held private corporations have a legal right to refuse to comply with provisions of the ACA that require them to provide certain contraceptive coverage to employees (*Burwell v. Hobby Lobby Stores, Inc.*, 2014). (A closely held corporation is one that has a limited number of shareholders; in the *Burwell v. Hobby Lobby* case, the plaintiffs were two private, for-profit companies owned by members of a single family—Hobby Lobby Stores [owned by Evangelical Christians] and Conestoga Wood Specialties [owned by Mennonites].) In a 5–4 decision, the Court

majority determined that the ACA's contraception mandate imposed a significant enough burden on the plaintiff companies' exercise of their beliefs so as to violate RFRA. Just a year later, the Supreme Court ruled that subsidies available under the ACA to help individuals and small businesses buy insurance were available whether the insurance was purchased through a state-run or federally facilitated insurance exchange (*King v. Burwell*, 2015, discussed earlier in this chapter).

Just a year later, the Supreme Court heard a case that was an offshoot of its earlier decision in *Burwell v. Hobby Lobby* (*Zubik v. Burwell*, 2016). After the *Burwell v. Hobby Lobby* decision, the Obama administration offered an accommodation to religious entities that objected to the requirement to provide contraceptive coverage without cost-sharing: The religious organization could simply inform HHS of its objection and identify its insurer, at which point HHS would take responsibility for ensuring that contraceptive services are provided by the insurer without the involvement of the religious organization. The accommodation, however, was not acceptable to a number of religious entities, which filed their own RFRA lawsuits. Over time, nine federal appellate courts ruled that the accommodation did not substantially burden the entities' exercise of religion; however, one appellate court ruled the opposite way, creating a division that the Supreme Court wanted to clear up. Eventually, the Supreme Court—likely split 4–4 on the merits by this time (after Justice Scalia died and the Senate failed to hold hearings on his replacement), and perhaps hoping to spark a compromise among the litigants—remanded the cases to the lower courts without a definitive answer.

In 2018, the Trump administration issued rules offering any for-profit or nonprofit employer or insurer that objected to contraceptives for religious or moral reasons an absolute exemption (i.e., without the need to notify the government or insurers) from providing contraceptive coverage to its employees. The rules were set to go into effect in January 2019 but were blocked by multiple federal courts, leaving the Obama-era contraceptive mandate accommodation in place. The Trump administration and another plaintiff asked the Supreme Court to lift the injunctions. As noted earlier, in July 2020 the Supreme Court ruled 7–2 in favor of the Trump administration's expanded exemptions (the consolidated cases of *Little Sisters of the Poor v. Pennsylvania* and *Trump v. Pennsylvania*, 2020). In a nutshell, the Court majority determined that under the ACA, the federal government had the authority to adopt broad religious and moral exemptions to the contraceptive mandate. As a result, employers that object to the coverage of contraceptives for religious or moral reasons can decline to cover contraceptives for employees or students, without the need for an accommodations process that would otherwise make these services available to affected individuals.

Many women who were receiving no-cost contraception through their employer will now be forced to find these services—if they can find them at all—from another source, and likely at some expense. Soon after the *Little Sisters* decision was handed down, the attorneys general in multiple states initiated *separate* lawsuits targeting the same Trump administration rules, this time contending that the rules are "arbitrary and capricious" under the federal Administrative Procedures Act. At its core, their argument maintains that the rules fail to adequately balance women's health with religious freedom, and that this failure violates the prior Supreme Court decisions pertaining to the ACA's contraceptive mandate. A Massachusetts federal district court was the first to weigh in on the "arbitrary and capricious" issue, ruling against the state's attorney general. That decision has been appealed to the Court of Appeals for the First Circuit but, as of the time of this writing, has been put on hold by the court.

The most recent Supreme Court ACA decision came in the case of *California v. Texas*. This lawsuit was originally brought by 20 Republican-led states and effectively contended that given the repeal of the individual mandate financial penalty (discussed previously), the entire ACA must fall. On what basis did Texas and its counterparts reach this conclusion? They argued that absent the monetary fine for not having health insurance, the requirement to buy insurance has no legal basis, and because the insurance mandate is central to the ACA architecture, the entire law should be thrown out.

As if the lawsuit itself was not enough of a threat to the ACA, a different type of threat emerged in June 2018, when the Trump administration alerted the federal trial court that was hearing the case that it would not defend the ACA in court. Politically speaking, this might not seem like a big deal to most readers; however, this decision represents a dramatic break from the tradition of the federal executive branch in defending existing statutes. Even though the Justice Department's filing with the trial court acknowledged that the decision not to defend an existing law deviates from history, it contended that its decision was not unprecedented. In turn, Democratic state attorneys general from 21 states and the District of Columbia were allowed over the course of the litigation to intervene in the case to defend the ACA. (Also, after 2018 mid-term election wins for the Democratic party in Wisconsin and Maine, those two states dropped out as plaintiffs in the case.)

Many legal scholars across the political spectrum viewed the plaintiffs' argument in *California v. Texas* as absurd, given that plaintiffs effectively argued that a single provision in the ACA that now literally does nothing should render the entire ACA unlawful. Early on, however, the legal rulings were favorable to the plaintiffs, in no small part because the legal arguments have been heard almost exclusively by very conservative judges. Judge Reed O'Connor, the sole judge overseeing the litigation in the federal trial court, ruled in 2018 that the entire ACA must be overturned because the individual mandate could not be "severed" from the rest of the law (in other words, the individual mandate could not be struck down while leaving the rest of the ACA intact).

The defendants appealed to the U.S. Court of Appeals for the Fifth Circuit. At that stage, the federal government abandoned its laissez-faire approach to the lawsuit and argued in support of the trial court's decision. In 2019, in a 2–1 decision, two Republican-appointed judges on the Fifth Circuit Court of Appeals affirmed the unconstitutionality of the individual mandate, setting the stage for Supreme Court intervention.

Finally, in June 2021, the Supreme Court ended this rather weak attempt to undo the entire ACA, although it did so without ever reaching the merits of the arguments. Instead, the Court, in a 7–2 decision, ruled that the Republican-led states and private individuals who had sought to strike down the ACA lacked the standing—a specific injury to their own legal interests—to bring the lawsuit in the first place.

As of summer 2021, there is one additional ACA-specific lawsuit that particularly seems to be causing headaches for ACA supporters (space limitations prevent us from discussing all ongoing ACA litigation, but various websites do this well). The case is called *Kelley v. Becerra*, and it targets several of the ACA provisions that regulate which types of preventive care must be covered, without cost-sharing requirements, by health insurers. There are now approximately 80 items on the preventive services list, including things like birth control drugs and devices, vaccinations, HIV medications, and cancer screenings. The individuals targeting this list are religious conservatives who, according to their lawsuit, would prefer to be able to purchase health insurance policies that do not cover some of the required preventive services. If successful, this lawsuit could potentially undo insurers' responsibility to cover preventive services (think back to religious conservatives' success in the *Little Sisters of the Poor* litigation), or perhaps allow insurers to charge copayments for them. Because the case has yet to be heard by even a federal trial court, there is no clear way to know what is in store for the

ACA's preventive services requirement; stay tuned. Given the seemingly relentless nature of ACA lawsuits, it is clear that, more than a decade after its passage, the Supreme Court and lower federal courts will continue to shape the contours of the ACA for years to come. As you watch these lawsuits unfold, keep in mind just two of the many enormous consequences that would result from a decision that tears down the ACA. First, some 30 million people would immediately become uninsured (in addition to the 30 million who are already uninsured, and that number would likely continue to rise for as long as the COVID-19 pandemic wreaks havoc). Second, the healthcare market in the U.S. would revert back to its pre-ACA days, when millions of people with preexisting conditions could be charged more for their health insurance, or simply be denied coverage altogether.

Conclusion

After decades of trying, and against the predictions of numerous experts, in 2010 the U.S. Congress passed a health reform law that provides insurance coverage on a more universal scale than ever before, includes protections for individuals who have been historically excluded from the insurance market, and shows a concern for improving healthcare quality and access to preventive care. From a philosophical perspective, the ACA moves the United States toward becoming a society where (almost) everyone is expected to have adequate access to affordable health insurance. Under this perspective, health insurance is considered both an obligation and a right: Individuals are required to obtain insurance, and the government is obligated to make it affordable and accessible.

At the same time, there remains in some quarters strong philosophical and political opposition to the ACA, which continues to be challenged both legislatively and in the courts. Republican opposition to the ACA has been consistent and forceful, suggesting challenges and changes to the law will remain a political priority for years to come. Democrats are not unified about the best approach to improving the healthcare system, with some preferring to focus on the ACA while others support a complete overhaul. Nevertheless, the growing popularity of the ACA, the Republicans' inability to repeal and replace the law when they had control of Congress, and a closely divided Congress suggest the ACA will remain part of our healthcare landscape. Whether the ACA will continue to limp along or be used to improve our healthcare system remains to be seen.

References

Abraham, J., & Royalty, A. B. (2017, January 19). *How has the Affordable Care Act affected work and wages?* Penn LDI. https://repository.upenn.edu/ldi_issuebriefs/114/

Abrams, M. K., Nuzum, R., Zezza, M. A., Ryan, J., Kiszla, J., & Guterman, S. (2015, May 7). *The Affordable Care Act's payment and delivery reforms: A progress report at five years.* Commonwealth Fund. https://www.commonwealthfund.org/publications/issue-briefs/2015/may/affordable-care-acts-payment-and-delivery-system-reforms

ACAwise. (n.d.). *State individual mandate: ACA reporting requirements for 2021.* https://www.acawise.com/state-individual-mandate-aca-reporting-requirements/

Affordable Health Care for America Act of 2009, H.R. 3962, 111th Cong. (2009).

Agiesta, J. (2017, March 7). *CNN/ORC poll: Public splits on revoking individual mandate.* CNN. https://www.cnn.com/2017/03/07/politics/health-care-replacement-poll/index.html

American Health Care Act of 2017, H.R. 1628, 115th Cong. (2017).

American Recovery and Reinvestment Act of 2009, Pub. L. No. 111-5, 123 Stat. 115 (2009).

Andrews, M. (2014, September 16). *Health law tempers new state coverage mandates.* Kaiser Family Foundation. https://khn.org/news/health-law-tempers-new-state-coverage-mandates/

Andrews, M. (2018, April 24). *4 New exemptions to the tax penalty for lacking health insurance.* NPR. https://www.npr.org/sections/health-shots/2018/04/24/605007498/4-new-exemptions-to-the-tax-penalty-for-lacking-health-insurance

Antonisse, L., Garfield, R., Rudowitz, R., & Artiga, S. (2018, March 28). *The effects of Medicaid expansion under the ACA: Updated findings from a literature review.* Kaiser Family Foundation. http://files.kff.org/attachment/Issue-Brief-The-Effects-of-Medicaid-Expansion-Under-the-ACA-Updated-Findings-from-a-Literature-Review

Aron-Dine, A. (2017, May 30). *CBO correctly predicted historic gains under ACA.* Center on Budget and Policy Priorities. https://www.cbpp.org/blog/cbo-correctly-predicted-historic-coverage-gains-under-aca

Artiga, S., Corallo, B., & Pham, O. (2020, August 17). *Racial disparities in Covid-19: Key findings from available data and analysis.* Kaiser Family Foundation. https://www.kff.org/report-section/racial-disparities-in-covid-19-key-findings-from-available-data-and-analysis-issue-brief/

Barrett, T., Bash, D., Glass, E., Malveaux, S., Silverleib, A., Walsh, D., & Cohen, T. (2010, January 21). *Pelosi: House won't support Senate health care bill, at least for now.* CNN. https://www.cnn.com/2010/POLITICS/01/21/pelosi.health.care/index.html

Bartsch, S., Ferguson, M., McKinnell, J., O'Shea, K., Wedlock, P., Siegmund, S., & Lee, B. (2020, April 23). The potential health care costs and resource use associated with COVID-19 in the United States. *Health Affairs, 39*(6), 927–935. https://doi.org/10.1377/hlthaff.2020.00426

Better Care Reconciliation Act of 2017, H.R. 1628, 115th Cong. (2017).

Biden, J. (2020, May 7). *Statement by Vice President Joe Biden on birth control case before the U.S. Supreme Court.* Medium. https://medium.com/@JoeBiden/statement-by-vice-president-joe-biden-on-birth-control-case-before-the-u-s-supreme-court-fe16addb28d4

Bipartisan Policy Center. (2020, February). *A bipartisan Rx for America's health care: A practical path for reform.* https://bipartisanpolicy.org/wp-content/uploads/2020/02/WEB_BPC_Future-of-Health-Care-Report_R01-1.pdf

Blake, C. H., & Adolino, J. R. (2001). The enactment of national health insurance: A Boolean analysis of twenty advanced industrial countries. *Journal of Health Politics Policy and Law, 26*(4), 670–708. https://doi.org/10.1215/03616878-26-4-679

Blendon, R. J., Altman, D. E., Benson, J. M., Brodie, M., Buhr, T., Deane, C., & Buscho, S. (2008). Voters and health reform in the 2008 presidential election. *New England Journal of Medicine, 359*(19), 2050–2062. https://doi.org/10.1056/NEJMsr0807717

Blumberg, J., Holahan, J., & Buettgens, M. (2014, May 9). *Why not just eliminate the employer mandate?* Urban Institute. https://www.urban.org/research/publication/why-not-just-eliminate-employer-mandate

Blumberg, J., Holahan, J., Buettgens, M., & Wang, R. (2018a, December 1). *A path to incremental health reform: Improving affordability, expanding coverage, and containing costs.* Robert Wood Johnson Foundation. https://www.rwjf.org/en/library/research/2018/12/a-path-to-incremental-health-care-reform.html

Blumberg, J., Holahan, J., Karpman, M., & Elmendorf, C. (2018b, July 11). *Characteristics of the remaining uninsured: An update.* Urban Institute. https://www.urban.org/research/publication/characteristics-remaining-uninsured-update

Blumenthal, D., & Morone, J. A. (2009). *The heart of power: Health and politics in the Oval Office.* University of California Press.

Boston Globe Editorial Board. (2021, March 21). Stop the filibuster's stranglehold on civil rights. *Boston Globe.* https://www.bostonglobe.com/2021/03/21/opinion/stop-filibusters-stranglehold-civil-rights/

Brodie, M., Hamel, E., Kirzinger, A., & Altman, D. (2020). The past, present, and possible future of public opinion on the ACA. *Health Affairs, 39*(3), 462–470. https://doi.org/10.1377/hlthaff.2019.01420

Brown, C. B., & O'Connor, P. (2010, January 21). *The fallout: Democrats rethinking health care bill.* Politico. https://www.politico.com/story/2010/01/fallout-dems-rethinking-health-bill-031693

Bryan, A., Diuguid-Gerber, J., Davis, N., Chokshi, D., & Galea, S. (2020, July 2). Moving from the five whys to the five hows: Addressing racial inequities in COVID-10 infection and death. *Health Affairs.* https://www.healthaffairs.org/do/10.1377/hblog20200625.389260/full/

Bureau of Labor Statistics. (2020, June 19). *State employment and unemployment (monthly) new release.* https://www.bls.gov/news.release/archives/laus_06192020.htm

Bursztynsky, J. (2019, July 5). *Biden vows to bring back Obamacare's individual mandate penalty for not having health insurance.* CNBC. https://www.cnbc.com/2019/07/05/joe-biden-vows-to-bring-back-obamacare-individual-mandate-penalty.html

Burwell v. Hobby Lobby Stores, Inc., 134 S. Ct. 2751 (2014).

California v. Texas, No. 19-10011 (5th Cir. 2019).

Cancryn, A. (2020, February 19). *Politico–Harvard Poll: Health care costs are top priority heading into elections.* Politico. https://www.politico.com/news/2020/02/19/poll-health-care-election-115866

Center for Consumer Information and Insurance Oversight, Centers for Medicare and Medicaid Services. (2018, April 9). *Guidance on hardship exemptions from the individual shared responsibility provision for persons experiencing limited issuer options or other circumstances.* https://www.cms.gov/CCIIO/Resources/Regulations-and-Guidance/Downloads/2018-Hardship-Exemption-Guidance.pdf

Center for Responsive Politics. (n.d.). *Reelection rates over the years.* OpenSecrets.org. https://www.opensecrets.org/overview/reelect.php

Center on Budget and Policy Priorities. (2021, February 2). *Sabotage watch: Tracking efforts to undermine the ACA.* https://www.cbpp.org/sabotage-watch-tracking-efforts-to-undermine-the-aca

Centers for Medicare and Medicaid Services. (n.d.). *Information on essential health benefits (EHB) benchmark plans.* https://www.cms.gov/CCIIO/Resources/Data-Resources/ehb

Centers for Medicaid and Medicare Services. (2017, March 17). *State effective rate review programs.* https://www.cms.gov/CCIIO/Resources/Fact-Sheets-and-FAQs/rate_review_fact_sheet

Centers for Medicare and Medicaid Services. (2020a, March 12). *FAQs on essential health benefits coverage and the coronavirus (COVID-19).* https://www.cms.gov/CCIIO/Resources/Fact-Sheets-and-FAQs/Downloads/EHB-Benchmark-Coverage-of-COVID-19.pdf

Centers for Medicare and Medicaid Services. (2020b, March 18). *FAQs on catastrophic plan coverage and the coronavirus disease 2019 (COVID-19).* https://www.cms.gov/CCIIO/Resources/Files/Catastrophic-Coverage-of-COVID-19.pdf

Cochrane, E., & Tankersley, J. (2020, March 14). Here's what's in Congress's emergency coronavirus bill. *The New York Times.* https://www.nytimes.com/2020/03/14/us/politics/congress-coronavirus-bill.html

Coll, S. (2008, December 11). Obama's priorities. *The New Yorker.* https://www.newyorker.com/news/steve-coll/obamas-priorities

Collins, S., & Gunja, M. (2019, September 26). *What do Americans think about their health coverage ahead of the 2020 election?* Commonwealth Fund. https://www.commonwealthfund.org/publications/issue-briefs/2019/sep/what-do-americans-think-health-coverage-2020-election

Commercial Insurance. (2012, July). *Self-insured plans under health care reform.* http://www.ciswv.com/CIS/media/CISMedia/Documents/Self-Insured-Plans-Under-Health-Care-Reform-070312_1.pdf

Condon, S. (2010, January 20). *Scott Brown win shakes up health care fight.* CBS News. https://www.cbsnews.com/news/scott-brown-win-shakes-up-health-care-fight/

Congressional Budget Office. (2017a). *American Health Care Act: Cost estimate.* https://www.cbo.gov/system/files?file=115th-congress-2017-2018/costestimate/americanhealthcareact.pdf

Congressional Budget Office. (2017b). *Better Care Reconciliation Act of 2017: Cost estimate.* https://www.cbo.gov/publication/52941

Congressional Budget Office. (2017c). *Federal subsidies under the Affordable Care Act for health insurance coverage related to the expansion of Medicaid and nongroup health insurance: Tables from CBOs January 2017 baseline.* http://acasignups.net/sites/default/files/CBO-2017-01-healthinsurance.pdf

Congressional Budget Office. (2018). *Federal subsidies for health insurance coverage for people under age 65: Tables from*

CBOs spring 2018 projections. https://www.cbo.gov/system/files?file=2018-06/51298-2018-05-healthinsurance.pdf

Congressional Budget Office. (2019a). *Federal subsidies for health insurance coverage for people under age 65: 2019–2029.* https://www.cbo.gov/publication/55085

Congressional Budget Office. (2019b). *How CBO and JCT analyzed coverage effects of new rules for association health plans and short-term plans.* https://www.cbo.gov/system/files/2019-01/54915-New_Rules_for_AHPs_STPs.pdf

Congressional Budget Office. (2020, September). *Federal subsidies for health insurance coverage for people under age 65: 2020–2030.* https://www.cbo.gov/system/files/2020-09/56571-federal-health-subsidies.pdf

Congressional Budget Office. (2021, February). *The budget and economic outlook: 2021 to 2031.* https://www.cbo.gov/system/files/2021-02/56970-Outlook.pdf

Congressional Research Service. (2021, February 9). *Medicaid disproportionate share hospital (DSH) reductions.* https://crsreports.congress.gov/product/pdf/IF/IF10422

Corallo, B., & Rudowitz, R. (2021, July 20). *Analysis of recent national trends in Medicaid and CHIP enrollment.* Kaiser Family Foundation. https://www.kff.org/coronavirus-covid-19/issue-brief/analysis-of-recent-national-trends-in-medicaid-and-chip-enrollment/

Coverage of Certain Preventive Services Under the Affordable Care Act, 78 Fed. Reg. 127, 29870–29899 (July 2, 2013).

Cox, C., Amin, K., Claxton, G., & McDermott, D. (2021, April 7). *The ACA family glitch and affordability of employer coverage.* Kaiser Family Foundation. https://www.kff.org/health-reform/issue-brief/the-aca-family-glitch-and-affordability-of-employer-coverage/

Dunn, A. (2019, July 26). *Democrats differ over best way to provide health coverage for all Americans.* Pew Research Center. https://www.pewresearch.org/fact-tank/2019/07/26/democrats-differ-over-best-way-to-provide-health-coverage-for-all-americans/

Editors of Encyclopaedia Britannica. (n.d.). United States presidential election results. In *Britannica.com* https://www.britannica.com/topic/United-States-Presidential-Election-Results-1788863

Eibner, C., & Nowak, S. (2018, July 11). *The effect of eliminating the individual mandate penalty and the role of behavioral factors.* Commonwealth Fund. https://www.commonwealthfund.org/publications/fund-reports/2018/jul/eliminating-individual-mandate-penalty-behavioral-factors

Elflein, J. (2021, January 7). *Uninsured U.S. non-elderly people percentage and rate by age 2019.* Statista. https://www.statista.com/statistics/498532/percentage-and-rate-of-us-non-elderly-without-health-insurance-by-age/

Emergency Economic Stabilization Act of 2008, Pub. L. No. 110-343, 122 Stat. 3765 (2008).

Employee Retirement Income Security Act of 1974, Pub. L. No. 93-406, 88 Stat. 829 (1974).

Exchange Establishment Standards and Other Related Standards Under the Affordable Care Act, 177 Fed. Reg. 11718, 2012.

Feder, J. (2004). Crowd-out and the politics of health reform. *Journal of Law, Medicine, and Ethics, 32*(3), 461–464. https://doi.org/10.1111/j.1748-720X.2004.tb00158.x

Fehr, R., McDermott, D., & Cox, C. (2020, May 13). *Individual insurance market performance in 2019.* Kaiser Family Foundation. https://www.kff.org/private-insurance/issue-brief/individual-insurance-market-performance-in-2019/

Fiedler, M. (2020). The ACA's individual mandate in retrospect: What did it do and where do we go from here? *Health Affairs, 39*(3), 429–435. https://doi.org/10.1377/hlthaff.2019.01433

Finegold, K., Conmy A., Chu, R., Bosworth, A., & Sommers, B. (2021, February 11). *Trends in the U.S. uninsured population.* Assistant Secretary for Planning and Evaluation. https://aspe.hhs.gov/sites/default/files/private/pdf/265041/trends-in-the-us-uninsured.pdf

Fise, P. (2017, June 8). *Cost sharing reduction subsidies: What happens if they aren't paid?* Bipartisan Policy Center. https://bipartisanpolicy.org/blog/cost-sharing-reduction-subsidies-what-happens-if-they-arent-paid/

Ford, T., Reber, S., & Reeves, R. (2020, June 16). *Race gaps in COVID-19 deaths are even bigger than they appear.* Brookings. https://www.brookings.edu/blog/up-front/2020/06/16/race-gaps-in-covid-19-deaths-are-even-bigger-than-they-appear/

Galewitz, P. (n.d.). *HHS targets young adults for Obamacare enrollment.* WebMD. https://www.webmd.com/health-insurance/news/20160621/hhs-targets-young-adults-in-2017-obamacare-enrollment-plan

Galewitz, P. (2019, September 10). *Breaking a 10-year streak, the number of uninsured Americans rises.* Kaiser Family Foundation. https://khn.org/news/number-of-americans-without-insurance-rises-in-2018/

Gangopadhyaya, A., & Garrett, B. (2020, April). *Unemployment, health insurance, and the COVID-19 recession.* Robert Wood Johnson Foundation & Urban Institute. https://www.urban.org/sites/default/files/publication/101946/unemployment-health-insurance-and-the-covid-19-recession_1.pdf

Garfield, R., Orgera, K., & Damico, A. (2021, January 21). *The coverage gap: Uninsured poor adults in states that do not expand Medicaid.* Kaiser Family Foundation. https://www.kff.org/medicaid/issue-brief/the-coverage-gap-uninsured-poor-adults-in-states-that-do-not-expand-medicaid/

Garrett, T. A. (2011, October 19). State balanced-budget and debt rules. *Economic Synopses, 33.* https://files.stlouisfed.org/files/htdocs/publications/es/11/ES1133.pdf

Giovannelli, J., Lucia, K. W., & Corlette, S. (2014, October 31). *Implementing the Affordable Care Act: Revisiting the ACA's essential health benefits requirements.* Commonwealth Fund. https://www.commonwealthfund.org/publications/issue-briefs/2014/oct/implementing-affordable-care-act-revisiting-acas-essential

Glied, S., Collins, S., & Lin, S. (2020). Did the ACA lower Americans' financial barriers to health care? *Health Affairs, 39*(3), 379–386. https://doi.org/10.1377/hlthaff.2019.01448

Gonzales v. Raich, 545 U.S. 1 (2005).

Gonzalez, D. (2020, May 6). *Hispanic adults in families with non-citizens disproportionately feel the economic fallout from COVID-19.* Urban Institute. https://www.urban.org/research/publication/hispanic-adults-families-noncitizens-disproportionately-feel-economic-fallout-covid-19

Goodnough, A., Abelson, R., Sanger-Katz, M., & Kliff, S. (2020, March 23). Obamacare turns 10. Here's a look at what works and doesn't. *The New York Times.* https://www.nytimes.com/2020/03/23/health/obamacare-aca-coverage-cost-history.html

Gordon, C. (2003). *Dead on arrival: The politics of health care in twentieth-century America.*: Princeton University Press.

Gorlick, A. (2017, August 7). Stanford economists find Affordable Care Act not hindering the U.S. labor market. Stanford University. https://news.stanford.edu/2017/08/07/aca-not-hindering-u-s-labor-market/

Gunja, M. Z., Aboulafia, G. N., & Collins, S. R. (2019, October 31). *What young adults should know about open enrollment.* Commonwealth Fund. https://www.commonwealthfund.org/blog/2019/what-young-adults-should-know-about-open-enrollment

Guttmacher Institute. (2021a, July 1). Insurance coverage of contraceptives. https://www.guttmacher.org/state-policy/explore/insurance-coverage-contraceptives

Guttmacher Institute. (2021b, July 1). An overview of abortion laws. https://www.guttmacher.org/state-policy/explore/overview-abortion-laws

Hamel, L., Firth, J., & Brodie, M. (2014, April 29). *Kaiser health tracking poll: April 2014.* Kaiser Family Foundation. https://www.kff.org/health-reform/poll-finding/kaiser-health-tracking-poll-april-2014/

Healthcare.gov. (n.d.). *Grandfathered health insurance plans.* https://www.healthcare.gov/health-care-law-protections/grandfathered-plans/

Health Insurance Issuers Implementing Medical Loss Ratio Requirements Under the Patient Protection and Affordable Care Act, 75 Fed. Reg. 74864 (2010).

Health Insurance Premium Tax Credit, 77 Fed. Reg., 30377 (2012, May 23).

Heart of Atlanta Motel, Inc. v. United States, 379 U.S. 241 (1964).

HHS Notice of Benefit and Payment Parameters for 2019. 83 Fed. Reg. 74, 16930–17071 (2018, April 17).

Hui, K. (2021, January 21). *What is Biden's plan for reproductive health care?* https://www.verywellhealth.com/reproductive-health-biden-plan-5096100

Johns Hopkins University & Medicine. (2020, July 11). *The Demographics of COVID.* https://coronavirus.jhu.edu/data/racial-data-transparency

Jones, J. M. (2010, October 26). *Economy top issue for voters: Size of gov't may be more pivotal.* Gallup. https://news.gallup.com/poll/144029/economy-top-issue-voters-size-gov-may-pivotal.aspx

Jost, T. S. (2004). Why can't we do what they do? National health reform abroad. *Journal of Law, Medicine, and Ethics, 32*(3), 433–441. https://doi.org/10.1111/j.1748-720X.2004.tb00154.x

Jost, T. S. (2013). Implementing health reform: Exemptions from the individual mandate. *Health Affairs.* https://www.healthaffairs.org/do/10.1377/hblog20130627.032474/full/

Jost, T. S. (2017, May 15). CMS announces plans to effectively end the SHOP exchange. *Health Affairs.* https://www.healthaffairs.org/do/10.1377/hblog20170515.060112/full/

Kaiser Family Foundation. (n.d.). *Health reform FAQs.* https://www.kff.org/health-reform/faq/health-reform-frequently-asked-questions/#question-who-is-eligible-for-marketplace-premium-tax-credits

Kaiser Family Foundation. (2008, October 20). *Findings of Kaiser health tracking poll: Election 2008: October 2008.* https://www.kff.org/health-reform/poll-finding/kaiser-health-tracking-poll-election-2008-october/

Kaiser Family Foundation. (2009a, August 1). *Kaiser health tracking poll—August 2009.* https://www.kff.org/health-costs/poll-finding/kaiser-health-tracking-poll-august-2009/

Kaiser Family Foundation. (2009b, November 1). *Chartpack: Kaiser health tracking poll—November 2009.* https://www.kff.org/health-costs/poll-finding/chartpack-kaiser-health-tracking-poll-november-2009/

Kaiser Family Foundation. (2019, September). *Employer health benefits 2019 annual survey.* https://www.kff.org/health-costs/report/2019-employer-health-benefits-survey/

Kaiser Family Foundation. (2020, May 27). *Public opinion on single-payer, national health plans, and expanding access to Medicare coverage.* https://www.kff.org/slideshow/public-opinion-on-single-payer-national-health-plans-and-expanding-access-to-medicare-coverage/

Kaiser Family Foundation. (2021a, June 3). *KFF health tracking poll: The public's views on the ACA.* https://www.kff.org/interactive/kff-health-tracking-poll-the-publics-views-on-the-aca/#?response=Favorable--Unfavorable&aRange=twoYear

Kaiser Family Foundation. (2021b, July 23). *Status of state Medicaid expansion decisions: Interactive map.* https://www.kff.org/medicaid/issue-brief/status-of-state-medicaid-expansion-decisions-interactive-map/

Kaiser Family Foundation. (2021c). *Average marketplace deductible.* https://www.kff.org/other/state-indicator/average-marketplace-deductible/?currentTimeframe=0&sortModel=%7B%22colId%22:%22Location%22,%22sort%22:%22asc%22%7D

Kaiser Family Foundation. (2021d, June 3). *KFF health tracking poll: The public's views on the ACA.* https://www.kff.org/interactive/kff-health-tracking-poll-the-publics-views-on-the-aca/#?response=Favorable--Unfavorable&group=Party%2520ID::Democrat::Independent::Republican&aRange=twoYear

Kahn, H. (2010, January 22). *Health care bill aftermath: Rep. Patrick Kennedy hails dad's dream: Sen. John McCain sees "heavy price."* ABC News. https://abcnews.go.com/GMA/Health Care/health-care-congress-passes-landmark-reform-obama-sign/story?id=10167139

Kamal, R., Cox, C., Fehr, R., Ramirez, M., Hortsman, K., & Levitt, L. (2018, October 26). *How repeal of the individual mandate and expansion of loosely regulated plans are affecting 2019 premiums.* Kaiser Family Foundation. https://www.kff.org/health-costs/issue-brief/how-repeal-of-the-individual-mandate-and-expansion-of-loosely-regulated-plans-are-affecting-2019-premiums/

Keith, K. (2018a, April 10). Unpacking the 2019 final payment notice (part 1). *Health Affairs.* https://www.healthaffairs.org/do/10.1377/hblog20180410.631773/full/

Keith, K. (2018b, April 11). Unpacking the 2019 final payment notice (part 2). *Health Affairs.* https://www.healthaffairs.org/do/10.1377/hblog20180411.618457/full/

Keith, K. (2018c, July 19). States' lawsuit over cost-sharing reductions is dismissed. *Health Affairs.* https://www.healthaffairs.org/do/10.1377/hblog20180719.822849/full/

Keith, K. (2019, December 19). ACA provisions in the new budget bill. *Health Affairs.* https://www.healthaffairs.org/do/10.1377/hblog20191220.115975/full/

Keith, K. (2020a, March 26). Latest coverage proposals in Congress. *Health Affairs.* https://www.healthaffairs.org/do/10.1377/hblog20200526.769681/full/

Keith, K. (2020b, April 2). Final marketplace enrollment data for 2020. *Health Affairs.* https://www.healthaffairs.org/do/10.1377/hblog20200402.109653/full/

Keith, K. (2020c, April 28). Supreme Court rules that insurers are entitled to risk corridor payments: What the Court said and what happens next. *Health Affairs.* https://www.healthaffairs.org/do/10.1377/hblog20200427.34146/full/

Keith, K. (2020d, May 7). Supreme Court: No clear consensus on contraceptive mandate rules. *Health Affairs.* https://www.healthaffairs.org/do/10.1377/hblog20200507.225892/full/

Keith, K. (2020e, May 21). ACA round-up: NH 1332 waiver, risk adjustment, and quality reporting. *Health Affairs.* https://www.healthaffairs.org/do/10.1377/hblog20200521.609605/full/

Keith, K. (2020f, July 9). Supreme Court upholds broad exemptions to contraceptive mandate—for now. *Health Affairs.* https://www.healthaffairs.org/do/10.1377/hblog20200708.110645/full/

Keith, K. (2021a, March 9). Section 1332 pass-through funding for 2021, new health plan guidance. *Health Affairs.* https://doi.org/10.1377/hblog20210309.706522

Keith, K. (2021b, April 29). Biden's first 100 days: The ACA and the American Families Plan. *Health Affairs*. https://www.healthaffairs.org/do/10.1377/hblog20210429.417119/full/

Keith, K., & Jost, T. (2017, October 7). Trump administration regulatory rebalancing favors religious and moral freedom over contraceptive access. *Health Affairs*. https://www.healthaffairs.org/do/10.1377/hblog20171021.317078/full/

King v. Burwell, 135 S. Ct. 2480 (2015).

Kirzinger, A., Muñana, C., & Brodie, M. (2019, November 27). *6 Charts about public opinion on the Affordable Care Act*. Kaiser Family Foundation. https://www.kff.org/health-reform/poll-finding/6-charts-about-public-opinion-on-the-affordable-care-act/

Kornreich, L. (2007, September 21). *Obama talks about mother's cancer battle in ad*. CNN. http://politicalticker.blogs.cnn.com/2007/09/21/obama-talks-about-mothers-cancer-battle-in-ad/

Lantz, P., & Rosenbaum, S. (2020, October). The potential and realized impact of the Affordable Care Act on health equity. *Journal of Health Politics, Policy, and Law, 45*(5), 831–845. https://doi.org/10.1215/03616878-8543298

Lawrence, Q. (2020, April 15). *Public Health Service poised to create a ready reserve to fight the coronavirus*. NPR. https://www.npr.org/2020/04/15/834235294/public-health-service-poised-to-create-a-ready-reserve-to-fight-the-coronavirus

Levey, N. (2019, May 2). Health insurance deductibles soar, leaving Americans with unaffordable bills. *The Los Angeles Times*. https://www.latimes.com/politics/la-na-pol-health-insurance-medical-bills-20190502-story.html

Lewis, C., Abrams, M., Seervai, S., & Blumenthal, D. (2020, April 1). *Evidence from a decade of innovation: The impact of payment and delivery system reforms of the Affordable Care Act*. Commonwealth Fund. https://www.commonwealthfund.org/evidence-decade-innovation-impact-payment-and-delivery-system-reforms-affordable-care-act

Lieberman, T. (2021, June 16). *Is Biden opting out of a 'public option' for the Affordable Care Act?* Center for Health Journalism. https://centerforhealthjournalism.org/2021/06/15/biden-opting-out-public-option-affordable-care-act

Liptak, K., Luhby, T., & Mattingly, P. (2017, October 13). *Trump will end health care cost sharing subsidies*. CNN. https://www.cnn.com/2017/10/12/politics/obamacare-subsidies/index.html

Little Sisters of the Poor v. Pennsylvania, Docket No. 19-431 (S. Ct. 2020).

Lopez, G. (2021, June 3). *The 6 reasons Americans aren't getting vaccinated*. Vox. https://www.msn.com/en-us/money/news/the-6-reasons-americans-arent-getting-vaccinated/ar-AAKDBSD

Luhby, T. (2017, March 12). *What CBO got right—and wrong—on Obamacare*. CNN. https://money.cnn.com/2017/03/09/news/economy/cbo-obamacare/index.html

Luhby, T. (2021, June 7). *Biden has paused a public option. Nevada is about to try its own*. CNN. https://www.cnn.com/2021/06/07/politics/public-option-nevada-biden/index.html

Magness, J. (2017, March 30). *America's opposition to repealing Obamacare grows, particularly among Republicans*. McClatchy DC. https://www.mcclatchydc.com/news/politics-government/article141562849.html

Mann, C. (2020, April 15). *The COVID-19 crisis is giving states that haven't expanded Medicaid new reasons to reconsider*. Commonwealth Fund. https://www.commonwealthfund.org/blog/2020/covid-19-crisis-giving-states-havent-expanded-medicaid-new-reconsideration

McDermott, D., & Cox, C. (2021, April 12). *Data note: 2021 medical loss ratio rebates*. Kaiser Family Foundation. https://www.kff.org/private-insurance/issue-brief/data-note-2021-medical-loss-ratio-rebates/

Medicaid, CHIP Payment and Access Commission. (n.d.). *Medicaid enrollment changes following the ACA*. https://www.macpac.gov/subtopic/medicaid-enrollment-changes-following-the-aca/

Morone, J. A. (2010). Presidents and health reform: From Franklin D. Roosevelt to Barack Obama. *Health Affairs, 29*(6), 1096–1100. https://doi.org/10.1377/hlthaff.2010.0420

Murse, T. (2019, July 13). *Do members of Congress ever lose re-election?* ThoughtCo. https://www.thoughtco.com/do-congressmen-ever-lose-re-election-3367511

National Academy for State Health Policy. (2019, January 14). *State reinsurance programs lower premiums and stabilize markets: Oregon and Maryland show how*. https://www.nashp.org/state-reinsurance-programs-lower-premiums-and-stabilize-markets-oregon-and-maryland-show-how/

National Association of Insurance Commissioners. (2020, April 17). *Short-term limited-duration health plans*. https://content.naic.org/cipr_topics/topic_short_term_limited_duration_health_plans.htm

National Federation of Independent Business v. Sebelius, 132 S. Ct. 2566 (2012).

Newport, F. (2009, July 31). *Americans on health reform: Top 10 takeaways*. Gallup. https://news.gallup.com/poll/121997/americans-healthcare-reform-top-takeaways.aspx

Nicholson, H., & Wile, M. (2021, March 17). *Health and human services funding in the American Rescue Plan*. National Conference of State Legislators. https://www.ncsl.org/ncsl-in-dc/publications-and-resources/health-and-human-services-provisions-in-the-american-rescue-plan-magazine2021.aspx

Norris, L. (2019, September 23). *ACA's cost-sharing subsidies: Key takeaways*. Healthinsurance.org. https://www.healthinsurance.org/obamacare/the-acas-cost-sharing-subsidies/

Norris, L. (2021a, March 26). *The ACA's cost-sharing subsidies*. Healthinsurance.org https://www.healthinsurance.org/obamacare/the-acas-cost-sharing-subsidies/

Norris, L. (2021b, May 5). *What type of health insurance exchange does my state have?* Healthinsurance.org. https://www.healthinsurance.org/faqs/what-type-of-health-insurance-exchange-does-my-state-have/

Norris, L. (2021c, June 1). *Can small businesses use the ACA's health insurance marketplaces (exchanges)?* Healthinsurance.org. https://www.healthinsurance.org/faqs/ive-heard-a-lot-about-health-insurance-exchanges-but-what-are-shop-exchanges/

ObamaCareFacts.com. (2020, September 22). *Out-of-pocket maximums and deductible limits for 2021*. https://obamacarefacts.com/out-of-pocket-maximums-and-deductible-limits-for-2021/

Oberlander, J. (2010). Long time coming: Why health reform finally passed. *Health Affairs, 29*(6), 1112–1116. https://doi.org/10.1377/hlthaff.2010.0447

Office of Assistant Secretary for Planning and Evaluation. (2021). *U.S. federal poverty guidelines used to determine financial eligibility for certain federal programs*. https://aspe.hhs.gov/topics/poverty-economic-mobility/poverty-guidelines/prior-hhs-poverty-guidelines-federal-register-references/2021-poverty-guidelines#main-content

Ollove, M. (2021, June 1). *Obamacare prices continue to fall*. PEW. https://www.pewtrusts.org/en/research-and-analysis/blogs/stateline/2021/06/01/obamacare-prices-continue-to-fall

Patient Protection and Affordable Care Act of 2010, 42 U.S.C. § 18001 (2010).

Pew Research Center. (2008, August 21). *More Americans question religion's role in politics*. https://www.people-press

.org/2008/08/21/more-americans-question-religions-role-in-politics/

Pew Research Center. (2016, July 7). *2016 Campaign: Strong interest, widespread dissatisfaction.* https://www.people-press.org/2016/07/07/2016-campaign-strong-interest-widespread-dissatisfaction/

Pollitz, K., Long, M., Semanskee, A., & Kamal, R. (2018, April 23). *Understanding short-term limited-duration health insurance.* Kaiser Family Foundation. https://www.kff.org/health-reform/issue-brief/understanding-short-term-limited-duration-health-insurance/

ProCon.org. (2020, March 9). *Top issues for voters.* https://2020election.procon.org/view.resource.php?resourceID=007111

Rao, P., & Nowak, S. (2019). *Effects of alternative insurer responses to discontinued federal cost-sharing reduction payments.* RAND Corporation. https://www.rand.org/pubs/research_reports/RR2963.html

Rosenbaum, S., Teitelbaum, J., & Hayes, K. (2011). Crossing the Rubicon: The impact of the Affordable Care Act on the content of insurance coverage for persons with disabilities. *Notre Dame Journal of Law, Ethics, and Public Policy, 25*(2), 527–562. https://scholarship.law.nd.edu/cgi/viewcontent.cgi?article=1066&context=ndjlepp

Saad, L. (2008, November 10). *Obama and Bush: A contrast in popularity.* Gallup. https://news.gallup.com/poll/111838/obama-bush-contrast-popularity.aspx

Segers, G. (2021, March 18). *Senators spar over eliminating the filibuster to pass Democratic priorities.* CBS News. https://www.cbsnews.com/news/filibuster-senate-elimination-debate-democratic-priorities/

Scott, D. (2018, April 13). *A requiem for the individual mandate.* Vox. https://www.vox.com/policy-and-politics/2018/4/13/17226566/obamacare-penalty-2018-individual-mandate-still-in-effect

Scott, D. (2021, June 17). *The public option is now a reality in three states.* Vox. https://www.msn.com/en-us/news/politics/the-public-option-is-now-a-reality-in-3-states/ar-AAL9acb

Shapiro, I. (2010). State suits against health reform are well grounded in law—and pose serious challenges. *Health Affairs, 29*(6), 1229–1233. https://doi.org/10.1377/hlthaff.2010.0449

Sheen, R. (2021, April 8). *Recapping on Biden's ACA reforms, what employers need to know.* https://acatimes.com/recapping-on-bidens-aca-reform

Starr, P. (1982). *The social transformation of American medicine: The rise of a sovereign profession and the making of a vast industry.* Basic Books.

Steinhauer, J. (2017, July 17). Old truths trip up G.O.P. on health law: A benefit is hard to retract. *The New York Times.* https://www.nytimes.com/2017/07/17/us/politics/republican-party-health-care-law-obamacare.html

Stolberg, S. (2020, July 13). Millions have lost health insurance in pandemic driven recession. *The New York Times.* https://www.nytimes.com/2020/07/13/us/politics/coronavirus-health-insurance-trump.html

Swanson, E., & Alonso-Zaldivar, R. (2020, June 8). *Poll: Pandemic does little to alter US views on health care.* AP News. https://apnews.com/12c5c9873cfd9e8a5cd5787694204b9f

Swartz, K. (2017, August 14). *"Reinsurance" program critical to shoring up the ACA.* Harvard School of Public Health. https://www.hsph.harvard.edu/news/features/reinsurance-aca/

Tax Cut and Jobs Act of 2017, Pub. L. No. 115-97, 131 Stat. 2054 (2017).

Tax Policy Center. (n.d.). *Briefing book: What is reconciliation?* https://www.taxpolicycenter.org/briefing-book/what-reconciliation

Taylor, A., Saenz, A., & Levine, M. (2015, June 25). *Supreme Court upholds Obamacare subsidies, president says ACA is "here to stay."* ABC News. https://abcnews.go.com/Politics/supreme-court-upholds-obama-health-care-subsidies/story?id=31931412

Tobin-Tyler, E., & Teitelbaum, J. (2019). *Essentials of health justice.* Jones & Bartlett Learning.

Trump v. Pennsylvania, Docket No. 19-454 (S. Ct. 2020).

Trust for America's Health. (n.d.). *The Prevention and Public Health Fund backgrounder: Preventing disease and reducing long-term health costs.* https://www.tfah.org/report-details/prevention-and-public-health-fund-detailed-information/

Trust for America's Health. (2019, April). *The impact of chronic underfunding on America's public health system: Trends, risks, and recommendations, 2019.* https://www.tfah.org/wp-content/uploads/2020/03/TFAH_2019_PublicHealthFunding_07.pdf

Trust for America's Health. (2021, May). *The impact of chronic underfunding on America's public health system: Trends, risks, and recommendations, 2021.* https://www.tfah.org/wp-content/uploads/2021/05/2021_PHFunding_Fnl.pdf

United States v. Lopez, 514 U.S. 549 (1995).

U.S. Census Bureau. (2010). *Income, poverty, and health insurance coverage in the United States: 2009.* Current Population Reports, P60-238. U.S. Government Printing Office.

U.S. Census Bureau. (2019). *Health insurance coverage in the United States: 2018.* Current Population Reports, P60-267(RV). U.S. Government Printing Office.

U.S. Constitution, Article I, § 8.

Volpe, K. (2021, March 15). *Overcoming Covid-19 vaccine hesitancy in minority communities.* Clinical Advisor. https://www.clinicaladvisor.com/home/topics/vaccine-information-center/overcoming-covid-19-vaccine-hesitancy-minority-communities/

Weissert, C. S., & Weissert, W. G. (2002). *Governing health: The politics of health policy* (2nd ed.). Johns Hopkins University Press.

West, D. M., Heith, D., & Goodwin, C. (1996). Harry and Louise go to Washington: Political advertising and health care reform. *Journal of Health Politics, Policy, and Law, 21*, 35–68. https://doi.org/10.1215/03616878-21-1-35

White House. (2009a, June 3). *Letter from President Obama to Chairmen Edward M. Kennedy and Max Baucus.* Office of the Press Secretary.

White House. (2009b, September 9). *Remarks by the President to a joint session of Congress on health care.* Office of the Press Secretary.

White House. (2010, January 27). *The 2010 State of the Union address.* Office of the Press Secretary.

Wickard v. Filburn, 317 U.S. 111 (1942).

Wihbey, J. (2014, October 1). *Midterm Congressional elections explained: Why the president's party typically loses.* Journalist's Resource. https://journalistsresource.org/studies/politics/elections/voting-patterns-midterm-congressional-elections-why-presidents-party-typically-loses/

Wynn, B. (2017, March 27). Five lessons from the AHCA's demise. *Health Affairs.* https://www.healthaffairs.org/do/10.1377/hblog20170327.059388/full/

Zubik v. Burwell, 136 S. Ct. 1557 (2016).

CHAPTER 12

Healthcare Quality Policy and Law

LEARNING OBJECTIVES

By the end of this chapter you will be able to:

1. Discuss licensure and accreditation in the context of healthcare quality
2. Describe the scope and causes of medical errors
3. Describe the meaning and evolution of the medical professional standard of care
4. Identify and explain certain state-level legal theories under which healthcare professionals and entities can be held liable for medical negligence
5. Explain how federal employee benefits law often preempts medical negligence lawsuits against insurers and managed care organizations
6. Describe efforts to measure and incentivize high-quality health care

Introduction

This chapter steps away from the topics of healthcare access and coverage to focus on healthcare quality. As with access and coverage, healthcare quality has various dimensions, and the topic of healthcare quality has increasingly been a focal point of researchers, analysts, health professionals, and consumers. For instance, in the span of only a couple of years, the influential National Academy of Medicine (NAM, formerly the Institute of Medicine) released two major reports pertaining to healthcare quality: *To Err Is Human: Building a Safer Health System* (Kohn et al., 2000), which focused on the specific quality concern of patient safety, and *Crossing the Quality Chasm: A New Health System for the 21st Century* (Committee on Quality of Health Care in America, 2001), which described how the healthcare delivery system should be overhauled to improve care.

Like healthcare access and coverage issues, healthcare quality is a key concern in health policy and law. For example, long-standing problems related to the administration of health care—like racial and ethnic health disparities, and the geographical variation in the amount or type of care provided to patients—have drawn responses from policymakers and the legal system. Furthermore, policy and legal responses are often needed, because healthcare quality is affected by changes in the marketplace or by advances in medical technology. For instance, institutional payers for healthcare services—traditional insurers, employers, and managed care companies—are more involved in healthcare practice now than was the case historically (Furrow et al., 2001, p. 26), a fact that spurred policymakers and courts to reconsider traditional notions of healthcare quality and liability.

The role of law as a monitor of the quality of health care was on display in the context of the no-duty-to-treat principle and the case of *Hurley v. Eddingfield* (1901). Indiana's physician licensure law was described as a filter to weed out individuals without the requisite skills to safely and adequately practice medicine. In theory, licensure provides a second healthcare quality function—it allows state regulators to monitor the conduct of medical practitioners even after they have been licensed—although, as discussed later, this function has not been performed with much vigor over the years.

Holding healthcare professionals and entities liable for substandard care is another (and perhaps the most well-known) legal tool used to promote quality in health care. Physicians have no legal duty to accept a patient into their practice or to provide care upon request, except in limited circumstances. However, a doctor's decision to treat a patient establishes a legally significant physician–patient relationship, under which the physician owes the patient a reasonable duty of care. Failure to meet what is termed the *professional standard of care*—the legal standard used in medical negligence cases to determine whether health professionals and entities have adequately discharged their responsibility to provide reasonable care to their patients—can result in legal liability for reasonably foreseeable injuries.[a] This potential liability is on display in **Box 12.1**.

As you will soon discover, the laws and legal principles that define the circumstances under which aggrieved individuals can successfully sue an MCO for substandard care or coverage determinations are complex. This complexity stems from multiple facts.

First, the legal framework applied to medical negligence cases was developed long before the advent of managed care. Second, the hybrid nature of managed care (combining as it does the financing and delivery of care) defies easy categorization and makes application of the legal framework challenging. And third, a federal law (Employee Retirement Income Security Act, or ERISA) pertaining to employee benefit plans preempts (i.e., precludes) many typical state-level legal claims against MCOs.

The next section of this chapter provides a brief overview of healthcare licensure and accreditation in the context of healthcare quality. The chapter then turns to an overview of errors in health care. Although medical errors are only one small component of the broad subject of healthcare quality, they are commonly included in the quality discussion and serve as a jumping-off point for a discussion of healthcare liability. The chapter then turns to a full discussion of the professional standard of care and its evolution, followed by a description of some of the state legal theories under which hospitals, traditional insurers, and MCOs can be held liable for substandard medical professional conduct. It then explores the complex area of how ERISA preempts lawsuits premised on these same legal theories. Finally, the chapter describes the concepts of measuring and incentivizing healthcare quality.

Quality Control Through Licensure and Accreditation

The licensing of healthcare professionals and institutions is an important function of state law. As noted previously, healthcare licensure is centrally about filtering out those who may not have the requisite knowledge or skills to practice medicine; in other words, states exercise their police powers when applying licensure laws in order to protect residents from being subjected to substandard health care. State licensure laws both define the qualifications required to become licensed and the standards that must be met for purposes of maintaining and renewing licenses (Rosenbaum et al., 2012).

As important as the licensing function is, however, historically it has been used in the promotion of healthcare quality in only the bluntest sense. This stems from the fact that in most states, the only method by which to promote quality through licensure is, simply, the granting or denial of the license to practice medicine. In other words, there exists no

> 📝 **Box 12.1** VIGNETTE   Michelina Bauman was born on May 16, 1995, in New Jersey. The managed care organization (MCO) through which her parents received healthcare coverage had precertified coverage for 1 day in the hospital post-birth, and both Michelina and her mother were discharged from the hospital 24 hours after Michelina was born. The day after the discharge, Michelina became ill. Her parents telephoned the MCO, but they were neither advised to take Michelina back to the hospital nor provided an in-home visit by a pediatric nurse as promised under the MCO's "L'il Appleseed" infant care program. Michelina died that same day from meningitis stemming from an undiagnosed strep infection.

middle ground between being granted a license and not being granted (or renewed for) a license, no ongoing monitoring or application of standards intended to promote quality and ensure competence in the face of evolving medical care practices. In designing licensing laws, most state legislatures assume that medical professional trade associations (e.g., the American Medical Association) and/or accrediting bodies have sufficient ethical and practice standards to effectively regulate healthcare practitioners and that the purpose of licensure as a quality control measure is to identify and deal with a relatively small number of cases of individual provider deviation from those standards (Rosenbaum et al., 2012). This assumption is correct, to a point; private professional and industry standards do indeed exist, although their effect on day-to-day quality is debatable. Some commentators maintain that accreditation amounts to little more than self-serving indicia of individual or institutional exceptionalism, while others argue that accreditation plays an important and useful role alongside licensure. There are many examples of healthcare accreditation bodies: The Joint Commission (formerly the Joint Commission on Accreditation of Healthcare Organizations), which may be best known for its review and accreditation of hospitals; the National Committee for Quality Assurance, which accredits MCOs; the Healthcare Facilities Accreditation Program; the Commission on Accreditation of Rehabilitation Facilities; the Community Health Accreditation Program; the Utilization Review Accreditation Commission; and others.

A second historical fact related to licensure's effect (or lack thereof) on healthcare quality—one that plays into detractors' claims about the self-serving nature of today's industry-designed accreditation processes—is that state licensing schemes were designed not with healthcare quality, per se, in mind, but rather with an eye toward protecting the medical professions from unscrupulous or incompetent providers and bad publicity. Thus, the laws tended to focus on preventing relatively rare instances of grossly poor-quality care, rather than on long-term promotion of high-quality care.

One final topic pertaining to licensure that bears mentioning is the immensely important role it plays in defining the permissible "scope of practice" of the various types of healthcare providers. It is one thing for state legislators to define the meaning of practice for various broad medical fields (e.g., there is not so much overlap between, say, medicine and dentistry as to cause a huge number of policy and legal disputes), but quite another for legislators to define the lawful activities of doctors as compared to physician assistants as compared to nurses, and even more specifically of advanced practice nurses as compared to licensed practical nurses as compared to registered nurses. It is in delineating permissible scopes of practice within fields and subspecialties that fierce policy disputes take place.

Yet, it is not surprising that these disputes take place. Licensure laws define who has the power to engage in medical practice, who gets to practice specific types of health care, and how and when professional standards of conduct are enforced. In short, licensure laws have the power to determine who is in, as they say, and who is out. Some states are relatively more inclusive in their approach to the licensing of healthcare professionals, whereas others hew closely to a more traditional approach in which physicians are granted broad scope of practice powers while other professionals (e.g., nurses) have far less ability to diagnose and treat patients. The latter approach is being hotly contested, as nurses and other nonphysician healthcare professionals decry their inability to practice to their full education and training, particularly in light of the healthcare workforce shortages that plague the nation (Iglehart, 2013) and the large number of individuals who were newly able to access health insurance (and thus more likely to seek care) under the Patient Protection and Affordable Care Act (ACA).

Medical Errors as a Public Health Concern

Notwithstanding licensure laws and accreditation standards, medical errors are bound to, and often do, occur. And while medical errors are obviously not a new problem, framing the issue as a public health problem is a relatively new phenomenon, and healthcare providers, public health professionals, and policymakers have in recent years committed increased attention to the problem of medical errors.

The regularity with which medical errors occur and the resulting extent of adverse health outcomes and mortalities indicate that the problem is not confined to one ethnic or racial population, socioeconomic group, or geographical area. One study indicates that medical errors in hospitals and other healthcare facilities may now be the *third-leading* cause of death in the United States (Makary & Daniel, 2016), behind only heart disease and cancer. This prevalence suggests that factors such as unskilled or poorly trained doctors and poor communication systems within facilities contribute to more deaths annually than do respiratory disease, accidents, strokes, Alzheimer disease, diabetes, flu and pneumonia, kidney disease, and suicide, which round out the top 11 causes of death (Makary & Daniel, 2016). The negative effects of medical errors on individual patients and on society as a whole—including associated reductions in work productivity, lost income, and the costs associated with correcting injuries resulting from errors—support the conclusion that medical errors are properly classified as a public health problem requiring a strong response from policymakers and the legal system.

Medical errors have various causes. Some causes are, relatively speaking, concrete, such as failure to complete an intended medical course of action, implementation of the wrong course of action, use of faulty equipment or products in effecting a course of action, failure to stay abreast of one's field of medical practice, or health professional inattentiveness. For example, according to the previously mentioned NAM reports, errors in the prescribing, administering, and dispensing of medications result in at least 1.5 million injuries or deaths annually in the United States (Kaufman, 2006). Furthermore, "mistakes in giving drugs are so prevalent in hospitals that, on average, a patient will be subjected to a medication error each day he or she occupies a hospital bed" (Kaufman, 2006). Yet according to the NAM reports, "at least a quarter of the injuries caused by drug errors are clearly preventable" (Kaufman, 2006). Some of the errors are spawned by something as simple as name confusion among pharmaceuticals; for example, it is easy to see how physicians, nurses, and pharmacists could easily confuse the arthritis drug Celebrex, the anticonvulsant drug Cerebyx, and the antidepressant drug Celexa when prescribing, administering, and filling medications (Nordenberg, 2000).

There are more abstract causes of medical errors, as well. For example, they can result from the fact that "much of medical treatment is still primitive: the etiologies and optimal treatments for many illnesses are not known [and] many treatment techniques, such as cancer chemotherapy, create substantial side effects" (Furrow et al., 2001, p. 30). Also, many people argue that the culture of medicine, including its history of elitism, its focus on memorization in both diagnosing and treating illness, and its dedication to secrecy when adverse medical outcomes occur, helps to explain the extent of medical errors.

Just as there are multiple causes of medical errors, so too are there various strategies—some broad and systemic, others more incremental—for preventing and reducing their occurrence. For instance, hospitals usually employ two vehicles to minimize medical errors and assure quality care for patients: risk management programs and peer review processes. Risk management programs monitor risks associated with nonphysician personnel and with facilities under the direct control of hospital administrators; peer review processes entail a secretive evaluation of hospital-based physician practices by physicians themselves. Most physicians encounter the peer review process when they apply for "staff privileges" at a hospital, which grant doctors the ability to use the hospital for their own private practice, including the ability to admit patients and use the hospital's resources in treating patients. Once doctors are granted such privileges, they are subject to ongoing peer review. Many analysts maintain that the secretive manner in which the peer review process is conducted stifles meaningful improvements to patient safety and that it is too reactive—responding to errors only after they have occurred.

Recently, public and private policymakers have begun shifting their attention to medical error reforms that are less reactive and more centered on error prevention and patient safety improvements. There are two primary objectives of these reforms: (1) to redesign healthcare delivery methods and structures to limit the likelihood of human error, and (2) to prepare in advance for the inevitable errors that will occur in healthcare delivery regardless of the amount and types of precautions taken. Medical error reform could entail various approaches, including improving standardization of medical procedures, enforcing mandatory reporting of medical errors, reducing reliance on memory in medical care, increasing and improving medical information technology systems, encouraging patients to be more participatory in their own medical care, and establishing a national focus on the topic of patient safety (Furrow et al., 2001, pp. 43–64). For example, the federal Patient Safety and Quality Improvement Act (PSQIA) was signed into law in 2005 in response to the *To Err Is Human* report. PSQIA created a system for use by healthcare providers to anonymously report medical error data for systematic analysis. The hope is that by aggregating, analyzing, and disseminating the data analyses to healthcare providers nationwide, healthcare professionals and entities will increase their knowledge about what leads to adverse medical outcomes and alter their practice methods accordingly. Before turning to the next section, consider the discussion questions in **Box 12.2**.

What do you think of the term *medical error* as a descriptor of adverse medical outcomes? After all, there are many medical procedures (e.g., invasive surgeries) and treatments (e.g., chemotherapy) that not only are inherently risky, but also cause painful and dangerous (and often unpreventable) side effects (i.e., that lead to "adverse" medical results). Given this fact, is it conceivable that the healthcare delivery system could ever operate free of "error"? Can you think of other terms that better (or more fairly) convey the range of adverse outcomes attending healthcare practice?

Promoting Healthcare Quality Through the Standard of Care

Not all medical errors rise to the level of being contrary to law. This section details the measure used by the legal system to determine which errors trigger legal protections: the professional standard of care. The standard of care is key both to the provision of high-quality health care and to legal claims that a health professional's, hospital's, or MCO's negligence in rendering medical care resulted in injury or death. This type of liability falls under the law of *torts*, a term that derives from the Latin word for "twisted" and that applies to situations where the actions of an individual or entity "twist away" from being reasonable and result in harm to others. Generally speaking, proving tort liability is not easy, and this task is no less difficult in the specific context of medical care. A patient seeking to hold a health professional or entity responsible for substandard care or treatment must demonstrate the appropriate standard of care, a breach of that standard by the defendant, measurable damages (e.g., physical pain or emotional suffering), and a causal link between the defendant's breach and the patient's injury.[b]

The Origins of the Standard of Care

The professional standard of care has its origins in 18th-century English common law. Courts in England had established that a patient looking to hold a physician legally accountable for substandard care had to prove that the doctor violated the *customs of his own profession*, as determined by *other professionals within the profession*. In other words, no objective standard was used by courts to measure the adequacy of physician practice.[c] Furthermore, courts were not in the habit of making searching analyses of whether the customs and standards proffered by the profession as defensible were at all reasonable. This type of physician deference was incorporated into America's legal fabric, as policymakers and courts delegated key decisions about medical practice—including determinations as to whether a specific practice undertaken in the treatment of a particular patient was acceptable or negligent—to the medical profession itself.

The law's reliance on health professionals to determine the appropriate standard of medical care was not without its problems. In effect, this laissez-faire approach made it virtually impossible for an injured patient to successfully recover monetary damages from a negligent doctor, because the patient was required to find another health professional willing to testify that the doctor's treatment violated the customary standard of care. (This type of testimony was certainly uncommon, as health professionals rarely openly questioned the practices of other members of the profession.) Moreover, using professional custom as the touchstone for determining legal liability had the effect of thwarting the modernization of medical care, because practicing physicians knew they would be judged, in essence, based on how other physicians customarily practiced.

Furthermore, establishing a violation of professional custom was not the only hurdle injured patients had to clear in their effort to hold their physicians legally accountable for substandard care. English courts also developed what became known as the "locality rule," which held that testimony provided on behalf of a patient as to whether a physician's actions met the standard of care could come only from physicians who practiced *within the same or similar locality* as the physician on trial. Thus, not only did aggrieved patients need to find a physician willing to testify that a fellow member of the profession violated customary practice, they needed to find this expert witness within the (or a similar) locality in which the defendant-doctor actually practiced. As they did with the professional custom rule, U.S. courts gradually adopted the English locality rule. For example, the Supreme Judicial Court of Massachusetts ruled that a small-town physician was bound to possess only the skill that physicians and surgeons of ordinary ability and skill, practicing in similar localities with opportunities for no larger experience, ordinarily possess, and that he was not bound to possess the high degree of art and skill possessed by eminent surgeons practicing in larger cities and making a specialty of the practice of surgery (*Small v. Howard*, 1880).

Courts' application of the locality rule severely limited patients' ability to bring medical malpractice actions against their physicians. Indeed, some injured patients were prevented from even initially mounting a case, because they were unable to convince a "geographic colleague" of their own physician to serve as an expert witness. (This problem was particularly acute in rural communities where there were fewer doctors to begin with, and where collegiality was the norm.) Furthermore, the locality rule likely resulted in at least a few local medical standards that were set by doctors who were less than completely skilled. The rule had another effect, as well: It led to a gulf among localities and cities in the standard of medical care practiced, and thus to different standards of care for similarly situated patients. Imagine, for example (notwithstanding the fact that the professional custom rule generally discouraged advancements in the standard of medical care), that physicians in a large town or city upgraded their practice techniques to reflect new medical technologies. Small-town practitioners had little incentive to model their big-city colleagues in the improvement of their own practice techniques, because the locality rule limited testimony as to the reasonableness of a physician's care to practitioners in the same or similar locality as the doctor on trial and their own actions would never be measured against the elevated techniques of their big-city counterparts.

By the 1950s, policymakers and courts grew wary of a healthcare system effectively in charge of policing itself; not surprisingly, this view was reflective of society more broadly, which during the civil rights era adopted a set of values heavily influenced by social justice and circumspect of concentrated institutional power. It also reflected the fact that no matter how chilling the effects of the professional custom and locality rules, the practice of medicine—particularly the dissemination of medical research findings—had obviously evolved from the 1800s. These facts both vastly altered the law's approach to measuring physician care and promoted higher-quality health care (Rosenbaum et al., 2012).

The Evolution of the Standard of Care

Under the law's modernized approach to the standard of care, both legal pillars of the physician autonomy era—the professional custom rule and the locality rule—were more or less razed.

The Professional Custom Rule

Courts no longer defer to professional custom as solely determinative of whether a physician's actions reached the accepted standard of care. Instead, courts now analyze whether the custom itself is reasonable in light of existing medical knowledge and technology.[d] Although evidence of professional custom remains probative in determining whether the standard of care has been met, courts consider a range of other relevant evidence as well. Thus, the benchmark that courts employ today to determine whether a health professional's treatment of a particular patient rose to the standard of care is whether it was *reasonable given the "totality of circumstances."*

Furthermore, it is no longer the case that evidence as to what is and is not customary medical practice is limited to what medical professionals themselves testify. Although evidence as to medical custom may still be introduced by medical professionals, objective clinical and scientific evidence—such as scientific research and clinical trial results—are now considered relevant in determining medical negligence. For example, the well-known case of *Helling v. Carey* (1974) shows how advances in medical knowledge can obliterate long-standing medical customs and replace them with new requirements. In *Helling*, a 32-year-old woman sought treatment from a series of ophthalmologists for glaucoma-type symptoms. The ophthalmologists, however, refrained from screening the patient for glaucoma, on the ground that professional custom called for the screen only in patients beyond the age of 40 years because the incidence of glaucoma in younger people was low. The State of Washington's Supreme Court ruled that notwithstanding the fact that the ophthalmologists had properly adhered to accepted custom, the *custom itself* was outdated based on current medical knowledge and was therefore unreasonable. The court effectively determined that a new treatment standard was required of the ophthalmology profession and held that the defendant-physicians were liable for the patient's blindness.

The key legal principle at work in *Helling* is that courts can (and do, in rare circumstances) determine for an entire industry (medical or otherwise) what is legally required of them, despite long-standing industry practices. This principle is premised on the famous case of *T. J. Hooper v. Northern Barge Corp.* (1932), in which the U.S. Second Circuit Court of Appeals held that a tugboat company was liable for damages to cargo it was shipping because the company failed to maintain radio-receiving equipment that could have warned the crew of a storm that battered the boat.

The company argued that it should not be liable for the damage because at the time it was not typical practice in the tugboat industry to carry radio equipment. In response, the court wrote the following:

> There are, no doubt, cases where courts seem to make the general practice of the calling the standard of proper diligence. . . . Indeed in most cases reasonable prudence is in fact common prudence; but strictly it is never its measure; *a whole calling may have unduly lagged in the adoption of new and available devices.* It never may set its own tests, however persuasive be its usages. *Courts must in the end say what is required;* there are precautions so imperative that even their universal disregard will not excuse their omission. (*T. J. Hooper v. Northern Barge Corp.*, 1932)

Essentially, the court determined that the tugboat company was not acting reasonably under the circumstances, but was instead hewing too closely (and foolishly) to what should have been considered an outmoded industry practice. This same view appeared to drive the court in *Helling v. Carey.* Indeed, the idea that the quality of health care provided by a health professional should be measured by an objective standard based on reasonableness under the circumstances, rather than by other professionals cloaked in the protections of outright autonomy, is today considered the norm. Furthermore, this view extends to big cities and small towns alike, and to both well-off and indigent patients.

The Locality Rule

Just as professional custom was transformed by the courts from being conclusive evidence of proper medical practice to being merely one piece of the evidentiary puzzle, so too was the locality rule mostly undone by more modern judicial thinking. Based in part on the fact that medical education and hospital-based care were becoming increasingly standardized under national accreditation efforts, courts stopped restricting evidence regarding the appropriate standard of care to the locality in which a physician practiced. Instead, most states have adopted what could be termed the "reasonably competent physician" standard, described as

> that degree of care and skill which is expected of a reasonably competent practitioner in the same class to which he belongs, acting in the same or similar circumstances. Under this

standard, advances in the profession, availability of facilities, specialization or general practice, proximity of specialists and special facilities, together with all relevant considerations, are to be taken into account. (*Shilkret v. Annapolis Emergency Hospital Ass'n*, 1975)

Under this revised standard, the practice of medicine nationally is key, because for purposes of determining medical liability, a physician's actions are now measured objectively against those of a reasonably prudent and competent practitioner under similar circumstances, not against the actions of physicians who practice within a particular defendant's locality. Thus, in the eyes of most state laws, local medical practice customs have properly given way to higher expectations where health quality is concerned.

At the same time, some states still retain the locality rule as the appropriate standard for the admissibility of medical evidence, and some states use a modified rule that takes into account local resources and other factors in determining whether a defendant-doctor was able to meet the standard of care. For an example of the latter point, see *Hall v. Hilbun* (1985), in which the Mississippi Supreme Court determined that the locality rule still had relevance to the extent that the physician's imperfect care resulted not from his substandard medical knowledge and skills, but from the fact that he did not have access to needed resources and equipment. In this type of situation, the court reasoned, health professionals who genuinely attempt to meet the requisite standard of care should not be held legally responsible when factors outside their control prevent them from doing so. The court in *Hall* went on to explain that under these circumstances, a physician is required to be aware of extant limitations and to actively demonstrate an effort to assist patients as best he or she can by, for example, referring them to doctors and facilities better able to care for them.

For purposes of determining legal liability for substandard treatment, the notion of distinguishing between medical knowledge and skills on the one hand and medical resources and outside factors on the other has particular relevance when the treatment involves an indigent patient whose care implicates broad contextual problems, such as poor living conditions or insufficient access to providers. Here, again, many courts look to see whether the treating physician's actions demonstrate an understanding of the proper level of care and a sincere effort to reach that level. However, do not confuse the fact that the law does not generally hold physicians liable for the consequences of resource problems attending

Give some thought to the term *national standard of care*. What do you think it means, from both a healthcare quality and legal (i.e., evidentiary) perspective? Are you aware of any national body—governmental or otherwise—that determines the efficacy of new diagnostic protocols or treatment modalities? In the absence of such an entity, how are health professionals put on notice that a new medical care standard for a particular procedure or treatment has emerged?

the healthcare system, or of poverty, with the idea that different standards of care exist for the well-off and for the poor. As far as the law is concerned, there is a unitary standard of care to be applied regardless of a patient's socioeconomic status, and physicians can certainly be held legally responsible for mistreating an indigent patient.

Together, the revamped legal rules pertaining to medical custom and local practice were combined to create what is called the *national standard of care*. Before turning to the discussion of how this standard is applied to healthcare institutions and insurers, consider the discussion questions in **Box 12.3**.

Tort Liability of Hospitals, Insurers, and MCOs

Just as physicians are now held to a national standard of care in cases challenging the quality of their care and treatment, so too have courts moved to apply this same standard to hospitals, traditional health insurers, and MCOs. The following sections consider each party's liability considerations in turn.

Hospital Liability

By the early 1900s, the healthcare industry began to rely much more heavily than had been the case previously on hospitals (as opposed to physicians' offices or patients' homes) as a focus of patient care. As with all healthcare settings, hospital-based medical practice created circumstances that led patients to challenge the quality of care provided. Out of necessity, the legal system (specifically, state-level courts) responded to these challenges by applying theories of liability, premised on the national standard of care, meant to hold hospitals accountable for negligence that occurred within their walls. Two theories—one

premised on hospitals' relationship with doctors and one based on the actions and decisions of hospitals themselves—dominate the field of hospital liability. The former theory is called vicarious liability; the latter is termed corporate liability.

Vicarious Liability

The concept of vicarious liability, which maintains that one party can be held legally accountable for the actions of another party based solely on the type of relationship existing between the two parties, is premised on the long-standing principles of "agency" law. Under this field of law, where one party to a relationship effectively serves (or is held out to society) as an agent of another party, a court can assign legal responsibility to the other party where the agent's actions negligently result in injury to a person or damage to property. For example, vicarious liability allows a hospital to be held responsible in some situations for the negligent acts of the doctors that practice medicine under its roof—not because the hospital itself somehow acted negligently, but rather because the doctor is (or is viewed as by the law) an agent of the hospital.

One relatively easy way for a plaintiff to win a lawsuit premised on vicarious liability is to establish through evidence that the two parties at issue are engaged in an employer–employee relationship, and that the employee (i.e., the agent) was acting within the normal scope of professional duties when the act of negligence occurred. In these instances, courts frequently look to the employer to adequately supervise the employee while on the job and hold the employer responsible when an employee's negligent acts occur within the parameters of the employee's job responsibilities.

However, many "agents" of the companies they are hired to work for are not formal employees; rather, they are hired as independent contractors. Indeed, this is true of most hospital–physician relationships. Historically, agency law respected hiring entities' decisions to hire individuals as independent contractors rather than as employees, and the general legal rule is that employers are not accountable for the illegal actions of these contractors. Nonetheless, there are exceptions to this rule, and courts have developed theories of vicarious liability—such as *actual agency*, *apparent agency*, and *nondelegable duty*—that are more concerned with the scope of an employer–independent contractor relationship than with the formal characterization of the relationship as determined by the parties themselves. In other words, employers cannot avoid legal liability simply by labeling a hired worker as an independent contractor, because courts will analyze the relationship to determine whether it operates at the end of the day like a typical employer–employee relationship.

Actual agency exists, and the negligence of an independent contractor can be imputed to the employer when the employer exercises de facto supervision and control over the contractor. Thus, for example, agency can be shown to exist between a healthcare corporation and a health professional when the particular facts pertaining to the relationship reveal that the corporation actually exercises control over the professional, even though the professional is not technically an employee. Similarly, the doctrine of apparent agency (also called ostensible agency) is another exception to the general rule that employers should not be legally exposed for the negligence of their independent contractors. In the context of health care, this type of agency exists, for example, when a patient seeks care from a hospital emergency department (rather than from any particular physician working in that department) and the hospital has led patients to believe that physicians are employees of the hospital, such as via a billboard extolling the skills of the physicians who practice in its emergency department (*Mehlman v. Powell*, 1977). Finally, courts have also associated the doctrine of vicarious liability with certain duties considered so important to society as to be legally "nondelegable." For example, the importance of a hospital's obligation to maintain control over the care provided in its emergency department led one court to rule that it would be improper for the hospital to claim immunity from vicarious liability when its independent contractor furnished substandard medical care (*Jackson v. Power*, 1987).

Corporate Liability

As opposed to vicarious hospital liability, which is predicated on the negligence of individual health professionals, corporate liability holds hospitals accountable for their own "institutional" acts or omissions. In other words, a hospital can also be held liable when its own negligent acts as a corporation cause or contribute to a patient's injury. Several general areas give rise to litigation around hospitals' direct quality of care duties to patients: failure to screen out incompetent providers (i.e., negligence in the hiring of clinicians), failure to maintain high-quality practice standards, failure to take adequate action against clinicians whose practices fall below accepted standards, and failure to maintain proper equipment and supplies (Rosenbaum et al., 2012).

The most famous hospital corporate liability case is *Darling v. Charleston Community Memorial Hospital* (1965). In *Darling*, the Illinois Supreme Court found Memorial Hospital liable for negligent treatment provided to plaintiff Dorrence Darling, an 18-year-old who suffered a broken leg while playing in a college football game. The poor treatment Darling received by the hospital's emergency department staff—his leg cast was not properly constructed and its application cut off blood circulation—ultimately resulted in amputation of Darling's leg below the knee. The court held the hospital liable not for the actions of the emergency department staff, but for *its own* negligence. According to the court, Memorial Hospital did not maintain a sufficient number of qualified nurses for post–emergency department bedside care (when Darling's leg became gangrenous), and it neither reviewed the care provided by the treating physician nor required the physician to consult with other members of the hospital staff.

Insurer Liability

Like hospitals, conventional (i.e., indemnity) health insurers historically were not susceptible to being sued under tort principles; rather, they were subject mainly to breach of contract lawsuits when they failed to reimburse medical claims for services covered under beneficiaries' health insurance policies. This protection from tort liability stemmed from two related facts: first, normative insurer practice was to leave medical judgments and treatment decisions in the hands of doctors, meaning it was rare for an insurer-related action to lead to the type of injury covered by tort law; second, to the extent that an insurer did deny a beneficiary's claim for insurance coverage, it did so retrospectively—in other words, *after* the beneficiary received needed diagnostic tests, treatments, medications, and so on. This effectively meant that when beneficiaries sued their health insurer, they did so not because they had been physically or emotionally injured by the insurer's decision to deny an insurance claim, but because there was a dispute as to whether the insurer was going to pay for the already-received medical care.[e] Thus, although coverage denials had potentially enormous economic implications for affected beneficiaries, they did not tend to raise healthcare access or quality issues.

In the years following the *Darling* decision, however, courts began to apply tort liability principles to traditional indemnity insurers when their coverage decisions were at least partially responsible for an individual's injury or death,[f] which had the effect of opening insurers to a fuller range of potential damages (e.g., pain and suffering) than had been the case previously (when, under breach of contract principles, insurers were liable only for the actual cost of care they had initially declined to cover). This increased exposure to liability grew out of the fact that insurers were becoming more aggressive in their use of *prospective* coverage decisions, and courts were aware of how these types of coverage determinations could impact access to and the quality of health care. The advent of managed care as the primary mechanism for delivering and financing health care only magnified this concern, given managed care's use of techniques such as utilization review, and opened the door to one of the most contentious aspects of health services quality today—the extent to which patients can sue MCOs for negligent coverage or treatment decisions.

Managed Care Liability

Just as state courts were important in the extension of tort principles to health professionals, hospitals, and insurers, so too did they inaugurate application of these principles to MCOs. Modern MCOs are complex structures that heavily regulate the practices of their network physicians. Indeed, perhaps the most defining aspect of managed care is its oversight of physician medical judgment through various mechanisms—utilization review, practice guidelines, physician payment incentives, and so on.

A function of managed care's oversight of physician practice is that there is no longer any doubt that application of the professional standard of care for the purpose of determining negligence extends beyond the literal quality of health care delivered and reaches the very *coverage* of that care. This is because managed care has so altered coverage decision-making practices to focus on prospective decisions; where this type of coverage determination used to be the exception, it is now the rule. Instead of coverage denials leading to disputes over who was going to pay for an already-received medical service, prospective managed care coverage decisions more or less determine whether an individual receives treatment at all (Rosenbaum et al., 1999).

Needless to say, the negative impact of prospective coverage decisions on individuals' ability to access necessary, high-quality care is no small policy matter. At the same time, in one critical legal sense it does not particularly matter whether a dispute between an MCO and one of its beneficiaries is framed as one of negligence in healthcare *quality* or healthcare *coverage*; either way, the key issue is whether the medical judgment exercised by the MCO met the professional standard of care. In applying this standard, courts have had little trouble finding MCOs liable under state law both for the negligence of their network physicians and for their own direct negligence. (However, as discussed in the next section, these court decisions presume the nonapplicability of ERISA, a federal law that often precludes individuals from suing their managed care company under state tort laws.)

There have been a number of cases in which courts have determined that MCOs can be held vicariously liable for the negligent actions of their network physicians where a patient can prove an agency relationship under one of the theories (actual agency, apparent agency, or nondelegable duty) described previously. In these cases, courts perform an exhaustive examination of the facts to determine the specific relationship between the treating physician and the MCO or the ways in which the MCO portrays and obligates itself to its beneficiaries. For example, in the case of *Boyd v. Albert Einstein Medical Center* (1988), a Pennsylvania court closely analyzed the literature of a health maintenance organization (HMO) for evidence of a contractual relationship to its beneficiaries to determine whether the HMO could be held vicariously liable under a theory of apparent agency for the treatment of a woman who died after physicians negligently treated her for a lump in her breast. Among other things, the court noted that the HMO's contract with its beneficiaries agreed to "provide healthcare services and benefits to members in order to protect and promote their health" and that the patients' contractual relationship was with the HMO, not with any individual physician in the HMO's network. In the end, the court determined that because the patient looked to the HMO itself for care and the HMO held itself out as providing care through its network physicians, the HMO was vicariously liable for the patient's negligent treatment.

Similarly, courts have applied the doctrine of corporate liability to MCOs. Courts have given various reasons for subjecting MCOs to this type of liability—at least in their role as arrangers or providers of health care, MCOs are much like hospitals; MCOs have the resources to monitor and improve the quality of healthcare delivery; and MCOs maintain tremendous authority over the makeup of their physician networks. The case of *Jones v. Chicago HMO Ltd. of Illinois* (2000) is a good example of the application of corporate liability principles to managed care. In *Jones*, the plaintiff called her MCO-appointed physician (Dr. Jordan) after her 3-month-old daughter (Shawndale) fell ill with constipation, fever, and other problems.

Box 12.4 DISCUSSION QUESTIONS

What do you think about the role and success of tort law in promoting high-quality health care? Does it help to deter errors? If not, why?

Both an assistant to Dr. Jordan and, eventually, Dr. Jordan himself explained that Shawndale should not be brought to the physician's office but should instead be treated at home with castor oil. A day later, Shawndale was still sick and her mother took her to a hospital emergency department, where she was diagnosed with bacterial meningitis secondary to an ear infection. Shawndale was permanently disabled as a result of the meningitis. It emerged through pretrial testimony that the defendant MCO had assigned 4500 to 6000 patients to Dr. Jordan, far more than its own medical director deemed acceptable under the professional standard of care. The Illinois Supreme Court agreed, ruling that MCOs breach a legal duty as a corporate entity by assigning an excessive number of patients to any single network physician, because doing so can affect the quality of care provided to beneficiaries.

This section provided a general review of the application of the professional standard of care to hospitals, insurers, and MCOs and described certain state-level theories of liability that are implicated when patients claim that the care they received fell short of this standard. However, as alluded to earlier, ERISA often preempts (i.e., supersedes) these kinds of state law liability claims against insurers and MCOs. Complete this section by reflecting on the questions in **Box 12.4**; then, turn to the discussion of ERISA and its preemptive force in the next section.

Federal Preemption of State Liability Laws Under ERISA

Generally speaking, ERISA prohibits individuals from recovering damages for death and injuries caused by substandard medical professional conduct to the extent that the individuals receive their health coverage through a *private employer–sponsored* benefit plan. (Among others, individuals who work for federal, state, and local public employers are not covered by ERISA's rules.) Because approximately 150 million workers and their families in the United States receive this type of health coverage, and because managed care represents the dominant structure of healthcare

delivery, the issue of whether individuals with private employer–sponsored managed care coverage can recover damages for substandard medical professional conduct is paramount.

Overview of ERISA

One of the most complex areas of federal civil law, ERISA[g] was established in 1974 mainly to protect the employee pension system from employer fraud. However, the law was drafted in such a way as to extend to all of the benefits offered by ERISA-covered employers, including health benefits. Because ERISA does not distinguish among employers based on size, essentially all employees in this country who receive health and other benefits through a private employer can be said to work for an "ERISA-covered" employer.

ERISA employs two main devices to protect employee pensions and other benefits. First, it imposes "fiduciary" responsibilities on those individuals or entities that administer various types of employer-sponsored benefit plans (in the case of health benefits, these are often conventional insurers or MCOs, or the employers themselves). A person or entity with fiduciary responsibilities is analogous to a trustee, who is expected to act primarily for another's benefit in carrying out his or her duties. Put differently, a fiduciary is one who manages money or property (like a pension fund or healthcare benefit) for another person and who is expected to act in good faith in that management. One critical fiduciary responsibility is to act with an eye toward the best interests of the person who has placed trust in the fiduciary, rather than seeking personal enrichment through trustee activities.

The second tool used by Congress in ERISA to regulate employee benefits is a set of uniform, nationwide rules for the administration of employee benefits. However, although ERISA closely regulates the structure and operation of pension plans, the law includes few substantive standards governing the design or administration of health (or other) employee benefits. This stems mainly from the fact that Congress's main purpose in passing ERISA was to confront the employer fraud and underfunding evident in the pension system in the early 1970s (after all, the title of the law hints that its purpose is to specifically protect employee *retirement income*), not to regulate all employee benefit plans. However, the language used by ERISA's drafters is both broad and ambiguous, and courts have interpreted the statute as applying well beyond the field of pensions (Rosenbaum et al., 2012). As a result of the dearth of substantive standards pertaining to employee health benefits, employers enjoy discretion under ERISA to decide whether to offer health benefits at all and, if they do, to offer a benefit package of their choosing. This discretion allows the employer to design the benefit plan itself or buy an "off the shelf" insurance policy from a health insurer. If the employer chooses the latter, it also must decide whether to use a conventional insurer or a managed care company; if using a managed care company, it must decide whether to include physician incentive schemes in its benefit plan.

ERISA's lack of substantive health benefit regulations is compounded by the fact that the law contains few avenues for employees to remedy negligent benefit plan administration, including substandard conduct in the administration of health plan benefits. As mentioned, ERISA precludes the recovery of monetary damages under state law theories of liability when employer-sponsored benefits are improperly denied; Congress was of the opinion in fashioning ERISA that payment of these types of damages would drain employer benefit plans of needed resources. However, one might assume that when Congress broadly displaces state laws aimed at remedying negligence (as it did with ERISA), it would put in place meaningful enforcement provisions in the federal law. Yet the remedies available under ERISA are dramatically more limited than those available under state law. Under ERISA (1974), employees and their beneficiaries are effectively limited to suing to prospectively force a plan administrator to grant a covered benefit, to recover payment retrospectively when a covered benefit was improperly denied, and to enforce a plan administrator's fiduciary responsibilities. The upshot of these rights is that they allow employees injured by an action or decision of their benefit plan to recover *nothing beyond the actual cost of the benefit due in any event*.

Furthermore, in *Pilot Life Insur. Co. v. Dedeaux* (1987), the U.S. Supreme Court held that ERISA's enforcement provision constituted not merely *a* remedy for negligent administration of an employee benefit plan, but rather the *exclusive* remedy. This means that all other state remedies generally available to individuals to remedy corporate negligence are preempted (and thus not available) to employees whose health benefits are provided through an ERISA-covered plan.

ERISA Preemption

To ensure the uniform regulation and administration of employee pension plans (and, as it turned out,

other employee benefits) across the nation, Congress included in ERISA one of the most sweeping preemption provisions ever enacted under federal law. The uniqueness of the scope of ERISA's preemptive force is underscored by the fact that the states in America's governmental structure maintain broad authority to regulate many fields (including the fields of health care and health insurance) as they see fit, and federal law generally supplements, but does not replace, state law.

Furthermore, ERISA actually implicates two different types of preemption. The first, known as "conflict preemption," occurs when specific provisions of state law clearly conflict with federal law, in which case the state law is superseded. The second form of preemption triggered by ERISA is "field preemption," which the courts employ when they interpret federal law to occupy an entire field of law (e.g., employee benefit law), irrespective of whether there are any conflicting state law provisions (this is the type of preemption at work in ERISA's remedial provisions, described earlier). The practical import of this second type of preemption is that a wide range of state laws are preempted by ERISA even though they do not directly conflict with it. All in all, it is little wonder that ERISA is considered to function as a "regulatory vacuum."

The length of ERISA's conflict preemption provision belies its preemptive scope, and its wording belies the enormous amount of litigation it has engendered. The substantive entirety of the preemption clause reads: "[ERISA] shall supersede any and all State laws insofar as they may now or hereafter relate to any employee benefit plan." Courts have grappled with the meaning of this language for decades. For example, the term *relate to* has been interpreted by the U.S. Supreme Court to include any state law that has "a connection with or reference to" an employee benefit plan (*Shaw v. Delta Air Lines, Inc.*, 1983), but not those that have only a "remote and tenuous" relationship to benefit plans (*New York State Conference of Blue Cross & Blue Shield Plans v. Travelers Insur. Co.*, 1995). Thus, the former types of state laws are preempted, while the latter are not. The Supreme Court has also weighed in on the meaning of "employee benefit plan" (*Fort Halifax Packing Co. v. Coyne*, 1987).

In addition to the preemption clause itself, however, there are two additional pieces to the ERISA conflict preemption puzzle that only add to the law's complexity. The second piece is referred to as the "insurance savings" clause, which says that the preemption clause shall not "be construed to exempt or relieve any person from any law of any State which regulates insurance." This essentially means that even where a state law relates to an employee benefit plan, it is saved from preemption if it regulates insurance (*Metropolitan Life Insur. Co. v. Massachusetts*, 1985). The Supreme Court has interpreted this provision to mean a state law is saved from preemption if it is specifically directed toward entities engaged in insurance and substantially affects the risk-pooling arrangement between an insurer and its beneficiaries (*Kentucky Ass'n of Health Plans, Inc. v. Miller*, 2003). The practical effect of the savings clause, then, is to narrow the reach of the preemption clause, because state laws that meet the "regulates insurance" test fall outside the scope of ERISA preemption.

The final element of ERISA conflict preemption is the "deemer" clause, which addresses the distinction between fully insured and self-insured employee health benefit plans. A fully insured health plan (sometimes referred to simply as an insured plan) is one in which an employer purchases health insurance coverage (i.e., pays premiums) to a conventional insurance company or MCO, and in return the insurance company or MCO accepts the financial risk of paying claims for covered benefits. A self-insured health plan (also called a self-funded plan) exists when an employer retains some or all of the financial risk for its employees' claims for covered benefits. Nearly one-half of all U.S. employers self-insure their health benefit plans.

ERISA's deemer clause reads in pertinent part: "An employee benefit plan shall [not] be deemed to be an insurance company or other insurer, . . . or to be engaged in the business of insurance . . . for purposes of any law of any State purporting to regulate insurance companies." The purpose of this clause is to prohibit states from deeming employee benefit plans as the functional equivalent of health insurers, and its practical effect is critical for the tens of millions of employees who receive their health benefits under self-insured plans: The deemer clause prevents state laws that meet the "regulates insurance" test from applying to self-insured employee health benefit plans (*Metropolitan Life Insur. Co. v. Massachusetts*, 1985). In other words, even state laws "saved" from preemption do not apply to self-insured plans because under ERISA these types of plans are "deemed" not to be insurance companies. The ultimate result of the deemer clause's application is to *exempt completely* self-funded employee benefit plans from state insurance law. This exemption allows sponsors of self-funded plans enormous discretion to design the plans as they choose.

The Intersection of ERISA Preemption and Managed Care Professional Medical Liability

The final matter to discuss in the context of ERISA preemption has been one of the most unstable over the past several years: the extent to which ERISA preempts state tort law claims by individuals against managed care companies for negligent coverage decisions and substandard provision of care. This issue has played out over a series of federal court decisions attempting to define with some precision ERISA's application in the context of employer-sponsored managed care plans.

In the 1992 case of *Corcoran v. United HealthCare, Inc.*, the Fifth Circuit Court of Appeals ruled that Florence Corcoran's state law claim against United HealthCare for the wrongful death of her fetus had to be dismissed under ERISA, regardless of any medical negligence on the part of the MCO. The court held that even if the company improperly denied coverage of preterm labor management services for Mrs. Corcoran, her state lawsuit seeking damages for a negligent coverage decision was preempted because the company's determination was, in the language of ERISA, sufficiently "related to" Mrs. Corcoran's employee benefit plan.

Three years later, the Third Circuit Court of Appeals ruled in *Dukes v. U.S. Healthcare, Inc.* (1995) that although individuals in ERISA-covered health benefit plans may not be able to sue under state law for an MCO's negligent coverage denial (i.e., for a company's decision as to the *quantity* of care covered under the plan), they can seek state law damages where a managed care company's negligence is connected to the *quality* of care actually provided. The Third Circuit essentially ruled that Congress did not intend in passing ERISA to supersede state laws aimed at the regulation of healthcare quality, historically a subject area under the states' purview. Instead, according to the court, federal policymakers enacted ERISA to alleviate national companies' concerns over abiding by many different state pension and employee benefit laws and to instead subject them to a uniform set of funding and administration rules. Whatever Congress meant by a "state law that relates to an employee benefit plan," the *Dukes* court did not interpret ERISA's preemption provision to sweep in laws pertaining to the quality of medical care provided to beneficiaries of employer-sponsored health benefit plans.

In the 5 years after *Dukes* was decided, federal court decisions applying ERISA to managed care plans more or less subscribed to this quantity/quality distinction.

However, the Supreme Court stepped into the fray in 2000 in the case of *Pegram v. Herdrich*, seemingly altering the approach lower courts had been taking when analyzing ERISA preemption of state law negligence claims against MCOs. The main issue in *Pegram* was whether physician incentive arrangements were violative of the fiduciary responsibility rules contained in ERISA (incidentally, the court ruled they were not). However, the court included several paragraphs in its decision about the role of the treating physician in the case, who also happened to be one of the owners of the managed care company being sued for negligently failing to order a diagnostic test. In so doing, the court described two different kinds of decisions made by MCOs:

> What we will call pure "eligibility decisions" turn on the plan's coverage of a particular condition or medical procedure for its treatment. "Treatment decisions," by contrast, are choices about how to go about diagnosing and treating a patient's condition: given a patient's constellation of symptoms, what is the appropriate medical response? *These decisions are often practically inextricable from one another.* . . . This is so not merely because . . . treatment and eligibility decisions are made by the same person, the treating physician. It is so because a great many *and possibly most* coverage questions are not simple yes-or-no questions, like whether appendicitis is a covered condition (when there is no dispute that a patient has appendicitis), or whether acupuncture is a covered procedure for pain relief (when the claim of pain is unchallenged). The more common coverage question is a when-and-how question. Although coverage for many conditions will be clear and various treatment options will be indisputably compensable, physicians still must decide what to do in particular cases. . . . In practical terms, these eligibility decisions cannot be untangled from physicians' judgments about reasonable medical treatment. (*Pegram v. Herdrich*, 2000)

Importantly, the court went on to suggest that these intertwined decisions fall beyond ERISA's reach and that state laws implicated when these decisions are negligently made are not preempted, although the court provided no clear guidance as to when managed care decisions tipped sufficiently toward coverage or care to pull them out of the realm of being "mixed." Following the decision, many federal courts faced with ERISA's application to claims by managed care beneficiaries adopted *Pegram*'s approach over the one developed in *Dukes*. Courts favored *Pegram*'s approach because it opened the door to state law remedies for individuals (like Florence Corcoran) who were injured as a result of managed care negligence but who otherwise had no way to recover for their loss.

In the 2004 case of *Aetna Health, Inc. v. Davila*, however, the Supreme Court appeared to close the door it seemed to open in *Pegram*, suggesting that lawsuits premised on the intertwined or "mixed" decisions made daily by MCOs escape ERISA's preemptive force only when the decisions include actual treatment by an MCO medical employee. The *Davila* decision actually represented a pair of cases (the other one originally called *Cigna v. Calad*) consolidated by the court due to the similarity of the respective plaintiffs' claims. Both Juan Davila and Ruby Calad were members of ERISA-covered employee health benefit plans. Davila was injured when Aetna chose to substitute a less expensive medication for the one he normally took to control his arthritis pain; Calad suffered complications after being prematurely discharged from the hospital subsequent to Cigna's decision to cover just 1 day of hospitalization post-surgery. Rather than filing appeals directly with their insurance companies, Davila and Calad sued under a state law called the Texas Health Care Liability Act. They argued that their respective insurer's decision breached a duty under the Texas law to exercise reasonable care in healthcare decision-making and that the breach caused their injuries.

In rejecting both plaintiffs' claims, the Supreme Court ruled that ERISA preempts lawsuits for damages against ERISA-covered plans for negligent healthcare coverage decisions, even when the coverage decision was predicated on flawed medical judgment. Thus, *Davila* makes clear that when an individual covered by an ERISA plan complains only of negligent coverage decision-making (including the wrongful denial of a benefit) on the part of an MCO, ERISA shields the MCO from liability beyond the actual value of the benefit itself.[h] However, the Supreme Court in *Davila* also explained that notwithstanding ERISA, MCOs remain liable under state tort laws for negligence when acting in their capacity as providers or arrangers of health care. Although this ruling sustains the general distinction made by the federal court of appeals in the *Dukes* decision, its effect on the legal remedies available to injured patients is likely to be limited, given that policymakers and courts still view coverage decision-making, rather than the provision of health care, as the primary aim of MCOs. Before moving on, consider the questions posed in **Box 12.5**.

The critical intersection between health care and health insurance as exemplified by the *Davila* decision leads to an important question: Is it reasonable to treat a healthcare coverage decision as having nothing to do with health care itself? Put another way, given the expense of health care today, do you believe that individuals and families can afford necessary health care if there is no third party responsible for covering at least some of the cost?

Measuring and Incentivizing Healthcare Quality[i]

We turn now to the final topics in this chapter—what exactly is meant by healthcare "quality," how is it measured, and how should policy be designed in order to encourage and reward it? Given the explosive growth in healthcare costs in the United States over the past few decades, combined with evidence from leading researchers and experts[j] that collectively points to the disconnect between high spending and healthcare quality and to serious deficiencies in healthcare quality overall, these are important questions.

To analyze these questions, focusing on the Medicare program is particularly instructive. As the single largest payer (in terms of dollars spent) in the U.S. health system, Medicare is a major national driver of policy in other markets (both public and private). Therefore, how the Medicare program addresses issues pertaining to quality is not only important to Medicare beneficiaries and providers but also to other purchasers and stakeholders whose policies and procedures are often driven, or at least influenced, by Medicare policy. The remainder of this section will focus on how the Medicare program, as authorized by federal legislation, is working to improve the quality and lower the cost of healthcare delivery. It also addresses similar efforts of other payers and stakeholders, including the role of health information technology in facilitating quality improvement.

Traditionally, the Medicare program has paid for healthcare services on a fee-for-service (FFS) basis, with the exception of inpatient hospital services, which are paid based on diagnosis-related groups under the prospective payment system (PPS), and the Medicare Advantage and Prescription Drug plans, which are paid on a capitated basis. All payment systems (public

and private) tend to incentivize something; in the case of FFS, it is indiscriminate increases in the volume of treatments and services, while in case-based or capitation systems, it is indiscriminate reductions in volume. Whatever the payment arrangement, the challenge is to promote both quality and value while also apportioning financial risk appropriately. However, because Medicare has historically lacked a program-wide and deliberate approach to promoting quality and value, and because it has relied principally on an FFS approach to payment for physician and other services, the program has experienced incredible growth in the volume of services for which it pays.

Over the years, Congress has passed a series of laws designed to move both the Medicare and Medicaid programs from passive purchasers of volume-based health care to active purchasers of high-quality, high-value health care based in large part on successful demonstration projects. For example, as authorized under the Medicare Prescription Drug, Improvement, and Modernization Act of 2003 (MMA) and extended by the Deficit Reduction Act of 2005 (DRA), hospitals that reported on specific quality measures receive the full annual payment update, while failure to participate resulted in a decrease in the annual payment update. Similarly, as authorized by the Tax Relief and Health Care Act of 2006 (TRHCA) and extended by the Medicare, Medicaid, and SCHIP Extension Act of 2007 (MMSEA), and made permanent by the Medicare Improvements for Patients and Providers Act of 2008 (MIPPA), the Physician Quality Reporting System (PQRS) offered bonus payments to Medicare physicians who reported on specific quality measures. The Health Information Technology for Economic and Clinical Health (HITECH) Act, enacted as part of the American Recovery and Reinvestment Act of 2009 (ARRA), provided significant financial incentives to Medicare and Medicaid providers for "meaningfully using" electronic health records to improve the quality of care delivery.

The ACA also focused on incentives to improve the quality of Medicare-covered care. The ACA set forth a broad vision for quality measurement, reporting, and financial incentives in Medicare, including quality measure development, quality measurement and payment incentives, public reporting, and value-based purchasing. The ACA also called for other payers and stakeholders to align their efforts with federal efforts. In short, the ACA greatly expanded the existing efforts noted previously, while introducing new tools for the Medicare program to identify, measure, and pay for high-quality care, and it encouraged other payers and stakeholders to do the same. The ACA also moved the country toward implementing a "national quality strategy" that would work to align quality improvement and value-based purchasing initiatives among and across payers, both public and private. To realize this goal, the ACA required the U.S. Department of Health and Human Services (HHS) to establish a National Strategy for Quality Improvement in Health Care, which functions as a strategic plan to improve the quality of healthcare delivery and, as a result, the health of the U.S. population.

Since passage of the ACA, several other pieces of healthcare-related legislation have extended and refined its quality improvement initiatives. The American Taxpayer Relief Act of 2012 (ATRA) made several changes to quality- and utilization-based payment adjustments created or modified by the ACA, revised reporting requirements under the PQRS, and established a commission to develop a plan for delivering high-quality long-term care services. The Improving Medicare Post-Acute Care Transformation Act of 2014 (the IMPACT Act) required that long-term care hospitals, skilled nursing facilities, home health agencies, and inpatient rehabilitation facilities report specific, standardized data on quality and resource-use measures. Most notably, the Medicare Access and CHIP Reauthorization Act of 2015 (MACRA) established the Quality Payment Program (QPP), which established two payment methodologies to reward Medicare providers for quality improvement or the adoption of an alternative value-based payment model. MACRA also provided additional funding for quality measure development and expanded the availability of Medicare data to support public and private quality improvement efforts.

Quality Measure Development

Residing at the core of public and private efforts to improve the quality of care in the United States are measures used to evaluate the quality of providers' clinical care. But what constitutes quality clinical care? The answer to this question varies by stakeholder. A patient is likely focused on a good outcome and good relationship with his or her provider. A health plan is likely focused on whether the provider achieved a good outcome at the lowest cost (based on time and resources used). A provider is likely focused on whether the desired outcome was achieved and payment was made. Given the diversity of stakeholders involved in healthcare delivery, there is great variation in the definition of quality, even between and among different types of providers (e.g., primary care physicians and specialists).

To address the varying perspectives on quality, HHS uses a multistakeholder approach to design and approve quality measures that are specific to provider types (e.g., hospital-specific measures). This approach, mandated by the ACA and MACRA, requires that HHS select an organization (currently the National Quality Forum, or NQF) to convene multistakeholder groups to provide consensus-based input on quality measures; together, these stakeholders are part of the NQF Measure Applications Partnership (MAP), a group of over 60 private stakeholders and representatives from nine different federal agencies that meets annually to provide input on measures for several Medicare quality programs. HHS considers the measures endorsed by the NQF when selecting quality and efficiency measures for use in public reporting, performance-based payment, and other programs applicable to Medicare and Medicaid providers. Most public and private quality improvement efforts also use the measures that are approved by the NQF. More than 65 different developers, representing specific types of providers and other stakeholders, design quality and performance measures applicable to their members prior to NQF review; these include the Ambulatory Quality Alliance (AQA), Pharmacy Quality Alliance (PQA), National Committee for Quality Assurance (NCQA; health plan measures), Physician Consortium for Performance Improvement (PCPI), and Hospital Quality Alliance (HQA).

The ACA also provided some clarification for defining quality measures. It defines a "quality measure" as a "standard for measuring the performance and improvement of population health or of health plans, providers of services, and other clinicians in the delivery of healthcare services." The NQF, in its capacity as the organization designated to review and endorse quality measures, is required to identify gaps where no quality measures exist and any existing quality measures that need to be improved, updated, or expanded for use in federal healthcare programs (including Medicare, Medicaid, and CHIP). Identified gaps are reported on a publicly available website, and the HHS Secretary provides grants to organizations to develop, update, or expand quality measures. Priorities for new measures include those that assess outcomes, functional status, care coordination across episodes, shared decision-making, use of health information technology, efficiency, safety, timeliness, equity, and patient experience. The Secretary also develops (and updates) outcome measures for acute and chronic diseases and primary and preventive care for hospitals and physicians.

Quality Measurement

The ACA reauthorized and developed quality measurement programs for multiple types of providers participating in the Medicare program. For example, the ACA reauthorized incentive payments under the PQRS through 2014 and mandated participation in PQRS for all eligible physicians beginning in 2015. In 2017, the Centers for Medicare and Medicaid Services (CMS) introduced the Merit-Based Incentive Payment System (MIPS), a system created under MACRA to replace the PQRS and two other performance-related programs. One of the two QPP options, MIPS streamlined multiple Medicare incentive programs into a single system designed to enable providers to better monitor their performance and reward high-quality and cost-effective care delivery. Provider performance under MIPS is evaluated across four categories:

- Quality (the category that replaced the PRQS)
- Improvement activities (a new category created under the MIPS program)
- Promoting interoperability (which replaced the Medicare EHR Incentive Program, or Meaningful Use program)
- Cost (which replaced the Value-based Payment Modifier [VM] Program)

Beginning in 2017, participation in MIPS was mandatory for all eligible providers, who are required to report on specific performance measures within the four MIPS performance categories. Beginning in 2019, payment to providers is adjusted up (a bonus) or down (a penalty) to reflect their reported performance relative to the median performance of all participating providers. By 2022, provider reimbursements will be adjusted by up to 9%, based on performance under MIPS. MACRA also provides funding for development and selection of MIPS quality measures and requires that selected measures address several quality domains (clinical care, safety, care coordination, patient and caregiver experience, and population health and prevention), with priority given to outcome, patient experience, care coordination, and resource utilization measures, emphasizing outcome measures where feasible. The ACA required the HHS Secretary to provide feedback to eligible professionals on their performance on reported quality measures under PQRS, and MACRA similarly requires the Secretary to provide feedback on performance related to selected quality measures and resource utilization.

Public Reporting

In addition to informing providers about the quality of care they deliver, quality information enables consumers to make more informed provider choices. The CMS currently posts a significant amount of quality and cost of care information on their suite of *Compare* websites (e.g., Hospital Compare[k]). The ACA also expanded required public reporting to Medicare physicians and several other provider types, including long-term care hospitals, inpatient rehabilitation hospitals, psychiatric hospitals, hospice programs, and non-PPS cancer hospitals. Information reported must include the quality measures as well as assessments of patient health outcomes, risk-adjusted resource use, efficiency, patient experience, and other relevant information deemed appropriate by the HHS Secretary. Beginning in 2013, CMS also made several changes to their data release policy, publishing data sets containing physician-identifiable information on utilization and payment in the Medicare Part B and Part D programs. As of early 2018, CMS further enhanced transparency by providing Medicare Part C program claims data to researchers upon request; in mid-2020, they began to make some Medicaid and CHIP encounter and claims data publicly available.

Value-Based Purchasing

The quality improvement programs described previously focused on developing provider-specific quality measures and incentivizing providers to report specific quality information. Typically, the programs began with providers collecting and reporting information to CMS and then transitioned to linking incentive payments to the reporting. While these "pay for reporting" programs have been successful in encouraging providers to assess the quality of care they are delivering through the reporting mechanisms, they do not take into account individual patient outcomes or population health outcomes (i.e., they do not "pay for *performance*"). However, CMS's End-Stage Renal Disease Quality Incentive Program (ESRD QIP) began reducing payments to facilities that do not meet or exceed certain performance benchmarks in 2012. In addition, as authorized by the DRA, CMS has implemented a similar type of payment program that reduces payments to hospitals that have the highest rates of certain hospital-acquired conditions (HACs)—HACs stand in contrast to conditions that were present on admission. It is worth noting that these programs are not unique to the Medicare program; many state Medicaid programs and private payers have also developed and implemented similar programs.[l]

Until passage of the ACA, CMS was not able to move beyond "pay for reporting" programs or the HAC Reduction Program because it did not have the necessary legal authority to vary payments based on actual provider performance. Specifically, the ACA required the implementation of Medicare value-based purchasing programs for most hospitals subject to the inpatient PPS. Value-based purchasing programs for home health agencies and skilled nursing facilities were respectively implemented in 2016 and 2018, and, as required by the ACA, a program for ambulatory surgical centers was developed in 2018 (although it has yet to be implemented). These value-based programs require the Medicare program to financially reward and penalize providers based on their performance on specified quality measures and other indicators, such as rates of readmission and HACs. For example, through the hospital value-based purchasing program, eligible hospitals began receiving incentive payments for discharges after October 1, 2012, that met certain performance standards. Quality domains on which hospital performance is evaluated include patient- and caregiver-centered experience (based on the hospital's HCAHPS score, which stands for Hospital Consumer Assessment of Healthcare Providers and Systems), clinical process of care, patient safety (measured by rates of certain healthcare-associated infections), and efficiency and cost reduction (based on spending per Medicare beneficiary). Information regarding the performance of individual hospitals under the program is available online through the Hospital Compare website.

The ACA authorized a physician and physician practice group VM Program that provided differential payments to physicians and physician practice groups based on the quality of care furnished compared to cost. As noted previously, MACRA's QPP has replaced the VM Program for physicians participating in the MIPS track with the "cost" performance category. The MIPS cost category evaluates physician performance on cost of care and resource utilization measures relevant to specific episodes of care.

In early 2015, HHS announced its goals of making 30% of FFS Medicare payments to alternative payment models (APMs), such as accountable care organizations (ACOs) or bundled payment arrangements, and of tying 85% of FFS payments to quality or value through programs such as hospital value-based purchasing and hospital readmissions reduction by the end of 2016. It achieved both goals ahead of schedule in early 2016 and announced its intention to make 50% of payments to APMs and to tie 90% of payments to quality or value by the end of 2018. These new goals were revised in late 2019 by the Health Care Payment Learning and Action Network (LAN), a public–private group launched by HHS in 2015 to provide support and advice on the shift toward APMs. The LAN established new and ambitious goals for different programs—most notably, to tie 100% of Medicare payments to certain types of APMs by 2025. Similarly, MACRA's QPP includes the APM participation track, which offers an incentive payment to physicians participating in certain alternative payment models who meet volume-based thresholds.

National Quality Strategy

As previously noted, the ACA required that HHS develop a national quality strategy to better align quality improvement initiatives across payers and to improve the delivery of healthcare services, patient health outcomes, and population health. HHS released its initial report to Congress, titled "National Strategy for Quality Improvement in Health Care," in March of 2011, outlining aims and priorities for quality improvement. The Strategy was updated in 2014 with levers representing core business functions, resources, and/or actions that stakeholders could use to align to the Strategy. What follows is a summary of the updated Strategy (Agency for Healthcare Research and Quality [AHRQ], 2016):

- **Adopting national aims:** The National Quality Strategy will pursue three broad aims that will be used to guide and assess local, state, and national efforts to improve healthcare quality. These aims include the following:
  - Better care: Represents efforts to improve the overall quality of health care by making care more patient centered, reliable, accessible, and safe.
  - Healthy People/Healthy Communities: Encompasses efforts to improve the health of the population by supporting interventions that address behavioral, social, and environmental determinants of health.
  - Affordable care: Seeks to reduce the cost of quality health care for individuals, families, employers, and government.
- **Setting priorities:** To advance these three aims, the strategy focuses on six priorities:
  - Making care safer by reducing harm caused in the delivery of care.
  - Ensuring that each person and family is engaged as partners in his or her care.
  - Promoting effective communication and coordination of care.
  - Promoting the most effective prevention and treatment practices for the leading causes of mortality, starting with cardiovascular disease.

- Working with communities to promote wide use of best practices to enable healthy living.
- Making quality care more affordable for individuals, families, employers, and governments by developing and spreading new healthcare delivery models.

- **Using levers to achieve improved health and health care:** In addition to adopting one or more of these aims and priorities, stakeholders can align to the National Quality Strategy using any of the following nine levers:
  - Payment: Payment arrangements should reward and incentivize high-quality, patient-centered care.
  - Public reporting: Public reporting initiatives compare costs, treatment outcomes, and patient experience for consumers.
  - Technical assistance: These efforts foster learning environments that offer training, resources, tools, and guidance to help organizations achieve quality improvement goals.
  - Certification, accreditation, and regulation: These activities ensure that providers adopt or adhere to approaches to meet safety and quality standards.
  - Consumer incentives and benefit designs: These are designed to help consumers adopt healthy behaviors and make informed decisions.
  - Measurement and feedback: These activities provide performance feedback to plans and providers to improve care.
  - Health information technology: These tools improve communication, transparency, and efficiency for better coordinated health and health care.
  - Workforce development: These activities involve investing in people to prepare the next generation of healthcare professionals and support lifelong learning for providers.
  - Innovation and diffusion: This lever aims to foster innovation in health care, in quality improvement, and within and across organizations and communities.

Annual reports have provided an update on quality improvement in the national tracking measures and highlighted public and private accomplishments in the six priority areas at the federal, state, and local levels. For the Strategy's fifth anniversary update in 2016, the annual report was combined with the annual National Healthcare Quality and Disparities Report to describe the nation's progress toward improving healthcare access, quality, and disparities. The report found that while quality had continued to improve since adoption of the National Quality Strategy, wide variation existed across its six priorities (the annual reports are available on the AHRQ website). In addition to the National Quality Strategy, multiple HHS agencies, as well as several state health departments, have their own quality strategies, many of which use the National Quality Strategy as their foundation.

In 2020, the Trump administration released Executive Order 13877, which mandated that HHS develop a National Health Quality Roadmap to recommend numerous reforms to the federal quality enterprise. The Roadmap urged greater private stakeholder involvement in establishing and overseeing quality measures, called for significant investment in quality infrastructure, and recommended focusing on quality measures that matter most to industry stakeholders.

Private Payer Efforts

While the federal government drives much of the quality improvement activity in the United States, private payers also make significant contributions to quality measurement and improvement and to related payment initiatives. For example, payers have created set payments for care during specific periods (i.e., a modified global payment arrangement) that connect payments to quality goals and provide bonuses to participants that meet or exceed set benchmarks. Others use NQF, NCQA, and similar measures to assess providers' performance and resource consumption; providers achieving set thresholds in both metrics are designated as high-quality performers online, for consideration by beneficiaries and other stakeholders. These are not unique examples; most payers post quality information about their network providers to enable their enrollees to make more informed decisions. Other efforts focus on incentives to ensure patient satisfaction, such as offering refunds to any patient who reports a negative healthcare encounter, or aim to achieve compliance with best practice guidelines, such as agreeing to bear the costs of any care associated with complications arising after a procedure. Organizations develop, implement, refine, and expand on these innovative approaches, which can encourage others to adapt and adopt successful models and methods of quality improvement.

It is important for private payers to be involved in quality improvement initiatives. Absent common standards across payers for provider quality and value, systemwide delivery and payment reform will be hampered. Because providers typically contract with federal payers (e.g., Medicare) as well as multiple private payers, they will likely be subject to different definitions of quality and different requirements for demonstrating value. This makes it a challenge for providers to align their quality improvement efforts. Multipayer efforts enable more efficient quality measurement and validate the importance of systemwide quality improvement.

Underscoring the importance of multistakeholder involvement, in 2015 HHS established the LAN, a public–private partnership tasked with, among other efforts, proposing strategic goals to advance the adoption of APMs. The LAN virtually convenes thousands of stakeholders (including payers, providers, employers, patients, states, and consumer groups) to set goals related to payment reform, share best practices, and decrease variation in payment methodologies. Interested individuals and organizations can register to participate in the network via the CMS Innovation Center's website.

In addition, across the country, multistakeholder collaboratives and community groups are partnering with employers, payers, providers, and consumers to further public–private efforts to improve quality. For example, Aligning Forces for Quality, a signature Robert Wood Johnson Foundation initiative from 2007 to 2015, established alliances in 16 communities across the United States. These multistakeholder alliances collected and reported provider performance data, tested new care delivery and payment reform models, and disseminated best practices. Providers used the information provided by the alliances to improve quality of care for the nearly 40 million residents of those 16 communities, demonstrating the value of multistakeholder partnerships in healthcare delivery transformation.

Role of Health Information Technology

Health information technology, or health IT, provides critical support for quality improvement and payment reform. Health IT includes electronic features that facilitate care delivery, such as decision support tools, electronic health records, and electronic prescribing functions. Health IT enables instant sharing of health information throughout a facility, among providers in different locations, and with the patient. Health IT can prevent clinical errors that may have dire consequences, such as by alerting providers of potential adverse drug interactions or treatment contraindications. These features facilitate quality improvement across clinical settings. Beyond clinical functions, health IT can also facilitate quality improvement efforts by collecting and analyzing data related to outcomes and process measures for use by

a provider in required reporting or conducting quality improvement initiatives. However, connecting health IT systems and allowing providers to communicate across different health IT systems remains a challenge. HHS's Office of the National Coordinator (ONC) for Health Information Technology is working with other stakeholders to foster a health IT environment where patient information can be shared electronically across the entire care spectrum, regardless of the technology used.

The value of health IT is demonstrated through federal efforts to encourage its adoption. For example, the Meaningful Use program, created in 2009 by the HITECH Act, established incentives for providers and hospitals to adopt electronic health records. The Center for Medicare and Medicaid Innovation (CMMI), established by the ACA, tests new payment and delivery models and must consider whether a model uses technology in making its selections. MACRA's QPP phased out the Meaningful Use program and replaced it with the Promoting Interoperability Performance Category for MIPS-participating providers. This category requires use of certified electronic health record technology (CEHRT) and provides performance-based incentive payments for achieving measures related to use of CEHRT to engage patients and exchange health information.

Conclusion

This chapter introduced the concept of healthcare quality generally, briefly described the concepts of licensure and accreditation, discussed the specific quality concern of medical errors, detailed the topic of legal liability for substandard healthcare provision and decision-making, and covered measurement of healthcare quality. While the majority of the chapter was dedicated to legal accountability for negligence in healthcare delivery, this is of course just one method used to promote high-quality care. Policymakers, health services researchers, the health professions themselves, and others have proposed or implemented several additional strategies (e.g., related to the healthcare system's organizational structure, or to evidence-based medicine, or to information technology) aimed at remedying existing quality concerns and improving the quality of care going forward, some of which are reflected in federal legislation. Many of these strategies have yet to take hold on a national scale, however, and finding effective ways to mesh them with existing legal rules—and navigating the legal system's responses to them—are issues with which the country will continue to grapple.

References

Aetna Health, Inc. v. Davila, 542 U.S. 200 (2004).

Agency for Healthcare Research and Quality. (2016). *National Strategy for Quality Improvement in Health Care*. https://www.ahrq.gov/workingforquality/about/agency-specific-quality-strategic-plans/nqs3.html

Boyd v. Albert Einstein Med. Ctr., 547 A. 2d 1229 (Pa. Super., 1988).

Canterbury v. Spence, 464 F.2d 772 (D.C. Cir. 1972).

Committee on Quality of Health Care in America. (2001). *Crossing the quality chasm: A new health system for the 21st century*. National Academy Press.

Corcoran v. United Healthcare Inc., 965 F.2d 1321 (5th Cir. 1992).

Darling v. Charleston Cmty. Mem. Hosp., 211 N.E.2d 253 (Ill. 1965).

Dukes v. U.S. Healthcare, Inc., 57 F. 3d 350 (3d Cir. 1995).

Employee Retirement Income Security Act of 1974, 29 U.S.C. §§ 1132, 1144(a)-(b)(2)(A) & (B) (1974).

Fisher, E., Goodman, D., Skinner, J., & Bronner, K. (2009). *Health care spending, quality and outcomes: More isn't always better*. http://www.dartmouthatlas.org/downloads/reports/Spending_Brief_022709.pdf

Fisher, E. S., Wennberg, D. E., Stukel, T. A., Gottlieb, D. J., Lucas, F. L., & Oinder, E. L. (2003). The implications of regional variations in Medicare spending. Part 1: The content, quality, and accessibility of care. *Annals of Internal Medicine, 138*, 273–287.

Fort Halifax Packing Co. v. Coyne, 482 U.S. 1 (1987).

Furrow, B. R., Greaney, T. L., Johnson, S. H., Jost, T. S., & Schwartz, R. L. (2001). *Health law: Cases, materials and problems*. West Group.

Gruenberg v. Aetna Insur. Co., 510 P. 2d 1032 (Cal. 1973).

Hall v. Hilbun, 466 So.2d 856 (Miss. 1985).

Helling v. Carey, 519 P.2d 981 (Wash. 1974).

Hurley v. Eddingfield, 59 N.E. 1058 (Ind. 1901).

Iglehart, J. K. (2013). Expanding the role of advanced nurse practitioners: Risks and rewards. *New England Journal of Medicine, 368*, 1935–1941.

Jackson v. Power, 743 P. 2d 1376 (Alaska, 1987).

Jones v. Chicago HMO Ltd. of Illinois, 730 N.E. 2d 1119 (2000).

Kaufman, M. (2006, July 21). Medication errors harming millions, report says. *Washington Post*. http://www.washingtonpost.com/wp-dyn/content/article/2006/07/20/AR2006072000754.html

Kentucky Ass'n of Health Plans, Inc. v. Miller, 538 U.S. 329 (2003).

Kohn, L. T., Corrigan, J. M., & Donaldson, M. S. (Eds.). (2000). *To err is human: Building a safer health system*. National Academy Press.

Kuhmerker, K., & Hartman, T. (2007). *Pay-for-performance in state Medicaid programs: A survey of state Medicaid directors and programs*. https://www.commonwealthfund.org/publications/fund-reports/2007/apr/pay-performance-state-medicaid-programs-survey-state-medicaid

Makary, M. A., & Daniel, M. (2016, May 3). Medical error—The third leading cause of death in the U.S. *BMJ, 353*, i2139. https://www.bmj.com/content/353/bmj.i2139

McGlynn, E. A., Asch, S. M., Adams, J., Keesey, J., Hicks, J., DeCristofaro, A., & Kerr, E. (2003). The quality of health care delivered to adults in the United States. *New England Journal of Medicine, 348*, 2635–2645.

Mehlman v. Powell, 378 A. 2d 1121 (Md. 1977).

Metropolitan Life Insur. Co. v. Massachusetts, 471 U.S. 724 (1985).

New York State Conference of Blue Cross & Blue Shield Plans v. Travelers Insur. Co., 514 U.S. 645 (1995).

Nordenberg, T. (2000). *Make no mistake: Medical errors can be deadly serious*. https://permanent.access.gpo.gov/lps1609/www.fda.gov/fdac/features/2000/500_err.html

Patient Protection and Affordable Care Act (Pub. L. 111-148) § 3013 (2010), adding Public Health Service Act § 931.

Patient Safety and Quality Improvement Act of 2005, 42 U.S.C. § 299 et seq. (2005).

Pegram v. Herdrich, 530 U.S. 211 (2000).

Pilot Life Insur. Co. v. Dedeaux, 481 U.S. 41 (1987).

Rosenbaum, S., Frankford, D. M., Law, S. A., & Rosenblatt, R. E. (2012). *Law and the American health care system* (2nd ed.). Foundation Press.

Rosenbaum, S., Frankford, D. M., Moore, B., & Borzi, P. (1999). Who should determine when health care is medically necessary? *New England Journal of Medicine, 340*(3), 229–233.

Shaw v. Delta Air Lines, Inc., 463 U.S. 85 (1983).

Shilkret v. Annapolis Emergency Hospital Ass'n, 349 A. 2d 245, 253 (Md. 1975).

Slater v. Baker and Stapleton, 95 Eng. Rep. 860, 862 (King's Bench 1767).

Small v. Howard, 128 Mass. 131 (1880).

T. J. Hooper v. Northern Barge Corp., 60 F.2d 737 (2d Cir. 1932).

Van Vector v. Blue Cross Ass'n, 365 N.E. 2d 638 (Ill. App. Ct., 1977).

Wennberg, J. (Ed.). (1996). *The Dartmouth atlas of health care in the United States 1996*. American Hospital Publishing.

Wennberg J. E., Fisher, E. S., & Skinner, J. S. (2002). Geography and the debate over Medicare reform. *Health Affairs, 21*(Suppl. 1), W96–W114. https://doi.org/10.1377/hlthaff.W2 96

Endnotes

a. For example, in the lawsuit stemming from the facts described at the outset of this chapter, the parents of the infant who died alleged that their MCO's decision to precertify only 24 hours of hospital care coverage did not meet the requisite standard of care in several healthcare quality respects: (1) it was not medically appropriate and was motivated by financial profit, not Michelina's health and well-being; (2) it forced Michelina's premature discharge from the hospital; (3) it was made despite the MCO's knowledge that newborns are particularly at risk for developing illnesses; and (4) it discouraged physicians participating in the MCO's provider network from readmitting infants to the hospital when problems arose after discharge.

b. Because the law's evolving view of the standard of care closely mirrors its view of the medical profession more generally, it is worth pausing for a moment to reflect on the health policy and law conceptual framework that is focused on historical, social, political, and economic views. This framework includes three perspectives: professional autonomy, social contract, and free market. The first perspective, dominant from about 1880 to 1960, argues that physicians' scientific and medical expertise leaves them in the best position to determine whether care rendered to patients is of adequate quality, and thus that legal oversight of the medical profession should be driven by the profession itself. The second perspective guided policymaking and legal principles for roughly 20 years beginning around 1960 and maintains that healthcare delivery and financing should be governed by enforcement of a "social contract" that generally elevates patient rights and societal values over physician autonomy and control. The free market perspective—dominant since the 1990s—contends that healthcare services are most efficiently delivered in a deregulated marketplace controlled by commercial competition. Bear in mind the first two perspectives specifically as you read this section.

c. One of the most commonly cited English cases for this rule is *Slater v. Baker and Stapleton* (1767), in which the court ruled that the appropriate legal standard for determining a surgeon's liability was "the usage and law of surgeons . . . the rule of the profession" as testified to by practicing surgeons.

d. An example of this shift can be seen in the case of *Canterbury v. Spence* (1972), which is often discussed in the context of a patient's right to make informed healthcare decisions. The *Canterbury* court ruled that a professional-oriented standard for measuring the legality

of a physician's disclosure of information to a patient should be replaced by an objective standard predicated on what a reasonable patient would need to be told to effect the aforementioned right.

e. For example, see *Van Vector v. Blue Cross Ass'n* (1977).

f. For example, see *Gruenberg v. Aetna Insur. Co.* (1973).

g. Even citations to ERISA are complicated, because the law's section numbers in the U.S. Code (where much of ERISA can be found under Title 29) do not always correspond to the section numbering in the original act as written by Congress. For a helpful website effectively decoding where ERISA provisions are located in the U.S. Code, go to http://benefitslink.com/erisa/crossreference.html.

h. Note how this outcome can reasonably be viewed as incentivizing ERISA plans to arbitrarily deny patients' claims for healthcare coverage, because even in the event that plans are found to have acted negligently, they are responsible for paying only the cost of the denied benefit, but nothing more.

i. We are deeply grateful to professors Jane Thorpe and Elizabeth Gray, our colleagues in the Department of Health Policy and Management and experts in healthcare quality promotion, for the drafting of this section.

j. There is extensive literature on this topic. See, for example, Fisher et al., 2003; Fisher et al., 2009; McGlynn et al., 2003; Wennberg, 1996; Wennberg et al., 2002.

k. Go to www.medicare.gov/care-compare/?providerType=Hospital&redirect=true to see the hospital comparisons and to www.medicare.gov/ to access other Compare websites.

l. See, for example, Kuhmerker & Hartman, 2007.

CHAPTER 13

What Is Public Health Emergency Preparedness?

Suzet McKinney

Mary Elise Papke

LEARNING OBJECTIVES

Public health emergency preparedness is a highly specialized area of public health practice. In order to effectively appreciate the importance of public health preparedness in keeping populations healthy following a large-scale public health emergency, the basic foundations of public health practice must be placed into context with emergency and disaster situations. By the end of this chapter you will be able to:

1. Explain the role of public health in emergency preparedness
2. Describe the role of state and local governments in preparedness and response
3. Describe the Incident Command System (ICS) and the importance of a centralized command structure during response operations
4. Articulate the premise of the "whole community" approach to preparedness and response
5. Describe key legal considerations in emergency preparedness planning

What Is Public Health?

In its groundbreaking report, *The Future of Public Health*, the National Academy of Medicine defines public health in terms of its mission to "fulfill society's interest in assuring conditions in which people can be healthy," and the report further depicts public health's "aim to generate organized community effort to address the public interest in health by applying scientific and technical knowledge to prevent disease and promote health" (publishing as Institute of Medicine, 1988, p. 7). Unlike traditional medical care, public health employs policies and interventions to minimize disease and improve health outcomes for populations, as opposed to narrowly focusing on how

to address the health of an individual. Public health is "measured in terms of improved health status, diseases prevented, scarce resources saved and improved quality of life" (Turnock, 2012, p. 2). Improvements in health due to public health advancements, such as the use of vaccines and sanitation practices to prevent the spread of disease, are distinct scientific interventions. However, the public typically does not link public health's work with its achievements.

The three core functions of public health—assessment, policy development, and assurance—characterize and shape how public health practitioners approach their work. Assessment deals with the collection and analysis of health status information for communities. Policy development deals with the development of policies and the determination of appropriate interventions to address the problems in health. Finally, assurance deals with the responsibility of public health to implement strategies and interventions to promote health. Similarly, emergency preparedness as a discipline utilizes a systematic approach, the preparedness cycle, to preparing for emergencies and disasters. The steps of hazard/vulnerability assessment, planning, and mitigation/response can be likened to the three core functions of public health.

What Is Emergency Preparedness?

Public health emergency preparedness is the ability to prevent, prepare for, protect against, respond to, and recover from health emergencies. Public health emergencies are emergencies whose "scale, timing, or unpredictability threaten to overwhelm routine capabilities" to provide health care (Nelson et al., 2007, p. S9). These emergencies are characterized by their high severity, inability to be managed with routine resources, and tendency to cause increased illness, injury, or death. Public health emergencies span a broad range of emergency and disaster situations, including natural hazards, acts of terrorism, and large-scale infectious disease outbreaks. The 2021 Western United States wildfires; the terrorist attacks of September 11, 2001; and coronavirus-19 infectious disease (COVID-19) pandemic are examples of these types of emergency situations.

History of Preparedness Programs and Preparedness Funding

Public health preparedness programs in the United States started in the late 1990s. In 1999, the U.S. Centers for Disease Control and Prevention (CDC) established the "Public Health Preparedness and Response for Bioterrorism Program." This program was narrowly focused on preparing for a biological terrorism attack on the United States. At that time, the threat was considered to be remote, and as such, little funding was allocated to public health for this effort. Public health agencies across the United States conducted planning for a response to a bioterrorism attack; however, the sense of urgency in this preparation was limited, as bioterrorism was thought to be a high-impact, but low-probability threat. The World Trade Center attacks in New York City on September 11, 2001 (9/11), and the subsequent anthrax attacks on the United States in October of 2001 changed this thinking. With these two events came the sharp realization that the United States could not properly respond to a large-scale bioterrorism attack. This was due in large part to the severely depleted infrastructure of the U.S. public health system. As a result, Congress appropriated $1 billion to public health in order to build the public health infrastructure in a manner that would strengthen the country's ability to respond to a bioterrorism attack. **Figure 13.1a** and **Figure 13.1b** illustrate funding levels since the

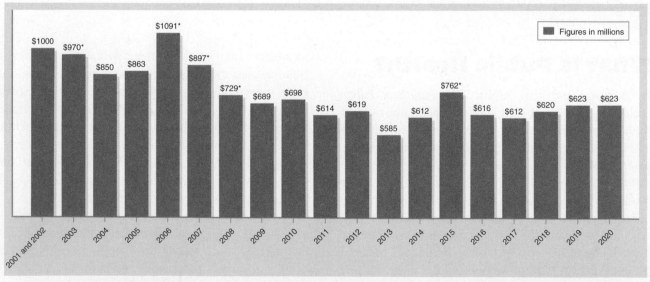

*Asterisk denotes increase in PHEP awards due to emergency supplemental funding (2003 for smallpox; 2006, 2007, and 2008 for pandemic influenza; and 2015 for Ebola). The FY2008 total includes $24 million for pandemic influenza preparedness projects that were from a different, competitive funding opportunity announcement.

Figure 13.1a Public Health Emergency Preparedness (PHEP) Cooperative Agreement Funding

Data from Centers for Disease Control and Prevention. Office of Public Health Preparedness and Response.

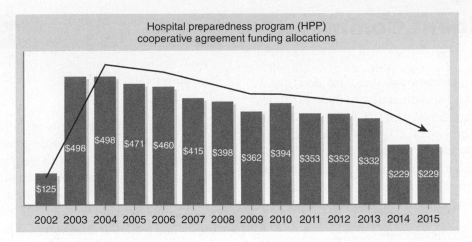

Figure 13.1b HPP Cooperative Agreement Funding

Data from U.S. Department of Health and Human Services. Office of the Assistant Secretary for Preparedness and Response.

beginning of the Public Health Emergency Preparedness (PHEP) Cooperative Agreement and the Hospital Preparedness Program (HPP) Cooperative Agreement funding. Funding was allocated to 62 public health awardees, including the state health departments in all 50 states, 8 territories, and 4 directly funded cities. These directly funded cities—Chicago, New York City, Los Angeles County, and the District of Columbia—were considered to have the highest risk of a terrorist attack and thus the need to be funded separately from their states.

The initial work of the expansion of bioterrorism programs in the United States focused the role of public health as being a critical leader in the country's response to a terrorist attack (CDC, 2000). This work focused on seven areas: preparedness planning and readiness assessment (focus area A), surveillance and epidemiology capacity (focus area B), laboratory capacity—biological agents (focus area C), laboratory capacity—chemical agents (focus area D), health alert networks/communications and information technology (focus area E), risk communication and health information dissemination (focus area F), and education and training (focus area G). Jurisdictions conducted planning activities around these focus areas, as well as cross-cutting areas that were integrated with hospital preparedness benchmarks and requirements funded by the Health Resources and Services Administration (HRSA; CDC, 2004). (The HPP Cooperative Agreement was moved from HRSA to the Office of the Assistant Secretary for Preparedness and Response when this office was created in 2006 by the Pandemic and All-Hazards Preparedness Act, or PAHPA.)

In the years after 9/11, public health has used preparedness funding to plan and prepare for the aftereffects of a bioterrorism attack. However, since that time, preparedness programs have evolved from the original focus on bioterrorism attacks. This evolution of focus is not to negate the possibility of a biological, chemical, or other form of terrorist activity; however, the emergence of large-scale infectious disease outbreaks and the increase in catastrophic natural disasters have led public health toward an "all-hazards" approach to public health preparedness. There is now a greater recognition and understanding that most emergencies are not acts of terrorism, but are instead most likely to be natural disasters, such as floods, hurricanes, and tornadoes, or large-scale infectious diseases such as the 2009 H1N1 influenza and COVID-19 pandemics, or severe respiratory infections and zoonotic diseases, such as severe acute respiratory syndrome (SARS) and Ebola.

Public health has also become an integral component of the emergency response community as an accepted first responder. Public health's role as a first responder was initiated by the 9/11 attacks and subsequent anthrax attacks in 2001. This new role represented a culture shift for both public health and traditional first responders. For public health professionals, integration into the first responder community has been an enormous learning curve. One example is the Incident Command System (ICS) and the National Incident Management System (NIMS) and the new language that public health first responders had to learn in order to communicate with other first responders when working alongside them during response operations. Before moving on to the next section, please review **Box 13.1**.

💡 Box 13.1 DISCUSSION QUESTIONS

What is public health emergency preparedness? Describe the incidents that led to the creation and/or expansion of public health emergency preparedness programs in the United States.

The Incident Command System

The ICS is an organizational structure designed to assure an organized, coordinated, rapid, and seamless response to an emergency. The ICS was created in the early 1970s by the National Fire Service as a means of managing the response to forest fires in California. Developed to manage emergencies of various sizes and scopes, the ICS provides a mechanism for managing personnel, facilities, equipment, and communications (U.S. Department of the Interior, National Park Service, n.d.). Additionally, the ICS provides a common language among multiple responders, clearly identifies the chain of command and reporting structure, is cost-effective and flexible to meet the needs of emergencies of various scales, and can be used for routine operations as well as emergencies.

Today, the ICS is used by the Federal Emergency Management Agency (FEMA) and emergency management agencies across the country. Hospitals and healthcare systems have also adopted a form of ICS that is modified to suit their needs. The Hospital Incident Command System (HICS) applies the structure of ICS within hospitals and healthcare systems to enhance preparedness and response capability within healthcare institutions (HICS, n.d.). Like the application of ICS to public health, this system also proved to have a considerable learning curve for healthcare professionals. Nevertheless, it has increased coordination not only within the healthcare sector, but also among officials in local and state governments.

In public health, we use what many have termed the Public Health Incident Command System (PHICS). The PHICS has become critically important to public health. Since the recognition of public health as a first responder, public health has struggled with this new role. Public health officials and other first responders have been challenged to work in concert, in both planning and response to emergencies (Werner et al., 2005). This increased coordination, the need to forge new partnerships, and the need to integrate with other public safety partners represented a struggle for public health; however, public health responders have found that the system provides everyone with a common language and that this facilitates coordination and communication across disciplines.

The traditional ICS structure includes the incident commander and four functional sections: planning, logistics, operations, and finance/administration. Surveillance and epidemiological response efforts are usually included as a fifth functional section or as a

component of the operations section. This is important in public health response efforts because surveillance drives public health response, particularly where disease occurrence is the identified threat. Surveillance enables public health to apply the science of epidemiology to determine the causative agent of disease and track the disease trends to limit the spread (**Figure 13.2**). Before moving on to the next section, please review **Box 13.2**.

Presidential Policy Directive-8 (PPD-8) and the Whole Community Approach to Preparedness

Preparedness is a shared responsibility, and as such, preparedness activities should be undertaken using a "whole community" approach (FEMA, 2011). While many preparedness efforts will be coordinated and led by government agencies, those agencies should engage individuals, communities, private-sector businesses, hospitals, and healthcare systems in planning and other preparedness activities. These critical stakeholders can bring great value not only during the planning process, but they can also assist government officials during an emergency response by fostering community and institutional recovery following a disaster. Disasters that are significantly large in their scale and scope may require response assistance from state and federal government partners, as all levels of government have a role in emergency response. However, all emergencies are inherently local first. This means that local governments must be prepared to initiate emergency responses and have the capability to maintain those responses for a minimal amount of time, generally 72 hours. Engagement of the whole community can help ensure a more comprehensive, robust response. The concept of this shared responsibility is further strengthened by PPD-8. Enacted in March 2011 by President Barack Obama, PPD-8 calls for a systematic approach to preparedness for all-hazards threats and disasters. Based on the tenet that all people possess abilities that can contribute to the nation's security, PPD-8 further calls upon the federal government to

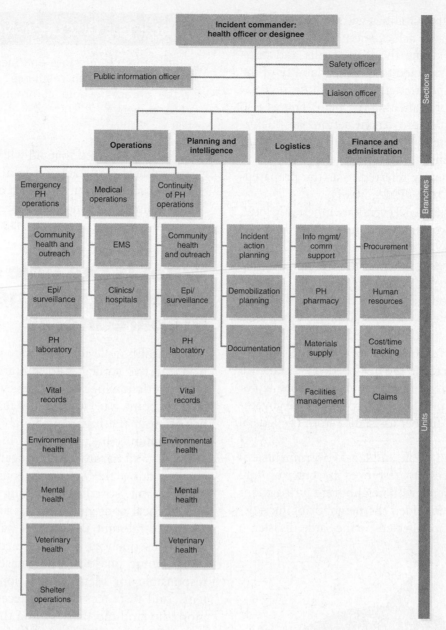

Figure 13.2 Public Health Incident Command Chart

Reproduced from Rottman, S., Shoaf, K., & Dorian, A. (2005). *Writing a disaster plan: A guide for health departments.* www.ualbanycphp.org/pinata/phics/guide/fig02.cfm

develop a national preparedness goal and core capabilities to guide activities and ensure a systemwide approach to preparedness (Department of Homeland Security, 2014).

Role of State and Local Governments in Preparedness and Response

More than the management of a single emergency or disaster event, emergency preparedness is a process. It is the process of assessing jurisdictional hazards

and vulnerabilities to determine which threats are most likely to occur within a given area (community, jurisdiction, city, county, region, state). Once the most likely hazards have been identified, operational plans are developed to describe actions that will be undertaken to mitigate the hazards identified during the assessment. Preparedness plans should employ an all-hazards approach, with specific details given to the most likely threats, as identified by the hazard vulnerability assessment. Plans need to be scalable, flexible, and operationally sound in order to be viable during a response. Preparedness plans should be living, breathing documents. This means no good plan is ever final. Instead, the plan is reviewed with regularity, generally on an annual basis.

Those with responsibilities within the plan need to be trained to ensure achievement of the necessary competencies to execute the plan. Drills and exercises should be conducted to test the viability of the plan, and finally, the strengths and weaknesses analyzed as a means of evaluating the plan. This is also the point at which improvement actions are identified and documented. This entire process of hazard identification, planning, training, exercising, and evaluation is frequently referred to as the preparedness cycle (**Figure 13.3**; FEMA, 2014).

As previously stated, all events are inherently local, and local jurisdictions must ensure that they have the capability to properly respond to emergency events and sustain themselves for, at minimum, 72 hours. This is not to say that assistance will not be available prior to 72 hours; however, this is the generally accepted time frame for self-sustainment. Once local resources have become exhausted, localities should request assistance from state-level entities. State governments are expected to provide needed assistance to localities until the state resources are overwhelmed or exhausted. At this point in the response, state governments can request further assistance from the federal government.

Prior to an event, state and local governments can augment their access to resources by entering into mutual aid agreements with neighboring jurisdictions or other partners. Provided the neighboring jurisdiction or partner is not affected by the same disaster, it

Box 13.3 DISCUSSION QUESTIONS

What is the role of state and local governments in preparedness and response? What is meant by the phrase "whole community approach to preparedness"?

is reasonably expected that aid will be provided. This is one strategy that state and local governments can employ to achieve a longer period of self-sustainment before additional assistance is requested from the state or federal government. See **Box 13.3**.

What Is the Role of Public Health in Emergency Preparedness?

Public health's role in emergency preparedness is to plan effective strategies to minimize morbidity and mortality following an emergency or disaster. As a starting point, public health is responsible for participation in the hazard vulnerability assessment of the community or jurisdiction. In the identification of threats and hazards, public health officials should be evaluating the expected consequences of the hazard event, specifically looking to identify health and medical consequences that are likely to occur. Once the relevant threats and hazards, along with their consequences, are identified, work moves to the planning phase. In this phase, public health is responsible for identifying actions, strategies, systems, and resources that are necessary to minimize morbidity and mortality should the hazard or threat occur. Potential actions that public health officials might identify include the initiation of surveillance and epidemiological investigations to determine the source and spread of the disease or other hazard as well as the determination of potential treatment options, including laboratory testing, medical countermeasures, and the appropriateness of quarantine and isolation measures or other nonpharmaceutical interventions. Strategies to limit the spread of disease and illness frequently involve efforts to isolate the disease and implement targeted measures aimed at mitigating the threat.

Often in emergency preparedness, public health officials become overwhelmed when planning for particularly complex hazards and threats. This sense of becoming overwhelmed is spurred by a misperception that public health is responsible for all aspects of threat mitigation. In fact, public health is not

Figure 13.3 Preparedness Cycle

Federal Emergency Management Agency. *Preparedness cycle.* www.fema.gov/media-library/assets/images/114295#

responsible for all aspects of emergency response; it is only responsible for engaging the appropriate stakeholders and partners that hold specific expertise that will aid in the emergency response or those who may also play a role in the response effort. Engagement of community and social service partners who can lend expertise in planning for the needs of individuals with access and functional needs (i.e., individuals who have physical, developmental, or intellectual disabilities; chronic conditions; or limited English proficiency) is critical. Faith-based organizations hold strong trust relationships with community members and have an in-depth knowledge of the needs of the community. Thus, they are uniquely positioned to provide support and assistance not only during the planning phase but also in response.

Public health is also responsible for engagement and coordination with the healthcare system, namely, hospitals, community clinics, long-term care facilities, specialty providers, and other public health entities. Other healthcare system partners could include, but are not limited to, blood banks, dialysis centers, mental health providers, and home healthcare providers. Public health has a unique role in healthcare system coordination—that of coordinating collaboration among the multiple healthcare partners and ensuring that healthcare partners are equipped with supplies, equipment, and other resources that foster preparedness capability across the healthcare system. For example, during the initial February 2020 COVID-19 outbreak (caused by the novel SARS-CoV-2 virus) in a Seattle-area nursing home, Public Health-Seattle and King County, along with CDC staff, worked closely with the nursing home to investigate the outbreak, conduct surveillance and contact tracing, and implement quarantine and isolation measures (McMichael et al., 2020). The local health department and CDC staff also worked with facility staff to review and refine infection prevention and control plans (McMichael et al., 2020).

Just as no good plan is ever complete, neither is public health's role in emergency preparedness. Public health's planning and coordination role should continuously evolve, employing lessons learned from drills, exercises, and real events to validate and improve mitigation strategies; engaging new partners; and refining a system's approach to emergency response. Indeed, public health's experience with the COVID-19 pandemic offers a unique opportunity at the local, state, and national levels to assess outcomes, describe lessons learned, and enhance emergency plans with existing and new partners.

Importance of Public Health Infrastructure and Capacity Building

To effectively fulfill its role in emergency preparedness and response, public health needs to maintain a strong infrastructure. Public health infrastructure includes maintenance of core public health capabilities and relationships that can aid emergency response efforts. The most important of these core public health capabilities is surveillance and epidemiology. As the study of diseases and injuries in human populations, disease patterns, and the frequency of occurrence, epidemiology is considered to be the basic science of public health (Dworkin, 2011). Epidemiologists conduct outbreak investigations to determine the origin of outbreaks, identify the populations at risk, and characterize the modes of disease transmission. Findings from these investigations are then used to initiate the efforts to control the outbreak and to prevent similar occurrences from happening in the future. Public health surveillance is the mechanism by which diseases and other health conditions are tracked. This too is an important core public health capability. Surveillance data can provide public health officials with important information that can be used to determine the subsets of the population who are affected by a particular condition. An important illustration of the use of surveillance data to identify disparities among different populations is local, state, and national analysis of COVID-19 cases, hospitalizations, and mortality data. Health and county officials in Milwaukee, Wisconsin, were among the first to call attention to inequities in patterns of cases in communities of color in Milwaukee County (Spicuzza & Dirr, 2021). Local and state public health agencies across the country have taken action to implement strategies for testing and vaccinating by working with leaders and organizations connected to communities that are disproportionately affected by COVID-19. Public health surveillance and epidemiological investigation are cornerstones in public health responses to emergencies. Public health systems must have the ability to maintain and support routine surveillance and investigation processes, and to expand these efforts in response to incidents of public health significance.

While epidemiology and surveillance provide critical data and information that fuel public health response, there are many other capabilities that public health agencies must develop in order to ensure full capacity to respond to emergency events. These capabilities describe the training, skills, equipment, and other resources that public health must have, or have access to, in order to properly respond to an emergency or disaster.

Other important aspects of public health infrastructure include human resources and financial management systems. These systems are needed during an emergency response in order to maintain employee records, track employee time, and appropriately compensate employees for time worked. Inventory management and communication systems are also necessary to ensure appropriate tracking of equipment, supplies, and staff.

Federal Response Structure: National Response Plan (NRP), National Response Framework (NRF)

The NRP was developed in December of 2004 and established a single, comprehensive framework for the management of domestic incidents (FEMA, 2004). More specifically, the NRP established a progressive approach to emergency response, dictating that emergency response begin locally, flow to the state government once local resources are exhausted, and then flow to the federal government at the point that state resources become overwhelmed or are exhausted. The NRP also established multiple coordinating structures, which are designed to effectively guide and coordinate site-specific incident management activities, as well as provide coordination for management of disasters with national significance. In 2008, the NRP was replaced by the NRF, which is a more comprehensive guidance that incorporates lessons learned from several events of national significance, most notably Hurricane Katrina (FEMA, 2008a).

The NRF builds on the NIMS and strives to guide national response to emergencies and improve coordination among all response partners. The NRF aligns key roles and responsibilities to foster response partnerships at all levels of government with nongovernmental organizations and the private sector. In doing so, the NRF further promotes the "whole community" approach to preparedness and response, as established by PPD-8, and thus should be used by the whole community for emergency preparedness and response. The priorities of the NRF are to "save lives, protect property and the environment, stabilize the incident and provide for basic human needs" (FEMA, 2008b, p. i). To meet these priorities, the NRF establishes a response vision through five key principles:

1. **Engaged partnership:** All levels of government and the whole community must develop shared response goals and align capabilities to ensure that no one entity is overwhelmed in times of crisis.
2. **Tiered response:** Incidents must be managed at the lowest possible jurisdictional level (local) and supported by additional capabilities when needed.
3. **Scalable, flexible, adaptable operational capabilities:** As incidents change in size, scope, and complexity, the response must adapt to meet these changing requirements.
4. **Unity in response through unified command:** Respect the chain of command of participating organizations and ensure seamless coordination across jurisdictions in support of common objectives.
5. **Readiness to act:** Ensure the best response possible that is grounded in a clear understanding of potential risks and decisive actions.

The NRF is composed of multiple components that can be used together or independently, based on the nature, scope, and scale of the emergency. Those components include the base document, Emergency Support Function (ESF) Annexes, Support Annexes, and Incident Annexes (**Figure 13.4**).

As indicated in the guidance document, the annexes provide detailed information to assist with the implementation of the NRF. ESF Annexes describe the federal coordinating structures that group resources and capabilities into functional areas that are most frequently needed in a national response. Support Annexes describe the essential supporting processes and considerations that are most common to the majority of incidents. Incident Annexes describe the unique response aspects of incident categories.

Figure 13.4 Structure of the National Response Framework

Federal Emergency Management Agency (2008). *National response framework.* www.fema.gov/media-library-data/20130726-1914-25045-1246/final_national_response_framework_20130501.pdf

The Public Health Workforce and Development of Preparedness Competencies and Association of Schools and Programs of Public Health Core Competencies

Ensuring the public health workforce develops and maintains the appropriate skills, knowledge, and competencies for responding to emergency events is a critical component of the development of emergency preparedness capability. For many years, specific preparedness competency remained a mystery. Early iterations of preparedness competency were developed by staff at the Columbia University School of Nursing, Center for Health Policy. PAHPA called for a comprehensive, competency-based training program that is responsive to the needs of state, local, and tribal public health organizations and that emphasizes public health security capabilities. In response to the call for the development of a comprehensive competency framework for educational programs in public health emergency preparedness, the Association of Schools and Programs of Public Health (ASPPH) developed the master's Public Health Preparedness and Response Model (ASPPH, n.d.). This model was designed for use by graduate-level education programs to ensure that students obtain the necessary knowledge, skills, and attitudes associated with public health emergency preparedness and response. Under this model, students should gain competency in roles and relationships, communication and information management, planning and improvement, assessment, and incident management. The model's framework is based on a series of tenets that are designed to build competency in future generations of the public health workforce with particular expertise in preparedness and response.

Legal Issues in Public Health Emergency Preparedness

Most observers consider the United States to be an extraordinarily legalistic country. Law is something of a rudder for American social life, and an important one at that. It establishes frameworks, creates formal relationships, and articulates guidelines. It prescribes and proscribes. Law is perhaps the clearest and most obvious expression of public policy.

Public health law as a whole and emergency preparedness law in particular focus on protecting the health and safety of the population. Law of this sort is so important that it constitutes a major part of the public health infrastructure (Turnock, 2012). Statutes, regulations, and judicial decisions are crucial in emergency preparedness. These statutes, regulations, and judicial decisions related to emergency preparedness can be found at the local, state, and federal levels. The laws vary from jurisdiction to jurisdiction, and the relationships among the laws at these levels of government have evolved over time for a variety of reasons (Turnock, 2012, pp. 166–167). As a result, there are many laws in each of the states that address public health matters and emergency preparedness specifically.

One venerable but particularly controversial variety of emergency preparedness law that illustrates the variation and the changing relationships among different laws involves isolation and quarantine. Local and state governments are empowered through their police powers, as defined in state constitutions, to protect the public's health and safety. Typically, powers to protect the public's health lie with the local public health authority. Isolating and quarantining those with communicable diseases in specified circumstances is one way to safeguard the public's health and safety. State statutes specify a list of diseases that must be reported to state health departments and to the CDC, which maintains a national surveillance system of notifiable diseases.

The controversial nature of quarantine as a state legal power was dramatically illustrated in the states of New Jersey and Maine in 2014. A nurse named Kaci Hickox returned in October from Sierra Leone in West Africa, where she had been working with Doctors Without Borders treating patients suffering from Ebola. Upon her arrival at the Newark Airport in New Jersey, she was ordered by Governor Chris Christie to face a mandatory 21-day quarantine in New Jersey (**Box 13.4**).

Hickox challenged the quarantine order, as she had no symptoms and had tested negative for Ebola. She was then allowed to travel to Maine, where Governor Paul LePage issued a quarantine order that confined Hickox to her home. She defied that order on a bike ride near her home, and with national media focused on Maine, a judge ruled in her favor against the state. In his ruling (**Exhibit 13.1**), Judge Charles LaVerdiere stated, "The State has not met its burden at this time to prove by clear and convincing evidence that limiting Respondent's movements to the degree requested is 'necessary to protect other individuals from the dangers of infection,' however. According to the information

Box 13.4 Challenging a State Quarantine Order

In an interview with CNN on October 26, 2014, Kaci Hickox described her feelings on being placed in quarantine at a New Jersey hospital after returning from West Africa. "This is an extreme that is really unacceptable, and I feel like my basic human rights have been violated."

Data from Crowley, C. (2014, October 26). *Quarantined nurse slams new policy*. State of the Union with Candy Crowley. CNN Press Room.

Exhibit 13.1 Court Decision—*Mayhew v. Hickox*, State of Maine; Ebola Quarantine Case, Judge Charles LaVerdiere; October 31, 2014

STATE OF MAINE   DISTRICT COURT
AROOSTOOK, SS.   Location: Fort Kent
                                        Docket No: CV-2014-36

Mary C. Mayhew, Commissioner   )
State of Maine Department of Health   )
and Human Services,   )
          Petitioner,   )   Order Pending Hearing
        v.   )
Kaci Hickox,   )
          Respondent.   )

The State has requested that the court issue an order restricting Respondent's activities pending the final hearing on its Verified Petition for a Public Health Order. This decision has critical implications for Respondent's freedom, as guaranteed by the U.S. and Maine Constitutions, as well as the public's right to be protected from the potential severe harm posed by transmission of this devastating disease. Given the gravity of these interests, the Court yesterday entered a temporary order maintaining the status quo until a further hearing could occur this morning. It was imperative that the court take the necessary time to review in detail the parties' submissions, the arguments of counsel, and the cases cited by counsel regarding the necessity of entering an order pending the final hearing in this matter.

Maine Law authorizes a court to "make such orders as it deems *necessary to protect other individuals from the dangers of infection*" pending a hearing on a petition for a public health order. 22 M.R.S. § 811(3) (2014) (emphasis added). At this point in time, the only information that the Court has before it regarding the dangers of infection posed by Respondent, who has potentially but not definitely been exposed to the Ebola virus, derives from the Affidavit of Shiela Pinette, D.O., Director of the Maine Center for Disease Control and Prevention, together with the attachments from the U.S. Centers for Disease Control. In her affidavit, Dr. Pinette averred, *inter alia:*

8. Ebola Virus Disease is spread through direct contact with the blood, sweat, vomit, feces and other body fluids *of a symptomatic person*. It can also be spread through exposure to needles or other objects contaminated with the virus.
. . .

12. Transmission of Ebloa is usually through direct contact with the blood, sweat, emesis, feces and other body secretions of an infected person, or exposure to objects (such as needles) that have been contaminated with infected secretions.
. . .

14. *Individuals infected with Ebola Virus Disease who are not showing symptoms are not yet infectious.* Early symptoms of Ebola are non-specific and common to many other illnesses.

15. Symptoms usually include: fever, headache, joint and muscle aches, weakness, diarrhea, vomiting, stomach pain, and lack of appetite. *Ebola may be present in an individual who does not exhibit any of these symptoms, because they are not yet infectious.*

16. The incubation period for the virus, before it can be determined that a person does not have Ebola virus, is 21 days ("the incubation period"). A person who is infected with Ebola virus can start to show symptoms of the disease (become infectious) at any point during the incubation period. A person can test negative for Ebola virus in the early part of the incubation period and later become infectious and test positive.

17. The Respondent remains at risk of being infected with Ebola, until the 21-day time period has assed. The most common time of developing symptoms is during the second week after last exposure. Respondent entered that second week starting October 28, 2014. The surest way to minimize the public health threat is direct active monitoring and additional restrictions on movement and exposure to other persons or the public until a potentially exposed person has passed the incubation period. For Respondent that period expires November 10, 2014.

18. Symptoms usually appear 8 to 10 days after exposure and 90% of cases develop symptoms within the first 14 days of exposure. So the time of greatest risk of showing symptoms and becoming infectious is within the first 14 days of the incubation period. Once someone is displaying symptoms and is actually infected with Ebola, they become increasingly infectious and extremely ill, requiring attendance for basic daily needs within a matter of a few days. There is no known cure for Ebola.

. . .

27. Respondent is asymptomatic (no fever or other symptoms consistent with Ebola), as of the last check pursuant to her direct active monitoring this morning. Therefore the guidance issued by US CDC states that she is subject to Direct Active Monitoring. Health care workers in the "some risk" category require direct active monitoring for the 21-day incubation period.

28. Direct active monitoring means the MeCDC provides direct observation at least once per day to review symptoms and monitor temperature with a second follow-up daily by phone. The purpose of direct active monitoring is to ensure that if individuals with epidemiologic risk factors become ill, they are identified as soon as possible after symptoms onset so they can be rapidly isolated and evaluated. Once a person is symptomatic they become contagious to others, and their infectiousness increases very quickly.

. . .

(10/30/2014 Aff. of Dr. Pinette, at 2-4).

Based on the information in this affidavit with attachments and arguments of counsel, the Court finds by clear and convincing evidence that an order is necessary. With regard to the contents of the order, the court finds that ordering Respondent to comply with Direct Active Monitoring and to engage in the steps outlined below is "necessary to protect other individuals from the dangers of infection." The Court is aware that Respondent has been cooperating with Direct Active Monitoring and intends to continue with her cooperation. While this Court has no reason to doubt Respondent's good intentions, it is nevertheless necessary to ensure public safety that she continue to comply with Direct Active Monitoring until a hearing can be held on the State's Petition. The State has not met its burden at this time to prove by clear and convincing evidence that limiting Respondent's movements to the degree requested is "necessary to protect other individuals from the dangers of infection," however. According to the information

(Continues)

presented to the court, Respondent currently does not show any symptoms of Ebola and is therefore <u>not</u> infectious. Should these circumstances change at any time before the hearing on the petition—a situation that will most quickly come to light if Direct Active Monitoring is maintained—then it will become necessary to isolate Respondent from others to prevent the potential spread of this devastating disease.

For the foregoing reasons, the Court hereby ORDERS that, pending the hearing on the petition, Respondent shall:

1. Participate in and cooperate with "Direct Active Monitoring" as that term is defined by the United States Centers for Disease Control in its October 29, 2014 *Interim U.S. Guidance for Monitoring and Movement of Persons with Potential Ebola Virus Exposure* and in paragraph 28 of Dr. Pinette's October 30, 2014 affidavit.

2. Coordinate her travel with public health authorities to ensure uninterrupted Direct Active Monitoring; and

3. <u>Immediately</u> notify public health authorities and follow their directions if <u>any</u> symptom appears.

This Order is intended to and does supersede the Temporary Order entered on October 30, 2014 in this matter.

The Court pauses to make a few critical observations. First, we would not be here today unless Respondent generously, kindly and with compassion lent her skills to aid, comfort, and care for individuals stricken with a terrible disease. We need to remember as we go through this matter that we owe her and all professionals who give of themselves in this way a debt of gratitude.

Having said that, Respondent should understand that the court is fully aware of the misconceptions, misinformation, bad science and bad information being spread from shore to shore in our country with respect to Ebola. The Court is fully aware that people are acting out of fear and that this fear is not entirely rational. However, whether that fear is rational or not, it is present and it is real. Respondent's actions at this point, as a health care professional, need to demonstrate her full understanding of human nature and the real fear that exists. She should guide herself accordingly.

Further, since Respondent has waived her right to confidentiality pursuant to 22 M.R.S. § 811(6)(E), it is hereby ORDERED that all filings, orders, and hearings in this matter shall be open to the public.

This Order shall be incorporated into the docket by reference pursuant to M.R.Civ. P. 79(a).

Dated: October 31, 2014

Charles C. LaVerdiere
Chief Judge, Maine District Court

State of Maine Judicial Branch. *High profile cases*: State of Maine Department of Health and Human Services v. Kaci Hickox. *Order pending hearing.* www.courts.maine.gov/news_reference/high_profile/hickox.shtml

presented to the court, Respondent currently does not show any symptoms of Ebola and is therefore *not* infectious" (Dexter, 2016). The judge's ruling confirms the fine line between safeguarding individual rights and protecting the health of the public (Cornish, 2014).

The federal government is also legally authorized to use isolation and quarantine. This would be most likely if someone with a communicable disease crossed state lines or entered the United States from an international destination. In 2007, the federal government isolated Andrew Speaks in Atlanta after he had been diagnosed with a dangerous form of tuberculosis that is resistant to antibiotics (XDR TB) and returned from Europe to the United States via Montreal and New York.

Examples of the ways in which various levels of government utilize their police powers to assure the public's health are distributed throughout this text. The focus here is on key laws, regulations, and directives related to public health emergency preparedness and response. The goal is to highlight the important features of these laws, regulations, and directives while also underscoring the political, ethical, and practical reality of this legal landscape. As this overview illustrates, roles and responsibilities of local, state, and national governments have evolved over time as the nature of public health threats has changed since the early 2000s. Local jurisdictions and the states are responsible for the health and safety of their residents through their police powers, and states do have some authority for emergency preparedness. Yet, the authority for prevention, response, mitigation, and recovery is shaped by federal mandates that guide local and state planning, establish standards, influence relationships, and direct funding (Landesman, 2012). The events of 9/11, coupled with the global threats of SARS, H1N1, Ebola, and now COVID-19, have underscored the federal government's emphasis on national security as an important dimension of public health emergency preparedness. The response to public health emergencies is always local initially, but what local plans look like and how jurisdictions relate to each other during a public health emergency are, in part, driven by federal laws and regulations.

There are legal tools that enable local and state governments to prepare for and anticipate certain responses during an emergency through planning. Local jurisdictions and states use mutual aid agreements and memoranda of understanding in planning so that they can define what they and/or specific agencies will do following a presidential declaration of a major disaster or emergency through the Stafford Act. The purpose of these documents is to identify resources that may be needed from neighboring jurisdictions when local resources have been exhausted and to provide a framework for addressing the important issues such as logistics, liability, and costs for supplies, equipment, and personnel. If there is no presidential declaration, whether a jurisdiction provides assistance to another jurisdiction during recovery from a public health emergency is voluntary (Landesman, 2012, p. 50).

Emergency Management Assistance Compact

The EMAC (Public Law No. 104-321) is a nongovernmental interstate mutual aid agreement. Signed into law in 1996, EMAC is administered by the National Emergency Management Association (NEMA), and the 50 states, the District of Columbia, and three territories—the U.S. Virgin Islands, Puerto Rico, and Guam—are part of the Compact (EMAC, 1996). The Compact enables states to share resources, equipment, and personnel, including National Guard

members, with a neighboring state once the president has declared a major disaster or emergency. The state requesting assistance is obligated to reimburse the state that provided assistance (Kershner, 2014). The EMAC traces its roots to initiatives within the Southern Governors Association to support each other during hurricanes, with Hurricane Andrew in 1992 the major impetus for formalizing these relationships (EMAC, 1996). The largest mobilization of resources occurred in 2005 for Hurricanes Katrina in August and Rita in September. EMAC deployed about 66,000 emergency personnel and 46,500 National Guard members over 90,000 square miles, providing helicopter and air support, communications, and advance team, security, and search and rescue personnel, among other resources (Copple, 2006).

Of note, the COVID-19 pandemic was an incident of national significance. In other words, all states and local jurisdictions were affected to the point of widespread supply and resource exhaustion. In cases such as these, an activation of any mutual aid agreement is not considered appropriate when all parties to the agreement are affected and thus unable to provide aid. While this is reasonable and should be obvious, it is important to understand that there are situations that arise that will prohibit a jurisdiction from providing aid or cause a jurisdiction to decline to provide aid even when a resource is available (U.S. Department of Justice, 2005).

Emergency Use Authorization

The Emergency Use Authorization (EUA) is codified in Section 564 of the Federal Food, Drug, and Cosmetic Act. Under this law, the Secretary of Health and Human Services (HHS) may authorize the FDA to allow the use of a particular drug or device in an emergency situation for which it is not approved. The Secretaries of HHS, Homeland Security, and Defense need to establish that there is a significant risk from a chemical, biological, radiological, or nuclear (CBRN) event before the Secretary of HHS declares that an EUA is necessary. Given the potential threat to national security in such an event, both the 2006 Pandemic and All-Hazards Preparedness Act and the 2013 PAHPRA reaffirmed the importance of the development of countermeasures, including drugs and vaccines for pandemics, and fostered conditions to promote the research, development, and manufacturing of such products. Most recently, the FDA issued EUAs for three COVID-19 vaccines in the ongoing effort to mitigate the pandemic's effects on the social and economic life of the country. Between December

2020 and February 2021, the FDA authorized the Pfizer-BioNTech, Moderna, and Janssen vaccines and approved the Pfizer-BioNTech vaccine in August 2021 (U.S. Food and Drug Administration, n.d.).

There has been much debate, public concern, public scrutiny, and even politicization of the COVID-19 vaccines. Many believe the EUAs for the three COVID-19 vaccines were issued too quickly to market these countermeasures against COVID disease (Institute of Medicine, 2010). In fact, the EUAs offer public health and healthcare officials a valuable tool to provide a countermeasure for protection against a specific threat when no other countermeasure is available. An EUA can be issued not only because a drug (or other countermeasure) is new, but also because the drug may have another approved use, other than the use for which the EUA is issued. An example would be a drug that is approved for use as a cancer treatment being used as a treatment for an autoimmune disorder, even though the drug was not approved for use against the autoimmune disorder. See **Box 13.5**.

Quarantine and Isolation

Local jurisdictions, states, and the federal government have the authority to issue quarantine and isolation orders to protect the health and safety of residents. These orders restrict the movement of people who have been exposed to a communicable disease (quarantine) or who have symptoms and are presumed to have the communicable disease (isolation). At the local and state levels, this authority is codified in state statutes. At the federal level, this authority is codified in Sections 311, 361, and 362 of the Public Health Service Act. Federal regulations address interstate and foreign quarantine. The list of diseases for which people can be confined, dating from 1983, includes cholera, diphtheria, tuberculosis, plague, smallpox, yellow fever, and viral hemorrhagic fevers (CDC, 2014). Since 2003, three executive orders have modified the list of communicable diseases for which quarantine

Box 13.5 DISCUSSION QUESTIONS

Read several articles from different sources about the Emergency Use Authorizations (EUAs) for the three COVID-19 vaccines. Why was the EUA such an important public health measure or tool in the effort to control COVID-19? What surprised you about the EUA process? How would you explain the EUA process to someone who has been hesitant to receive a COVID-19 vaccine and is looking for reassurance about this approach?

Box 13.6 DISCUSSION QUESTIONS

Review the information about the quarantine case involving the nurse who returned to the United States from treating West African patients with Ebola in October 2014. Do you agree with her decision to challenge both the New Jersey and Maine quarantine orders? Why or why not? Do you agree with Judge Charles LaVerdiere's decision in the Maine case? Why or why not?

and isolation may be used. Executive Order 13295 in 2003 added SARS, and Executive Order 13375 in 2005 added influenza viruses that have the potential to cause a pandemic. Finally, Executive Order 13674, in 2014, clarified the reference to SARS.

Protecting the public from communicable diseases is an essential public health service, yet implementation of an isolation or quarantine order is sometimes controversial and raises ethical concerns. At the state level, the 2014 Ebola quarantine case discussed earlier in this chapter highlighted the tension between protecting the public's health and respecting individual rights. Without any symptoms of Ebola, it was hard for the nurse returning from West Africa to accept the Maine quarantine order (see **Box 13.6**).

As noted earlier, an example of the federal government using its power in this arena came in 2007 when the CDC placed a citizen with a severe form of drug-resistant tuberculosis who had traveled out of the country in isolation upon his return (Altman, 2007). The individual disregarded both a restriction not to leave the country and an order not to travel back to the country from Europe, given his disease. While he later acknowledged that his travel may not have been the best decision, he raised questions about how he was to have been treated in Italy (Katz, 2013; Schwartz, 2007).

Legal Preparedness

The term *legal preparedness* describes the idea that practitioners and organizations have the knowledge regarding legal authorities for public health practice in their jurisdictions and the capability to act in appropriate ways based on existing laws and regulations. The expectation is that laws would be clear, lines of communication open, and actions needed in response to a particular public health event apparent. The reality is that legal issues involving the public's health are complex, and laws and statutes vary greatly among the states. During public health emergencies, this lack of coordination and standards is particularly problematic when lives and damage to property and the environment are at stake. As part of a broader initiative to strengthen public health systems, the Robert Wood Johnson Foundation (RWJF) and the W.K. Kellogg Foundation funded the Turning Point program, which included a national collaborative on modernization of public health statutes (RWJF, 2008). The model statute that local, state, and tribal governments could use to enhance their legal preparedness was issued in 2003, and as of August 2007, 48 out of 133 bills in 33 states had passed (Centers for Law and the Public's Health, 2008). This work reflects a concerted effort to address what was acknowledged to be a gap in the public health infrastructure.

Particularly since 9/11, public health emergency legal preparedness has taken on more urgency. Our experience since 2001 with diseases such as SARS, H1N1, Ebola, and, most recently, COVID-19 underscores the importance of clear lines of authority and mechanisms for assistance across jurisdictions. The Model State Emergency Health Powers Act was issued in 2001, and as of July 2006, 38 states had passed 66 bills that adopted language from the Act (Centers for Law and the Public's Health, 2008). This work prompted considerable discussion about the role of the federal and state governments during public health emergencies, as well as the need to balance the rights of individuals during periods of crisis when the health and safety of the public are of paramount importance (Katz, 2013).

Along with work to modernize statutes related to public health emergency legal preparedness, efforts have been underway more generally to define gaps in legal preparedness for emergencies and to identify the key components of legal preparedness and the competencies necessary for the public health workforce. Four core elements were identified in a 2007 summit designed to address legal preparedness: laws and legal authorities, competency in using laws effectively, coordination of legal interventions across jurisdictions and sectors, and information on laws and best practices (Benjamin & Moulton, 2008). These core elements provide a framework for public health practitioners and local and state leaders to examine local practices and conditions, identify gaps, and create solutions to enhance legal preparedness during public health emergencies. To assist jurisdictions in this work, the National Association of County and City Health Officials (NACCHO) has developed an emergency preparedness training kit (NACCHO, 2012).

With respect to competencies for educating and training the public health workforce to know how to use the laws effectively, the CDC and ASPPH developed the Public Health Emergency Law Competency Model in 2008 for mid-tier professionals (CDC Public Health Law Program, 2014). The competencies address three domains: (1) systems preparedness and response, (2) management and protection of property and supplies, and (3) management and protection of persons. Of particular importance is the focus on a systems approach to emergency legal preparedness, as reflected in Domain 1. Having the knowledge and information about laws related to emergencies, coordinating and communicating with partners, and acting within the scope of the specific legal authorities are essential in all phases of public health emergency preparedness planning, prevention, response, and recovery.

Conclusion

Public health emergency preparedness is the ability to prevent, prepare for, protect against, respond to, and recover from health emergencies. As the scope, size, and scale of public health emergencies continue to increase, it is more and more important for public health to maintain the ability to respond to threats and hazards that impact the public's health. While public health preparedness programs date back to the late 1990s, those early programs were narrowly focused. These programs became top of mind for many Americans following the 2001 anthrax attacks in New York City, Florida, and Washington, D.C., yet they remained narrowly focused on biological threats. With the increased occurrence of different types of threats, the focus of preparedness programs has now adjusted to include all-hazards emergencies.

The NIMS and the ICS provide responders with a coordinated framework within which to operate during emergency response efforts. Although difficult for public health workers to grasp initially, these concepts are now widely accepted and used as the standard framework for managing disasters of all sizes, with participation by multiple agencies and jurisdictions.

In the U.S. history of public health emergency response to both man-made and natural disasters, legislation, regulations, and presidential directives reflect the federal government's evolving policies toward prevention, mitigation, response, and recovery. While the response to disasters has always been driven at the local level, the federal government's role in the face of external events has become more centralized with respect to the articulation of a national preparedness goal and a national response plan for all phases of an emergency event. Initially, federal assistance was provided during only the recovery phase, as local jurisdictions managed to the best of their capabilities during the event. Various revisions to disaster declaration legislation now provide governors the opportunity through the Robert T. Stafford Act to request aid during the response to a disaster. Organizational structures changed over time as leaders struggled with how best to manage the response and to support recovery with logistics and financial assistance. From the establishment of FEMA in 1979 via Executive Order 12127, to the creation of the Department of Homeland Security in the Homeland Security Act of 2002 and FEMA's more prominent role in disaster management, the federal government has sought a more unified vision for ensuring domestic security and safety. Emergency preparedness planning was mandated at all levels, sometimes with specific approaches in mind. Pets and service animals, for example, were the priority in the PETS Act of 2006 following the experiences of Hurricane Katrina in 2005. The PAHPRA of 2013 mandated that protection of children and vulnerable populations be addressed in grantees' All-Hazards Public Health Emergency Preparedness and Response plans.

No one law, executive order, regulation, or directive can anticipate all of the possible outcomes from either a man-made or natural disaster. The timing, scope, and complexity of each event affect the nature of response and recovery at all levels. The events of 9/11, the anthrax letters, and Hurricanes Katrina, Rita, and Sandy marked significant turning points in how the United States addresses emergency preparedness. Now, the experience with COVID-19 over the past year and a half has underscored just how much

 Box 13.7 DISCUSSION QUESTION

Considering that the ultimate responsibility for implementing measures to protect the public health lies with local officials, what are your thoughts about the measures to pull back public health powers related to masking and shut-downs during COVID-19 by some state legislators as described in the September 15, 2021, article titled "Over Half of States Have Rolled Back Public Health Powers in Pandemic" by Lauren Weber and Anna Marie Barry-Jester (Kaiser Health News, https://khn.org/news/article/over-half-of-states-have-rolled-back-public-health-powers-in-pandemic/)?

the country continues to learn about emergency preparedness, especially in the context of heightened social, economic, and political tensions at the local, state, tribal, and national levels (see **Box 13.7**). There will always be a need to evaluate how laws work and what plans need further coordination and practice. While the federal government seeks an integrated approach to response and recovery using a whole-of-government and whole community framework, public health law is an integral part of the infrastructure. Although the mission of public health embodies a social justice lens, the realities of the social, political, and economic environment at the local, state, and federal levels mean that legal preparedness needs to be a part of our ongoing approach to ensure a fair and equitable, coordinated, and comprehensive approach to prevention, response, mitigation, and recovery from man-made or natural disasters.

References

Altman, L. K. (2007, May 30). TB patient isolated after taking two flights. *New York Times.* http://query.nytimes.com/gst/fullpage.html?res=9403E5DA1430F933A05756C0A9619C8B63

Association of Schools & Programs of Public Health. (n.d.). *Public health preparedness & response model.* https://www.aspph.org/teach-research/models/public-health-preparedness-response

Benjamin, G. C., & Moulton, A. D. (2008). Public health legal preparedness: A framework for action. *Journal of Law, Medicine & Ethics, 36,* 13–17. https://doi.org/10.1111/j.1748-720X.2008.00254.x

Centers for Disease Control and Prevention. (2000). Biological and chemical terrorism: Strategic plan for preparedness and response. *MMWR, 49*(RR04), 1–14. http://www.cdc.gov/mmwr/preview/mmwrhtml/rr4904a1.htm

Centers for Disease Control and Prevention. (2004). *Continuation guidance for cooperative agreement on public health preparedness and response for bioterrorism—budget year five program announcement.* http://www.cdc.gov/phpr/documents/coopagreement-archive/FY2004/guidance_intro.pdf

Centers for Disease Control and Prevention. (2014). *Quarantine and isolation.* https://www.cdc.gov/quarantine/index.html

Centers for Disease Control and Prevention Public Health Law Program. (2014). *The Public Health Emergency Law Competency Model.* https://www.cdc.gov/phlp/publications/topic/phel-competencies.html

Centers for Law and the Public's Health, Collaborative at Johns Hopkins and Georgetown Universities. (2008). *The Turning Point Model State Public Health Act (MSPHA).* http://www.publichealthlaw.net/ModelLaws/MSPHA.php

Copple, A. (2006). EMAC overview. [Slide 31]. https://www.fema.gov/media-library-data/20130726-1726-25045-0915/060802emac.pdf

Cornish, A. (2014, October 30). Is it legal to quarantine someone who's not sick? *National Public Radio.* http://www.npr.org/2014/10/30/360179363/is-it-legal-to-quarantine-someone-whos-not-sick

Department of Homeland Security. (2014). *Presidential policy directive/PPD-8: National preparedness.* http://www.dhs.gov/presidential-policy-directive-8-national-preparedness

Dexter, B. (2016). *Mayhew v. Hickox*: Balancing Maine's public's health with personal liberties during the Ebola "crisis." *Maine Law Review.* www.mainelawreview.org/volume-68-no-1-2016/mayhew-v-hickox/

Dworkin, M. (2011). *Cases in field epidemiology: A global perspective.* Jones & Bartlett Learning.

Emergency Management Assistance Compact. (1996). https://www.emacweb.org/index.php/learn-about-emac/emac-history

Federal Emergency Management Agency. (2004). *National response plan* [Brochure]. http://www.dhs.gov/xlibrary/assets/NRP_Brochure.pdf

Federal Emergency Management Agency. (2008a). *National response framework.* https://www.fema.gov/national-response-framework

Federal Emergency Management Agency. (2008b). *National response framework.* https://www.fema.gov/media-library-data/20130726-1914-25045-1246/final_national_response_framework_20130501.pdf

Federal Emergency Management Agency. (2011). *A whole community approach to emergency management: Principles, themes, and pathways for action.* http://www.fema.gov/media-library-data/20130726-1813-25045-0649/whole_community_dec2011__2_.pdf

Federal Emergency Management Agency. (2014). *National preparedness cycle.* https://www.fema.gov/national-preparedness-cycle

Hospital Incident Command System. (n.d.). *The center for HICS education and training.* http://hicscenter.org/SitePages/Mission.aspx

Institute of Medicine. (1988). *The future of public health.* National Academy Press.

Institute of Medicine Forum on Medical and Public Health Preparedness for Catastrophic Events. (2010). *Medical countermeasures dispensing: Emergency Use Authorization and the Postal Model, workshop summary.* National Academies Press.

Katz, R. (2013). *Essentials of public health preparedness.* Jones & Bartlett Learning.

Kershner, S. (2014). *Selected federal legal authorities pertinent to public health emergencies.* Centers for Disease Control and Prevention, Public Health Law Program. https://www.cdc.gov/phlp/docs/ph-emergencies.pdf

Landesman, L. Y. (2012). *Public health management of disasters: The practice guide* (3rd ed.). APHA Press.

McMichael, T. M., Currie, D. W., Clark, S., Pogosjans, S., Kay, M., Schwartz, N. G., Lewis, J., Baer, A., Kawakami, V., Lukoff, M. D., Ferro, J., Brostrom-Smith, C., Rea, T. D., Sayre, M. R., Riedo, F. X., Russell, D., Hiatt, B., Montgomery, P., Rao, A. K., Chow, E. J., … Public Health–Seattle and King County, EvergreenHealth, and CDC COVID-19 Investigation Team. (2020). Epidemiology of Covid-19 in a long-term care facility in King County, Washington. *New England Journal of Medicine, 382*(21), 2005–2011. https://doi.org/10.1056/NEJMoa2005412

National Association of County and City Health Officials. (2012). *Public health and the law: An emergency preparedness training kit.*

Nelson, C., Lurie, N., Wasserman, J., & Zakowski, S. (2007). Conceptualizing and defining public health emergency preparedness. *American Journal of Public Health, 97*(S1), S9–S11.

Robert Wood Johnson Foundation. (2008, May 13). *Turning point: Collaborating for a new century in public health.* http://www.rwjf.org/content/dam/farm/reports/program_results_reports/2008/rwjf69892

Schwartz, J. (2007, June 2). Tangle of conflicting accounts in TB patient's odyssey. *New York Times.* http://www.nytimes.com/2007/06/02/health/02tick.html

Spicuzza, M., & Dirr, A. (2021, April 16). Milwaukee puts race front and center as it tracks Covid-19's toll, helping shape a national conversation on racism as a public health crisis. *Milwaukee Journal Sentinel.* https://www.jsonline.com/story/news/local/milwaukee/2021/04/16/milwaukee-helped-expose-covid-19-s-toll-black-latino-communities/6907736002/

Turnock, B. (2012). *Public health: What it is and how it works* (5th ed.). Jones & Bartlett Learning.

U.S. Department of Justice. (2005). *Mutual aid: Multijurisdictional partnerships for meeting regional threats.* https://www.ojp.gov/pdffiles1/bja/210679.pdf

U.S. Department of the Interior, National Park Service. (n.d.). *Fire and aviation management, incident command system.* https://www.nps.gov/fire/wildland-fire/learning-center/fire-in-depth/incident-command-system.cfm

U.S. Food and Drug Administration. (n.d.). *COVID-19 vaccines.* https://www.fda.gov/emergency-preparedness-and-response/coronavirus-disease-2019-covid-19/covid-19-vaccines

Werner, D., Wright, K., Thomas, M., & Edgar, M. (2005). An innovation in partnership among first responders and public health: Bridging the gap. *Public Health Report, 120*(S1), 64–68. http://www.ncbi.nlm.nih.gov/pmc/articles/PMC2569990/pdf/phr120s10064.pdf

PART III

Basic Skills in Health Policy Analysis

Parts I and II covered fundamental concepts of health policy and law and engaged in a substantive discussion of essential issues in health policy. This analysis of the content of health policy and law is complemented by Part III, which focuses on key skills for policy students and professionals. Chapter 14 provides a tutorial covering one of the most important skills in the field of health policy—writing a health policy analysis. Chapter 15 then provides a practical discussion regarding the role of advocacy in policymaking.

The Art of Structuring and Writing a Health Policy Analysis

LEARNING OBJECTIVES

By the end of this chapter you will be able to:

1. Understand the concept of policy analysis
2. Analyze a health policy issue
3. Write a health policy analysis
4. Develop descriptive and analytic side-by-side tables

Introduction

Imagine you work for the governor of a state that recently received a large sum of federal money for antibioterrorism efforts and your boss asks you how it should be spent. How will you respond? Or, assume you are an assistant to the director of a state nutrition program for low-income children and the program's budget was slashed by the legislature. The program's director needs to reduce costs and turns to you for help. How will you approach this problem? Finally, pretend you work in the White House as a domestic policy advisor and the president is considering revising the administration's methane emissions guidelines. What guidance will you offer?

While the *substance* of health policy and law has been discussed in detail up to this point, this chapter teaches you what policy analysis is and the *skill* of addressing complex health policy questions through a written policy analysis.

We use the following definition to describe a policy analysis: *an analysis that provides informed advice to a client that relates to a public policy decision, includes a recommended course of action/inaction, and is framed by the client's powers and values.* We briefly review each element of this definition in this chapter.

Policy Analysis Overview

In this section we define what a policy analysis is, and then we review the purposes for developing one. In the following section, we provide a step-by-step process detailing how to create a written health policy analysis.

Client-Oriented Advice

The client is the particular stakeholder that requests the policy analysis, and the analysis must be developed to suit the client's needs. (The client, for example, could be a policymaker who hires you, a fictional policymaker in an exercise developed by your professor, or an employer who asks you to analyze a problem.) In general, a stakeholder refers to an individual or a group that has an interest in the issue at hand. There may be many stakeholders related to a particular policy issue. Of course, the client requesting an analysis is also a stakeholder because that person or entity has an interest in the issue. However, to avoid confusion, we refer to the person or group that requests the analysis as the client and the other interested parties as stakeholders.

Informed Advice

Providing informed advice means the analysis is based on thorough and well-rounded information. The information included in the analysis must convey all sides of an issue, not just the facts and theories supporting a particular perspective. If a decision maker is presented with evidence supporting only one course of action or one side of a debate, it will be impossible for the client to make a well-informed decision. In addition, to be effective in persuading others to favor the recommended policy, your client must be able to understand and, when necessary, refute alternative solutions to the problem.

Public Policy Decision

Policy analyses involve public policy decisions. A public policy problem goes beyond the individual sphere and affects the greater community.

Providing Options and a Recommendation

A key component of any policy analysis is providing the client with several options to consider, analyzing those options, and settling on one recommendation. In other words, a policy analysis is not simply a background report that identifies a variety of issues relating to a particular problem; instead, it gives the client ideas about what steps to take to address the problem and concludes by recommending a specific course of action.

Your Client's Power and Values

Finally, the analysis should be framed by the client's power and values. Framing the analysis based on the client's *power* is fairly straightforward and uncontroversial: The options presented and the recommendation made must be within the power of the client to accomplish. On the other hand, the notion of framing an analysis according to the client's *values* is more

controversial. In most conceptualizations of policy analysis, including the one discussed later in this chapter, the process is roughly the same: Define the problem and provide information about it, analyze a set of alternatives to solve the problem, and implement the best solution based on the analysis (Patton & Sawicki, 1993, p. 3). As new information is uncovered or the problem is reformulated, analysts may move back and forth among these steps in an iterative process (Stone, 2002, p. 47). However, although there is general agreement that politics and values play a role in policy analysis, there is disagreement over the stage of the analysis at which they come into play.

To understand this controversy, it is necessary to discuss two models of policy analysis: the rational model and the political model. The rational model was developed in an attempt to base policy decisions on reason and science rather than the vagaries of politics (Stone, 2002, p. 7). In the traditional rational model, the analyst does not consider politics and values. Instead, he or she should recommend the "rational, logical, and technically desirable policy" (Stone, 2002, p. 51). According to the rational model, the *decision maker* infuses the analysis with politics and values once the analyst's work is complete.

Professor John Kingdon and others have moved away from the rational model and toward a political model. Kingdon suggests that policy analysis occurs through the development of three streams: problems, policies, and politics (Kingdon, 1995). The problem stream is where problems are defined and noticed by decision makers. The policy stream is where solutions are proposed. These proposals may be solutions to identified problems, but they are often favored projects of policymakers or advocates that exist separate from specific problems that have garnered attention. Finally, the political stream refers to the ever-changing political mood. As a general matter, these streams develop separately, only coming together at critical junctures when the problem reaches the top of the agenda, the solutions to that problem are viable, and the political atmosphere makes the time right for change (Weissert & Weisser, 2002, p. 87).

Kingdon's approach discusses occurrences the rational model does not consider, such as why some problems are addressed and others are not, why some solutions are favored even if they are not technically the best approach, and why action is taken at some junctures but not at others (Kingdon, 1995). In addition, the rational model refers to only one cycle of problems. As Kingdon and others have noted, solutions to one problem often lead to unintended consequences that create other problems to be addressed, resulting in an ongoing policy analysis cycle instead of an event with a start and a finish (Weissert & Weissert, 2002, p. 260).

Professor Deborah Stone also focuses on the role of politics and values in analysis (Stone, 2002, pp. 1–4). She argues that the idea of the rational policy analysis model misses the point because "analysis itself is a creature of politics" (Stone, 2002, p. 8). According to Stone, every choice, from defining a problem, to selecting analytic criteria, to choosing which options to evaluate, to making a recommendation, is political and value laden. As she states, "Rational policy analysis can begin only after the relevant values have been identified and . . . these values change over time as a result of the policymaking process" (Stone, 2002, p. 32). She contends that policy analysis should do the very things that the rational model does not permit—allow for changing objectives, permit contradictory goals, and turn apparent losses into political gains (Stone, 2002, p. 9). The goal of the rational model founders—to divorce analysis from the vagaries of politics—is simply not possible in Stone's view.

Having differentiated these models, we now return to our definition of policy analysis: *an analysis that provides informed advice to a client that relates to a public policy decision, includes a recommended course of action/inaction, and is framed by the client's powers and values.* You can see that this definition follows Stone's political model of policy analysis, requiring the analysis to be developed with a particular client's values in mind. After reviewing the numerous examples provided in the following section, it will be evident that client values permeate all aspects of a policy analysis. Only after you take into account your client's values, combine it with the information you have gathered, place it in the prevailing political context, and understand your client's powers, can you make an appropriate policy recommendation.

Multiple Purposes

The ultimate product of a policy analysis is a recommendation to a specific client about how to address a problem. However, a policy analysis has several other purposes as well. It provides general information necessary to understand the problem at hand and may be an important tool to inform stakeholders about a policy problem. In addition, the analysis may be a vehicle for widespread dissemination of ideas and arguments. Although your analysis is targeted to the client requesting advisement, it may also be used to inform and persuade other supporters, opponents,

the media, the general public, and others. Finally, it will help you, the policy analyst, learn how to think through problems and develop solutions in an organized, concise, and useful way.

Policy analyses can take many forms—a memorandum, an oral briefing, a report, and so on—and, correspondingly, have varying degrees of formality. This chapter explains how to construct a *short, written* analysis because it is a commonly used, highly effective, and often practical way to provide a policy analysis to your client. In addition, the principles embedded in a policy analysis can then be used in whatever other format(s) your client prefers. Whether you are aiding a governor, the director of a state program, the CEO of a private business, or any other decision maker, you often will not have the opportunity to discuss issues in person or for a significant length of time. Furthermore, given time pressures, the demands on high-level policymakers, the need for rapid decision-making, and the variety of issues most policymakers deal with, many clients will not read a lengthy analysis. That is why it is essential for anyone who wants to influence policy to be able to craft a clear and concise written analysis.

Structuring a Policy Analysis

We now turn to a five-step method for writing a thorough yet concise policy analysis. Regardless of the subject matter, you can use this structure to analyze the question your client is considering. As you review each part of the analysis, notice the various disciplines and tools that may be part of writing an effective policy analysis. Analysts draw from a variety of disciplines—law, economics, political science, sociology, history, and others—and use a number of quantitative and qualitative tools when explaining issues, analyzing options, and making recommendations.

Although policy analyses come in various formats and use different terminology, they will all contain the following essential elements:

- **Problem identification:** Defines the problem addressed in the analysis
- **Background:** Provides factual information needed to understand the problem
- **Landscape:** Reviews the various stakeholders and their concerns
- **Options:** Describes and analyzes several options to address the problem
- **Recommendation:** Offers one option as the best action to pursue

The following sections discuss each of these elements in detail.

Problem Identification

Define the Problem

The first step in writing a policy analysis is to clearly define the problem you are analyzing. A problem identification should be succinct and written in the form of a question that identifies the problem addressed in the analysis. It usually consists of a single sentence, although it may be two sentences if you are analyzing a particularly complex issue. Although a problem identification is simple to define, it is often one of the most difficult parts of the analysis to do well. It is also one of the most important.

The problem identification is the key to your analysis because it frames the problem at hand. Indeed, some policy battles are won or lost simply by how the problem identification is crafted. For example, consider the different questions asked in these problem identifications:

Problem identification 1:
What type of tax credit, if any, should the president include in the next budget proposal?

Problem identification 2:
What type and size of health insurance tax credit should the president include in the next budget proposal?

The first problem identification asks what type of tax credit, if any, should be considered. One possible answer to that question is that no tax credit of any kind should be considered. Another answer could involve a tax credit, but not one related to health insurance. The second problem identification suggests that the option of not proposing a health insurance tax credit is unacceptable. Instead, the second problem identification lends itself to an analysis of identifying the pros and cons of various health insurance tax credit options. In other words, one option that may be considered based on the first problem identification (no tax credit) is excluded based on the second problem identification.

Consider another example:

Problem identification 1:
Which health issue should be the governor's top priority?

Problem identification 2:
Should the governor's priority of reducing the number of obese residents be accomplished by relying on currently existing programs?

Again, the first problem identification asks an open-ended question about identifying the governor's top priority. The answer may be obesity, but it may be any other health issue as well. The second problem identification starts with the governor committed to reducing the obesity rate and asks how to best accomplish that goal. These two problem identifications lead to very different analyses and (most likely) different recommendations.

It is possible that your client's values will be evident from the way the problem identification is phrased. For instance, in the second example, the second policy statement clearly reflects the governor's desire to reduce the obesity rate. Consider another example: You have been asked to write a policy analysis about the merits of importing low-cost prescription drugs from Canada. How might the problem identification differ if your client is a pharmaceutical lobbying group versus if your client is an elder rights association? Here are two possible problem identifications.

An acceptable way to identify the problem for the pharmaceutical lobbying firm:
How can this firm help improve medical care quality in the United States by reducing the importation of dangerous prescription drugs from Canada?

An acceptable way to identify the problem for the elder rights association:
How can this association help seniors obtain low-priced prescription drugs from Canada?

The vast differences in these problem identifications reflect differing viewpoints regarding the importation of prescription drugs. A pharmaceutical lobbying firm is more likely to be concerned about reduced profits for its drug company clients and therefore would want to deter or restrict importation, which could lead to more competition in the market. One way to accomplish that goal is to phrase the issue as a safety/quality-of-care concern. An elder rights association is more likely to be concerned with high-priced prescription drugs in the United States and would therefore want to promote drug importation (assuming, of course, there is no actual safety concern with the drugs). One way to accomplish that goal is to phrase the issue as one of cost reduction.

It is also possible to identify the problem in a neutral manner. From the immediately previous example, analysts for both groups could use the following phrasing.

Neutral problem identification:
What action should [the client] take in response to recent congressional proposals

relating to importing prescription drugs from Canada?

Neutral wording is not necessarily better or worse than value-driven phrasing. The value-driven phrase provides additional information about the direction of the policy analysis and clearly limits some of the options that might otherwise be considered. Neutral wording is often broader, leaving more options on the table at the outset. Yet, even if neutral phrasing is used, the options the analyst considers and the recommendation the analyst makes will still be constrained by the client's values and needs.

Because it is possible to identify problems numerous ways for any issue, how do you develop the best one? In general, you want to use the one that provides the best fit for your analysis. If you decide to focus on all safety-related concerns, for example, the pharmaceutical lobbying firm example would be a good fit. If, however, the firm chose to have one safety-related option, one state government-focused option, and one convenience-centered option, then you would want a broader problem identification that allows for all types of options. For example, "How can this firm help improve consumers' experience purchasing prescription drugs?" would allow for various types of options. In addition, you want to make sure your problem identification is analytically manageable and does not include your recommendation.

Make the Problem Identification Analytically Manageable

Acceptable phrasing can be broad or narrow. One is not better than the other; they suit different purposes. Policy analyses with broad problem identifications may require more diverse information in terms of background and may consider a wider range of issues in the paper's landscape section. Also, the recommendations may promote "big picture" changes instead of specific and tailored ideas. Narrower wording may require less extensive background and landscape information, but it may not capture big picture, systemic concerns relating to the problem under consideration.

Reflect on the following examples. They both may be acceptable problem identifications, depending on the needs of your client.

A broad problem identification:
What action should the U.S. Department of Health and Human Services take to avoid another flu vaccine shortage?

A narrow problem identification:
How can the U.S. Department of Health and Human Services create incentives for additional manufacturers to supply flu vaccine to the United States?

The first one could result in a variety of recommendations, such as improving surveillance to lower the incidence of flu in the future, developing new vaccines that have longer-lasting immunity, or finding ways to entice additional manufacturers to provide supplies to the United States. It is a broad problem identification that will lead to an analysis that could recommend a wide variety of actions. The second one focuses on one particular way to decrease a flu vaccine shortage—increasing the number of suppliers. Although the analysis will also provide a number of options, all of the options will address the specific issue of increasing suppliers. Again, there is no single right or wrong way to phrase a problem. Whether it is more useful to have a broad or narrow problem will depend on the needs and concerns of your client.

However, it is possible to make a problem identification so vague that it will be impossible to write a sound policy analysis. Unfortunately, there is no easy way to differentiate an acceptably broad problem phrasing from an unmanageably vague one when you begin your analysis. You will know your wording is too vague, however, if you find it impossible to write a *complete and concise* policy analysis and you can think of too many diverse options to include (if you can think of 5 to 10 possible options your statement is probably workable; if you can think of 15 or more options, your statement is probably too broad). Your paper will require too much information in the background and landscape sections if you draft an overly vague problem identification. In addition, you will find that you cannot devise a coherent series of options addressing the problem because the problem identification is too broadly defined. Instead of a concise and useful policy analysis, you will end up with a lengthy and unfocused paper.

If you believe your problem identification may be so vague that it is analytically unmanageable, ask yourself if you are addressing one specific problem that may be countered with a few specific options. If you are having trouble narrowing your problem identification, you can try including limitations based on geography (e.g., refer to a particular state or city), time (e.g., focus on the next year or over the next 5 years), or numerical boundaries (e.g., use a goal of reducing a figure by a certain percentage or a budget by a specific dollar amount). Consider this example:

An unmanageably vague problem identification:
What is the best use of the Centers for Disease Control and Prevention's resources to improve the health status of our citizens?

This phrasing is not analytically manageable. It is extremely broad and unfocused. Using this problem identification, your analysis could address any health issue, such as access to care problems, the need to improve vaccination rates, racial disparities in health care, or many others. The list is endless and your policy analysis will be as well.

A manageable problem identification:
What preventive health issue should be the top priority for the Centers for Disease Control and Prevention next year?

This one is analytically manageable. It is focused on preventive measures specifically and is limited to determining the top priority. In addition, the problem is focused on what can be done in the upcoming year. This second problem identification allows for a much more concise and directed policy analysis.

Do Not Include the Recommendation in Your Problem Identification

Another pitfall when identifying problems is crafting a problem in a way that suggests a particular solution to the issue. A problem identification should define a specific problem; it should not indicate how that problem should be solved. If the answer is preordained, why bother with the analysis? When phrasing your problem, ask yourself if you can imagine four, five, or six potentially viable options to address the problem. If you cannot, then you have not defined the problem well.

For example, assume you have been asked to address how to reduce medical malpractice insurance premiums. Here is a problem identification that leads the reader to one conclusion:

A leading problem identification:
To what extent should jury awards be limited in malpractice cases in order to reduce malpractice premiums?

This phrasing leads to one very specific solution (limiting jury awards) as a way to counter a broad problem (reducing malpractice premiums). The only question presented by this problem identification is what the award limit should be. It does not provide a range of options for reducing malpractice premiums

(one of which may be limiting jury awards) for your client to consider. (Of course, if you were specifically asked to address how to limit jury awards in malpractice cases, this would be an appropriate problem identification.) A better way to word the problem would be, "What action should be taken to stem the rise in malpractice premiums nationwide?"

This problem identification lends itself to an analysis that considers several options. Possible alternatives include limiting jury awards, enacting regulations that limit the amount insurance companies can increase premiums each year, and a host of other options. This wording also narrows the focus of the analysis to national solutions.

Once you have written your concise and precise problem identification, you have set the framework for your analysis. Every other section of the analysis should relate directly to the problem you identified. Remember that writing a policy analysis is an iterative process; you must review, revise, and tighten the information and arguments throughout the writing process. As you review the other components of your policy analysis, it may become evident that what you thought was the best way to describe the problems can be further improved. There is nothing wrong with revising your wording as you craft your analysis, as long as you remain true to your client's values and power.

The Background Section

The first substantive information your analysis provides is in the background section. The background informs the reader why the particular problem has been chosen for analysis. This section should make clear why the issue is important and needs to be addressed now. In addition to providing general information about the topic, your background and landscape (discussed next) sections provide the information necessary to assess the options you lay out.

Much of the information in the background will be relevant regardless of who assigned the analysis. However, because the background provides information necessary to understand the problem, it is essential to understand the knowledge level of your client when constructing the background. For example, assume you are writing an analysis relating to state preparedness planning for smallpox vaccination in the event of a bioterror attack. Regardless of your client, your background would likely include information about why a smallpox attack is a threat, including (but not limited to) the following:

- Reference to the September 11, 2001, attacks on the World Trade Center and subsequent events
- The belief that although smallpox has been eradicated as a natural disease, it is likely that samples of the virus still exist
- Reference to any information provided by the federal government or other sources relating to the possibility of a bioterror attack

If your client does not have knowledge relating to smallpox, you would also include details about smallpox transmission, the effects of the disease, the vaccination procedure, and the risks associated with vaccination.

In addition, your background should include whatever factual information is necessary to fully assess the options discussed. Remember, your client needs a complete picture, not just the information that supports the recommended action or your client's viewpoint. By the time the reader reaches your paper's options section, all of the information necessary to evaluate the options should have been presented in your background or landscape.

For example, assume one of your options for the smallpox vaccination state preparedness analysis is immediate compulsory vaccination of all first responders and establishment of a protocol for vaccinating the remaining population if there is a smallpox outbreak. In that case, your background (and possibly the landscape) should provide information regarding who first responders are, where they are located, how many there are, legal issues relating to compulsory vaccination, and so on.

Because the background section is an informational—not analytic—part of the analysis, the material provided in it should be mostly factual. The tone of the background is not partisan or argumentative. It should simply state the necessary information.

The Landscape Section

Together, the background and landscape sections frame the context of the analysis for your client. Whereas the background provides factual information to assist the client in understanding what the problem is and why it is being addressed, the landscape provides the overall context for the analysis by identifying key stakeholders and the factors that must be considered when analyzing the problem. In the following discussion, you will read about numerous types of people, groups, and issues that might be included in a landscape. These examples are meant to provide suggestions and provoke thought about what should be included in an analysis. It would be impossible to include everything discussed here in any single landscape section. It is the job of the policy analyst to choose among these options—to be able to identify whose views and which factors are the most salient ones in creating a complete landscape.

Identifying Key Stakeholders

Up to this point, the policy analysis discussion has focused on just one stakeholder: the client who asked for the policy analysis. The landscape brings in other stakeholders who have an interest in the issue. Although it is often impossible to include every possible stakeholder in a single analysis, it is necessary to identify the key stakeholders whose positions and concerns must be understood before a well-informed decision can be made.

How do you identify the key stakeholders particular to your issue? Unfortunately, there is no magic formula. The best approach is through research and thinking. Also, bear in mind that the stakeholders and issues discussed in the landscape must relate to your overall policy analysis. Your options must address the problem identified initially, and all of the information necessary to assess the options must be presented in the background and landscape. As you learn about the problem to be analyzed and think about options for addressing the problem, it should become apparent which stakeholders have a significant interest in the issue.

For example, assume your analysis relates to proposed legislation regulating pharmacists and pharmaceuticals. Who are possible key stakeholders regarding this issue? They may include several parties:

- Democratic and Republican politicians (you might need to distinguish among those in Congress, state legislatures, and governors)
- Pharmaceutical industry
- Health insurance industry
- AARP and other elder rights groups
- Advocacy groups for the disabled
- Pharmacists' lobby
- Foreign pharmaceutical companies
- Internet-based pharmaceutical companies

Can you think of others?

Deciding which stakeholders *must* be included in an analysis depends on the exact problem being analyzed and which options are included in the analysis. For example, assume you are writing an analysis about requirements relating to how pharmacists inform consumers about their medications. If your problem deals with face-to-face encounters only, Internet-based pharmaceutical companies would not be a key stakeholder. Alternatively, if the problem definition deals with purchasing limitations over the Internet, Internet-based pharmaceutical companies must be included in the analysis. If one of your options focuses on comprehension among older adults, elder rights groups should be included in the analysis. If your client is someone running for public office in a county where the health insurance industry is a major employer, the views of those companies would be essential to include. In other words, although it is possible to make a generic list of the types of individuals and groups that could be included, the specific list for any policy analysis will depend on the client for whom the analysis is being written, the specific problem being addressed, and the options being considered.

Identifying Key Factors

Once you have settled on a list of key stakeholders, it is necessary to analyze their position on the issue at the center of the analysis. Earlier, we described the landscape as the portion of the analysis that provides the overall context of the issue. The "overall context" refers to the mix of factors that are relevant when any decision is being made. These factors are used to analyze stakeholder positions. Although there is not one comprehensive list of context factors and not all factors are relevant to all analyses, the list in **Box 14.1** includes some common factors that could be discussed.

Box 14.1 Possible Factors to Include in a Landscape Section

Political Factors
What is the political salience of the issue?
   Is this a front-burner issue?
   Is this a controversial issue?
   Are your client, legislators, and the general public interested in addressing this issue?
   Has this or a similar healthcare issue been addressed recently?
   Do key constituents, opponents, interest groups, or other stakeholders have an opinion about the issue? Who is likely to support or oppose change?
   Is there bipartisan support for the issue?
   Is there a reason to act now?
   Is there a reason to delay action?

Social Factors
Who is affected by this problem?
   According to the client who assigned the analysis, are influential or valued people or groups affected by this problem?
   Is there a fairness concern relating to this issue?
   Is there a stigma associated with this issue?

Economic Factors
What is the economic impact of addressing this problem? Of not addressing it?
   Are various people or groups impacted differently?
   Are there competing demands for resources that relate to this issue?
   What is the economic situation of the state or nation? How does this affect the politics relating to this issue?
   How will addressing this issue affect healthcare costs/healthcare spending?

Practical Factors
Is it realistic to try to solve this problem?
Do others need to be involved to be able to solve this problem?
   Is the technology available to solve this problem?
   Would it be more practical to solve this problem later?
   Are other people in a better position to solve this problem?
   What do we know about solutions that do or do not work?
   If this problem cannot be solved, is it still necessary (politically, socially) to act in some way to address the problem?
   Is evidence available to support potential solutions?

Legal Factors
Are there legal restrictions affecting this problem?
   Is there a need to balance public health concerns and individual legal rights?
   Are there legal requirements that impact the analysis?
   Is new legislative authority necessary to solve the problem?
   Is there legal uncertainty relating to this problem?
   Is future litigation a concern if action is taken?

Quality-of-Care Factors
Does this problem address quality-of-care issues?
   Do some solutions focus on quality of care more than others?
   Do quality-of-care concerns vary based on which provider is involved?
   Is evidence available about the best ways to improve quality of care?
   Has the client already taken any actions to improve quality of care?

The list of factors in Box 14.1 is by no means exhaustive, but rather is intended to provide a sense of the types of questions that are often relevant to understanding the context of a problem. Just as it would be impossible to discuss every stakeholder who might be connected to the problem, it would be impossible to include in a concise analysis all the issues raised by the six factors listed in Box 14.1. It is the policy analyst's job to identify not only which key stakeholders must be included, but also which key factors must be discussed.

Consider again the example relating to limiting prescription drug purchases made over the Internet. The following key factors would likely be included:

- **Political factor:** Who supports or opposes the limitation and how influential are they?
- **Economic factor:** Would it be costly to implement this limitation or costly to key constituents who may need more prescription drugs than are allowed by the limit? Would it provide an economic benefit to some stakeholders?
- **Practical factor:** Is it possible to implement and enforce a restricted purchasing system over the Internet?
- **Legal factor:** Are there legal barriers to limiting Internet prescription drug purchases?

For each factor, the analysis should discuss relevant views of the stakeholders you included in your analysis. For example, when discussing economic factors, the analysis might explain that Internet-based pharmaceutical companies would experience a loss of revenue, some consumers would pay more for prescription drugs if they needed more than the limited amount, and storefront pharmaceutical companies would make money because consumers probably would have to fill more of their orders in person. Depending on the political situation, the analysis might explain that the client's most influential constituents are older adults who use many prescription drugs and are likely to oppose any restriction, or that storefront pharmaceutical companies are large campaign contributors and would support a restriction.

Structuring the Landscape Section

The landscape may be organized by stakeholder or by factor. In other words, it is acceptable to identify stakeholder 1 and then describe that stakeholder's views based on various concerns, and then identify stakeholder 2 and describe that stakeholder's views, and so on. Alternatively, the landscape could be structured based on factors described in Box 14.1. Within that structure, the landscape would address one set of factors (e.g., economic), then another set (e.g., social), and so on. Some stakeholders may not have relevant views for all of the factors, but each stakeholder must be addressed as often as necessary to convey his or her policy position. For example, the economic factors section would identify various stakeholders and their views based on economic concerns. It would include information such as "Canadian companies would oppose regulating Internet pharmacies because it would increase the cost of doing business with Americans, while U.S. storefront pharmacists would support regulating Internet pharmacies because it may increase prices for their competitors' products."

When you discuss a particular view, it is important to identify which stakeholders hold that view. At the same time, do not insert opinions unattached to individuals or groups. For example, it would not be helpful to write, "Some oppose legislation regulating Internet pharmacies." Such a statement does not identify *who* opposes the legislation or *why* they oppose the legislation. If your client will be able to assess the political, practical, and ethical feasibility of taking a particular action, the client needs to understand where the various groups stand and why they hold those views. Thus, a more helpful sentence would be: "RxData, a large software company that assists Internet pharmacies and is a major employer in your congressional district, opposes legislation regulating Internet pharmacies because it will add costs to its business and may result in future employee layoffs." That sentence tells your client who is opposed to the legislation, why they are opposed to it, and why they are a key stakeholder.

The tone of the landscape should be neutral and objective. The landscape is not an argumentative section to persuade the reader that one view is better than another. Its purpose is to identify all of the key stakeholders and their concerns so the decision maker is well-informed before assessing options.

The Options Section

Once your client finishes reading the background and landscape sections, he or she should have a thorough understanding of the policy problem and the overall context in which a decision will be made. The time has come for the client to consider what action to take. This is where your paper's options section comes in, providing three to five alternatives for your client to consider. This section is more than a recitation of various choices; it provides an analysis of each option by stating the positive and negative aspects of pursuing each path.

Identifying Options

The first step to writing your options section is to identify the various options you could analyze. Although you may develop a new option not previously considered by others, it is likely that you will find numerous possibilities that others have already suggested. Some places to find already-considered options include the following:

- Media
- Scholarly articles
- Interest group recommendations
- Think tanks/experts in the field
- Congressional testimony
- Legislation (passed or proposed)
- Agency reports

Another approach to developing options is to consider several major actions that policymakers often take to deal with a policy problem. For example, depending on the circumstances, the following actions could be added, eliminated, or altered by a policymaker in response to a policy problem:

- Taxes
- Subsidies
- Grants
- Laws
- Regulations
- Programs
- Government organizations
- Information
- Outreach

Once you have compiled a list of options, how do you choose the best three to five options to include in the analysis? As always, the guiding principle underlying your decision is to base your decision on your client's values and powers. You should not suggest an option that clearly violates your client's values because your client will not seriously consider that option. For example, if your client has rejected spending new state money to solve a problem, you should not include an option that would cost the state money (or if you do, you would need to be clear about how these funds would be offset). Also, it is important to remember the extent of your client's power. For example, on one hand, an analyst might recommend that a member of Congress introduce or sponsor a bill, or that an interest group submit a comment as part of the public notice and comment period before a regulation is finalized. On the other hand, an analyst should not recommend that a member of Congress force a state to pass a particular law, because that action is not within Congress's power (the responsibility of passing

state laws falls to state legislatures). Similarly, an interest group cannot issue an executive order or force an administrative agency to craft a regulation in a particular way. In other words, any option you include must be within the ability of your client to undertake.

In addition, you will probably want to include in your analysis any major proposals that are currently being considered. You may also choose to include proposals backed by key allies and constituents. Even if your client does not act on these proposals, it is important to be able to explain why "mainstream" options are being rejected. Also, it may be appropriate to consider the status quo (the "do-nothing" approach) as an option. The status quo option works best when there is a specific reason for waiting to act; otherwise, it may appear to be an option because the analyst ran out of ideas. For example, if there is an evaluation underway of a key program, a valid status quo option would be to wait until the evaluation is complete and then reconsider the issue based on the findings. Simply suggesting to do nothing without a rationale is not acceptable. Even when considering the do-nothing tactic, it is necessary to evaluate the pros and cons of this option. In addition, your options should be different enough from one another to give your client a real choice. For example, if all of your options involved creating a big, new federal program and your client does not prefer that strategy, then the analysis is not useful. There is one final rule to follow: Whichever alternative you ultimately recommend must be analyzed in the options section of your analysis.

All of the options included in the analysis must directly address the problem identified in your problem identification. For example, if your problem identification involved ways to reduce the number of uninsured individuals, an option that promotes increasing access to care for insured residents would be inappropriate because it does not directly address the problem. Indeed, everything in your analysis must flow from your problem identification, from what is included in the background and the issues discussed in your landscape, to the alternatives suggested in the options section, and (as discussed later) your final recommendation.

Assessing Your Options

Your options analysis must include a discussion of the pros (what is useful) and the cons (what is problematic) of each option. Although policymakers often seek a "silver bullet" that solves a problem without any negative effects, it is highly unlikely that such an option exists. As a result, an analysis must include the positive and negative aspects of an option. Also, all options must be analyzed equally. Do not provide more analysis for the option you decide to recommend even though it is your preferred option. Your client can make a fully informed decision only if you analyze what is both good and bad about each proposal.

To draft your pros and cons, you must identify the appropriate criteria for the analysis of the pros and cons and apply each criterion to all of the options. Many possible criteria could be used, so you must pick the ones that best fit your client's values and that address the key issues relating to the policy problem. Sometimes your client will provide you with criteria; other times you must deduce the correct criteria based on what you know about your client and the problem. Generally, you should choose between three and five criteria for your evaluation of the pros and cons in this type of analysis. Typically, fewer than three will not allow for a full analysis, and more than five are difficult to assess in a relatively short analysis.

Your choice of criteria should reflect the concerns discussed in the landscape, where you identified the key factors relating to the problem. For example, if economic burden was an important aspect of the issue being considered, costs should be one of the criteria used to analyze the options. If the need for quick action was an important aspect of the issue, timeliness and administrative ease might be important criteria to consider. In general, cost and political feasibility are usually important criteria to include in your analysis. However, the specific criteria that are best for your analysis will depend on your client, the specific problem identification being addressed, and the landscape of the issue. **Box 14.2** provides some criteria that could be considered when analyzing options. Can you think of others?

Structuring the Options Section

When structuring your options section, you may find it helpful to use headings or bullets delineating each option. Your headings should clearly label each option. Also, it is generally useful to separate out the options by paragraph instead of having a continuous page or two assessing all of the options. The first sentence or two of each options paragraph should be a clear description of that option so the client understands what is being proposed and exactly what action your client would be taking; then assess the pros and cons of the option based on the criteria you identified. You should explicitly state the criteria prior to your options description.

For example, assume you are writing a policy analysis for the Secretary of the Department of Health and Human Services about how to increase access

---

Box 14.2 Sample Options Criteria

Cost: How much does this option cost? (You may have to break this down: how much does it cost the federal government, state government, individuals, etc.?)

Cost–benefit: How much "bang for the buck" does this option provide? (This is a difficult criterion to assess in shorter, less complicated policy analyses because you often do not have the information necessary to make this determination.)

Political feasibility: Is this option politically viable? Is it likely to become law? Even if it is not likely to become law, is it likely to help your client politically?

Legality: Is this option legal? If so, are there any restrictions?

Administrative ease: Does this option have steep implementation hurdles?

Fairness: Are people affected by this option treated fairly/equally?

Timeliness: Can this option be implemented in an appropriate or useful amount of time?

Targeted impact: Does this option target the population/issue involved?

Effectiveness: How well does this option accomplish the goal set out in the problem identification?

Healthcare-specific criteria: Does this option improve quality of care, lower healthcare spending, reduce the incidence of a particular disease, etc.?

---

to care for immigrants. After drafting the necessary background and landscape information, you decide to assess the following options: (1) creating a public education campaign, (2) providing grants to states, and (3) increasing funding to community health centers. You decide the best criteria to use are cost to the federal government, political feasibility, and degree of increase in the number of immigrants who seek care. In your options section, you would have three different parts—one for each option—assessing the pros and cons based on the criteria you chose. Although the structure of the analysis may vary, you might have a paragraph looking something like this:

Option 1: Create a Public Education Campaign. The Secretary of the Department of Health and Human Services should order the Centers for Disease Control and Prevention to create a public education campaign to alert immigrants to the various ways they can access health care in their area. The campaign will be delivered in English and the most common immigrant languages in the area and will occur on television, over the radio, and in public (e.g., billboards). In these difficult economic times, this is a relatively low-cost option (although if immigrants access more care, the cost of providing care will increase). In addition, the political feasibility is somewhat high because this option does not call for any policy changes, but rather merely alerting individuals to policies that already exist. On the other hand, the political feasibility is tempered because the option focuses on helping immigrants, a group that has been under attack politically in recent times. The most significant disadvantage of this option is that it may not be very effective in increasing the number of immigrants who access care because it does not increase access points, reduce the cost of care, or address concerns in the immigrant community about being deported if they participate in public programs.

You would write a similar analysis for each of the options under consideration.

Side-by-Side Tables

You may choose to assess your options with the help of a side-by-side table. This table may be descriptive or analytic. A descriptive table would provide a description of each option but not provide any analysis. An analytic table would assess the options based on the criteria chosen. In either case, the table should be appropriately labeled and easy to read. As a general matter, a side-by-side table should supplement, not replace, your textual analysis because it is difficult to provide sufficient information within the space provided by a table. However, a table is a useful visual aid that may enhance the reader's understanding of your options and overall analysis. **Table 14.1** and **Table 14.2** provide examples of side-by-side tables.

As you can see from both tables, additional information is necessary for a complete analysis. In the text of your options section, you would need to provide a more complete explanation of each option. It is difficult (but not impossible) to provide sufficient depth of analysis in a chart without creating a busy, difficult-to-read table.

Although the second table uses the terms *low*, *medium*, and *high* to assess the options, other terms or symbols (e.g., +, –) may be used. In addition, you may choose to include phrases instead of single words or symbols. Whatever choice you make, be sure that it is clear which assessment is positive and which is negative. When necessary, provide a legend explaining your terms. Also, some people prefer to use numerical assessments (e.g., 1 = low, 2 = medium, 3 = high). Although debates exist regarding the value of this type of quantitative assessment in a side-by-side chart, we strongly discourage it. Policy analysis is both an art and a science, and using a numerically based table can obscure that balance. An attempt to use quantitative measures may lead readers to assume a simple summation will suffice—just add up the columns and choose the best one. Overall, reducing the analysis to numerical labels hides the value judgments that are part of every analysis, fails to address whether certain criteria should be weighted more than others, and makes the optimal solution appear more certain than it probably is.

Table 14.1 Descriptive Side-by-Side Table

Increasing Access to Care for Immigrants—Options Description

	Public Education Campaign	Grants to States	Health Center Funding
General description	Campaign on radio, television, and public areas	Federal government provides funds to states to increase access to care for immigrants	Federal government provides funding to health centers for services
Populations affected	All will hear, focus on immigrants in community	Only immigrants in the state	All health center patients, including immigrants
Length of option	1 year	5 years, subject to annual appropriations	2 years
Payer	Federal	Federal	Federal

Table 14.2 Analytic Side-by-Side Table

Increasing Access to Care for Immigrants—Options Assessment

Options Criteria	Public Education Campaign	Grants to States	Health Center Funding
Cost to federal government	Low	Medium	High
Political feasibility	Medium	Low	High
Increase in access for immigrants	Low	High	Medium

The Recommendation Section

The time has finally arrived in your policy analysis to make a recommendation. You should choose *one* of your options as your recommendation. Although it is possible to make more than one recommendation or a hybrid recommendation of multiple options, we discourage those approaches. Making multiple recommendations might make it necessary for your client to conduct further analysis to choose among the options, and making a hybrid recommendation (a combination of two or more options) is not appropriate unless the hybrid option was analyzed separately as a single option. In general, it is the analyst's job to organize and clarify the issues and place them in the context of the client's views and power. Ultimately, this approach should result in one path that you believe best suits your client.

The recommendation section should begin by clearly identifying which option is favored and why this option is preferred over the other ones. As mentioned in the options section, every alternative will have pros and cons. The recommendation section does not simply repeat the analysis in the options section. Instead, this portion of the analysis must explain why, despite the drawbacks, this is the best action to take based on your client's values and power. In addition, the recommendation section identifies what, if any, actions may be taken to mitigate or overcome the negative aspects of your recommendation.

Conclusion

You now have a basic understanding of what policy analysis is and an introduction to the tools necessary to analyze a policy problem. Additionally, thinking through the process described in this chapter should train you to evaluate your options when *you* become the decision maker. The checklist in **Box 14.3** provides examples of what should be included in each section of a written policy analysis.

Box 14.3 Checklist for Writing a Policy Analysis

1. **Problem Identification**
   Is my problem written as one sentence in the form of a question?
   Can I identify the focus of my problem?
   Can I identify several options (but not too many) for solving the problem?

2. **Background**
   Does my background include all necessary factual information?
   Have I eliminated information that is not directly relevant to the analysis?
   Is the tone of my background appropriate?

3. **Landscape**
   Does the landscape identify all of the key stakeholders?
   Are the stakeholders' views described clearly and accurately?
   Is the structure of the landscape consistent and easy to follow?
   Is the tone of the landscape appropriate?
   Does the reader have all the information necessary to assess the options?

4. **Options**
   Do my options directly address the issue identified in the problem identification?
   Did I assess the pros and cons of each option?
   Did I apply all of the criteria to each option's assessment?
   Are the options sufficiently different from each other to give the client a real choice?
   Are all of the options within the power of my client?

5. **Recommendation**
   Is my recommendation one of the options assessed?
   Did I recommend only one of my options?
   Did I explain why this recommendation is the best option, despite its flaws?

References

Kingdon, J. (1995). *Agendas, alternatives, and public policies* (2nd ed.). Addison-Wesley Educational Publishers.

Patton C. V., & Sawicki, D. S. (1993). *Basic methods of policy analysis and planning* (2nd ed.). Prentice Hall.

Stone, D. (2002). *Policy paradox: The art of political decision making.* W. W. Norton.

Weissert, C. S., & Weissert, W. G. (2002). *Governing health: The politics of health policy* (2nd ed.). Johns Hopkins University Press.

CHAPTER 15

Federal Policy Advocacy: Advancing Policy Goals

Naomi Seiler

Katie Horton

LEARNING OBJECTIVES

By the end of this chapter you will be able to:

1. Understand the concept of policy advocacy
2. Differentiate policy advocacy and policy analysis
3. Identify the relevant problem, policy solution, and decision maker for a policy advocacy campaign
4. Apply the four key tools of policy advocacy campaigns—policy research, direct lobbying and coalition building, grassroots and grasstops advocacy, and communications and media

Introduction: What Is Policy Advocacy?

Policy advocacy includes a wide range of activities designed to influence decision makers. It involves taking a policy proposal and, working with multiple tools of advocacy, getting a decision maker to take ownership of and advance your policy idea. Enacting new policies is a major task, and persuasion and support from advocates is often crucial to motivating action. Without policy advocacy, it is unlikely that Congress would have passed most of the major health laws of recent decades, such as the Patient Protection and Affordable Care Act in 2010, the Children's Health Insurance Program in 1997, the Mental Health Parity and Addiction Equity Act in 1996, and the Health Insurance Portability and Accountability Act in 1996.

Policy advocacy is about finding solutions for systemic or community problems. Instead of solving a problem for one person at a time, or simply raising awareness about a problem, policy advocacy analyzes the causes of a problem and develops policy-based solutions to effect systemic change. While this chapter focuses on federal policymaking, a policy advocacy campaign can be designed to influence state and local issues as well. These policy changes may occur via laws, regulations, executive orders, and/or ballot initiatives. Overall, policy advocacy efforts typically try to establish new policies, improve existing policies, or challenge the development of policies that create a difficulty or an injustice for specific groups in society.

Policy advocacy seeks to influence policy at the decision-making level, by focusing efforts on public officials, elected officials, and legislators. To be engaged in policy advocacy, organizations and individuals not only need to know how to identify problems, but also how to isolate causes, analyze evidence, understand and apply research, and develop viable policy options.

A number of key terms and definitions are central to policy advocacy:

- **Advocacy:** The most basic meaning of advocacy is to represent, promote, or defend some person, interest, or opinion. Advocacy is the application of *pressure* and *influence* on the people and institutions that have the power to give you what you want. Advocacy includes actions designed to persuade decision makers to implement public policies and practices that benefit the affected group. Advocacy is used to promote an issue to influence policymakers and encourage social change. Advocacy in public health plays a role in educating the public, swaying public opinion, and influencing policymakers.
- **Policy advocacy campaign:** A policy advocacy campaign is a *strategic, multicomponent*, long-term set of advocacy activities targeting a decision maker and aiming to result in a specific policy change.
- **Policy analysis:** Policy analysis provides informed advice to a client that relates to a public policy decision, includes a recommended course of action/inaction, and is framed by the client's powers and values. In the context of policy advocacy, policy analyses may be used to develop an advocacy goal. This topic is discussed in detail in Chapter 14, "The Art of Structuring and Writing a Health Policy Analysis."

After reviewing these definitions, you can see that there are many similarities and differences between policy advocacy and policy analysis. Both activities rely on research, evidence, and political intuition to identify possible solutions to systemic policy problems. For advocates, the overarching task is to convince a policymaker to adopt the advocate's preferred solution. For analysts, as discussed in this text, the overarching task is to help the client/policymaker identify their own preferred solution.

Planning an Advocacy Campaign

Placing a public health issue onto the policy agenda and into the policymaking process requires a well-planned, strategic advocacy campaign. Three key questions to ask at the start of a campaign are

1. What is the problem?
2. What policy change will help solve it?
3. What individuals or institutions have the power to make the policy change?

Identify a Problem

Putting together a strong policy advocacy campaign starts with identifying a problem that needs a policy solution. Policy problems are identified in a number of ways and from a variety of sources, such as the following:

- Individual members of Congress or staff
- Constituents
- Press
- Executive branch agencies
- States and localities
- Stakeholder organizations
- Policy research

Issues will often rise to the attention of policymakers through multiple routes. For example, if a problem at a manufacturing plant for a commonly used drug is receiving heightened attention in the press, legislators may also be receiving calls from concerned constituents or relevant patient organizations.

Select a Policy Solution

Once a policy problem has been identified, the process of developing a policy solution begins. In advocacy, it is often easier to identify problems than it is to identify solutions. Some policy solutions, for example, may require extensive time spent on research to identify a clear policy-based solution. For other policy solutions, there may already be significant research on a topic, and a potential policy response may be more readily identifiable.

In deliberating your policy options, consider the following:

- What policy solution will be most effective?
- Will Congress need to pass a bill to make the change, or can the problem be addressed through administrative action in an Executive Branch agency?
- What is politically feasible given the existing landscape?
- Can you make the solution sound plausible in a way that would attract policymakers?

In a sense, this process mirrors the policy analysis process (discussed in Chapter 14, "The Art of Structuring and Writing a Health Policy Analysis"). Although there is not necessarily a "client" involved, advocates will think through the same issues when developing a policy solution around which the campaign will be centered.

Developing effective policy options requires three key elements, all of which are discussed in detail in this chapter:

1. Developing and using a sound evidence base. This results from solid issue identification, problem analysis, and research.
2. Understanding the political landscape. This includes how and where decisions are made.
3. Being able to describe and communicate complicated issues in a clear and compelling way.

The ultimate goal of an advocacy campaign is the policy change your campaign is trying to achieve, and this often reflects the positive outcome that will occur for those who have been affected by the problem. For example, policy campaigns could have the goal of reducing childhood obesity, improving access to health insurance, or reducing tobacco use. However, if you walk into a meeting with congressional staffers and say, "My organization would like to end childhood obesity," the staffers will want to know, specifically, what action you want them to take. Therefore, with end goals in mind, advocates need to identify the specific policy objectives of their campaign. So, for the examples given earlier, specific policy objectives could be, respectively:

- For Congress to create a new program at the Centers for Disease Control and Prevention to address childhood obesity by funding afterschool sports programs
- For Congress to pass a law encouraging more states to expand Medicaid
- For FDA to issue regulations to limit the sale of certain types of tobacco products

Identify the Decision Makers and Who Influences Them

Decision makers are the people with the power and/or authority to approve or implement the change that you want to achieve. The decision makers affecting your advocacy campaign will depend on your issue of focus and your objective. For example, some policy changes can only be made by changing federal law, and therefore will require lobbying Congress. Other changes can be made by a federal agency, and will therefore require a different approach, such as drafting comments to affect the regulatory process.

To understand who to target in an advocacy campaign, an in-depth understanding of how the policymaking process works is critical. An advocate must know how legislation is passed, how regulations are informed, and how policy is implemented (for a fuller discussion of these topics, see Chapter 2, "Policy and the Policymaking Process"). Power mapping is a process used in advocacy campaigns to analyze the political environment and to understand key decision makers, policy processes, and opposition viewpoints relevant to a policy goal. Power mapping takes time, resources, and knowledge regarding the relationships between stakeholders, but the more comprehensive the mapping, the better prepared you will be to carry out a strong campaign. A variety of tools exist to help an advocate conduct power mapping (for example, see Global Road Safety Partnership, n.d.).

The Four Key Tools of Policy Advocacy Campaigns

Advocacy campaigns typically rely on four key tools, all of which are used to help persuade the decision maker(s) to enact the desired policy change. These tools are as follows:

1. Policy research
2. Direct lobbying and coalition building
3. Grassroots and grasstops campaigns
4. Communications and media

There is no one-size-fits-all blueprint for every advocacy campaign. While an advocacy campaign typically begins with policy research, the framework is dynamic, and each of the four components can be used strategically at different times throughout a campaign to accomplish certain objectives.

Policy Research

All policy advocacy campaigns must use and be supported by policy research. Policy research is the process of conducting research on, or analysis of, a problem or issue. It provides policymakers with action-oriented recommendations for addressing the policy problem.

Policy research is the foundation of a policy advocacy campaign. It documents the policy problem, helps define the policy solution, and drives the message around which a policy advocacy campaign is developed. Assessing the state of existing literature and evidence related to an advocacy goal is one of the first steps in a campaign.

The Role of Policy Research

Research is the foundation of policy analysis and is vital to developing a well-supported advocacy campaign. This is discussed in depth in Chapter 14, "The Art of Structuring and Writing a Health Policy Analysis." Policy research can support an advocacy campaign at multiple levels as follows:

1. **To substantiate the problem.**

    The first element of persuading your decision maker is demonstrating that there is a problem. At the simplest level, a campaign needs data to illustrate the scope of the underlying health policy issue. For example, a campaign related to diabetes would require information about the prevalence of diabetes in the United States. Advocates should then consider what additional facets of the problem are relevant to the policy they are supporting. For example, data on specific disparities in the burden of diabetes in the United States could support a policy directed at diabetes and health equity. These data should come from peer-reviewed sources and established nonpartisan bodies, such as federal agencies and respected professional societies.

2. **To justify the policy proposal.**

    Once the decision makers understand the scope of the underlying problem, they also need to be persuaded that the proposed policy solution is likely to be effective. One way to illustrate the effectiveness of a particular approach is to corral data from jurisdictions that have implemented similar policies. For example, data on tobacco-control interventions enacted at the city and state level can be used to argue for analogous policies at the federal level. Similarly, evidence on the effectiveness of earlier policy decisions at the federal level, such as the impact of past tobacco tax increases on smoking, could be used to argue for further such changes.

    Like data on health conditions generally, the best kind of research to use on policy effectiveness would be peer-reviewed publications. In some cases, particular jurisdictions conduct or fund analyses of the impact of their policies; although not peer reviewed, these may be useful resources. For some policies, specific impact analyses may not be available, but it could be useful to cite models or projections.

3. **To illustrate public opinion.**

    Decision makers, particularly elected officials, are sensitive to the opinions of their constituents and of the public broadly. If data are available showing public support for a campaign's policy proposal, that should be highlighted.

Where the Evidence Comes From

Campaigns should consider all available and relevant data. However, particularly when advocating to legislators, campaigns should identify all available evidence that is specific to key members' home districts or state. Members of Congress are highly responsive

to the needs of their constituents. They will be particularly interested in data on the health burdens their constituents experience, the potential impact of the proposed policy solution, and public opinion at home. For example, if proposing a new funding stream for federally qualified health centers (FQHCs) to address opioid use, advocates could quantify overdose rates in the target member's district or state and identify any FQHCs in the state or district. State data tend to be more readily available than district-specific information and can be useful with both senators and House members.

Filling in Policy Research Gaps

Sometimes, an advocacy campaign can start off with a robust body of peer-reviewed literature explaining the problem, justifying the policy solution, and illustrating public opinion. In other cases, minimal evidence may exist in one or more of these areas. When there is little data, particularly as to the scope of the problem or the effectiveness of the proposed solution, it may, in some cases, make sense to reassess the goals of the campaign. Are there other approaches that would be more strongly rooted in evidence, and more likely, if successful, to positively improve health?

In other cases, advocates can choose to engage in policy research to support their advocacy campaign. For example, if a policy has been enacted in states with no specific evaluations, advocates could carry out at least a qualitative assessment to determine the impact. This kind of research could be conducted internally or externally, depending on the expertise and capacity of the organization. Similarly, advocates can assess public opinion through focus groups, surveys, or other approaches to inform a policy campaign.

In addition, a campaign focused on a relatively novel policy approach can incorporate measures to closely evaluate progress. For example, say that advocates want to promote a promising approach to increasing rates of breast cancer screening. They could develop legislation to fund a pilot program that would include rigorous reporting and evaluation requirements. The results of that evaluation could help inform further expansion of the program.

Direct Lobbying and Coalition Building

Direct Lobbying

A key part of policy advocacy campaigns is direct lobbying of decision makers and those who influence them (see **Box 15.1**). This effort includes identifying key

Box 15.1 Understanding the Decision Maker

Advocates must do background research to understand what decision makers care about and what could influence them. Ask yourself the following questions:

- What motivates your key decision makers?
- Who among your allies has a relationship with those key decision makers?
- What do you know about your opposition?
- What is your opposition's influence on key decision makers?
- What is the political climate in which you are working?

It is important to know how much information, knowledge, or awareness the relevant decision makers have about the issue and how they feel about your policy goal. Your number one job is to make it *easy* for decision makers to give you what you want.

decision makers to inform and influence, and engaging in strategic meetings with policymakers. For example, advocates will want to know to which committees of jurisdiction a bill was referred, so that they can strategically target members of those committees (see Chapter 2, "Policy and the Policymaking Process," for key committees relevant to health policy issues). As a starting point, advocates would want to reach out and meet with staff for that committee and the personal staff of congressional members who sit on that committee.

Lobbying refers to the specific tactics you use to persuade your decision maker(s). There are many options when it comes to lobbying tactics, and part of building out your overall strategy is determining which lobbying tactics will advance your goal.

There are myriad ways to lobby Congress, including the following:

- Sending letters and emails to, or calling, representatives (House member or senator) or other relevant decision makers (e.g., committee chairs)
- Organizing a "fly-in" during which hundreds of grassroots volunteers visit their members of Congress to advocate on a particular issue
- Holding a congressional briefing on your policy goal and directing the media's attention to the policy issue at stake
- Encouraging members of Congress to write letters to the House and Senate appropriations committees in support of specific annual funding levels for target programs

To "lobby" federal agencies, advocates often focus on trying to influence the rulemaking process, through which agencies promulgate new regulations. There is a formal process that allows the public to comment on most draft regulations (see Chapter 2, "Policy and the Policymaking Process"). Advocates can also form ongoing relationships with agency officials and meet with them to discuss policy areas of concern.

Coalition Work

Policy advocacy is rarely a solo endeavor. Advocacy organizations frequently collaborate with other groups in order to achieve their policy goals. Working in a coalition has a number of substantial advantages, including, chiefly, the amplification of the message. A coalition of organizations has more financial and human resources, and, in many cases, an accumulation of more grassroots voices. In addition, policymakers appreciate hearing a clear, unified request from a community of advocates, which is far easier to act on than a disjointed set of competing or conflicting priorities.

Creating a coalition of like-minded partners is a powerful lobbying tactic used in advocacy campaigns. Working in coalition raises a host of choices and questions. Consider the following examples:

- How formal should the coalition be? Some coalitions are very informal—organizations may have a listserv where they communicate information and offer opportunities to support each other's goals, for example, by signing on to a letter. Others are very formal, with a specific entity created, and still others run the gamut in between.
- Should the coalition be long term, or is it specific to one advocacy campaign? Often, groups coalesce around a specific policy goal. They may stop collaborating after that campaign or continue to work around implementation or other policy goals.
- Who should lead the coalition? This issue can be contentious. It is helpful to establish clear lines of authority and communication to ensure that all organizations feel heard and that there is a process for resolving disagreements regarding policy or strategy.
- What will each member bring to the table? Are all members willing to activate their grassroots networks? How much time and resources can each contribute to the campaign?

Although coalition work can be challenging, it is typically well worth navigating these issues for the stronger persuasive power it brings (Center for Lobbying in the Public Interest, 2007). See **Box 15.2** for more information.

Box 15.2 Good Practices of an Advocate Leading a Coalition

Encourage participation: Allow others into the decision-making process of the campaign. For example, even if one organization is the leader of a coalition, there should be a process for shared decision-making to keep other coalition partners engaged and supportive.

Ensure legitimacy: Earn the trust of the policymakers and people you represent by consistently sharing valid, reliable information, and by always keeping close hold of information that you are asked not to share.

Be accountable: To both the organization you represent and to policymakers, report back on information (when permitted), and account for the actions of the coalition and your own organization.

Represent effectively: All advocacy groups should ensure that their policy goals are related to the real needs of the people affected by the health issue of concern. Develop strategy with the community or population you represent, informing them of risks and challenges as the advocacy campaign proceeds. Other modes of engagement include online community membership, surveys, focus groups, board representation, and other approaches.

Grassroots and Grasstops Advocacy

Grassroots advocacy means targeting an advocacy campaign message to a group of on-the-ground supporters who make up an organization's membership or follower base. The aim of reaching this group is to create a rapid groundswell that has the potential to spread the word about an advocacy issue among themselves and other like-minded individuals, and to reach out to advocacy targets to help inform and influence them. Grassroots advocacy is particularly effective when working with Congress, where representatives are influenced by knowing that a large number of their constituents care about an issue.

Grass*tops* advocacy is a term used for anyone within your supporter base who has a relationship with, or can bring extra influence on, decision makers. Grasstops advocates could include your organization's leadership and board members, or well-connected volunteers and donors. Some grasstops individuals have personal relationships with a decision maker and can reach out directly to request support.

Grassroots and grasstops supporters can be leveraged in a variety of ways, including the following:

- Letter writing to decision makers
- Phone calls to staff and decision makers
- In-person meetings with decision makers
- Providing expert opinion or firsthand accounts about the policy problem
- Testifying about your policy problem in a congressional hearing
- Writing op-eds and letters to the editor about your policy problem
- Participating in congressional fly-ins, where people from around the country come to meet with the representatives in Congress

It is not enough to simply identify grassroots and grasstops advocates—you need to make sure they are educated and prepared to communicate with legislators and other decision makers. There are many online tools to help manage and engage grassroots support. These tools will allow you to make it easy for your advocates to take action while giving them the opportunity to personalize their message to legislators. For example, various online tools can allow supporters to tell a personal story or to share details about how their lives have been impacted by an issue. Some organizations also hold trainings at the start of congressional fly-ins to make sure all grassroots and grasstops volunteers are prepared to advocate effectively.

Communications and Media

An effective advocacy campaign should incorporate an integrated communications approach that includes print, multimedia, and interactive content that is appealing and engaging to all stakeholders involved (see **Box 15.3** for additional considerations concerning timeline and budget). Media and communications are one of the best ways to gain the attention of decision makers, especially members of Congress.

Crafting the Campaign Message

Developing the campaign's core message is one of the most important steps and often relies on the policy research that was conducted for purposes of the advocacy campaign. The message should be clear, simple, and relevant to the decision maker. It should persuade decision makers that the policy proposal is in their interest, and in their constituents' interest too. For example, many elements of Medicare policy involve detailed, complicated legislative and regulatory provisions that lay out how the program reimburses various types of facilities and providers. Any kind of advocacy

Box 15.3 Campaign Timelines and Budgets

A critical part of advocacy campaign planning is establishing a timeline and budget for the campaign. Mapping out a timeline and incorporating specific tactics into your timeline help keep a campaign and its advocates on track. A simple timeline could be developed by month. Tactics and major events embedded in this simple timeline allow advocates to plan, implement, and assign responsibility for certain actions.

Also critical to any advocacy campaign is the budget. A number of questions should be considered, including how the campaign will be financed, what the expected costs will be, whether other coalition members will contribute funding, and what costs may be reduced or expanded depending on changes in the budget over time.

campaign related to such provisions needs to be able to clearly and succinctly explain what the proposed policy change would mean for how Medicare beneficiaries access care.

To achieve a core message, nearly every campaign integrates data and other evidence with personal stories. Data, as discussed previously, can intellectually persuade policymakers about the need for a policy response and of the rightness of a particular approach. However, lawmakers and their staff, as well as government agencies, grapple with hundreds of requests and issues every year. Therefore, adding personal stories to engage decision makers' empathy and imagination is crucial.

For legislators, personal stories from constituents are most effective. The most direct way to bring personal stories is through constituent visits, either in Washington, D.C., or at a congressperson's local district office. Constituent stories can also be brought to light in congressional hearings, with carefully identified individuals invited as witnesses.

The role of personal stories can be somewhat more complex for administrative agencies. In these cases, decision makers are typically scientists, thus more focused on data than on anecdotes. However, in some cases, individual stories can still be compelling. For example, the FDA has an adverse event reporting system to detect potential problems related to food allergies; event reports submitted from individuals with sesame allergies helped inform the agency's regulatory steps toward requiring allergen labeling for products containing sesame.

Types of Messaging Documents

Policy campaigns rely on a range of document types to support their advocacy. For direct meetings with policymakers, advocates may use any of the following:

- **Leave-behinds:** Leave-behinds are one- to two-page documents intended to be "left behind" at a lobbying visit. These documents should be clear, concise, and easy to read. Most importantly, a leave-behind should contain a succinct statement of the campaign's "ask," or request. For example, if the goal is to pass a specific piece of legislation in the House of Representatives, the leave-behind could be titled "Support H.R. [bill number], the [bill name]." It would then summarize the arguments for why policy action is needed and why the particular bill should be passed. Leave-behinds include information to allow recipients to follow up, such as the lead sponsor's contact information for other members who wish to cosponsor a bill.

- **Fact sheets:** Fact sheets are also brief, one- to two-page documents. Unlike leave-behinds, they do not focus on a specific policy proposal, but instead provide a key compilation of facts. A fact sheet can be a useful tool for legislative staffers when certain issues are at the top of their agenda. For example, if a committee is preparing a hearing on asthma, staffers would likely appreciate a well-cited fact sheet on asthma disparities. While this kind of document does not directly support a specific policy goal, it helps foster a staffer's trust in an advocacy group, strengthening the relationship and supporting ongoing access and communication. This trust in the evidence that an organization shares can translate into a stronger relationship and the ability to influence that staffer. Conversely, if an organization provides information that is clearly not evidence based—or, worse, that seems reliable but turns out to be inaccurate—a staffer is not likely to ever return to that organization for information or for policy input.

- **Issue briefs:** Issue briefs are somewhat longer, perhaps three to five pages. While many staffers will not read a document of this length, they can be useful explainers of complex subjects for some, such as committee staff, who will appreciate a deeper dive.

- **Dear Colleague letters:** Members of Congress can write and send (now electronically) communications called Dear Colleague letters. These are often used to encourage other members to cosponsor or vote for legislation they have introduced.

Advocates can work with congressional offices to help draft Dear Colleague letters to expand support for legislation.

Leveraging the Media

The advocacy campaign's message will also be conveyed to other audiences, particularly through the media. Most commonly, the goal is to persuade the public of a particular position so that they, in turn, make their opinion known to their elected representatives. In traditional press (both print and online), advocacy campaigns can attempt to place op-eds, as well as letters to the editor. Advocates can pay for messaging, through advertisements in print and other outlets. Campaigns can also attempt to get "earned media" exposure, working to get reporters to cover their campaign and the underlying issues. And, of course, advocates use social media—their own and that of other outlets—to create attention and generate dialogue. Just a few examples of the many ways that social media can be used in advocacy include the following:

- Updating a grassroots community on the progress of a campaign and motivating specific actions
- Engaging directly with policymakers' social media accounts
- Creating a "hashtag" around a policy campaign to gain awareness and momentum across multiple platforms

After the Advocacy Campaign

As advocacy campaigns unfold, it is essential to assess progress at regular intervals to identify both the strengths of the campaigns and areas where they can be improved. Some advocacy campaigns are clearly successful, whereas others are clear failures. Still others fall in the middle, with a goal partially achieved, or incremental progress made. Regardless, the end of a campaign requires a thoughtful assessment of the outcome and consideration of next steps (see **Box 15.4** for additional considerations).

Once Congress passes a bill, or an agency makes a decision that advocates requested, follow-up monitoring and advocacy are often necessary. For example, many health policy laws authorize funding for programs. Advocacy is subsequently needed each year after passage to ensure that the congressional

---

Box 15.4 Recognize and Reward

No matter the outcome of a campaign, it is important for advocates to pause and thank their allies. They should find ways to support and express thanks to members of Congress and their staff. In addition, they should inform their boards, donors, and grassroots communities about the outcome of the campaign; thank them for their efforts; and explain the status of any next steps. Engaging and recognizing the role of all allies is crucial for starting off the next campaign with strong support.

---

committees appropriate funds so that the program can be implemented and continued. Similarly, many bills direct agencies to issue detailed regulations to assist in the implementation of the legislative goals. Advocates will want to monitor and engage in the regulatory process to ensure that their priorities are addressed. In some cases, a victory in Congress or with an agency may be challenged in court, requiring a pivot to defense, as the scores of legal challenges to the Patient Protection and Affordable Care Act have illustrated.

If a campaign results in a partial victory, advocates need to decide on next steps. Will continuing the campaign potentially lead to further progress? Or is the outcome good enough, and should resources be shifted to other policy priorities?

If a campaign did not succeed, advocates can draw many lessons from the experience. Which decision makers seemed responsive to the message, and which did not? Did any unanticipated objections or opponents arise in the process? Do any actual or potential shifts in the political landscape point to the possibility of a different outcome if the campaign is revived in the next cycle?

Conclusion

Policy change is hard. Campaigns to change policy, whether through legislation or agency action, can take many years. It can be particularly challenging to advocate for policies to support communities with little political capital or for changes that are opposed by powerful industries. But the work is worth it. Well planned, thoughtful health advocacy is a critical strategy for improving the health of populations by addressing the systemic problems that challenge our public health and healthcare systems.

References

Center for Lobbying in the Public Interest. (2007). *Working in coalitions.* https://www.councilofnonprofits.org/sites/default/files/documents/07_coalitions.pdf

Global Road Safety Partnership. (n.d.). *Policy implementation toolkit – supporting tool: Political mapping for policy implementation.* https://www.grsproadsafety.org/wp-content/uploads/8-Tool-Political-Mapping.pdf

Glossary

accountable care organization (ACO) A group of healthcare providers that is collectively reimbursed for a single patient's care. This arrangement is meant to give providers an incentive to deliver high-quality, cost-effective care.

accreditation A process applied to healthcare institutions to ensure that all necessary and required processes, standards, competencies, ethics, and so on are up to par.

administrative law The body of law produced by executive (i.e., administrative) agencies of federal, state, and local governments.

Administrative Procedures Act A federal law that governs the way in which administrative agencies of the federal government may propose and establish regulations.

adverse selection A means of forming an insurance pool based on the idea that individuals with a higher-than-average risk of needing health care are more likely to seek health insurance coverage.

advocacy The representation, promotion, or defense of some person, interest, or opinion to the people and institutions that have the power to create or change policy.

annual aggregate limit A cap imposed by health insurance companies on the amount a policy will pay during a single year.

bioterrorism The threat or use of a biological agent, typically by a nonstate actor, to cause death or harm to humans, animals, or plants and specifically targeting civilian populations or resources.

block grant A large sum of money granted by the national government to a regional government with only general provisions as to how the money is to be spent.

bundling An arrangement by which providers are paid a predetermined amount for all services related to treating a specific condition, as opposed to compensating healthcare providers separately for every service performed. This arrangement is meant to give providers an incentive to deliver cost-effective care.

"Cadillac" healthcare plans Health insurance plans and other products whose value exceeds a stated annual dollar threshold.

cafeteria plans Employer-sponsored health benefit plans under which employees may set aside wages to be used for medical expenses not otherwise covered by their basic health insurance. Also referred to as flexible spending accounts (FSAs).

capitation A method of payment for health services in which a fixed amount is paid for each person served without regard to the actual number or nature of services provided.

catastrophic coverage A health insurance coverage option with limited benefits and a high deductible, intended to protect against medical bankruptcy due to an unforeseen illness or injury.

Centers for Disease Control and Prevention (CDC) The federal agency within the Department of Health and Human Services charged with disease prevention, education, and public health activities.

Centers for Medicare and Medicaid Services (CMS) The federal agency within the Department of Health and Human Services that administers the Medicare and Medicaid programs.

Children's Health Insurance Program (CHIP) A health insurance program targeted to low-income children, established in 1997 and reauthorized in 2009, that is administered by states and funded through a combination of federal and state payments.

COBRA The nickname for a law, enacted as part of the Consolidated Omnibus Budget Reconciliation Act of 1985, that allows individuals to continue to purchase employee health benefits for a period of 18 to 36 months following a "qualifying event" such as unemployment, death of a wage earner, divorce, or termination of minor dependent coverage.

coinsurance A form of beneficiary cost-sharing for covered health insurance benefits and services, expressed as a percentage of the approved payment amount for the benefit or service (e.g., 20% of the payable amount).

community health center A type of community clinic that provides a broad range of healthcare services and that charges on a sliding-scale fee basis. See also *federally qualified health center*.

community rating A method for setting a premium that requires health insurance providers to offer health insurance policies within a given territory at the same price to all persons without medical underwriting, regardless of individual health status.

comparative effectiveness research (CER) A type of health services research that compares different approaches to treating medical conditions in order to determine which methods are most likely to produce the best outcomes.

coordination of benefits A process by which health services are paid for by more than one health insurance plan.

For example, if a child is insured through both parents, one insurer is generally considered the primary policy, and the secondary policy reimburses for services not covered under the primary policy.

copayment A form of beneficiary cost-sharing for covered health insurance benefits and services, expressed as a flat dollar payment (e.g., $5.00 for a prescription drug).

cost-sharing A requirement that insured patients pay a portion of their medical costs, either as coinsurance or as a fixed copayment.

culturally and linguistically appropriate care A federal standard designed to eliminate ethnic and racial disparities in health care.

deductible The amount patients must pay out of their own pocket before their health insurance policy begins contributing to the cost of their care.

Department of Defense (DoD) A federal agency that, among other functions, administers healthcare programs for active military and their dependents through a publicly funded and privately administered health program called TRICARE.

Department of Health and Human Services (HHS) A federal agency that administers federal health and welfare programs and activities.

Department of Labor (DoL) A federal agency responsible for administration and enforcement of ERISA, a federal law that sets requirements for employer-provided health benefits that are not offered through state-licensed health insurance plans.

dependent coverage Health insurance coverage of a spouse, child, or domestic partner of an insured individual.

diagnostic-related group (DRG) A system used to classify patients (particularly under Medicare) for the purpose of reimbursing hospitals. Hospitals are paid a fixed fee for each case in a given category, regardless of the actual costs of providing care.

discrimination in health care Failure by providers to treat patients equitably for any of a number of reasons, including race, gender, age, ability to pay for care, or severity of illness. This term can also be used to describe the insurance company practice of medical underwriting and rating.

doughnut hole A gap in prescription drug coverage under Medicare Part D, for which beneficiaries pay 100% of their prescription drug costs after their total drug spending exceeds an initial coverage limit until they qualify for catastrophic coverage. The coverage gap will be gradually phased out under the Affordable Care Act by 2020.

dual eligibles Individuals who are eligible for both Medicaid and Medicare.

electronic medical record (EMR) An individual medical record that is stored electronically.

Employee Retirement Income Security Act (ERISA) A 1974 federal law that establishes standards governing both pension plans and "welfare benefit plans" (such as health benefits, dependent care benefits, and other types of benefits and services) and that is applicable to nonfederal employers, multiemployer arrangements, and union plans.

employer responsibility A requirement that employers assist in covering workers and their dependents, either through the provision of a health plan or through a contribution toward coverage that may be expressed as payment of a flat dollar charge (e.g., $500 per worker), a percentage of payroll, a percentage of an annual insurance premium, or some other amount. Also referred to as an "employer mandate."

employer-sponsored insurance (ESI) A health benefit plan offered by an employer to its employees (and often to employee dependents). Some employers purchase plans from a traditional insurance company, while other (primarily large) employers may choose to directly insure their employees through their own plan.

entitlement program An insurance program that guarantees access to benefits or services based on established rights or by legislation (e.g., the Medicaid program).

epidemic A situation in which new cases of a certain disease, in a given human population during a given period, substantially exceed what is expected based on recent experience.

epidemiology The study of patterns of health and illness and associated factors at the population level.

essential benefits A list of core benefits established under the Patient Protection and Affordable Care Act that must be included under any health insurance plan in order to meet minimum coverage requirements.

exchange-eligible employer An employer that is permitted to enroll in a health insurance exchange in order to offer health benefits to its employees.

exchange-eligible individual An individual who is permitted to obtain coverage through a health insurance exchange.

exchange-participating health benefit plan A health insurance plan offered to individuals and small employers through health insurance exchanges. They must meet federal insurance market and benefit requirements.

excise tax A tax on health insurance and health benefit plans whose annual dollar value exceeds a specified limit, as well as on the sale of specified healthcare items and services such as medical devices and equipment.

exclusion The practice by which an insurer or health benefit plan classifies certain otherwise-covered items and treatments as ineligible for coverage. Common exclusions include "experimental," "educational," and "cosmetic" treatments and services.

executive order A presidential directive, with the authority of a law, that directs and governs actions by executive officials and agencies.

fair marketing A term used to encompass a range of health insurance market reforms to protect consumers from medical underwriting and other practices designed to limit the amount an insurer pays for medical claims.

Federal Emergency Management Agency (FEMA) A federal agency responsible for responding to national emergencies, including natural disasters.

federalism A system of government in which sovereignty is constitutionally divided between a central governing authority and constituent political units (e.g., states), and in which the power to govern is shared between the national and state governments.

federally qualified health center (FQHC) A community health center that either receives funding under section 440 of the Public Health Service Act or has been certified as meeting the same criteria.

fee-for-service A method of paying for medical services under which doctors are paid for each service provided. Bills are paid by the patient, who then submits them to the insurance company for reimbursement.

fraud and abuse A range of wasteful healthcare activities, including billing for services not performed, billing for more expensive services than performed ("up-coding"), and performing inappropriate or unnecessary care.

gainsharing A system in which the government passes on savings from providing more-efficient care to insurers and providers.

guaranteed issue and renewal A rule that bars health insurers from denying or dropping an individual's coverage for any reason other than fraud or nonpayment of health insurance premiums. This rule is especially important to prevent insurance companies from denying coverage based on individuals' health status.

healthcare disparity A difference in access to healthcare services or to health insurance, or in the quality of care actually received.

healthcare/public health workforce A term used to define a range of health professionals in private and public practice who provide medical care and public health services such as primary care, disease diagnosis, and public education.

health disparity A situation in which one population group experiences a higher burden of disability or illness relative to another group.

health equity A situation in which everyone has the opportunity to attain his or her full health potential and no one is disadvantaged because of social conditions.

health information privacy and security Standards or procedures to ensure that personal health information is not compromised or disclosed in processing healthcare transactions.

health information technology (HIT) Technology that allows the comprehensive management of health information and enables its exchange among health professionals, healthcare providers, healthcare payers, and public health agencies.

health insurance exchanges Regulated marketplaces for the sale and purchase of health insurance established under federal law and operated in accordance with federal requirements.

health insurance exchange subsidies Federal subsidies made available on an income-related basis to exchange-eligible individuals for the purchase of health insurance coverage through health insurance exchanges.

health insurance issuers Entities that sell health insurance in the individual and employer-sponsored group markets.

Health Insurance Portability and Accountability Act (HIPAA) A federal law that regulates health insurers and health benefit plans in the group market and provides privacy protections for health information.

health maintenance organization (HMO) A type of health insurance plan that provides a coordinated array of preventive and treatment services for a fixed payment per month. Enrollees receive medically necessary services regardless of whether the cost of those services exceeds the premium paid on the enrollees' behalf.

health status All aspects of physical and mental health and their manifestations in daily living, including impairment, disability, and handicap.

health threat In the context of national or global security, an environmental, biological, chemical, radiological, or physical risk to public or community health.

high-risk insurance pool An insurance option for patients with existing medical conditions that make them expensive to insure.

homeland defense The protection of U.S. territory, populations, and infrastructure against external threats or aggression.

incidence The number of new cases of illness or disease during a specific period of time in a specific population.

Indian Health Care Improvement Act A federal law creating programs to strengthen healthcare options in Native American communities.

Indian Health Service A federal health program to provide health care to Native Americans and Alaska natives.

individual market The insurance market for individuals who are purchasing insurance for themselves and their families and are not part of a group plan, such as one offered by an employer. Also referred to as the nongroup market.

individual responsibility The requirement that all individuals must carry health insurance or pay a penalty. Also referred to as an individual mandate.

insurance pool A group of individuals whose premiums are used to pay all covered medical costs of its members. Insurance companies may charge higher premiums to a pool whose members are older or less healthy than other pools in order to cover the risk that its members may submit more medical claims.

interest group An organization that uses various forms of advocacy to influence public opinion and/or policy. Groups vary considerably in size, influence, and purpose. Also referred to as special interest groups, advocacy groups, or lobby groups.

International Health Regulations A 2005 international treaty obligating all Member States of the World Health Organization to detect, report, and respond to potential public health emergencies of international concern. These regulations are aimed at improving global health security through international collaboration and communication.

large group market The market for health insurance or health benefit plans among employers whose employee numbers exceed a specified threshold size (e.g., 100 full-time workers).

lifetime aggregate limits Provisions included in health insurance contracts designed to limit the total amount the policy will pay out in claims and benefits over the lifetime of the policy.

long-term care A set of healthcare, personal care, and social services provided to persons who have lost, or never acquired, some degree of functional capacity (e.g., the chronically ill, aged, or disabled) in an institution or at home, on a long-term basis.

managed care Health insurance arrangements that integrate the financing and delivery of services to covered individuals.

market failure A concept within economic theory in which the allocation of goods and services by a free market is not efficient.

Medicaid A program established in 1965 to provide health insurance to low-income families and individuals with certain disabilities. It is administered by the states and funded jointly with the federal government.

medical home A clinic focused on primary care and preventive services that offers a range of coordinated treatment services.

medical–legal partnership An approach to health that integrates the expertise of healthcare, public health, and legal professionals and staff to address and prevent health-harming social and civil legal needs for patients and populations.

medical underwriting The insurance industry practice of assessing the medical condition of individuals at the time that insurance enrollment is sought in order to identify existing physical or mental health conditions that may affect an individual's or group's eligibility for enrollment, the application of preexisting condition exclusions or waiting periods, or the price to be charged for coverage.

Medicare A federal program enacted in 1965 that provides government-sponsored health insurance to individuals ages 65 years and older and certain individuals younger than 65 years with disabilities that meet federal requirements.

Medicare Advantage Optional private insurance plans in which Medicare beneficiaries may enroll to receive their federal benefits.

Medigap coverage Supplemental health insurance designed to cover all or most of the charges that are not covered by Medicare, including the 20% copayment required for many outpatient services.

National Health Service Corps A commissioned corps of public health professionals employed by the federal Department of Health and Human Services. Members are assigned to settings that include clinics in underserved areas, state and local health departments, and federal agencies such as the Centers for Disease Control and Prevention.

National Institutes of Health A federal agency within the Department of Health and Human Services that is primarily responsible for conducting and supporting medical research.

notifiable disease A disease that, once diagnosed, must be reported under the law to a public health authority.

Office of Inspector General (OIG) Located within the federal Department of Health and Human Services, this office is charged with protecting the integrity of programs administered by the Department, protecting the health and welfare of program beneficiaries, and reporting problems to the Department Secretary and to Congress.

pandemic An infectious disease that spreads through human populations across a large region, over multiple continents.

parity A term generally used to require that large group insurers or plans pay equivalent benefits for different kinds of services. For example, federal law requires "mental health parity," which means that for health plans that include mental health benefits as well as medical ones, the services must be covered with the same financial requirements and treatment limitations.

Patient Protection and Affordable Care Act Also known as the Affordable Care Act or ACA, a major federal health reform law enacted in March 2010.

patient protections Laws establishing protections for patients, such as the right to health information, to choice of providers, to access to care, to file a grievance, or to appeal a denied health benefit claim.

pay-for-performance (P4P) A healthcare payment system in which providers receive incentives for meeting quality and cost benchmarks (or, in some cases, penalties for not meeting established benchmarks).

performance measurement A set of recommendations, requirements, or data used to determine whether plans, providers, or programs meet or exceed a standard of care.

policy advocacy campaign A strategic, multicomponent, long-term set of advocacy activities targeting a decision maker and aiming to result in a specific policy change.

policy analysis An analysis that provides informed advice to a client that relates to a public policy decision, includes a recommended course of action/inaction, and is framed by the client's powers and values.

population health The health outcomes of a group of individuals, including the distribution of such outcomes within the group.

preexisting conditions Health conditions that exist prior to or at the time of enrollment into a health insurance or health benefit plan.

preferred provider organization (PPO) A health insurance plan in which providers agree to provide care to covered individuals at a negotiated price. Covered individuals receive all medically necessary services regardless of whether the cost of the services exceeds the premium paid, although members do have cost-sharing obligations.

premium The amount a business or individual pays regularly to maintain health insurance coverage.

premium rating An insurance industry practice determining health insurance premiums based on factors including age, health status, gender, industry, geography, or other factors.

prevalence The total number of cases of a disease or illness in the population at a given time.

preventive services Measures taken to prevent the development of disease or to treat illnesses early so that they do not become more acute and expensive to treat. Examples include vaccination, weight-loss programs, and mammograms.

primary care provider (PCP) A healthcare provider, such as a physician engaged in the practice of internal medicine, pediatric care, or geriatric care, or a nurse practitioner, who provides general medical care and coordinates treatment.

public health emergency An acute event capable of causing large-scale morbidity and mortality, either immediately or over time. These events have the ability to overwhelm normal public health and medical care capabilities.

public health insurance A health insurance plan that is administered by the government either directly or through the use of private contractors. Medicare, Medicaid, and CHIP are considered forms of public health insurance.

public health preparedness The actions and policies associated with preventing, protecting against, responding to, and recovering from a major public health event.

quarantine The separation and restriction of movement of people or animals that may have been exposed to an infectious agent.

reinsurance A form of insurance that health insurers may purchase to protect themselves against losses that may occur should they underestimate how much they will pay out for medical claims in a year.

rescission A process by which an insurance company seeks to recover the amount paid out for covered services after discovering that information on a beneficiary's initial enrollment form was incomplete or incorrect.

retiree health benefits Health benefits provided by an employer to its retirees.

risk adjustment A tool for evaluating the relative risk of enrollees within insurance plans and providing for a financial transfer from plans with low-risk enrollees to plans with higher-risk enrollees.

safety net The collection of healthcare providers who serve patients regardless of patients' ability to pay for care. Providers include community health centers, public hospitals, local health departments, school- and church-based health clinics, and private physicians and nonprofit hospitals committed to serving uninsured and low-income, vulnerable patients.

skimming The insurance plan practice of enrolling predominantly healthy individuals in order to reduce the costs to the plan.

small group market The health insurance market for employers whose size is smaller than a specified threshold (e.g., 100 full-time workers).

social determinant of health (SDH) A factor outside of one's genetic predisposition that can cause or prevent poor health, as well as affect how disease can progress (or not) throughout one's lifetime. Examples include socioeconomic status, geographical birthplace, and housing quality.

stare decisis A Latin term that refers to the legal principle that prior case law decisions should be accorded great deference and should not be frequently overturned.

surge capacity The ability of clinical care facilities and laboratories to accommodate a sharp increase in patients and samples during a public health emergency.

telehealth The use of electronic information and telecommunications technologies to support long-distance clinical health care, patient and professional health-related education, public health, and health administration. Technologies may include videoconferencing, the Internet, store-and-forward imaging, streaming media, and terrestrial and wireless communications.

uncompensated care Services provided by physicians and hospitals for which no payment is received from the patient or from third-party payers.

underinsured Individuals with insurance policies that do not cover all necessary healthcare services, resulting in out-of-pocket expenses that exceed the ability to pay.

uninsured Individuals who lack public or private health insurance.

universal coverage The provision of at least basic or medically necessary health insurance for an entire population.

utilization review The examination, usually by an insurer or third-party administrator, of the necessity and/or appropriateness of healthcare services provided to a patient.

weapon of mass destruction (WMD) A weapon that causes large-scale destruction, generally through nuclear, radiological, chemical, or biological means.

wellness programs Special services and benefits offered by employers to employees in addition to health benefit plans, including nutrition classes, smoking-cessation programs, or gym memberships.

World Health Organization (WHO) The directing and coordinating authority for health within the United Nations system.

The following source was used, in part, in the compilation of this glossary:

Data from The Health Policy Institute of Ohio. (n.d.). *Glossary.* http://www.healthpolicyohio.org/tools/glossary/

Index

Page numbers followed by *f*, *t*, *b* and *n* indicate figures, tables, boxes and notes

options section, in policy analysis, 341,
351b
assessing options, 348–349
identifying options, 348
options section, 347–351
side-by-side tables, 350–351
structuring, 349–350
Organization for Economic Cooperation
and Development (OECD), 49,
138
originalism, 36
original jurisdiction, 45
out-of-pocket spending limits, 272t
oversight authority, 15

P

PAHPRA. *See* Pandemic and All-Hazards
Preparedness Reauthorization Act
of 2013 (PAHPRA)
Pandemic and All-Hazards Preparedness
Act (PAHPRA), 331
Pareto, Vilfredo, 177
Pareto-efficient, 177
Parmet, Wendy, 131
partial birth abortion, 123
Partial Birth Abortion Ban Act of 2003
(PBABA), 124
PAs. *See* physician assistants (PAs)
path dependency, concept of, 250–251
patient-centered medical home (PCMH),
66
patient-centeredness, in healthcare
system, 70
Patient-Centered Outcomes Research
Institute (PCORI), 280
patient dumping, 118
Patient Protection and Affordable Care
Act of 2010 (ACA). *See* Affordable
Care Act (ACA)
patient rights. *See* rights
Patient Safety and Quality Improvement
Act (PSQIA), 300
PBABA. *See* Partial Birth Abortion Ban
Act of 2003 (PBABA)
PCMH. *See* patient-centered medical
home (PCMH)
PCORI. *See* Patient-Centered Outcomes
Research Institute (PCORI)
PDPs. *See* private drug insurance plans
(PDPs)
peer review processes, 300
Pegram v. Herdrich case, 310
Pelosi, Nancy, 255, 258
Pennsylvania Abortion Control Act, 122
perfectly competitive market, 184
personal privacy, right to, 121–125
Personal Responsibility and Work
Opportunity Reconciliation Act of
1996 (PRWORA), 197

Pharmaceutical Research and
Manufacturers of America, 29,
257
Pharmacy Quality Alliance (PQA), 312
PHI. *See* private health insurance (PHI)
PHICS. *See* Public Health Incident
Command System (PHICS)
PHS. *See* Public Health Service (PHS)
physical and mental disability
discrimination, 127–128
physician assistants (PAs), 66, 67f
physician–patient relationship, 298
Physician Quality Reporting System
(PQRS), 311, 313
physician reimbursement, 234–235
physicians, shortages of, 66–67, 67f
Pilot Life Insur. Co. v. Dedeaux case, 308
*Planned Parenthood of Southeastern
Pennsylvania v. Casey* case,
122–123
Plessy v. Ferguson case, 46
"pocket veto," 18
point-of-service (POS) plans, 171
police powers, 4–5, 41, 129–130
policy advocacy
campaigns, 354
after, 360
coalition work, 357, 358b
communications and media,
358–360
direct lobbying, 356–357
grassroots and grasstops, 358
key tools of, 355–356
planning, 354–355
recognizing and rewarding, 360b
timeline and budgets, 359b
decision makers, identifying, 355
defined, 353–354
policy solution, selecting, 354–355
problem identification, 354
policy analysis, 354
art of structuring and writing,
339–351
defined, 339
overview
client-oriented advice, 339–340
client's power and values, 340–341
informed advice, 340
multiple purposes, 341
providing options and
recommendation, 340
public policy decision, 340
structuring, 341–351
background section, 344–345
landscape section, 345–347
options section, 347–350
problem identification, 342–344
recommendation section, 351
policy and policymaking process
defining policy
identifying public problems, 11–12
structuring policy options, 12–13
federal executive branch

administrative agencies, 23–26
presidency, 21–23
federal legislative branch
congressional budget and
appropriations process, 18–20
constituents of legislative branch,
20–21
passing laws, 18
health bureaucracy
federal government, 26–29
interest groups, 29–30
state and local governments, 29
public policymaking structure and
process, 13–26
state-level policymaking, 13–14
policy development, 92
policymakers, 178
policy options, structuring, 12–13
policy research, 355–356
filling policy research gaps, 356
identifying evidence, 356
role of, 355–356
illustrating public opinion, 356
justifying policy proposal, 356
substantiating problem, 356
policy research gaps, 356
policy solution, selecting, 354–355
political capital, 22
political model, of policy analysis, 340
population-level equity, 71
positive economics, 178
positive externality, 186
PPOs. *See* preferred provider
organizations (PPOs)
PPS. *See* prospective payment system
(PPS)
PQA. *See* Pharmacy Quality Alliance
(PQA)
PQRS. *See* Physician Quality Reporting
System (PQRS)
preferred provider organizations (PPOs),
63, 171, 223
pregnancy care, 8–9
premiums, 157
setting, 162–163
subsidies, 270–274
tax credits, 270–271, 271b, 272t
preparedness programs and preparedness
funding, 320–321
prescription drug benefits, through
Medicare, 225–227, 227b
presidency, 21–23
agenda setting, 22
constituents of executive branch, 23,
24f
presidential powers, 22–23
Presidential Policy Directive-8 (PPD-8),
322–323
presidential powers, 22–23
prevention, in public health approach,
100–102
National Prevention Strategy (NPS),
102